CURRENT THERAPY IN
DERMATOLOGY-2

Current Therapy Series

CURRENT THERAPY IN DERMATOLOGY-2

THOMAS T. PROVOST, M.D.

Noxell Professor and Chairman
Department of Dermatology
The Johns Hopkins Medical Institutions
Baltimore, Maryland

EVAN R. FARMER, M.D.

Associate Professor
Department of Dermatology and Pathology
The Johns Hopkins Medical Institutions
Baltimore, Maryland

1988
B.C. Decker Inc • Toronto • Philadelphia

Publisher

B.C. Decker Inc
3228 South Service Road
Burlington, Ontario   L7N 3H8

B.C. Decker Inc
320 Walnut Street
Suite 400
Philadelphia, Pennsylvania   19106

Sales and Distribution

United States and Possessions	**The C.V. Mosby Company** 11830 Westline Industrial Drive Saint Louis, Missouri 63146
Canada	**The C.V. Mosby Company, Ltd.** 5240 Finch Avenue East, Unit No. 1 Scarborough, Ontario M1S 5P2
United Kingdom, Europe and the Middle East	**Blackwell Scientific Publications, Ltd.** Osney Mead, Oxford OX2 OEL, England
Australia	**Harcourt Brace Jovanovich** 30–52 Smidmore Street Marrickville, N.S.W. 2204 Australia
Japan	**Igaku-Shoin Ltd.** Tokyo International P.O. Box 5063 1–28–36 Hongo, Bunkyo-ku, Tokyo 113, Japan
Asia	**Info-Med Ltd.** 802–3 Ruttonjee House 11 Duddell Street Central Hong Kong
South Africa	**Libriger Book Distributors** Warehouse Number 8 "Die Ou Looiery" Tannery Road Hamilton, Bloemfontein 9300
South America (non-stock list representative only)	**Inter-Book Marketing Services** Rua das Palmeriras, 32 Apto. 701 222–70 Rio de Janeiro RJ, Brazil

Current Therapy in Dermatology–2

ISBN 1–55664–023–4

Library of Congress catalog card number: 84–71742

10 9 8 7 6 5 4 3 2 1

This book is dedicated
to
Otis Field Jillson (1917 – 1986) and Israel Zeligman

Unique men with a zest for life:
kind, compassionate, master dermatologists, keen observers,
gifted teachers, good friends, and wise counselors.

CONTRIBUTORS

REGINA ANDERSON, M.D.

Assistant Professor, Department of Medicine, Division of Dermatology, University of Maryland School of Medicine; Chief, Department of Medicine, Division of Dermatology, Baltimore Veterans Administration Hospital, Baltimore, Maryland
Atypical Mycobacterial Infections

GRANT J. ANHALT, M.D.

Associate Professor, Department of Dermatology, The Johns Hopkins Medical Institutions, Baltimore, Maryland
Pemphigus
Cicatricial Pemphigoid

FRANK C. ARNETT, M.D.

Professor of Internal Medicine and Director, Division of Rheumatology, University of Texas Health Sciences Center, Houston, Texas
Reiter's Syndrome

NANCY BARNETT, M.D.

Assistant Professor of Pediatrics and Dermatology, The Johns Hopkins Medical Institutions, Baltimore, Maryland
Pityriasis Rosea

WILMA F. BERGFELD, M.D.

Head, Clinical Dermatology Research, Department of Dermatology and Head, Dermatopathology, Department of Pathology, Cleveland Clinic Foundation, Cleveland, Ohio
Hirsutism

BARBARA H. BJORNSON, M.D.

Assistant Professor, Boston University School of Medicine and Tufts University School of Medicine; Consulting Hematologist/Oncologist, University Hospital, Boston, Massachusetts
Hypereosinophilia

BARBARA L. BRAUNSTEIN-WILSON, M.D.

Assistant Professor, University of Virginia School of Medicine, Charlottesville, Virginia
Lichen Planus
Palmoplantar Pustulosis

JEFFREY P. CALLEN, M.D.

Associate Professor of Medicine (Dermatology), University of Louisville School of Medicine; Chief, Department of Dermatology, Veterans Administration Medical Center, Louisville, Kentucky
Sarcoidosis

WRIGHT CAUGHMAN, M.D.

Senior Staff Fellow, Dermatology Branch, National Cancer Institute, National Institutes of Health, Bethesda, Maryland
Epidermolysis Bullosa Acquisita

RICHARD A. F. CLARK, M.D.

Associate Professor of Dermatology and Medicine, University of Colorado School of Medicine; Director of Dermatology, National Jewish Center for Immunology and Respiratory Medicine, Denver, Colorado
Atopic Dermatitis

DONALD E. CLEMONS, M.D., COL., M.C., U.S.A.

Clinical Associate Professor of Dermatology, University of Texas Medical School; Staff Dermatologist and Dermatopathologist, Brooke Army Medical Center, San Antonio, Texas
Bowen's Disease

FRANK W. CROWE, M.D. (Deceased)

Formerly, Clinical Professor of Dermatology, Oregon Health Sciences University, Portland, Oregon; Clinical Professor of Medicine (Dermatology), University of Washington Medical School, Seattle, Washington; Active Staff, St. Luke's Hospital; Consultant in Dermatology, St. Alphonsus and Elk's Rehabilitation Hospitals, Boise, Idaho; Mt. Home AFB Hospital and Nampa State School and Hospital, Nampa, Idaho
Orf

PETER E. DANS, M.D.

Associate Professor of Medicine, The Johns Hopkins Medical Institutions; Active Staff, Department of Medicine and Director, Office of Medical Practice Evaluation, The Johns Hopkins Hospital, Baltimore, Maryland
Syphilis

JOHN J. DiGIOVANNA, M.D.

Expert Consultant, Dermatology Branch, National Cancer Institute, National Institutes of Health, Bethesda, Maryland
Pityriasis Rubra Pilaris
Xeroderma Pigmentosum

LEONARD M. DZUBOW, M.D.

Assistant Professor of Dermatology, University of Pennsylvania School of Medicine, Philadelphia, Pennsylvania
Keloids

DAVID E. ELDER, M.B., Ch.B., B.Med.Sc.,
F.R.C.P.A.

Associate Professor of Pathology and Laboratory
Medicine in Dermatology, University of Pennsylvania
School of Medicine; Attending Pathologist, The
Pigmented Lesion Group and Division of Surgical
Pathology, Hospital of the University of Pennsylvania,
Philadelphia, Pennsylvania
Malignant Melanoma

MERVYN L. ELGART, M.D.

Professor and Chairman, Department of Dermatology,
George Washington University School of Medicine;
Attending Physician (Medicine), George Washington
University Hospital and Chief, Dermatology Section,
Children's Hospital National Medical Center,
Washington, D.C.
Hyperhidrosis

DAVID J. ELPERN, M.D.

Assistant Clinical Professor, University of Hawaii John
A. Burns School of Medicine, Honolulu, Hawaii;
Active Staff, The Skin Department, Kauai Medical Group,
Lihue, Hawaii
Sunburn

EDWARD A. EMMETT, M.B., B.S., M.S.

Professor and Director, Division of Occupational
Medicine, The Johns Hopkins Medical Institutions; Active
Clinical Staff, The Johns Hopkins Hospital,
Baltimore, Maryland
Occupation Related Dermatoses
Phototoxic Dermatitis

BONNIE S. EPSTEIN, M.D.

Resident, Department of Dermatology, The Johns Hopkins
Medical Institutions, Baltimore, Maryland
Molluscum Contagiosum

JOHN H. EPSTEIN, M.D.

Clinical Professor of Dermatology, University of
California School of Medicine, San Francisco, California
Polymorphous Light Eruption

EVAN R. FARMER, M.D.

Associate Professor of Dermatology and Pathology, The
Johns Hopkins Medical Institutions, Baltimore, Maryland
Dermatophyte Infections
Cercarial Dermatitis
Sea Nettle Dermatitis

JAMES E. FITZPATRICK, M.D., Lt. Col., M.C.,
U.S.A.

Assistant Clinical Professor, Department of Dermatology,
University of Colorado School of Medicine, Denver;
Assistant Chief of Dermatology, Fitzsimons Army
Medical Center, Aurora, Colorado
Chancroid

THOMAS B. FITZPATRICK, M.D., Ph.D.

Professor and Chairman, Department of Dermatology,
Harvard Medical School; Chief, Dermatology Service,
Massachusetts General Hospital, Boston, Massachusetts
Hyperpigmentation and Vitiligo

NICHOLAS J. FIUMARA, M.D., M.P.H.

Clinical Professor of Dermatology, Tufts University
School of Medicine, Adjunct Professor of Dermatology,
Boston University School of Medicine, and Lecturer in
Dermatology, Harvard Medical School; Visiting
Dermatologist, New England Medical Center, University
Hospital, Boston City Hospital, and Massachusetts
General Hospital, Boston, Massachusetts
Lymphogranuloma Venereum

IRWIN M. FREEDBERG, M.D.

George Miller MaKee Professor and Chairman,
Department of Dermatology, New York University School
of Medicine; Director of Dermatology Departments,
Bellevue Hospital and New York University Hospital,
New York, New York
Ichthyosis and Palmoplantar Keratodermas

JAY S. GOODMAN, M.D.

Professor of Medicine, University of Maryland School of
Medicine; Chairman, Department of Medicine, Mercy
Hospital, Baltimore, Maryland
Rocky Mountain Spotted Fever

ERNESTO GONZALEZ, M.D.

Assistant Professor of Dermatology, Harvard Medical
School; Dermatologist, Massachusetts General Hospital,
Boston, Massachusetts
Photoallergic Contact Dermatitis

RICHARD D. GRANSTEIN, M.D.

Assistant Professor of Dermatology, Harvard Medical
School; Assistant in Dermatology, Massachusetts General
Hospital, Boston, Massachusetts
Photoallergic Contact Dermatitis

RUSSELL P. HALL III, M.D.

Assistant Professor, Department of Medicine, Duke
University School of Medicine, Durham, North Carolina
Dermatitis Herpetiformis

JOHN B. HARLEY, M.D., Ph.D.

Associate Professor, Department of Medicine, University
of Oklahoma Health Sciences Center and Affiliated
Associate Professor, Oklahoma Medical Research
Foundation; Clinical Investigator, Oklahoma City
Veterans Administration Medical Center,
Oklahoma City, Oklahoma
Hypereosinophilia

MARC C. HOCHBERG, M.D., M.P.H.

Associate Professor of Medicine, The Johns Hopkins Medical Institutions; Attending Physician, The Johns Hopkins Hospital and Good Samaritan Hospital, Baltimore, Maryland
Temporal Arteritis

ANTOINETTE F. HOOD, M.D.

Associate Professor, Department of Dermatology, The Johns Hopkins Medical Institutions, Baltimore, Maryland
Kaposi's Sarcoma
Acquired Immundeficiency Syndrome (AIDS)
Drug Reactions

EDWARD W. HOOK III, M.D.

Assistant Professor of Medicine, The Johns Hopkins Medical Institutions; Chief, STD Clinical Services, Baltimore City Health Department, Baltimore, Maryland
Gonococcal Infections

SHARON R. HYMES, M.D.

Assistant Professor of Internal Medicine and Dermatology, University of South Florida College of Medicine; Attending Dermatologist, Tampa General Hospital and H. Lee Moffitt Cancer Center, Tampa, Florida
Toxic Epidermal Necrolysis

DOUGLAS A. JABS, M.D.

Assistant Professor, Department of Ophthalmology, The Johns Hopkins Medical Institutions, Baltimore, Maryland
Cicatricial Pemphigoid

RISE M. JAMPEL, M.D.

Fellow (Dermatopathology), Department of Dermatology, The Johns Hopkins Medical Institutions, Baltimore, Maryland
Zinc Deficiency Syndrome: Acrodermatitis Enteropathica

ROBERT E. JORDON, M.D.

Professor and Chairman, Department of Dermatology, The University of Texas Medical School; Chief of Dermatology, The Hermann Hospital, Houston, Texas
Herpes Gestationis

WILLIAM P. JORDAN Jr., M.D.

Professor of Dermatology, Virginia Commonwealth University, Medical College of Virginia, Richmond, Virginia
Allergic Contact Dermatitis

JOHN A. KAZMIEROWSKI, M.D.

Clinical Associate Professor of Dermatology, Oregon Health Sciences University School of Medicine, Portland, Oregon
Erythema Multiforme

AMAL K. KURBAN, M.D.

Professor of Dermatology, Boston University School of Medicine; Director, Skin Clinic, Boston City Hospital, Boston, Massachusetts
Seborrheic Dermatitis

STANFORD I. LAMBERG, M.D.

Associate Professor of Dermatology, The Johns Hopkins Medical Institutions; Chief, Department of Dermatology, Francis Scott Key Medical Center, Baltimore, Maryland
Mycosis Fungoides and the Sezary Syndrome

W. CLARK LAMBERT, M.D., Ph.D.

Associate Professor, Departments of Pathology and Medicine, University of Medicine and Dentistry, Newark, New Jersey
Parapsoriasis

ALFRED T. LANE, M.D.

Assistant Professor of Dermatology and Pediatrics, University of Rochester School of Medicine and Dentistry, Rochester, New York
Staphylococcal Scalded Skin Syndrome

THOMAS J. LAWLEY, M.D.

Senior Investigator, Dermatology Branch, National Institutes of Health, Bethesda, Maryland
Cutaneous Vasculitis

HOWARD M. LEDERMAN, M.D, Ph.D.

Assistant Professor, Department of Pediatrics and Department of Molecular Biology and Genetics, The Johns Hopkins Medical Institutions, Baltimore, Maryland
Chronic Mucocutaneous Candidiasis

RONALD R. LITEPLO, M.D.

Assistant Clinical Professor of Medicine (Dermatology), Albert Einstein College of Medicine; Attending, Montefiore Medical Center, Bronx, New York
Infestations and Insect Bites

DONALD P. LOOKINGBILL, M.D.

Professor of Medicine, Division of Dermatology, Pennsylvania State University College of Medicine, Hershey, Pennsylvania
Leg Ulcers

FREDERICK D. MALKINSON, M.D., D.M.D.

Professor of Dermatology, Rush Medical College; Senior Attending Physician of Dermatology, Rush-Presbyterian-St. Luke's Medical Center, Chicago, Illinois
Erythropoietic Protoporphyria and Porphyria Cutanea Tarda

JAMES G. MARKS Jr., M.D.

Associate Professor of Medicine, Pennsylvania State University College of Medicine; Active Staff, Division of Dermatology, The Milton S. Hershey Medical Center, Hershey, Pennsylvania
Candidiasis

THOMAS A. MEDSGER Jr., M.D.

Professor of Medicine and Chief, Division of Rheumatology and Clinical Immunology, University of Pittsburgh School of Medicine; Attending Physician, Presbyterian-University Hospital, Pittsburgh, Pennsylvania
Scleroderma

HERMAN S. MOGAVERO Jr., M.D.

Assistant Clinical Professor of Medicine and Dermatology, State University of New York School of Medicine; Dermatologist, Buffalo Medical Group, Buffalo, New York
Exfoliative Dermatitis
Granuloma Inguinale

WARWICK L. MORISON, M.B., B.S., M.D.

Associate Professor, Department of Dermatology, The Johns Hopkins Medical Institutions, Baltimore, Maryland
Psoriasis

SAMUEL L. MOSCHELLA, M.D.

Clinical Professor of Dermatology, Harvard Medical School, Boston; Senior Consultant, Lahey Clinic, Burlington, Massachusetts
Leishmaniasis

DAVID B. MOSHER, M.D.

Instructor in Dermatology, Harvard Medical School; Clinical Associate, Massachusetts General Hospital, Boston, Massachusetts
Hyperpigmentation and Vitiligo

ANDREW M. MUNSTER, M.D., F.R.C.S.(Eng, Edin), F.A.C.S.

Professor of Surgery, The Johns Hopkins Medical Institutions; Director, Baltimore Regional Burn Center, Francis Scott Key Medical Center, Baltimore, Maryland
Thermal Injury

NOREEN HEER NICOL, R.N., M.S., F.N.C.

Nurse Dermatology Specialist, National Jewish Center for Immunology and Respiratory Medicine, Denver, Colorado
Atopic Dermatitis

LAWRENCE A. NORTON, M.D.

Associate Clinical Professor of Dermatology, Boston University School of Medicine, Boston, Massachusetts
Nail Disorders

HARISH P. PATEL, M.D.

Assistant Professor, Department of Dermatology, The Johns Hopkins Medical Institutions, Baltimore, Maryland
Bullous Pemphigoid

MADHUKAR A. PATHAK, M.B., Ph.D.

Senior Associate in Dermatology (Biochemistry), Harvard Medical School; Biochemist, Massachusetts General Hospital, Boston, Massachusetts
Hyperpigmentation and Vitiligo

JAMES W. PATTERSON, M.D.

Associate Professor of Pathology and Dermatology and Director of Dermatopathology, Virginia Commonwealth University, Medical College of Virginia, Richmond, Virginia
Lyme Disease (Erythema Chronicum Migrans)

GARY L. PECK, M.D.

Senior Investigator, Dermatology Branch, National Cancer Institute, National Institutes of Health, Bethesda, Maryland
Pityriasis Rubra Pilaris

PETER E. POCHI, M.D.

Professor of Dermatology, Boston University School of Medicine; Visiting Dermatologist, University Hospital, Boston, Massachusetts
Acne

THOMAS T. PROVOST, M.D.

Noxell Professor and Chairman, Department of Dermatology, The Johns Hopkins Medical Institutions, Baltimore, Maryland
Pyoderma Gangrenosum
Hidradenitis Suppurativa
Acne Rosacea
Acquired Immunodeficiency Syndrome (AIDS)

THOMAS H. REA, M.D.

Professor of Medicine (Dermatology), University of Southern California School of Medicine; Chairman of Dermatology, Los Angeles County-USC Medical Center, Los Angeles, California
Leprosy

GEOFFREY P. REDMOND, M.D.

Staff, Department of Endocrinology and Department of Pediatric and Adolescent Medicine, Cleveland Clinic Foundation, Cleveland, Ohio
Hirsutism

MORRIS REICHLIN, M.D.

Professor of Medicine and Chief, Combined Immunology Section, Department of Medicine, University of Oklahoma Health Sciences Center; Chief, Arthritis/Immunology Program, Oklahoma Medical Research Foundation; Attending Physician, Oklahoma Memorial Hospital and Veterans Administration Medical Center, Oklahoma City, Oklahoma
Mixed Connective Tissue Disease

HOWARD N. ROBINSON, M.D.

Instructor, Department of Dermatology, The Johns Hopkins Medical Institutions, Baltimore, Maryland
Granuloma Annulare

BARBARA M. ROCK, M.D.

Research and Clinical Postdoctoral Fellow, The Johns Hopkins Medical Institutions; Senior Clinical Fellow, The Johns Hopkins Hospital, Baltimore, Maryland
Warts

ROY S. ROGERS III, M.D.

Professor of Dermatology, Mayo Medical School; Consultant, Mayo Clinic and Attending Physician, Rochester Methodist and St. Marys Hospitals, Rochester, Minnesota
Recurrent Aphthous Stomatitis

STUART J. SALASCHE, COL., M.C., U.S.A.

Assistant Chief of Dermatology and Head, Dermatologic Surgery/Motts Surgery Unit, Brooke Army Medical Center, Fort Sam, Houston, Texas
Actinic Keratosis and Keratoacanthoma

MIGUEL R. SANCHEZ, M.D.

Assistant Professor, Department of Dermatology, New York University School of Medicine; Attending-in-Chief, Dermatology Outpatient Service, Bellevue Hospital and New York University Medical Center, New York, New York
Ichthyosis and Palmoplantar Keratodermas

MARK H. SAWYER, M.D.

Medical Staff Fellow, Medical Virology Section, Laboratory of Clinical Investigation, National Institute of Allergy and Infectious Diseases, Bethesda, Maryland
Herpes Simplex

JOHN W. SKOUGE, M.D.

Assistant Professor, Departments of Dermatology and Otolaryngology—Head and Neck Surgery and Director, Division of Cutaneous Surgery, The Johns Hopkins Medical Institutions, Baltimore, Maryland
Basal Cell and Squamous Cell Carcinoma
Hidradenitis Suppurativa

RICHARD D. SONTHEIMER, M.D.

Associate Professor of Dermatology and Internal Medicine, The University of Texas Southwestern Medical Center School; Staff Physician, Dermatology Consultation Service, Parkland Memorial Hospital, Children's Medical Center, and St. Paul Hospital, Dallas, Texas
Lupus Erythematosus

NICHOLAS A. SOTER, M.D.

Professor of Dermatology, New York University School of Medicine; Attending Physician, University Hospital, Bellevue Hospital, and Veterans Administration Hospital, New York, New York
Mastocytosis and Urticaria Pigmentosa

JENNY L. STONE, M.D.

Resident in Dermatology, Baylor College of Medicine, Houston, Texas
Sunburn

STEPHEN E. STRAUS, M.D.

Head, Medical Virology Section, Laboratory of Clinical Investigation, National Institute of Allergy and Infectious Diseases, Bethesda, Maryland
Herpes Simplex

RONALD J. SWEREN, M.D.

Clinical Assistant Professor of Dermatology and Pediatrics, University of Maryland Hospital, Baltimore, Maryland
Alopecia Areata

ROBERT A. SWERLICK, M.D.

Medical Staff Fellow, Dermatology Branch, National Institutes of Health, Bethesda, Maryland
Cutaneous Vasculitis

NORMAN TALAL, M.D.

Professor of Medicine and Microbiology, The University of Texas Medical School; Chief, Clinical Immunology Service, Audie L. Murphy Memorial Veterans Hospital, San Antonio, Texas
Sjögren's Syndrome

IRA N. TARGOFF, M.D.

Assistant Professor of Medicine, University of Oklahoma Health Sciences Center and Oklahoma Medical Research Foundation; Research Associate, Veterans Administration Medical Center, Oklahoma City, Oklahoma
Dermatomyositis

ROBERT M. TAYLOR, M.D.

Assistant Professor, Departments of Dermatology and Pathology, The Johns Hopkins Medical Institutions, Baltimore, Maryland
Granuloma Faciale
Bacterial Infections

BRUCE H. THIERS, M.D.

Associate Professor, Department of Dermatology, Medical University of South Carolina College of Medicine; Chief, Dermatology Service, Veterans Administration Medical Center, Charleston, South Carolina
Cutaneous Larva Migrans

MARCIA G. TONNESEN, M.D.

Assistant Professor, Department of Dermatology, University of Colorado School of Medicine; Chief, Dermatology Service, Veterans Administration Medical Center, Denver, Colorado
Pruritus

THEODORE A. TROMOVITCH, M.D.

Clinical Professor of Dermatology, University of California School of Medicine, San Francisco, California
Basal Cell and Squamous Cell Carcinoma

MARIA L. TURNER, M.D.

Professor of Dermatology, George Washington University School of Medicine, Washington, D.C.
Vulvar Dermatosis

MARK E. UNIS, M.D.

Assistant Clinical Professor, Department of Dermatology and Cutaneous Surgery, University of Miami School of Medicine, Miami, Florida; Chief of the Division of Dermatology, Department of Medicine, Holy Cross Hospital and North Ridge General Hospital, Fort Lauderdale, Florida
Erythema Nodosum

JOHN P. UTZ, M.D.

Professor of Medicine, Georgetown University School of Medicine; Attending and Consulting Physician, Infectious Disease Service, Georgetown University Hospital, Washington, D.C.
Systemic Mycoses

MARTIN D. VALENTINE, M.D.

Professor of Medicine, The Johns Hopkins Medical Institutions; Physician, The Johns Hopkins Hospital and Good Samaritan Hospital, Baltimore, Maryland
Chronic Urticaria

DAVID B. VASILY, M.D.

Consulting Dermatologist, St. Luke's Hospital and Chief, Dermatology Section, Muhlenberg Hospital Center, Bethlehem, Pennsylvania
Sweet's Syndrome

ROSEMARIE WATSON, M.D.

Assistant Professor, Department of Dermatology, The Johns Hopkins Hospital, Baltimore, Maryland
Subcorneal Pustular Dermatosis
Neonatal Lupus Erythematosus

FREDERICK M. WIGLEY, M.D.

Associate Professor of Medicine, The Johns Hopkins Hospital, Baltimore, Maryland
Raynaud's Phenomenon

JERRY A. WINKELSTEIN, M.D.

Professor of Pediatrics, The Johns Hopkins Medical Institutions, Baltimore, Maryland
Chronic Mucocutaneous Candidiasis

KIRK D. WUEPPER, M.D.

Professor of Dermatology, The Oregon Health Sciences University School of Medicine, Portland, Oregon
Erythema Multiforme

WILLIAM H. ZINKHAM, M.D.

Professor of Pediatrics and Professor of Oncology, The Johns Hopkins Medical Institutions; Director of Pediatric Hematology, The Johns Hopkins Hospital, Baltimore, Maryland
Cutaneous Histiocytosis

THOMAS M. ZIZIC, M.D., F.A.R.A.

Associate Professor, The Johns Hopkins Medical Institutions and Assistant Professor, University of Maryland School of Medicine; Associate Director of The Johns Hopkins Rheumatic Disease Unit at the Good Samaritan Hospital and Attending Rheumatologist, The Johns Hopkins Hospital, Baltimore, Maryland
Relapsing Polychondritis

JOHN J. ZONE, M.D.

Associate Professor of Medicine, Division of Dermatology, University of Utah Health Sciences Center, Salt Lake City, Utah
Chronic Bullous Dermatosis of Childhood

PREFACE

As we stated in the first edition of this text, standard textbooks of dermatology are helpful for understanding the basic information available about specific diseases, but customarily do not provide in-depth or up-to-date information about therapy. Specifically, textbooks rarely provide a basic approach to a problem in sufficient detail for practical management; neither do they supply alternative forms of therapy for complicated problems.

The emphasis of this book is on the current therapy of specific skin diseases. Common and somewhat unusual diseases were selected for inclusion, but as in the first edition, there was no attempt to cover all possible disorders. We believe this information will be useful for all clinicians who care for patients with skin disease.

The authors were selected for their clinical expertise in a given area and were asked to provide their personal approach to the management of a specific disorder. We asked them to recommend specific drugs, their dosages, and their routes of administration in detail, as well as alternative modes of therapy in order of preference with a rationale for the sequence. Complications of therapy and management of the complications were to be stressed. We realize that many of the modes of therapy given in this text have not been submitted to double-blind testing or may not even be mentioned in other textbooks, but they reflect the author's views and experience on what works and how to handle the problem at hand. Were they not given this freedom to discuss their approach, many of these ideas may not be widely available.

A second edition of a book implies not only acceptance and success of the first, but a promise of growth and improvement. Based on this premise, we have compiled this monograph to complement and succeed the first edition by increasing the number of diseases discussed, by replacing many authors to provide different points of view, and by updating the remaining chapters. As dermatology and all of medicine continues to evolve, we need this type of information at our fingertips to provide the best management for our patients. Who is better qualified to write on a specific disease than an expert in its treatment.

Thomas T. Provost

Evan R. Farmer

CONTENTS

PAPULOSQUAMOUS DISEASES

PSORIASIS

WARWICK L. MORISON, M.B., B.S., M.D.

We are all familiar with the concept of the "heartbreak" of psoriasis, although it is not clear whether the grief is felt by the physician, the patient, or both. The concept embodies the negative attitude toward treatment of the disease in so many patients and physicians. This negative attitude is unfounded because psoriasis can be successfully treated. However, to achieve this the physician must have a planned approach to the management of the disease. The plan must contain several key elements.

First, the physician must recognize, and explain to the patient, that psoriasis is a chronic disease that usually persists for years, that there is no quick fix or cure, but that there are some very successful treatments that can control the disease in most patients. Second, the initial visit must include a full evaluation of the patient and the disease. Sex, age, occupation, social environment, geographic location, and medical history are important factors in deciding upon the best treatment for the type and extent of disease present. This evaluation takes time, but is essential because the physician must know the patient, the disease, and how the patient feels about the disease. Third, the patient must be educated about the disease and all possible treatments; a handout is an invaluable addition but not a substitute for this explanation. Finally, the treatment program that is agreed upon with the patient must be tailored to the patient and to the disease. The patient must be "sold" on the treatment or it will not be used. The treatment must have a reasonable risk–benefit ratio and be effective for the type of disease being treated.

THERAPEUTIC AGENTS

Treatment modalities with antipsoriatic activity can be broadly divided into three groups: topical, ultraviolet radiation, and systemic. This sequence also roughly defines their risk–benefit ratios: topical agents are usually safest and of benefit only in limited disease, while systemic agents carry greatest risk and should be used only in extensive disease.

Topical Agents

Topically applied corticosteroids are the most frequently prescribed treatment for psoriasis, and this is probably more a tribute to advertising by drug companies rather than their true value as treatment. Only rarely do these agents convert psoriasis to normal skin, and as soon as the treatment is stopped, the psoriasis usually rapidly returns. Tachyphylaxis, permanent atrophy of the skin, and conversion of stable psoriasis to a more aggressive disease, are the chief problems associated with use of these agents. The introduction of clobetisol propionate and betamethasone dipropionate will undoubtedly add new adverse effects. Adrenal suppression and precipitation of generalized pustular psoriasis have been observed frequently in Europe with such potent agents. For all these reasons, corticosteroids should be used in psoriasis only as adjunctive treatment with other more effective agents, in special situations such as the treatment of nails, and in patients who will accept improvement rather than clearance of disease. Systemically administered corticosteroids have no place in the treatment of psoriasis, since rebound, spreading disease and serious adverse effects are almost inevitable.

There has been a resurgence of interest in using anthralin in the treatment of psoriasis, mainly because of the introduction of improved formulations and the discovery that its application for 30 minutes yields results as good as those from overnight application. Problems remain: Anthralin stains the skin a grayish color and this persists for several weeks. It also stains porcelain, and because this can be permanent, patients must be warned to wash it off in a fast flowing shower or to use a rubber basin for washing their hair. Anthralin is also a potent irritant and some patients cannot tolerate the treatment. Reducing the frequency of application and starting with a low strength are the main ways of minimizing the problems. However, despite these disadvantages, it has major advantages over topical corticosteroids: it can clear psoriasis, and remissions often last for months without treatment.

Tar is an effective antipsoriatic agent, but there are several reasons its use should be abandoned. First, it is only weakly effective. Second, it is messy and abhorrent to use. Third, it is carcinogenic in humans, and psoriatic patients are already exposed to enough other carcinogens and immunosuppressive agents. The so-called refined tar preparations appear to have little, if any, therapeutic effect.

1

Ultraviolet Radiation

The sun has probably been used in the treatment of psoriasis for as long as the disease has existed, since most patients know that they improve during the summer or a winter vacation in the tropics. The latter can be used as an effective and popular treatment in selected patients.

Phototherapy using ultraviolet B (UVB) radiation with prior application of a lubricant is an effective treatment for psoriasis. When erythemogenic doses of UVB radiation are used, about 95 percent of selected patients can be cleared in 20 to 30 treatments. This regimen requires, first, determining the minimal erythema dose, giving 70 percent of that dose as the first exposure dose, and then increasing the exposure dose by 17 percent each treatment. If there is significant disease on the limbs, the same dose is given as an extra exposure while the face and trunk are kept covered. Treatments are given three to five times each week. A lubricant must be applied to each psoriasis plaque that has a surface scale immediately before treatment, since this increases penetration of the radiation. Symptomatic erythema is the main short term problem. Over the long term this treatment is probably carcinogenic but the risk appears to be low. Photoaging of the skin is another long term problem. The main disadvantage of the treatment is the lack of a reasonable maintenance regimen. Twice-weekly treatment is usually necessary to maintain a clear state, and most patients find this frequency of treatment economically and socially unacceptable.

Low dose, nonerythemogenic UVB phototherapy has been used by some people with success. A starting dose well below an erythemal response is selected, and small increments are given with each treatment. A problem with this approach is that patients frequently finish a course of treatment tanned with psoriasis and, not surprisingly, unhappy.

Photochemotherapy, with ingestion of methoxsalen and subsequent exposure to ultraviolet A (UVA) radiation (PUVA therapy), is more effective than UVB phototherapy for both clearance and maintenance treatment. More than 95 percent of the patients with psoriasis can be cleared in 20 to 30 treatments. The treatment is given two to four times each week to clear disease, and the maintenance requirements vary from weekly to monthly treatments; most patients require two treatments each month.

The short term problems with this therapy are nausea and erythema. Nausea is due to methoxsalen and is dose related; reduction of the dose by 10 mg cures most people. Cataracts, skin cancer, and photoaging are the main long term concerns. Cataracts should not occur if patients wear ultraviolet-opaque glasses after ingesting methoxsalen. Skin cancer is a risk, especially if a patient has had superficial x-ray or grenz ray treatment, has had skin cancer, or is fair skinned. These risk factors must be evaluated in each patient. In addition, skin cancer is readily amenable to treatment provided the patient is carefully followed and regularly examined. The guidelines for PUVA therapy were published in the *Journal of the American Academy of Dermatology* (1979; 1:106).

Home phototherapy is useful in a few patients. A sunlamp from any drugstore can be used to augment topical treatment for localized psoriasis. Whole body treatment at home is not advisable for several reasons. First, it is not very effective, since patients frequently underdose or overdose themselves. Second, if the treatment is directed by a physician, he or she is taking some responsibility for its safety. Home built light boxes are unlikely to be electrically safe. Obviously if the physician supplies plans for the unit, he or she is even more involved. Finally, patients have a tendency to forget to come for follow-up examination until the first skin cancer appears.

The combination of the topical application of tar preparations and exposure to UVB radiation, the Goeckerman regimen, is still used in some centers. This treatment relies on the mild antipsoriatic effect of tar and the much more potent antipsoriatic effect of UVB radiation. On the positive side, the treatment is effective and safe. However, there is a negative side. The treatment is expensive, since it must be done in a hospital or a day care center. Second, because there is no provision for maintenance, the psoriasis gradually returns once the patient has been discharged. Finally, several studies have shown that tar given with UVB radiation is no more effective than a lubricant with UVB radiation; few patients have difficulty in choosing between a lubricant and a messy tar preparation.

Climatotherapy at the Dead Sea, a successful short term therapy for psoriasis, appears to involve a mixture of UVB phototherapy, psychotherapy, and topical treatment. The main component is phototherapy. Since the Dead Sea is below sea level, sunlight there passes through a greater thickness of atmosphere, which filters out the erythemogenic wavelengths shorter than 300 nm. Consequently, patients can expose themselves to sunlight for long periods each day and receive very high doses of radiation of wavelengths longer than 300 nm, which is more therapeutic for psoriasis. The psychotherapeutic effects of a vacation and association with other people with psoriasis, are also important factors. On the negative side, in many patients the disease does not clear completely, and the duration of a remission appears to be no longer than it is with the Goeckerman treatment. A winter vacation in the Caribbean is probably cheaper, more enjoyable, and equally effective.

Systemic Therapy

Methotrexate is the best systemically administered drug for the treatment of psoriasis. It is an excellent treatment, but it does have serious long term adverse effects. Therefore, this drug should be held in reserve until other less toxic therapeutic options have been exhausted and the patient has psoriasis of a sufficient severity to warrant taking the risks associated with the treatment. An exception is the short term use of methotrexate in combination with PUVA therapy or phototherapy.

Depression of the bone marrow is the main short term problem with methotrexate. The main long term problem is impairment of liver function, and this occurs in 25 to 40 percent of the patients. Methotrexate is teratogenic, and therefore it should not be used in women of child bearing age without adequate contraception during treatment and for 1 month after cessation of the drug. Another problem is that methotrexate appears to alter the nature of psoriasis, making it a more aggressive disease. Thus, a person may have had the ordinary plaque type of psoriasis but after receiving methotrexate for several years may develop unstable inflammatory psoriasis when an attempt is made to shift to another treatment. The guidelines for methotrexate therapy have been published in the *Journal of the American Academy of Dermatology* (1982; 6:145). Several different regimens are used, but the approach of dividing the weekly dose into 3 doses given at consecutive 12 hourly intervals appears to be the most effective and safest.

Retinoids have antipsoriatic activity. Etretinate is the preferred drug for the treatment of psoriasis because isotretinoin is much less effective. The main indications for etretinate are the erythrodermic and generalized pustular types of psoriasis, and in a daily dosage of 0.6 to 1 mg per kilogram of body weight this drug is equally as effective as methotrexate in the treatment of these two rare forms of the disease. Etretinate is not very useful in the treatment of the ordinary plaque type of psoriasis; in some patients the disease is partially controlled, but to achieve complete clearance, months of therapy are required. The major disadvantage of etretinate therapy is that it produces side effects in 100 percent of the patients. The most common adverse effects involve the skin and mucous membranes, and these are inconvenient rather than hazardous. However, hyperlipidemia, liver abnormalities, and calcification of tendons occur in 50 to 85 percent of the patients. The long term significance of some of these side effects is still unknown, and thus use of the drug should be restricted to the rare patient who is unresponsive to other less hazardous therapy. Etretinate is only slowly excreted over 12 to 18 months, and since it is markedly teratogenic, it should not be used in any women of child bearing age as it is impossible to guarantee contraception over such a long period.

Other Treatments

Trauma to the skin is a significant factor in inducing psoriasis, as evidenced by the Koebner phenomenon and localization of the disease to certain areas such as the elbows and knees. Telling patients to reduce the amount of trauma to the skin is good advice, but, except in specific instances, it is not a practical approach to treatment. Use of a condom in a person with psoriasis of the penis and protection of the hands, if they are affected, are two specific instances.

Emotional stress is also a trigger for psoriasis, but, again, telling patients to reduce the amount of stress in their lives is easy rather than practical advice. Perhaps the importance of emotional stress in exacerbating psoriasis is overemphasized. Certainly there are some patients who suffer a flare-up of disease whenever the social milieu becomes stormy. However, there are many other patients who

go through deaths, divorces, operations, and other stressful experiences without fluctuation of the disease or requirement for increased treatment to control the disease. Alcohol abuse is an issue that has been raised in psoriatic patients. Anecodotal comments have claimed that alcohol exacerbates psoriasis, but there is no evidence to support this comment. It is possible that patients drink because they have severe psoriasis rather than vice versa, if indeed they do consume more alcohol than other people.

Several medications can induce or exacerbate psoriasis and should be avoided by patients if possible. Lithium and the antimalarial drugs are the main offenders. Beta-blockers can induce a psoriasiform eruption as a rare side effect, and there are a few reports of the exacerbation of existing psoriasis.

Finally, providing information about the National Psoriasis Foundation can be a worthwhile therapeutic measure in some patients. These patients have a desire to "do something" about finding a cause and cure for their disease, and contact with this organization provides an outlet for these feelings. Furthermore, patients feel that they are being kept up to date about psoriasis through information in the foundation's newsletter.

THERAPEUTIC REGIMENS

Psoriasis Vulgaris

From a therapeutic stand point, plaque-form and papular psoriasis of the trunk and limbs can be divided into three categories: minimal psoriasis involving an area less than the surface area of two palms, moderate psoriasis involving an area less than the surface area of one upper limb, and extensive psoriasis involving a surface area greater than one upper limb. Although the extent of disease is usually the main factor dictating a choice of treatment, other characteristics of the disease or the patient may dominate the decision; this applies particularly to patients with moderate disease.

Mild disease localized to a few plaques or papules is best managed by topical therapy. Drithocreme is the linchpin of treatment because it can clear disease and provide a remission for weeks or months. In fair skinned patients treatment should be started with the 0.25 percent strength, whereas in dark skinned patients 0.5 percent is a safe preparation as initial therapy. The patient is instructed to apply the preparation daily for 30 minutes and then to wash it off in a shower. Treatment should be reviewed every two weeks, and if the cream is not causing any irritation, a higher strength preparation is prescribed. If the Drithocreme is causing marked irritation, the frequency of application should be reduced until this ceases to be a problem.

A second treatment to be used overnight should always be given in addition to the short term application of Drithocreme. Keralyt gel under occlusion with Saran Wrap is useful if plaques are thick and hyperkeratotic. Cordran tape, or a medium potency corticosteroid cream under occlusion can be used in other patients and is helpful for the control of irritation from anthralin. Vioform-hydrocortisone cream should be substituted for intertriginous areas. A moisturizing preparation, selected by the preference of the patient for a cream, lotion, or ointment, should be used during the day. Intralesional steroid treatment is sometimes useful in patients with a few small thick lesions, but its use should always be combined with anthralin because otherwise the psoriasis will rapidly return once the effect of the corticosteroid has dissipated.

This regimen for the treatment of minimal psoriasis will be successful only if the physician exhibits enthusiasm and involvement and goals are defined at the initiation of treatment. The patient should be seen at least every 2 weeks, and the aim is to clear the psoriasis in 6 to 8 weeks. Short duration, focused treatment breeds enthusiasm and succeeds, whereas treatment with absence of deadlines and infrequent follow-up is bound to fail.

Psoriasis of moderate extent is a difficult therapeutic problem for two reasons. First, it is an economic and physical logistic problem for the patient to use topical therapy over a moderately extensive area and succeed in clearing the disease. Second, if a more potent therapy is used, such as UVB phototherapy in the office, the patient is frequently unhappy with the end result. The reason for this is simple. Phototherapy usually achieves 95 percent clearance of disease but rarely achieves 100 percent clearance. The patient with moderate disease usually wants 100 percent clearance, whereas a patient with much more extensive disease is usually delighted with 95 percent clearance. Despite these problems, the treatment of choice is topical therapy, as for minimal psoriasis, supplemented in most instances with the use of a small sunlamp at home or a course of UVB phototherapy in the office. The selection of treatment depends on assessment of the disease and the patient. Psoriasis confined mainly to exposed areas and concern about appearance because of employment and social factors are characteristics that weigh in favor of UVB phototherapy. Short term maintenance UVB treatment for a couple of months is useful in this type of patient to ensure a reasonable remission.

There are a number of therapeutic regimens available for treating psoriasis covering an extensive area. UVB phototherapy in the office is the treatment of choice in the following cases: children, nursing and pregnant women, patients unwilling to use eye protection or take psoralen, patients who have sustained extensive solar damage or who have had significant exposure to grenz rays or superficial x-rays, and patients with psoriasis of recent onset. Whether long term maintenance treatment is given after clearance of disease is a decision reached after a full discussion with the patient, since usually weekly or more frequent treatment is necessary.

In all other patients the treatment of choice is PUVA therapy alone or in combination with methotrexate. PUVA therapy is effective in clearing disease in almost all patients and provides convenient maintenance treatment to prevent a recurrence. In the maintenance phase the frequency of treatment is gradually reduced, and if there is no significant flare-up of disease on monthly treatment, the therapy can be suspended. A methotrexate-PUVA combination treatment is useful in patients with very thick plaques, in patients with very active disease, and in those in whom the disease cannot be cleared with PUVA therapy alone. Methotrexate is given for 3 weeks before commencing PUVA therapy and is gradually withdrawn as clearing is achieved.

An alternative combination treatment is UVB phototherapy with PUVA therapy, and this combination is particularly useful in patients in whom methotrexate is contraindicated. Full doses of both treatments are given, exposure to the two wave bands being administered consecutively on the same day. These two combination treatments are very effective, and virtually all patients with psoriasis vulgaris can be cleared of disease using single or multiple treatments.

The main problem with the combination treatments is a high incidence of phototoxicity, but this is a short term effect that is easily corrected by modifying the exposure dose. Although most patients can be cleared of disease using ultraviolet radiation, a small number cannot be maintained in a clear state using PUVA therapy alone. A combination of low dose methotrexate and PUVA therapy is often a better treatment for these patients. In addition, there are patients in whom PUVA therapy is contraindicated, and long term methotrexate treatment must be considered in these cases.

Psoriasis of the Scalp

The scalp requires specific attention when it is involved, except in patients being treated with methotrexate or etretinate. PUVA and UVB therapy are not effective for the treatment of psoriasis on the scalp, but if it is first cleared with topical therapy, UV therapy is often effective in keeping the scalp free of disease without continuation of topical therapy.

The best topical treatment is anthralin as Drithoscalp cream, which is formulated for application to the scalp. The application time is 30 minutes daily or as often as tolerated. A tar shampoo is used, because although the therapeutic effect from this brief exposure to tar is probably minimal, such preparations are labeled for the treatment of psoriasis and thus are favored by patients.

A corticosteroid lotion, such as Lidex solution, is applied overnight for its effect in reducing irritation from the Drithoscalp cream and its antipsoriatic action. If a patient has the thick asbestos type of psoriasis of the scalp, Keralyt gel under occlusion should be used initially to remove all the scale.

Psoriasis of the Palms and Soles

The treatment of choice is oral PUVA therapy. There is the temptation to use topical application of psoralen for this localized disease, but there is a high frequency of blistering burns with that treatment. Between 20 and 30 treatments with oral PUVA therapy are usually required to achieve clearance of disease. The only adjunctive treatment required is application of a keratolytic agent in patients with hyperkeratotic lesions so as to reduce the barrier to radiation. Specialized hand and foot UVA radiators are available and are very efficient, but the door panel of a stand-up unit is almost as effective. Ordinary topical therapy is ineffective in the treatment of psoriasis of the palms and soles. Topical corticosteroid therapy usually produces some improvement, but because it is seldom sustained, the patient is left a virtual cripple in these socially and physically important areas of the body. UVB phototherapy is also without effect because this wavelength cannot penetrate the thick stratum corneum of the palms and soles.

Psoriatic Nail Disease

Involvement of the nail bed or nail matrix by psoriasis is a difficult therapeutic problem. Pitting or a more severe dystrophy can be treated by application of Cordran tape to the skin over the matrix, but the treatment must be continued for months and the incidence of success is low. Onycholysis does not appear to respond to intralesional steroids applied into the nail bed. Nail disease clears in about 50 percent of the patients treated with PUVA therapy, but it usually requires 4 to 6 months of treatment. Local PUVA treatment, with exposure of the dorsa of the hands and feet, is a useful treatment in patients with severe nail disease.

Erythrodermic and Generalized Pustular Psoriasis

These rare forms of psoriasis are usually an indication for hospitalization, since, particularly in the case of the von Zumbusch form of pustular psoriasis, they can be life-threatening. If an infection or metabolic disturbance is present, this must be treated. Patients with pustular psoriasis that has been triggered by the abrupt withdrawal of large doses of high potency corticosteroid preparations must be tested for adrenocortical suppression and given appropriate supplementation. Local care of the skin should be confined to wet dressings and moisturizers. Methotrexate and etretinate are the specific drugs of choice, methotrexate being preferred provided there are no contraindications to its use. When the patient is stabilized, PUVA therapy should be commenced using low doses of UVA radiation and treatment on consecutive days followed by a rest day. Once the lesions have cleared, PUVA therapy usually can be continued as the sole treatment.

Acute Guttate Psoriasis

This variant of psoriasis typically follows an upper respiratory tract infection with a delay of 10 to 14 days. Streptococcal infection used to be the most common cause, but viral infections now seem to be almost as common. A 2 week course of penicillin is indicated if a streptococcal organism grows from a throat swab culture. Many cases of acute guttate psoriasis are said to clear spontaneously, but certainly some do not and the condition can become chronic. Thus, the treatment of choice is a course of UVB phototherapy to ensure that all lesions do clear. Maintenance therapy is usually unnecessary.

Psoriatic Arthritis

There is a form of arthritis that is peculiar to patients with psoriasis and afflicts about 5 percent of the patients. Psoriatic arthritis is rheumatoid factor negative, is usually asymmetric, and affects the distal interphalangeal and sacroiliac joints. A severe form, arthritis mutilans, is fortunately rare. In most instances dermatologists or their patients elect to have an internist or rheumatologist manage the arthritis, but for several reasons the dermatologist should keep in close contact with the progress of therapy for the arthritis. The activities of the skin disease and the arthritis are usually independent of each other, and treatment of the skin seldom affects the arthritis; however, the reverse is not true. Nonsteroidal anti-inflammatory drugs occasionally may exacerbate the skin disease, although this is probably a rare event. Oral doses of corticosteroids should be avoided if at all possible, as has been mentioned. Finally, some internists are not aware that methotrexate is a very effective drug for treating arthritis. Thus, in a patient with significant skin disease and arthritis, methotrexate is often the treatment of choice for both problems. Preliminary reports suggest that etretinate is also effective for psoriatic arthritis, but the toxicity of the treatment may limit its usefulness.

CONCLUSIONS

It is obvious from meeting many patients and from published surveys that many patients with psoriasis are displeased with the management of their disease. There are several common reasons for their displeasure. First, they perceive a lack of interest or a feeling of resignation on the part of many physicians. The "try this; it is new and it might work" attitude is hardly likely to boost morale and engender enthusiasm in a patient with a chronic disease. Second, patients do not like many of the treatments that are frequently used. Tying oneself into a layer of Saran Wrap over a film of grease is not really the nicest way to retire for the evening. Anointing oneself with foul smelling black goop is not a pleasant experience. Third, patients do not like to have psoriasis, any psoriasis, and yet many treatments leave them with a significant level of disease for long periods of time. Topical corticosteroid treatment improves but seldom clears psoriasis. Hospital treatment often flattens psoriasis without clearing it, and then the patient has to endure months of disease until its severity warrants another admission to a hospital or day care center. Finally, many physicians regard psoriasis as being only a cosmetic disturbance. Offering a red, scaly hand for a handshake and leaving a confetti trail of scale behind are more than cosmetic problems; not to mention the soreness and pruritus that can be present.

All these sources of displeasure on the part of the patient must be kept in mind when treating psoriasis. A positive, interested attitude on the part of the physician can work miracles. Selection of a treatment that works, and yet does not totally disrupt the patient's life, is possible with the therapeutic modalities available today. The end result is a happy patient who stays with that physician.

PITYRIASIS RUBRA PILARIS

JOHN J. DIGIOVANNA, M.D.
GARY L. PECK, M.D.

Pityriasis rubra pilaris (PRP) is a chronic papulosquamous disorder characterized by hyperkeratotic follicular papules, palmar-plantar hyperkeratosis, and red-orange, finely scaling plaques. The extent of involvement varies from a few localized patches to generalized exfoliative erythroderma, both of which may contain islands of normal-appearing skin. The severity of the disease varies from patient to patient. The clinical course is of variable duration, as spontaneous remissions occur frequently but unpredictably.

Five clinical types have been described. In classic adult PRP, the most frequent type, spontaneous remissions occur in approximately 80 percent of the cases within 2 to 4 years. Patients with this type often have a rapid spread of scaling follicular papules leading to widespread erythema, which surrounds islands of spared skin. Palmar-plantar hyperkeratosis, ectropion, and nail changes can occur. Atypical adult PRP is clinically ichthyosiform and may include partial alopecia. Classic juvenile PRP is clinically similar to the classic adult type but begins in the first few years of life. Circumscribed PRP begins in childhood but does not become widespread. Atypical juvenile PRP begins in early childhood, is ichthyosiform in appearance, and may be familial. In this type, palmar-plantar keratoderma may be severe.

The value of any particular treatment of PRP is difficult to assess because of the rarity of PRP and its many subtypes, as well as the variable severity and variable natural duration of this disease. In addition, some of the therapies used, e.g., retinoids, have obvious side effects which preclude the possibility of doing long-term double-blind studies.

THERAPEUTIC ALTERNATIVES

Mild Disease

Mild, localized involvement with PRP may be adequately treated with topical therapy alone. While many topical therapies have been used for PRP, the most common include emollients, keratolytics, all-trans retinoic acid, and corticosteroids. Tar preparations alone or with ultraviolet light have also been used, but PRP has been reported to flare after sunlight and ultraviolet light exposure.

Topical emollients (e.g., petrolatum, Aquaphor) are safe and adequate symptomatic treatment for some patients whose disease is mild and localized. Liberal application, preferably after a bath, hydrates the skin and removes scale.

Keratolytics are agents that solubilize the stratum corneum. Salicylic acid (2 to 5 percent) in petrolatum or in a commercially available gel (Keralyt) may be useful to reduce hyperkeratosis, such as on the palms and soles. In more resistant cases, the gel can be applied with plastic occlusion for periods of 4 to 8 hours, possibly followed by application of a corticosteroid ointment. The possibility of salicylism from percutaneous absorption must be kept in mind, however.

Alpha-hydroxy acids, such as lactic acid and pyruvic acid, are thought to reduce epidermal hyperkeratosis by decreasing corneocyte cohesion preferentially at the lower, more newly formed, layers of the stratum corneum. After several days of topical treatment with alpha-hydroxy acids, a normal-appearing skin surface often appears abruptly after a sheetlike desquamation of the entire thickened stratum corneum. Lactic acid (2 to 10 percent) in a cream or ointment base may be applied one to four times daily. Twelve percent ammonium lactate lotion is commercially available (Lac-Hydrin) and in our experience is often well tolerated and more effective than other lactic acid preparations. Topical urea (10 to 20 percent) in a lotion or cream base, in contrast to the alpha-hydroxy acids, modifies abnormal stratum corneum by enhancing hydration and altering skin permeability.

The topical application of corticosteroid creams and ointments has been used in the treatment of PRP for years with variable effects. Mid- to high-potency fluorinated corticosteroid creams are of some benefit in mild to moderate PRP. However, frequent topical use of potent corticosteroid creams, especially on erythrodermic skin, can lead to cutaneous side effects, such as atrophy, and to systemic toxicity, such as adrenal suppression. Application of potent corticosteroid creams should be limited to two or three times daily. Bland emollients should be used with the topical corticosteroid creams for lubrication.

Topical all-trans retinoic acid can be especially useful on hyperkeratotic areas to produce a thinner, more normal-appearing skin. The main limitation to its use is the irritation that can occur, particularly if it is applied to erythematous skin.

Severe Disease

Patients with extensive involvement or severe symptoms may require systemic treatment. Emollients and other beneficial topical therapies may be continued in patients with severe cases of the disease in an effort to minimize the amount of systemic treatment required.

While psoralen and ultraviolet A light (PUVA) therapy has been used, PRP often flares after exposure to ultraviolet light. Consequently ultraviolet light therapy should be administered with caution, and patients should be monitored closely for adverse reactions.

Methotrexate has been extensively studied, but has yielded equivocal results in PRP. Candidates for methotrexate have generally been patients with widespread or generalized involvement, like patients with psoriasis who are given methotrexate. Prior to the initiation of methotrexate therapy, an assessment of renal, liver, and hematopoietic function should be made, including a complete blood count, urinalysis, serum creatinine level, liver function tests, and liver biopsy if indicated. These should be repeated periodically during methotrexate therapy. Appropriate measures must be taken to avoid conception during, and for at least 8 weeks following, methotrexate therapy. An initial test dose of 5 to 10 mg is administered 1 week prior to the initiation of therapy to detect any idiosyncracy. The dosage schedules employed are similar to those used for psoriasis, for example, 5 mg every 8 to 12 hours for three doses each week, up to a weekly dosage of about 30 mg for a 70 kg individual.

Although some patients have been reported to improve with systemic vitamin A (retinol) therapy in uncontrolled studies, its usefulness is limited because of toxicity. Two dosage schedules have been reported. Moderate doses of 150,000 to 200,000 IU per day have led to improvement in some patients with PRP. If no response occurs within 2 months, treatment with vitamin A should be discontinued. Even if a good response occurs, these doses of retinol should not be continued beyond 6 months. Adequate monitoring of clinical symptoms and laboratory parameters of hypervitaminosis A is necessary. Short-term use of high toxic doses of vitamin A (500,000 to 1,000,000 IU per day) has been reported to be beneficial for patients with severe, disabling PRP. Hospitalization of patients during treatment was required for close monitoring of erythroderma, neurologic symptoms, serum triglyceride levels, liver function tests, and clotting studies. These large doses of vitamin A produce generalized exfoliation. Although this desquamation may improve hyperkeratotic areas, the underlying eruption often remains.

Preferred Treatment

Although not yet approved by the Food and Drug Administration for this purpose, the synthetic retinoids, isotretinoin and etretinate, are considered the most consistently effective therapy for PRP. Chronic PRP, usually of childhood onset, characteristically responds dramatically to retinoid therapy and relapses on withdrawal. Relapse is not usually complete, allowing treatment-free intervals between courses of therapy. Adult-onset PRP may remain in remission after one or more courses of isotretinoin therapy. However, it is not clear that isotretinoin definitely induces these long-term remissions, since spontaneous resolution of classic adult-onset PRP is common.

The treatment of PRP with isotretinoin can begin at 0.5 to 1.0 mg per kilogram per day and may be increased by 0.5 mg per kilogram per day increments at weekly or biweekly intervals until either therapeutic effect or dose-limiting toxicity is observed. The usual therapeutic dose level is in the range of 0.5 to 2.0 mg per kilogram per day. Similarly, treatment with etretinate can begin at 0.25 to 0.5 mg per kilogram per day and be increased to a usual maximum dose of 1.0 mg per kilogram per day.

Using the above treatment schedules, we have treated eight patients with adult-onset PRP and five with childhood-onset PRP. Six of the eight patients with adult-onset PRP were treated with etretinate and two with isotretinoin. Four of six etretinate-treated patients and both isotretinoin-treated adult-onset PRP patients improved to varying extents, did not relapse during the post-treatment period, and cleared totally at various times up to 2½ years after retinoid treatment had been stopped. The other two patients, treated with etretinate, failed to clear totally even after 2 and 5 years of treatment.

In contrast to our patients with adult-onset PRP, four of the five patients with childhood-onset PRP responded well to retinoid therapy but relapsed afterward and have not had total clearing. The one child who cleared had a total disease duration of 6 years and cleared 2 years after stopping a 4 month course of therapy with isotretinoin.

Of the six adult-onset PRP patients who have cleared, the average total duration of the disease was 4 years (range: 20 months to 5 years). This is comparable to the clinical course of PRP without retinoid therapy.

We can draw several conclusions based on these patients' data. The synthetic retinoids improve PRP, but the response may be variable. As noted in other studies, the response to synthetic retinoids did not correlate with duration of disease prior to beginning therapy.

The role of the synthetic retinoids in the eventual total clearing that occurred after treatment was stopped is difficult to assess. Patients who cleared completely after retinoid therapy could have had spontaneous remissions. On the other hand, retinoid therapy, in addition to producing a partial clearing, may also have shortened the course of the disease.

RETINOID TOXICITY

The most common acute toxicities of the synthetic retinoids observed to date are well tolerated, not life-threatening, dose-dependent in incidence and severity, treatable with bland therapies, and reversible on discontinuation of treatment. Chronic toxicity, primarily involving the skeleton, has been observed after long-term therapy (longer than 6 to 12 months) with isotretinoin and etretinate. It is possible that additional chronic toxicities may become apparent after longer experience with these drugs.

Since many patients with PRP require prolonged therapy, they are at relatively higher risk of developing chronic toxicity than patients with cystic acne, for example, who usually obtain a long-term remission after a single 4 or 5 month course of isotretinoin therapy.

Acute Toxicity

The commonly observed acute toxic effects of the synthetic retinoids mimic some of the findings of vitamin A intoxication but are less severe and involve primarily the skin and mucous membranes. The major findings include cheilitis, facial dermatitis, conjunctivitis, xerosis with itching, dryness of the nasal mucosa with minor nosebleeds, dry mouth with thirst, excessive palmar-plantar desquamation, stratum corneum fragility (increased peeling with minor trauma), and hair loss. Rarely temporary corneal opacities due to isotretinoin have been reported. In addition to these mucocutaneous toxicities, systemic toxicities have been observed but appear in most patients to be limited to (1) transient, minor elevations in liver function test results that return to pretreatment levels without discontinuing therapy, (2) hyperlipidemia, with elevations primarily in the very low-density lipoproteins (VLDL) and occasionally low-density lipoproteins (LDL), (3) arthralgias, and (4) teratogenicity. Both etretinate and isotretinoin have led to birth defects in man.

As with vitamin A toxicity, the synthetic retinoids can alter tests of liver function. The levels most commonly elevated are those of the transaminases, but occasionally other test results (alkaline phosphatase, bilirubin) can also be abnormal. Elevations of the transaminase levels occur in approximately 15 percent of patients, usually return to normal within 2 to 4 weeks, and remain normal even with continued therapy with the retinoids.

Arthralgias have been seen in only a minority of patients treated with synthetic retinoids, and the arthralgias disappear after discontinuation of therapy. In contrast, etretinate has been reported to objectively improve psoriatic arthritis and chronic polyarthritis.

Another acute toxic effect common to both vitamin A and the synthetic retinoids has been triglyceride level abnormalities. The observed elevations of plasma triglyceride and VLDL levels have been dose dependent and reversible on discontinuation of therapy. In patients with normal pretreatment triglyceride levels, dosages of isotretinoin above 1.0 mg per kilogram per day are needed to induce elevations markedly beyond the normal range. One patient with a probable preexisting hyperlipoproteinemia developed eruptive xanthomas while being treated with isotretinoin at a dose of 2.5 mg per kilogram per day. Hypertriglyceridemia has also been observed with etretinate. Factors that predispose to the development of retinoid-induced hypertriglyceridemia include obesity, high alcohol intake, diabetes, and pretreatment hypertriglyceridemia. Certainly, if patients with pretreatment elevations in the plasma level of triglycerides are to be treated with retinoids, their condition must be monitored very closely. The long-term importance of this observation and the effect of dietary management of plasma triglyceride levels during therapy with retinoids remain to be determined.

Hair loss is an additional toxicologic finding that occurs both with hypervitaminosis A and with synthetic retinoid therapy.

Although retinoids at high doses may inhibit spermatogenesis in animals, semen analyses in men receiving oral doses of retinoids have revealed no abnormalities. It has recently been observed that a small number of patients with cystic acne treated with isotretinoin have developed more serious acute toxic effects including pseudotumor cerebri with impaired vision, regional ileitis, erythema nodosum, and diminished night vision. Acute toxic effects have generally been reversible after discontinuation of therapy.

The acute toxic effects of the two synthetic retinoids,

isotretinoin and etretinate, overlap but are not identical (Table 1). Under certain circumstances, the differences in relative toxicity could influence drug selection between the two retinoids in diseases in which the therapeutic effects are comparable, such as PRP.

Chronic Toxicity

There are several reports indicating that the synthetic retinoids induce chronic skeletal toxicity. The hazard of retinoid bone toxicity may be greater at a young age, when more rapid bone growth and remodeling occur than during adulthood. For instance, radiographic evidence of

TABLE 1 Comparative Acute Synthetic Retinoid Toxicities

Mucocutaneous
Common

  Cheilitis
  Blepharoconjunctivitis
  Dry nasal mucosa with minor nosebleeds
  Facial dermatitis*
  Xerosis, with pruritus*
  Palmoplantar peeling†
  Hair loss†
  Photosensitivity

Uncommon

  Paronychia†
  Stratum corneum fragility†
  Excessive granulation tissue or pyogenic granulomas
  Colonization of nares with *Staphylococcus aureus**
  Stickiness of skin with chills†
  Bruising
  Nail abnormalities†
  Inflamed urethral meatus*
  Dry mouth with thirst†
  Curly hair (pili torti)
  Retinoid dermatitis

Rare

  Corneal opacities or erosions*
  Erythema nodosum*
  Night blindness*
  Transient acute myopia*

Systemic
Common

  Arthralgias
  Teratogenicity
  Transaminase elevations
  Triglyceride elevations

Uncommon

  Headache
  Fatigue
  Mental depression
  Severe hepatotoxic reactions (including four deaths)†
  Stiff man syndrome†
  Exercise-induced bronchoconstriction
  Irregular menses
  Creatine phosphokinase elevations

* Increased incidence with isotretinoin
† Increased incidence with etretinate

partial closure of the proximal epiphysis of the right tibia, demineralization, and altered bone remodeling occurred in a 10-year-old boy with epidermolytic hyperkeratosis treated with high doses of isotretinoin for more than 4 years. Thinning of long bones due to shrinking of the medullary canal has been reported in a 7-year-old child suffering from chronic hypervitaminosis A and possibly in one etretinate-treated patient. The use of isotretinoin and etretinate in children is considered acceptable, but regular monitoring of the growth rate is necessary. In general, patterns of physical growth and development in children treated with retinoids, as monitored by sequential height and weight measurements, remain similar to pretreatment patterns.

Hypervitaminosis A in adult cats causes confluent exostosis formation in the cervical spine. Early retrospective studies of radiographs of the vertebral column in retinoid-treated patients showed that patients treated with isotretinoin for longer than 2 years at a minimum dosage of 1.5 mg per kilogram per day were at significant risk of developing vertebral osteophytes, anterior spinal ligament calcification, and bony bridging, similar to the findings of idiopathic skeletal hyperostosis and

hypervitaminosis A in the adult. More recent prospective studies of patients treated with isotretinoin at an average dosage of 2 mg per kilogram per day demonstrated that after 1 year, six of eight patients had developed small skeletal hyperostoses. In other studies in which lower doses were used in the treatment of acne, minimal spinal hyperostoses developed in about 10 percent of the patients.

Although short-term treatment with etretinate has not, to date, been associated with an increase in the prevalence of spinal hyperostoses, longer therapy (average 5 years) with moderate dosages (average 0.8 mg per kilogram per day) has been associated with a high prevalence (84 percent) of calcification in tendons and ligaments at extraspinal locations. Similarly, isotretinoin therapy (longer than 1½ years) has more recently been associated with a high prevalence of extraspinal tendon and ligament calcification. Identifying the exact nature, extent, and reversibility of retinoid bone toxicity will be important in determining the ultimate usefulness of chronic retinoid therapy. Our guidelines for the use and monitoring of retinoid therapy are given in Table 2 to facilitate careful patient management. It may become necessary to monitor further parameters if additional toxic effects are uncovered.

TABLE 2 Proposed Guidelines for Use of Synthetic Retinoid Therapy

Careful choice of patient

Management
  Administer lowest dose
  Combine with other treatment
  Insert retinoid-free intervals between courses of retinoids
  Avoid vitamin A supplementation

Monitoring acute mucocutaneous toxicity
  History and physical examination

Intervention for acute mucocutaneous toxicities
  Cheilitis—nonmedicated lip balms or lubricants; if severe, 1% hydrocortisone ointment
  Xerosis—nonmedicated lubricants; if severe, low or intermediate strength topical corticosteroid preparations
  Blepharoconjunctivitis—mild: (1) nonmedicated liquid tears, (2) avoid contact lenses; moderate or severe: (1) and (2) as for mild, (3) culture (often *Staphylococcus aureus*), (4) erythromycin ophthalmic ointment twice daily for 10 days
  Corneal opacities—discontinue therapy
  Dry nasal mucosa, nosebleeds—topical lubricants
  Paronychia—soaks, topical antibiotic therapy, topical or intralesional corticosteroid therapy

Monitoring for systemic toxicities
  History and physical examination
  Laboratory evaluation—pretreatment and at 1 to 2 month intervals during therapy: complete blood count with differential, liver function tests, serum calcium and phosphorus, fasting triglycerides and cholesterol (no solid or liquid food—including black coffee and gum—for 10 hours and no alcoholic beverages for 72 hours prior to phlebotomy), urinalysis
  Monitor growth and development in children anticipating long-term therapy: (1) height and weight measurements;

(2) pretreatment bone age x-ray studies; repeat if indicated

Intervention for systemic toxicities
  Joint—arthralgias: (1) mild analgesics, nonsteroidal anti-inflammatory agents, physical therapy; (2) radiologic examination of persistently painful joints
  Hepatotoxicity—transaminase elevations: (1) eliminate ethanol ingestion; (2) low-level elevations: can maintain therapy, levels should return to normal in 2 to 4 weeks; (3) high-level or persistent low-level elevations: reduce or stop therapy until normal values are obtained
  Lipids—triglyceride and cholesterol elevations: (1) insure proper fasting before phlebotomy; (2) reduce or discontinue therapy if lipid values exceed upper limit of normal by 2- to 3-fold; (3) dietary adjustment: strive for ideal weight, eliminate alcohol; then adjust ratio of ingested calories in favor of complex carbohydrates (starches) rather than simple sugars (e.g., sucrose)
  Bone—premature closure of epiphyses, periostitis, demineralization, hyperostosis of long bones (as seen with hypervitaminosis A), hyperostosis of spine, extraspinal tendon and ligament calcification, persistently painful joints: (1) radiologic examination of symptomatic area; (2) reduce or discontinue therapy
  Central nervous system—papilledema, persistent headache, visual disturbance or other evidence of pseudo tumor cerebri: (1) discontinue therapy; (2) appropriate consultation
  Gastrointestinal tract—inflammatory bowel disease: (1) discontinue therapy; (2) appropriate consultation
  Skin—hypersensitivity, erythema nodosum: discontinue therapy

Teratogenicity
  Contraception indicated in sexually active fertile women
  Use of etretinate is discouraged in women of child-bearing potential, conception permitted after discontinuation of isotretinoin for at least 1 month interval.

THE DECISION TO TREAT WITH RETINOIDS

It is in patients with severe PRP that the physician is inclined to initiate retinoid therapy, especially when educational, psychologic, or physical development may be compromised. As with other therapies, the ultimate determination of which, if any, retinoid is indicated in PRP must be based on an estimate of a current risk/benefit ratio. The degree of improvement and duration of disease response to retinoids may be the greatest determinants of benefit. In adult-onset PRP, in which the response may be dramatic and prolonged after discontinuation of therapy, and in which complete remission within a few years is the rule, only one treatment course or a few intermittent courses may yield substantial benefit. On the other hand, atypical and sometimes classic PRP may persist for many years, requiring greater retinoid exposure and an increased risk of developing chronic toxicity. In contrast, many patients with PRP undergo prolonged partial remissions after retinoid therapy, allowing the use of intermittent courses of therapy with prolonged treatment-free intervals.

The obvious major advantage of employing short or intermittent courses of therapy, as opposed to continuous therapy, is that one may minimize the likelihood of chronic toxicity. It appears logical to assume that the appearance of chronic toxicity would be dependent on the total dosage received and the total duration of therapy with the retinoids. In addition, a treatment-free period may allow recovery from subclinical insult, perhaps similar to the catch-up growth that occurs after cessation of systemic corticosteroid therapy or other growth insult during childhood.

The dose of retinoid required should also be considered. Use of lower doses in combination with emollients and possibly other treatments may eliminate some toxic effects that require a minimum or threshold dose. Other partially effective treatments interspersed between courses of retinoid therapy may be used to prolong retinoid-free intervals.

Retinoid teratogenicity entails special risks for female patients of child-bearing age. If a young female patient taking retinoids develops into a sexually active adolescent while being treated with retinoids, and is not adequately informed of the teratogenic potential or does not have the knowledge and means of contraception, an untimely pregnancy would involve the risk of teratogenicity. Although isotretinoin is rapidly cleared from the body within days, etretinate can be detected in the serum for months or even years after discontinuation of therapy. Thus, it is not known when it is safe to conceive after discontinuation of etretinate. In a female of child-bearing potential it may be wise to avoid exposure to etretinate.

Other disorders must be considered. Renal or hepatic compromise, preexisting hyperlipidemia, or a family history of hyperlipidemia or atherosclerotic cardiovascular disease should be considered in the therapeutic assessment. Patients with normal serum triglyceride and cholesterol levels but an underlying tendency toward developing hyperlipidemia may have this tendency unmasked by retinoids. A slight elevation of the serum triglyceride or cholesterol during short-term treatment should have little or no effect on the subsequent development of atherosclerosis. However, in patients who are genetically predisposed to develop elevated serum lipid levels during adulthood, the addition of lipid elevations throughout childhood and adolescence, as could be seen with chronic retinoid therapy, might increase their risk of atherosclerosis.

Assessing the risk/benefit ratio for a new drug that may require chronic use is difficult, especially because of the concern for unknown chronic toxicity. Widespread use, even of familiar drugs, can uncover unexpected toxic effects. Careful patient selection, minimizing the dose and duration of therapy, and close monitoring for toxic effects are necessary to ensure the safe and successful treatment of PRP with retinoids.

SEBORRHEIC DERMATITIS

AMAL K. KURBAN, M.D.

Seborrheic dermatitis is a chronic recurrent inflammation of the skin characterized by a rather distinctive morphologic appearance and sites of involvement. It is a pruritic scaly erythematous eruption involving the so-called areas of high sebaceous activity, and is not to be confused with dandruff, which is characterized by noninflammatory scaliness of the scalp and possibly itching. The main sites of involvement are the scalp, eyebrows, eyelashes (seborrheic blepharitis), nasolabial folds, external ears, ear canals, and behind the auricles. The presternal and interscapular areas may also be involved and occasionally the axillas, groin, and inframammary areas. Characteristically the individual lesion has well defined borders and produces greasy scales on the scalp, trunk, and body folds, whereas on the face the lesions are less well defined.

Seborrheic dermatitis appears in infancy (up to about 3 months of age) and in adulthood. The relationship between the two groups is unclear, notwithstanding a peak activity of the sebaceous glands occurring in both. Furthermore, it is not clear whether there is a relationship between seborrheic dermatitis and sebum production. Thus, the etiology of the disorder remains unknown, although several postulates have been advanced incriminating sebum, *Pityrosporon ovale*, and a psoriasis-like diathesis. There seems to be a constitutional predisposition to the disease, which is accentuated by emotional and physical stress, disorders affecting the basal ganglia (e.g., Parkinson's disease), spinal cord injuries, and acquired immunodeficiency syndrome (AIDS). Complications of seborrheic dermatitis are mainly secondary bacterial and candidal infections and contact dermatitis. The disease has to be differentiated mainly from psoriasis and atopic and contact dermatitis.

THERAPEUTIC ALTERNATIVES

In any disease of unknown etiology, especially if there is a constitutional predisposition (genetic or otherwise),

treatment is not curative. Because of the chronicity, the enthusiasm to accomplish near-cures is tempered by the realization of long-term dependency on medications. Consequently only medications with minimal side effects should be used; the patient's acceptability of the drugs ensures better compliance.

Treatments prescribed are aimed at controlling the scaliness and inflammation and at the same time preventing secondary infection or contact dermatitis. This can be accomplished with the use of shampoos, topical medications, and, if necessary, systemic antibiotic therapy.

PREFERRED APPROACH

Shampoos

Shampoos are available for controlling the scaliness of seborrheic dermatitis. These can also be used for dandruff. The active ingredients of these products are selenium sulfide, zinc pyrithione, tar, salicylic acid, or chloroxine (Table 1).

The shampoos are used primarily for treating scalp lesions. My preference is to begin with a salicylic acid–sulfur shampoo (e.g., Meted, Sebulex, Ionil, Vanseb). Once a response is achieved, follow with a shampoo containing 2.5 percent selenium sulfide (Selsun, Exsel, Iosel). Occasionally a patient responds initially and then relapses in spite of proper usage. In such cases it is useful to alternate the shampoos just mentioned with one containing 1 or 2 percent zinc pyrithione (e.g., Head and Shoulders, Zincon, Danex, DHS-Zinc). In instances of failure to respond to these shampoos and to topical treatment (see next section), tar containing shampoos (e.g., Ionil T, Pentrax, Sebutone, Zetar), which are also helpful in psoriasis, can be effective.

Initially the shampoo is used daily, and as improvement occurs, the frequency can be decreased to every other day. It is important to instruct the patient to apply the shampoo, leave it on for 2 to 5 minutes, and then rinse it off. When there are thick scales or crusts, the preshampoo application of mineral oil, olive oil, or any of the topical medications to be detailed is helpful. Best results are obtained if these are applied at least 2 hours before shampooing. Also effective is preshampooing with warm mineral oil or baby oil for 10 minutes.

TABLE 1 Shampoos for Seborrheic Dermatitis

Active Ingredient	Mode of Action	Brand Name
Chloroxine	Antibacterial	Capitol
Salicylic acid–sulfur	Keratolytic	Ionil, Meted, Sebulex, Vanseb
Selenium sulfide, 1 to 2.5%	Antimitotic	Selsun, Exsel, Iosel
Tar	Antimitotic	Pentrax, Ionil T Sebutone, Zetar
Zinc pyrithione, 1 to 2%	Cytotoxic, Antimicrobial	Head and Shoulders, Zincon, Danex, DHS-Zinc

It is important to remember that shampoos vary in smell, ease of lathering, and drying effect on the hair. Different brands should be tried, and patients should be involved in the final selection of the shampoos most acceptable to them.

Topical Medications

The topical use of medications is indicated when the scalp lesions show moderate to severe inflammation or when the lesions are present at sites other than on the scalp. The customary medications used for seborrheic dermatitis are topically applied corticosteroids. The strength of the steroid used depends on the severity of the dermatitis and the sites involved.

When corticosteroids are to be administered on the scalp, a lotion is preferred. A mild preparation such as 1 percent hydrocortisone lotion is advocated for the milder cases and 0.1 percent Valisone or Synalar lotion for the more severe forms. These are to be rubbed onto the scalp once or twice daily. As the dermatitis improves, the frequency of application is decreased to once daily or after shampooing. For seborrheic dermatitis on the face, 1 to 2.5 percent hydrocortisone cream or 0.025 percent Synalar cream is recommended twice daily until there is improvement. Thereafter the hydrocortisone cream is used once daily. Once the dermatitis has disappeared, the hydrocortisone cream is used, in decreasing frequency, to keep the inflammation under control; usually one application every 3 to 5 days suffices.

It is to be stressed that with a chronic condition like seborrheic dermatitis, the long-term use of potent corticosteroids on the face is discouraged because of their disfiguring side effects (telangiectasia, epidermal atrophy). For lesions other than those on the face corticosteroid creams are also effective. I prefer those with medium or low potency such as 0.1 percent triamcinolone cream. Other effective topically applied medications for seborrheic dermatitis contain sulfur, tar, or salicylic acid. A popular preparation is 3 percent precipitated sulfur in an ointment base. Recently topically applied antifungal drugs (clotrimazole or miconazole) have been used, but I am not convinced of their effectiveness. For seborrheic otitis externa, corticosteroid-containing eardrops are effective in controlling the disease; and for seborrheic blepharitis, sodium sulfacetamide solution is effective. The latter is used either alone (Sebizon) or in combination with prednisolone (Vasocidin, Sulfapred).

Systemic Use of Antibiotics

The need for systemic antibiotic therapy arises when there is clinical evidence of secondary bacterial infection. Patients with severe seborrheic dermatitis not infrequently have a superimposed infection, usually with *Staphylococcus aureus*. The choice of antibiotic depends on the antimicrobial sensitivity of the cultured organisms; if this information is unavailable, erythromycin or cloxacillin may be administered.

TREATMENT FAILURES AND COMPLICATIONS

Unresponsiveness or frequent relapses of seborrheic dermatitis are commonly due to:

1. Noncompliance. Patients either have not used the shampoos and topical treatment or have used them infrequently.

2. Inadequate shampoo-scalp contact. Either the shampoo is rinsed off immediately or, in patients with thick hair, the shampoo has not come in contact with the scalp. In these instances the patient should be reeducated, stressing the need for a 5 to 10 minute shampoo contact.

3. Exacerbating factors like emotional or physical stress.

4. Secondary infection. Impetiginization or folliculitis may appear. These are to be treated with topical or systemic doses of antimicrobial drugs. The secondary infection may not be overt but is to be suspected when the response to treatment is poor. In such instances antibiotics (e.g., neomycin, bacitracin, polymyxin) alone or in combination with steroids are applied topically. When the infection is more obvious, systemic antibiotic therapy is indicated. When candidiasis occurs, topical treatment with antiyeast-containing steroids is effective. My preference is for Mycolog, Vioform-hydrocortisone, or Lotrisone creams.

5. Contact dermatitis may result from any of the ingredients of the shampoos or from topical medications, cosmetics, or other contactants. Bacterial infection of eczematized seborrheic dermatitis is not infrequent and may necessitate the use of systemic corticosteroid therapy in addition to antimicrobial therapy.

6. Side effects of topical corticosteroids are encountered with the use of highly potent corticosteroids mainly on the face (telangiectasia, atrophy, rosacea-like lesions) (Table 2). In patients whose lesions are not easily controlled with topical corticosteroid therapy, other preparations (especially those containing sulfur) might be effective alone or in combination with the steroid.

SUMMARY

There are several alternatives available for the treatment of seborrheic dermatitis. The treating physician develops a preference for certain medications to be used,

TABLE 2 Precautions in the Topical use of Corticosteroids in Seborrheic Dermatitis

In general, the use of potent fluorinated corticosteroids on the face is discouraged.

For maintenance therapy use topical corticosteroid therapy sparingly and as infrequently as possible as long as the dermatitis is under control.

Monitor intraocular pressure in patients chronically treated with corticosteroids in or around the eyes.

Watch for bacterial or candidal infections.

TABLE 3   Management of Seborrheic Dermatitis—A Prototype

Site	Initial Treatment	Maintenance
Scalp:		
Mild cases	Meted shampoo daily for 2-3 weeks	Selsun alternating with Head and Shoulders shampoo
	Selsun shampoo or Head and Shoulders shampoo	
Severe cases	Shampoos as above. If no response, use Pentrax shampoo	Shampoos as above, 3 times weekly
	Hydrocortisone, 1% lotion daily	Hydrocortisone, 1% lotion after shampooing
	Mineral oil 2 hr before shampooing if scales are thick	
Face	Hydrocortisone, 2.5% cream daily	Hydrocortisone, 1% cream 1-5 times weekly
Other areas	Triamcinolone, 0.1% cream 2 times daily	Triamcinolone, 0.1% cream 1-3 times weekly
Any site: Bacterial infection	Erythromycin, 1 gm daily for 1-2 weeks	
Candidal infection	Mycolog cream b.i.d.	

a prototype of which is seen in Table 3. Familiarity with the alternative therapies allows for interchanges depending on responsiveness to, and complicance with, the treatment as well as any complications that might arise.

PARAPSORIASIS

W. CLARK LAMBERT, M.D., Ph.D.

Parapsoriasis is not a single entity, but rather a group of disorders created primarily as a part of an ancient, now long forgotten master scheme to reclassify all inflammatory dermatoses. Therapy of each of these disorders therefore has little or no relationship to treatment for the others. Since some of these diseases have the potential to develop into a lymphoma, whereas others do not, and since it is my opinion that this all-important complication can be delayed if not eliminated by treatment, it is critical that a correct diagnosis be made and treatment tailored accordingly. For this reason, some mention will be made here of the salient diagnostic features of these diseases, although the emphasis will be given to treatment. The reader is referred to dermatology texts for further discussion of the all-important question of diagnosis.

Parapsoriasis consists of three major entities, each of which consists of two or three variants, which certain authors may consider separate entities, so that, depending on one's opinions, there are as few as three or as many as seven entities within the group. The only important issue is that the three major entities be distinguished from each other; their treatments are quite different. These three entities are pityriasis lichenoides, small plaque parapsoriasis, and large plaque (atrophic) parapsoriasis.

PITYRIASIS LICHENOIDES

Pityriasis lichenoides consists of two variants, acute (pityriasis lichenoides et varioliformis acuta, PLEVA, PLVA, Mucha-Habermann disease) and chronic (pityriasis lichenoides chronica [Juliusberg]). Both consist of papular lesions occurring primarily over the trunk. In the acute form, the lesions tend to ulcerate and may undergo hemorrhage or vesiculation, whereas in the chronic form only scaling is noted. The most important diagnostic criterion is that the various lesions are, at a single time, all in varying stages of evolution. Individual lesions in the acute form last for 3 to about 6 weeks, with the entire process lasting weeks to months; the chronic form persists for months to years. The lesions, particularly in the acute form, may heal with scarring or pigmentary changes.

A biopsy of at least two lesions should be obtained in all cases of pityriasis lichenoides to confirm the diagnosis, since the disease shows a characteristic histologic picture, and to rule out the possibility that the patient may have lymphomatoid papulosis. In lymphomatoid papulosis, the clinical lesions are essentially identical with those observed in pityriasis lichenoides, but the inflammatory infiltrate is largely composed (usually about 40 percent or more of the lymphoid cells) of atypical lymphoid cells. It is important to bear in mind, when making this histologic diagnosis, that up to about 10 percent of the lymphoid cells in the inflammatory infiltrate of pityriasis

lichenoides may be atypical. Thus the clinician and the pathologist must be in close contact and work together in arriving at a final diagnosis. A small but significant proportion of patients with lymphomatoid papulosis develop lymphoma.

Pityriasis lichenoides may be treated using psoralen followed by long wavelength ultraviolet A (UVA) light (PUVA). The regimen should be precisely the same as that for psoriasis, and the reader is therefore referred to the chapter on psoriasis for details of management. Topical steroid therapy, tar preparations, and short wavelength (UVB) light do not appear to be effective. The results using PUVA are not uniformly good, and the disease may take months to clear. It may also recur following treatment. The best course may therefore be no treatment, giving reassurance to the patient but also warning him that scarring or pigmentary changes at sites of lesions may be sequelae. In particular, dark skinned individuals may show areas of leukoderma at sites of former lesions. H_1 antihistamine preparations are useful in alleviating lesional pruritus.

Severe cases, such as the ulceronecrotic form of the disease, may be treated with methotrexate in one single low oral dose (12.5 mg; at least 7.5 mg, up to 20 mg) once per week until the lesions clear. This differs from the regimen for psoriasis (three doses per week 12 hours apart) since, in pityriasis lichenoides, the growth kinetics of epidermal cells are not a factor. Periodic liver biopsies and weekly white blood counts 48 hours after administration of methotrexate should be obtained, although for short courses of treatment it may be possible to forego the liver biopsies. Systemic steroid therapy, prednisone up to about 30 mg per day, may also be given, with or without methotrexate. These treatments usually clear the lesions within 3 to 6 weeks, but recurrences are to be expected. Therefore, treatment should be reserved for the severe cases, and chronic pityriasis lichenoides probably should not be treated with either methotrexate or systemic steroid therapy. Treatment may be repeated with reexacerbations as necessary.

The methotrexate and steroid regimens just described are based on the rationale that an immune complex vasculitis is responsible for the lesions of pityriasis lichenoides. By no means has this been proved. The PUVA treatment is empiric. Based on the concept, completely unproved, that an infectious agent may be responsible for the disease, a treatment of tetracycline, 2 g per day, has been used by others with claims of success. I have had no experience with this treatment.

LYMPHOMATOID PAPULOSIS

The management of a biopsy proved case of lymphomatoid papulosis is identical to that for pityriasis lichenoides, except that it should be kept in mind that a small proportion of these cases progress to lymphoma. Therapeutic control of the lesions may lessen the likelihood of this complication, and thus the decision to treat or not to treat the patient should be made with this in mind. The patient should be followed closely, and frequent (biweekly to monthly) examinations for changes in the lesions, lymphadenopathy, or hepatosplenomegaly should be carried out for as long as the disease is active.

SMALL PLAQUE PARAPSORIASIS

Small plaque parapsoriasis consists of small (<5 cm) yellow to red-brown, well demarcated, flat plaquelike lesions over the trunk and proximal extremities. The lesions on the proximal extremities may be somewhat larger. The lesions on the trunk show a smooth regular border, which is not raised. Little or no scale is seen. In the variant, digitate dermatosis, the lesions are the same as those just described, but those on the trunk are palisaded in a manner following dermatomes. Xanthoerythrodermia perstans is digitate dermatosis in which the lesions have a yellow color. It is a superfluous term; lesions of small plaque parapsoriasis that are not palisaded may also be yellow. Biopsy of the lesions is not strictly necessary.

Treatment of small plaque parapsoriasis is strictly for cosmetic purposes; the disease has no known premalignant potential and there are no important sequelae. It thus may best be left untreated, except possibly with a lubricant. However, it does persist for years and may be an annoyance to the patient. The disease may be treated topically with a mild, clear tar preparation or ultraviolet B (UVB) light. Topical steroid therapy may be used sparingly. The risks associated with PUVA therapy, although not great, probably are not worth the limited benefits to be expected. Reassurance of the patient is important. One probably should see the patient at least every 3 to 12 months, mainly to be sure that the character of the process does not change, indicating an incorrect initial diagnosis.

LARGE PLAQUE (ATROPHIC) PARAPSORIASIS

Large plaque (atrophic) parapsoriasis is a potentially premalignant condition. About 10 percent of the cases eventuate in mycosis fungoides or, much less commonly, another form of lymphoma. Lesions of large plaque parapsoriasis occur mainly on the buttocks and adjacent areas of the groin, flanks, back, perineum, inguinal areas, and inferior abdomen. In women, lesions also characteristically occur on the breasts. The lesions are large (>10 cm), have poorly defined, irregular borders, and show atrophy of the epidermis. They are usually slightly erythematous with slight or no scale and may show a mottled bluish color. In the variant, retiform parapsoriasis (variegate parapsoriasis, parakeratosis variegata), lesions are extremely widespread, usually over the entire trunk, are confluent, and show a striking lacelike or netlike vascular pattern, sometimes with tiny (<1 mm) papules present.

Retiform parapsoriasis is extremely rare and appears to progress to lymphoma much more commonly than do other cases of large plaque parapsoriasis, perhaps in the majority of cases. In either form of large plaque parapsoriasis, induration, lymphadenopathy, and pruritus are signs that the disease may be progressing toward lymphoma. Rarely lesions clinically and histologically resembling pityriasis lichenoides may be seen within plaques of large plaque parapsoriasis. It is important that the more subtle lesions of large plaque parapsoriasis not be missed or, alternatively, that these lesions not be mistaken for induration indicating progression of the process to lymphoma. This point can be resolved by biopsy. Biopsy specimens in all cases of large plaque parapsoriasis should be obtained from at least two sites.

It has been my experience, not supported by a controlled clinical trial, that careful management of cases of large plaque parapsoriasis can have a marked beneficial effect on the likelihood of progression toward lymphoma. In this endeavor, the essential and important concept is very aggressive management with nonaggressive techniques. The two methods I favor are a high potency topical steroid therapy together with short wavelength ultraviolet B (UVB) light and PUVA, used alternatively rather than together. Use of UVB light should be carried out aggresively, with daily or thrice weekly treatments using large UVB units, gradually increasing the dosage over time, as tolerated, until the lesions clear. The PUVA regimen is the same as for psoriasis (see chapter on *Psoriasis*). These patients tend to be more light sensitive than patients with psoriasis, a factor that should be kept in mind when designing treatment regimens. It is important to use whatever special measures may be necessary to treat all body crevices.

Maintenance therapy, using either of the aforementioned methods, should be much more aggressive than in the treatment of psoriasis or other dermatoses in which cosmetic or palliative treatment is the goal. PUVA treatment, for example, should be given at least once per week. The lesions should be kept completely clear, if possible, or at least very nearly so. Etretinate, in doses as tolerated by the patient may be used in some as a valuable associated treatment to reduce the amount of other therapy required in some patients. The goal of treatment is to suppress the disorder to prevent occurrence of malignant disease; this should be carefully explained to the patient, if possible. Compliance is usually good once this has been done.

More aggressive methods of treatment, such as topical nitrogen mustard therapy and megavoltage electron beam radiotherapy, should be avoided in the treatment of large plaque parapsoriasis, not only because the possible complications are unwarranted, but also because the patient may need these modes of therapy later. At that point it would be a marked disadvantage to the patient to have become sensitized to nitrogen mustard or to have received a possibly compromising dose of radiation, such as to the bone marrow, owing to contaminating wavelengths associated with the electron beam radiotherapy.

Large plaque parapsoriasis has been known to persist for as long as 60 years before eventuating into a lymphoma. Treatment should be maintained for as long as lesions are present. Therapy may be discontinued from time to time to ascertain whether the disease is still present, but only at intervals of several years. The patient should be aggressively retreated as soon as a recurrence of lesions is noted.

In all cases of large plaque parapsoriasis, the patient

should be carefully examined at least every 6 to 12 months for evidence of progression toward lymphoma. This should include careful examination for lymphadenopathy, hepatosplenomegaly, and induration of lesions. Any suspicious lesion should be examined by biopsy.

The foregoing recommendations are based on my experience with large plaque parapsoriasis. I have had no personal experience in treating retiform parapsoriasis. Our understanding of all these diseases is progressing rapidly, and this may drastically alter management in the future.

PITYRIASIS ROSEA

NANCY BARNETT, M.D.

Pityriasis rosea is a papulosquamous eruption that is usually diagnosed because of a characteristic appearance, distribution, and evolution. Frequently there is a single plaque that is larger than 1 cm in diameter, oval or round, erythematous, and very slightly elevated with a "trailing" (inside the borders of the lesion) scale, which usually appears on the trunk up to 2 weeks before the appearance of other smaller lesions. The smaller plaques are typically ellipsoid, well demarcated, erythematous, slightly scaling lesions that follow skin lines and appear most prominently over the "nonexposed" skin surfaces (trunk and upper extremities). In children and black individuals the face and lower extremities may be involved. However, the palms and soles are generally spared, and this may help to distinguish the disorder from secondary syphilis in which palm and sole lesions frequently occur. A rapid plasma reagin (RPR) or Venereal Disease Research Laboratory (VDRL) test should be done to rule out secondary lues in adults, sexually active children, adolescents, and children with possible venereal contacts.

The lesions may last several months before resolving spontaneously. They are usually asymptomatic, although occasionally pruritus is a significant complaint. Bland emollients and lotions can help to decrease the scaling and pruritus. Oral antihistamine therapy is rarely indicated. The scale is not adherent or proliferative as in guttate psoriasis with which pityriasis rosea may be confused initially. Other entities to consider in the differential diagnosis are tinea versicolor, which can be distinguished by the short hyphae and spores seen on a potassium hydroxide preparation, and tinea corpis, which has long branched hyphae on potassium hydroxide preparations. Other disorders to be considered in the differential diagnosis of pityriasis rosea are asteatotic eczema, drug eruption, scabies, parapsoriasis, and autoeczematization.

Unusual varients of pityriasis rosea include a diffuse papular variety with only rare scattered ellipsoid but typical plaques, a hemorrhagic variant, typical pityriasis rosea without a preceding herald patch, a type limited in distribution to the "bathing trunk" area, one consisting of large lesions, and an almost urticarial inflammatory form with very red papules and plaques.

Except for the skin lesion appearance and mild pruritus, patients are otherwise well. Reassurance regarding spontaneous resolution without scarring may be all that is needed in many cases. However, in some, especially pigmented individuals, the inflammatory process clearly results in postinflammatory hyperpigmentation, leading to a disconcerting spotty pigmentation disorder. Ultraviolet B (UVB) exposure seems to shut off the inflammatory process, and this can be done with natural sunlight or phototherapy. Light box suberythemogenic UVB treatments three times per week for 1 to 2 weeks is usually sufficient to suppress new inflammation to prevent further pigment changes and to tan an individual so that older lesions are less noticeable.

The etiology of pityriasis is unclear. It is presumed to be an infectious exanthem because it occurs in small epidemics, primarily in the winter months. It does not seem to be caused by a highly virulent agent, perhaps a virus, because the rate of spread in household and frequent contacts is low. Once an individual has had pityriasis rosea, it is unlikely to recur but may in some 3 percent of the cases.

LICHEN PLANUS

BARBARA L. BRAUNSTEIN-WILSON, M.D.

Lichen planus is an inflammatory dermatosis of unknown etiology, which can involve the skin, hair, mucous membranes, and nails of both children and adults. Involvement of the skin may be localized or widespread, intensely pruritic or occasionally asymptomatic, and presents as scaly, violaceous, or hyperpigmented polygonal papules and plaques. The surface of the lesions may demonstrate a white, stippled, or reticulated pattern known as Wickham's striae. The Koebner phenomenon may be demonstrable and is responsible for linear lesions of lichen planus that develop at sites of trauma caused by scratching. When the lower extremities are involved, the lesions may be very hyperkeratotic and the condition is known as hypertrophic lichen planus. Other variants include atrophic, erosive, annular, and bullous lichen planus. Lesions usually resolve spontaneously over a period of months to years and can cause significant postinflammatory hyperpigmentation, especially in dark skinned individuals.

The mucous membranes may be involved alone or in association with cutaneous lesions. Oral lichen planus is frequently asymptomatic unless ulceration has occurred and appears clinically as a white reticulated or lacy eruption most often on the buccal mucosa, tongue or lips. The genital mucosa also may be involved. Ulcerated lesions of lichen planus on the mucous membranes can be extremely painful.

Involvement of the hair with lichen planus, known as lichen planopilaris, begins as pruritic, erythematous, follicular papules and gradually progresses to scarring alopecia. Lichen planus of the nails can involve only a few or all nails and may present as thinning, ridging, splitting, thickening, or discoloration of the nails. Pterygium formation (growth of the cuticle onto the nail plate) is a fairly characteristic finding in lichen planus of the nails. A lichen planus-like eruption, clinically identical to lichen planus, may be caused by various drugs and is called a lichenoid drug eruption (Table 1).

APPROACH TO THE PATIENT

A biopsy should be performed if other disorders, such as psoriasis, pityriasis rosea, nummular eczema, or cutaneous lupus, need to be ruled out. The possibility of a lichenoid drug eruption should be evaluated and, if suspected, the probable causative agent should be discontinued. The eruption should resolve upon cessation of the medication.

Treatment should be tailored to each patient and depends on the exact location of the disease, the degree of pruritus, and the cosmetic concern to the patient. Localized asymptomatic disease of the skin need not be treated unless desired by the patient. Symptomatic or extensive disease however, requires treatment. When involvement

TABLE 1   Drugs that Can Cause a Lichenoid Eruption

Captopril
Carbamazepine
Chlordiazepoxide
Chloroquine
Chlorpropamide
Ethambutol
Furosemide
Gold
Hydrochlorothiazide
Hydroxychloroquine
Mepacrine
Methyldopa
Para-aminosalicytic acid
Penicillamine
Phenothiazine
Practolol
Propanolol
Quinidine
Quinine
Tetracycline

is not extensive, lichen planus of the skin or hair should be treated initially with mid- to high-potency corticosteroids (e.g., 0.1 percent triamcinolone or 0.05 percent fluocinonide) applied topically three times daily. Retin A cream, 0.1 percent, alone or in combination with topical steroid therapy, has also been beneficial for some patients with lichen planus. Oral doses of antihistamines, such as Atarax, 25 to 50 mg three times daily, or Seldane, 60 mg twice daily, may help relieve pruritus but also cause drowsiness in some patients. If the foregoing regimen is not beneficial, corticosteroid impregnated tape (e.g., Cordran) or intralesional corticosteroid therapy can be used to treat individual lesions. The tape should be applied to the lesions for 12 to 18 hours a day. For intralesional therapy a small amount of triamcinolone suspension, 10 mg per cubic centimeter, is injected into individual lesions with a small-gauge needle. Up to 10 mg can be injected during one visit and can be repeated every 3 to 4 weeks as needed. Side effects of topical or intralesional steroid therapy include atrophy of the skin, telangiectasia, hypertrichosis, easy bruising, and systemic absorption with subsequent suppression of the hypothalamic-pituitary axis.

The treatment of choice for widespread or severe disease of the skin or hair is systemic steroid therapy. A recommended regimen is oral prednisone therapy, starting at a dosage of 40 to 60 mg daily and gradually decreasing to 5 or 10 mg daily over 4 to 6 weeks. One should use systemic steroid therapy with caution in diabetic and hypertensive patients.

An alternative therapy for extensive lichen planus of the skin or hair is a combination of oral 8-methoxypsoralen therapy with longwave ultraviolet A exposure (PUVA). The regimen is similar to that used to treat psoriasis (see the chapter on *Psoriasis*). However, in most instances maintenance therapy is not required. When the scalp is treated with PUVA, shaving of the hair may be required to permit adequate exposure of the scalp to the UVA light. Besides the usual side effects of PUVA, one can see an increase in the postinflammatory hyperpigmentation caused by lichen planus.

Asymptomatic nonerosive lichen planus of the mucous membranes need not be treated. Ulcerative lesions generally require treatment for the relief of pain. Potent topical steroid therapy or Retin A, 0.1 percent in Orabase, applied several times daily to the affected area may bring about significant improvement. Intralesional corticosteroid therapy may be administered as already described and frequently is beneficial. At times a tapering course of systemic steroid therapy is required, administered in a fashion similar to that used for the treatment of cutaneous lichen planus. Oral retinoids are helpful in some patients with ulcerative oral lichen planus; however, side effects with long-term therapy may contraindicate their use. Ulcers should be followed closely, and progressive lesions should be subjected to biopsy examination to rule out the possibility of squamous cell carcinoma.

Lichen planus of the nails is difficult to treat. Intralesional doses of corticosteroids can be injected around the base of the nail using a 30-gauge needle or Dermajet. The pain associated with this therapeutic modality is significant and frequently prohibitive. A tapering course of systemic steroid therapy as already described or PUVA therapy using a hand or foot unit may be helpful.

INFLAMMATORY DISEASES

EXFOLIATIVE DERMATITIS

HERMAN S. MOGAVERO Jr., M.D.

This entity, also known as erythroderma, is a cutaneous inflammation characterized by an intitial erythema with the subsequent development of pronounced scaling or exfoliation. Although often initially localized, the process typically has spread to the majority of the cutaneous surface at the time of presentation.

There are multiple etiologies for this disorder, recognizing both a primary de novo clinical presentation and secondary underlying causes. These can be conveniently compartmentalized into the following classification:

1. Idiopathic.
2. Generalized or widespread cutaneous disease states such as atopic, contact, or seborrheic dermatitis, psoriasis, lichen planus, pemphigus foliaceus, or pityriasis rubra pilaris.
3. Systemic diseases with cutaneous manifestations such as leukemias, lymphomas (of both the T and B cell types), and some solid tumors (i.e., lung or rectum).
4. Adverse cutaneous reactions to drugs. This reaction can involve many classes of drugs, including but not limited to antibiotics, anti-inflammatory drugs, anticonvulsants, and metallic compounds.

The diagnosis of a "preexisting" dermatitis in the erythrodermic patient relies on a detailed examination of the whole integument, looking for distinct areas of "typical" morphology isolated from the surrounding "sea of erythema." It is in these areas that there is the highest yield of diagnostic skin biopsy findings in specific dermatologic entities. In addition, skin biopsy can be helpful in the diagnosis of underlying leukemia or lymphoma and is indicated in the evaluation of all cases of erythroderma.

The objective cutaneous manifestations of exfoliative dermatitis can extend beyond the obvious erythema and scaling. There can be complete or partial alopecia, onychodystrophy, deep painful fissuring of the skin, and desquamation of the palms and soles in broad thick sheets. Mucous membrane involvement is distinctly unusual in erythroderma.

There are major systemic components of exfoliative dermatitis, and in most cases these features warrant hospitalization for appropriate diagnostic evaluation and splenomegaly. The distinction of lymphoma from dermatrophic lymphadenopathy often requires lymph node bitherapeutic intervention. Typically there are complaints referable to the inability to maintain thermostability. In spite of multiple layers of clothing the patient is unable to keep warm at ambient temperatures that are uncomfortable for others. The patient reports chills and shaking sensations. On examination there may be either fever or hypothermia. In the latter instance it is important to be sure that the device measuring the temperature can register below 96°F (36° C). The remainder of the physical examination must be complete, with special attention paid to assessing lymphadenopathy, hepatomegaly, and opsy as well. Other signs of secondary infection, hypervolemia, tachycardia, edema, and high output cardiac failure must be sought. The laboratory evaluation can parallel that used in a severe burn with prominent fluid and electrolyte abnormalities, including hypoalbuminemia and hypernatremia if increased transepidermal water loss is not corrected. Accurate weight measurements and daily monitoring of fluid intake and output are also required.

TREATMENT

The treatment of exfoliative dermatitis is focused on the diagnostic entity responsible. Elimination of an offending drug usually initiates resolution of the dermatitis. Treatment of the underlying systemic disease is necessary to control erythroderma secondary to neoplastic processes. In this setting a consultation with a hematologist or oncologist is appropriate for therapeutic intervention.

The approach in cases of erythroderma related to widespread cutaneous disease or idiopathic exfoliative erythroderma is initially conservative. The patient is often best served by hospitalization to allow for the aforementioned diagnostic studies and systemic monitoring and also to remove the patient from any negative environmental factors (e.g., atopic dermatitis).

The mainstay of therapy is frequent lubrication of the skin with colloidal baths and bland ointments such as Aquaphor or petrolatum. If pruritus is a component of the eruption, antihistamines are given. I routinely employ hydroxyzine as an H_1 blocker and increase the dosage to maximal tolerance (up to 100 mg orally every 6 hours) before adding additional H_1 blockers (cyproheptadine, 4 mg orally every 8 hours) or H_2 blockers (cimetidine, 300 mg orally three or four times daily).

The topical use of corticosteroid ointments is tempered by the realization that the widespread cutaneous inflammation and defective vasoconstriction allow for enhanced absorption percutaneously. I typically begin with 1 percent hydrocortisone ointment applied three times daily. If no response is noted after a brief period of time (while diagnostic studies are pending), one can advance to 0.1 percent triamcinolone ointment or its equivalents (class III or IV) three times daily. The topical use of more potent steroids (class I or II) is modulated by extent of the cutaneous eruption because widespread disease allows for pituitary-adrenal axis suppression. If the diagnosis of psoriasis has been excluded and the risk versus benefit of systemic treatment of severe seborrheic or atopic dermatitis is considered, a course of systemic corticosteriod therapy is warranted with initial doses of prednisone in the range of 1 to 1.5 mg per kilogram per day. The objective of therapy once control has been achieved is to consolidate to a single daily dose and then taper to alternate day, low dose steroid therapy to minimize the well known complications of daily systemic steroid therapy.

The introduction of retinoids has added greatly to the therapeutic tools available to the dermatologist. In cases of erythrodermic psoriasis, etretinate has proved very effective. In contrast to pustular psoriasis, the approach in erythrodermic psoriasis is to use a low dose of etretinate (25 mg orally each day) and to gradually increase if necessary. In a similar fashion, some refractory cases of pityriasis rubra pilaris have been responsive to isotretinoin in the 1 to 2 mg per kilogram daily dosage range.

The use of cytotoxic drugs to some extent has been displaced by the retinoids. Methotrexate in the usual dosage of 2.5 to 5.0 mg every 12 hours for three consecutive doses remains an alternative for cases of idiopathic exfoliative dermatitis that are refractory to the foregoing approach.

Mortality from exfoliative dermatitis has been a prominent feature in a number of retrospective studies. The metabolic complications of exfoliative dermatitis have been discussed. There must also be constant vigilance for complications of systemic infections (sepsis, pneumonia, cellulitis), venous thrombosis or embolism, as well as complications due to the underlying disease process or its treatment.

ALLERGIC CONTACT DERMATITIS

WILLIAM P. JORDAN Jr., M.D.

Contact dermatitis is either an immunologic or nonimmunologic exogenous disorder that produces inflammatory changes ranging from acute eruptions (eczematous) to chronic secondary skin lesions. Since many strong haptenes are also irritating on contact, some cases of contact dermatitis can represent nearly simultaneous immunologic and nonimmunologic injuries. The dermatitis that is delayed, specific, acquired through exposure(s), and transferable (by cells) is universally referred to as allergic contact dermatitis. Irritant contact dermatitis cannot be transferred to a recipient by cells or serum. Contacts with potential irritants can suggest immunologic contact dermatitis, because exposure concentrations and schedules for irritants can create the appearance of specificity in some patients. Distinguishing between the two forms of contact dermatitis, and appreciating that the two may coexist in the same patient, can be critical to the patient, employer, or a third party responsible for medical payment or compensations. The United States Department of Labor reported that 45 percent of all cases of occupational illness in 1977 were caused by skin disorders, most of which are called contact dermatitis.

Under certain circumstances all substances, including water, can produce an inflammatory nonimmunologic dermatitis, but not every substance can produce allergic contact dermatitis. Some haptenes require only one exposure under some test conditions. The dermatitis appears approximately 14 days later (range, 7 to 21 days) and without a deliberate second exposure. A residuum of the first dose, applied 14 days earlier, is sufficient to elicit the dermatitis after the critical induction period is over. This induction dose flare is rarely seen in the clinical setting from poison ivy or hair dying, but could occur with prodigious amounts of a haptene.

Haptenes causing weak to moderate reactions require a catalogue to name. They typically induce allergic contact dermatitis when repeatedly applied to skin that has pre-existing inflammation or loss of corneal barrier integrity.

Nearly all cases of allergic contact dermatitis stem from exposures that have just taken place 1 to 5 days prior to the dermatitis in previously sensitized subjects. The exposures are covert or overt eliciting exposures. The median time until well developed dermatitis develops is about 2 days. Dermatitis can be observed as early as 8 hours. The time until the onset of a grossly observable reaction is between 8 hours and about 5 days; the patient's sensitivity and haptene flux are critical in determining this range.

ACUTE IRRITANT CONTACT DERMATITIS

Cutaneous injury from contact with strong irritating chemicals is almost always a self-evident diagnosis. Workplace exposures to strong irritants are common, but homes and offices contain many utility substances that rival those used in heavy industry in the irritation they cause. These injuries require copious aqueous washings and supportive therapy. Oral or topical steroid therapy has no beneficial effects in cases of significant chemically induced cytotoxic injury. Vigilon provides a nontraumatic changeable protective dressing that helps to alleviate pain associated with skin injuries that expose the dermis to air. The physician must feel confident that no residual chemical from the injury will be trapped under this type of dressing. The hydrofluoric acid skin burn is an example of a severe chemical burn that could conceivably be trapped under this type of dressing. Some burns require hours of aqueous irrigation. Reports in literature tend to favor intradermal and subcutaneous injections of 10 percent calcium gluconate in and around the burned areas as a preferred treatment for this type of burn. The injection dose is 0.5 ml per square centimeter of burned area, the injection is extended about 0.5 cm into the normal surrounding tissue margins of the burn.

Topical steroid therapy can decrease the clinical signs and symptoms of mild intact epidermal injuries from chemicals.

Locally Severe or Generalized Acute Allergic Contact Dermatitis

Acute allergic contact dermatitis can be a dermatologic emergency, requiring timely and aggressive therapy. Definitive therapy requires the use of large systemic doses of corticosteroids. Initial oral dosages of prednisone should be in the range of 1 to 1.2 mg per kilogram daily. The daily dosage is tapered after the initial doses have brought about significant clinical improvement. The initial dosage is reduced over a 7 to 14 day period. Occasionally severe rhus dermatitis rebounds 10 to 14 days after a good initial clearing and an apparently adequate reduction phase. This scenario is common with oral steroid therapy in a dose pack. Abrupt steroid withdrawal is not contraindicated when clearing can be accomplished within 3 weeks. In acute self-limited cases, as in accurately diagnosed rhus dermatitis, dividing the total day's dosage (AM and PM) gives a more even 24 hour coverage for the short half-life of prednisone.

Intermittent cool wet soaks or dressing applied for 5 to 10 minutes and followed by enhanced tepid air drying with a hair blower dramatically curtails weeping. These wet to dry periods are 20 to 40 minutes in duration and ideally are frequent (three or four times a day). Tap water, isotonic saline, and Burow's solution are the wetting agents commonly used.

Oral antihistamine therapy is time honored but only a secondary treatment consideration in acute significant allergic contact dermatitis. Hydroxyzine or diphenhydramine may alleviate pruritus and can function as a sedative at bedtime. In adults I prefer the short acting drug triazolam (0.25 to 0.5 mg) to ensure sleep and offset any steroid insomnia. Daytime sedation from antihistamines (terfinidine is not sedating) can be a significant problem, and none are dramatically antipruritic in acute allergic contact dermatitis. More is accomplished with an appropriate dosage of prednisone and a good short acting hypnotic at bedtime.

Mild and Moderate Acute Contact Dermatitis with Limited Involvement

Class 1 topical steroids suppress the signs and symptoms of allergic contact dermatitis in patients judged to be in this category. Those seen in the very early phases of dermatitis can worsen in days, and the topical therapy suddenly appears to be "too little, too late." Because topical therapy with class 1 steroids is costly, next day communication with the patient can correct undertreated contact dermatitis. Wet to dry compresses, as already described, are employed if weeping is present. Clobetasol and betamethasone diproprionate (in an optimized release vehicle) are applied in the intervening periods between the soaks. The goal of topical therapy in acute self-limited dermatitis is to mimic the power of occlusive therapy without risking the increase in heat, maceration, and higher bacterial counts from a synthetic membrane. Frequently applied (topically every 3 to 4 hours), unoccluded, potent steroid therapy is a step in this direction, particularly in areas that are not easy to occlude. Some anatomic sites are suitable for occlusive dressings for 24 to 48 hours. Topical therapy can be reduced to twice daily applications after significant improvement occurs.

CHRONIC CONTACT DERMATITIS

Chronic contact dermatitis presents a different problem: the cause must be identified. Haptene removal or substitution stops the dermatitis. If allergic contact dermatitis is a complicating feature of intrinsic eczema, treatment will be more gratifying when a secondary disorder is eliminated. If this is not done, treatment is nearly impossible. A thorough history of exposures to irritants or allergens is paramount. Every part of the patient's day is suspect and all treatments must be questioned. Patients do not volunteer information about some of their temporizing self-treatments. A correct diagnosis may require patch testing, which should be performed by experienced persons knowledgeable in this technique. Many items suspected of causing allergic contact dermatitis by the patient, or physician, cannot be tested in the form or concentration that is suspected of causing the dermatitis. Poorly performed patch testing is worse than no patch testing, for it may give the physician a false sense of security and undeserved confidence in the diagnosis. Severe false positive reactions create more than just physician embarrassment.

Topical corticosteroid therapy is standard treatment and, like the treatment of chronic intrinsic eczema, is used judiciously. Hydrocortisone (1 to 2.5 percent) and tridesilon (creams or ointments) are preferred for the face and intertriginous areas. Fluorinated steroids must be carefully monitored when used in these areas. "How long?" has not been defined. Some patients are more susceptible than others to the well publicized adverse effects. Steroid atrophy, when recognized reasonably early, improves significantly when fluorinated steroid administration is discontinued.

Antihistamines should be offered to relieve pruritus in patients who believe that they are beneficial. Hydroxyzine and doxepin are good choices as a first offering. The patient will soon let it be known if one or the other is cost effective. Ice pack compresses relieve itching, but are not always available when needed.

OCCUPATION RELATED DERMATOSES

EDWARD A. EMMETT, M.B., B.S., M.S.

Occupational dermatoses are a set of rather diverse conditions either caused or aggravated by working conditions. Because of similar legal and social issues involved in the management of these conditions, they can be considered together. The range of possible occupational dermatoses is large, as illustrated in Table 1. Contact dermatitis accounts for over 90 percent of occupational skin diseases; many other conditions occur but are relatively rare. Other sections of this book should be consulted for the therapeutic management of the separate conditions. This section provides a general approach that can be used for most, if not all, occupational dermatoses.

This discussion is arranged to cover the subject under five major headings — the etiologic diagnosis, therapy, prevention, rehabilitation including return to work, and reporting and compensation requirements. These five topics should be considered in the management of all patients with occupational dermatoses. Finally, sources of assistance for the dermatologist are discussed.

The treating physician's objectives should be twofold: to control and eliminate the condition in the patient and to prevent recurrences both in the patient and in others exposed to similar hazards.

THE ETIOLOGIC DIAGNOSIS

The diagnostic assessment of a potential occupational dermatosis must include a determination as to whether the eruption is occupational and if so the identification of the etiologic factors. An etiologic diagnosis is the key to the subsequent management. Frequently multiple causal factors are involved; the better they can be identified and controlled, the greater the effectiveness of therapy and prevention.

From the history and physical examination causal factors likely to be playing a role are identified. In the case of suspected allergic contact dermatitis, patch testing should be performed whenever possible so that the offending allergen can be identified and sources of contact removed. In the case of irritant dermatitis, no specific confirmatory test is available; the judgement as to which irritants are playing a role is based on knowledge of the irritation caused by the contactants in question and the circumstances of exposure. Occupational dermatoses are frequently multifactorial. This is especially true of cumulative insult dermatitis. In this condition prolonged and frequent exposures to one or more marginal irritants, alternate drying and wetting cycles, low humidity, occlusion, abrasions, lacerations, extremes of temperature, preexisting dermatitis, atopic diathesis, and other factors may play a role. The identification of such factors and therefore their subsequent control may require a plant or worksite visit.

The plant visit may be made by the physician alone or if necessary with a professional industrial hygienist. The purpose of the plant visit is to identify hazardous conditions and to determine how they may be ameliorated as well as to become acquainted with the personnel and processes. Effective plant visits usually begin with interviews with appropriate management and union representatives if the plant is unionized, followed by a walk-through survey of the work areas, including change rooms and washing facilities. In conjunction with the walk-through

TABLE 1 Selected Occupational Dermatoses

Contact dermatitis	Occupational infection
Chemical burns	Viral
Irritant dermatitis	Fungal
Toxic insult	Rickettsial
Cumulative insult	Bacterial
Allergic contact dermatitis	
Photosensitivity dermatitis	Hyperpigmentation
Phototoxicity	Melanin
Photoallergy	Other pigments
Atopic dermatitis aggravated by occupation	Focal hypopigmentation
Fiberglass dermatitis	Miliaria
Indolent ulcerations (chromium, arsenic,	Vibration white finger
lime)	Acro-osteolysis
	Scleroderma (silica?)
Acne (coal tars, pitches, oils)	
Chloracne	
Folliculitis	
Alopecia	
Malignant and premalignant lesions	
Keratoses	
Basal cell carcinoma	
Squamous cell carcinoma	
Mycosis fungoides	
Malignant melanoma	
Bowen's disease	

survey, medical examinations of selected employees may be done. A final meeting is held to outline preliminary findings and recommendations, to reiterate requests for further information, and to discuss and agree about further steps.

Toxicologic information should be reviewed about the substances workers contact at the plant. Material safety data sheets describing each product, its toxicity, and handling precautions are now increasingly available to employers, employees, and physicians as a result of local and federal right-to-know regulations and laws. Although the data sheet may not contain all the information needed by the physician, it does identify the chemical nature of a product and provide basic toxicologic information. Since these data sheets are now available to employees, copies of these forms may be brought on clinic visits.

THERAPY

The pharmacologic and surgical treatment of occupational dermatoses does not usually differ from that of similar dermatoses of nonoccupational etiology.

Sometimes modification in work or therapy are necessitated, e.g., avoidance of antihistamines or other drugs with hypnotic effects in drivers, pilots, and heavy equipment operators and temporary changes in duties for laboratory workers exposed to potent pathogens if they have active dermatitis or are being treated with immunosuppressive drugs and for food handlers who have open lesions.

Sometimes modifications in a therapeutic regimen may be made to help protect the skin against workplace exposures. For example, I like to use steroid impregnated occlusive tape, such as Cordran tape, to treat local lesions, particularly of the fingers, since it provides protection for the affected area.

PREVENTIVE MEASURES

Preventive measures should be designed to protect both the affected patients and others who work at similar tasks.

Substitution and Use of Safer Agents

When occupational skin disease is due to chemical agents, attention should be given to the possibility that safer materials may be used. This is relatively simple when it is a matter of altering the soap, barrier cream, or moisturizer a patient is using. It is more difficult when a change in an industrial process is involved. However, on the basis of either toxicologic testing in animals or human experience, lists of potentially safer substances for various uses are becoming available. This substitution is particularly relevant in the case of allergens, for which process the term allergen replacement has been coined.

Engineering and Industrial Hygiene Controls

These should minimize contact of hazardous agents

with the skin. Measures include isolation of a process, careful cleaning of surfaces, use of splash shields and drip pans, avoidance of spills, ventilation to reduce airborne concentrations of contaminants, and control of hazardous radiation and excessive heat, cold, or humidity.

Personal Protective Clothing

Gloves, aprons, shoe covers, finger cots, or completely impervious suits can be worn. If clothing is designed to protect against chemical agents, it should be of a composition impervious to the agent in question. Chemically resistant gloves worn for long periods of time should have cotton linings or undergloves; soft leather gloves are appropriate for mechanical protection. Contaminated clothing should be appropriately cleaned or disposed of. Barrier creams are generally less effective than gloves but may assist, particularly in enabling soil to be removed relatively easily from the skin.

Personal Hygiene

The use of harsh abrasive cleansers and solvents should be minimized. Soap and water should be used whenever possible, sanitary conditions should be maintained, and washing facilities should be close to sites of contamination. Complete showering with a fresh change of clothes may be necessary at the end of a shift. Conversely some workers have irritant dermatitis as a result of overzealous washing. These people need guidance in gentle but effective skin cleansing.

Education

Workers and management personnel need education in skin care and avoidance of hazards. The increasing availability of material safety data sheets and educational programs in industry should facilitate this for the majority of employees.

RETURN TO WORK AND REHABILITATION

Depending on the severity, extent, and localization of disease and the need to avoid aggravating or inciting factors, the worker may need work restrictions or medical removal from work. Medical removal is usually necessary if the disease is extensive and acute. If work restrictions are imposed, they must be reasonable, be clearly spelled out, and be as specific as possible. For example, "avoid all chemicals" is a meaningless restriction. Often it is useful to discuss potential restrictions with worksite supervisors or the plant physician to ensure that they are practicable.

Care must always be taken on return to work to avoid recurrence or aggravation either by the original cause or by nonspecific factors (e.g., heat, marginal irritants, abrasion) acting on skin that is apparently healed but not yet physiologically readjusted to normal. If the worker will be unable to return to his original work, it is wise to seek rehabilitation counseling. A careful determination must be made in regard to new jobs to ensure that they will be free of the factors the worker cannot tolerate. In the case of specific allergies, the rehabilitation specialist must be given a list of allergens and cross reacting substances that need to be avoided, together with information about where these exposures are likely to occur.

REPORTING AND COMPENSATION REQUIREMENTS

Reporting requirements for occupational skin disease vary by state and jurisdiction; therefore, they are not discussed here in detail. In some localities the reporting of all occupational diseases to the authorities is mandatory.

Reports are commonly required from physicians for workmen's compensation purposes. Workmen's compensation laws vary by state or country, but there are some reasonably universal characteristics. Workmen's compensation is a no fault system designed to provide full medical care for accepted conditions and to protect the worker, at least in part, against income loss. Whether a condition is accepted as being caused by work usually depends on a determination that with a reasonable degree of medical certainty (i.e., more likely than not) it is caused or aggravated by the conditions of work. In some states a specific schedule or list of diseases is used to determine diagnoses that are compensable; occupational skin disease is usually included in these schedules.

The report of the attending physician serves either as the sole basis or as one of the bases for the determination of attributability. Thus such reports must be accurate and include necessary information. In complicated cases points that need to be addressed in such reports include sources of information other than the patient (previous case notes, reports from other physicians, inspection of place of work); the medical history, especially of skin disease and atopy; previous occupations; period of contact with assumed causal factors; description of the working process; other cases of dermatitis and standards of hygiene at the place of work; time and site of initial skin complaints, including previous injury at the initial site; progress, with approximate dates of gradual or sudden aggravation or improvement and the influence of vacations and weekends; degree of incapacity during the period of illness with dates of absence from work; therapy; clinical findings, including the present condition and degree to which this is influenced by current therapy such as steroids; special investigations — patch tests (positive and negative, method, site, vehicles, concentration), exposure tests, examinations for fungi; intercurrent diseases; diagnosis; and common knowledge of risk at the occupation in question. The conclusions should include the probable connection between occupational activity and the present pathologic condition, balanced against predisposing factors and contributory factors other than occupation, as well as the possibility of continuing in the previous occupatiion, necessity for rehabilitation, and probable prognosis.

If time off work and workmen's compensation payments to partially or completely replace lost wages are required, a determination of disability is required. The usual designations are of permanent or temporary disability; in either case the disability is either partial or total. Whereas it is usually fairly simple to make such a determination during an episode of acute illness, associated treatment, and convalescence, the assessment of permanent disability and its extent is more complex. The first step is usually to determine the extent of permanent impairment. Permanent impairment of the skin refers to a condition of the skin that persists following maximal medical treatment and rehabilitation and after a reasonable time has elapsed to permit optimal regeneration and other physiologic adjustments to occur. The degree of permanent impairment of the skin may not be static. Therefore, findings should be subject to review and the patient's impairment reevaluated at appropriate intervals. The degree of impairment is usually assessed in terms of functional loss as it affects personal efficiency in daily work and living. The assessment of impairment is a medical function. It is conveniently and reproducibly done using the AMA Guides to the Evaluation of Permanent Impairment (Order Department OP-298, American Medical Association, P.O. Box 821, Monroe, Wisconsin 53566).

However, permanent impairment is only one of the factors used to determine a patient's degree of disability (i.e., his actual or presumed abilty to engage in gainful employment in that community and at that time). The judgment of disability involves medical, behavioral, and societal factors. Disability depends on the degree of impairment, chronicity, expected response to treatment, intelligence, age, availability of work suitable for the patient, past work or school performance, influence of other physical defects, motivation, and other social and economic factors.

SOURCES OF ASSISTANCE FOR THE DERMATOLOGIST

Several sources of assistance and consultation are available to the physician in the United States. Some states and local health department personnel have expertise in occupational health. Nationally the Department of Labor through the Occupational Safety and Health Administration (OSHA) can provide consultation, although medical assistance is limited. The National Institute for Occupational Safety and Health (NIOSH) through its Hazard Evaluation and Technical Assistance Program responds to requests or complaints to determine whether toxic or hazardous workplace conditions are present. A NIOSH hazard evaluation can be initiated by the request of one or more workers (confidentiality is preserved), a union, or the plant management but not directly by a third party such as a physician.

A number of universities provide regional resources at comprehensive occupational and environmental health centers (e.g., Rutgers' Robert Wood Johnson Medical School in New Jersey, Northern and Southern California Occupational Health Centers, The Johns Hopkins University Center for Occupational and Environmental Health, Baltimore, Maryland), at NIOSH sponsored educational resource training centers (University of Alabama, University of Illinois, Harvard School of Public Health, University of Michigan, University of Minnesota, Mt. Sinai School of Medicine, University of North Carolina, University of Cincinnati, University of Texas School of Public Health, University of Utah, and University of Washington), or through divisions of occupational medicine or occupational dermatology units.

All the foregoing can provide referral or access to industrial hygiene and epidemiology capabilities and can direct the physician to useful guides and directories. Workmen's compensation insurance carriers and some larger employers may also assist in carrying out surveys and assisting with worker rehabilitation.

ATOPIC DERMATITIS

NOREEN HEER NICOL, R.N., M.S., F.N.C.
RICHARD A.F. CLARK, M.D.

Atopic dermatitis is a chronic relapsing pruritic skin disorder. The acute phase is characterized by intensely pruritic, erythematous papules and vesicles, often occurring on background areas of erythema. Localized or generalized exacerbations may be isolated or repetitive, occurring weekly or monthly. Repetition of exacerbations leads to subacute or chronic dermatitis with lichenification, scaling, and post-inflammatory hyper- or hypopigmentation. This condition usually occurs in patients with a personal or family history of one or more forms of atopy (allergic asthma, rhinitis, or conjunctivitis or food allergies). The health care team's understanding of each patient's disease pattern and his effectiveness in discovering and reducing exacerbating factors are crucial to effective management of this chronic disease. In addition, the treatment regimen must be individualized to effectively treat disease exacerbations because no one therapy is appropriate for all.

IDENTIFICATION AND ELIMINATION OF EXACERBATING FACTORS

Irritants

That atopic dermatitis is a condition of dry, sensitive, easily irritated skin should be stressed to patients and parents. Atopic disorders are thought to be susceptible to environmental factors owing to abnormal physiologic function of the skin, such as altered sweating and abnormal vascular responses. To prevent irritation, the use of soaps, solvents, and other drying compounds should be minimized. If soaps are to be used, they should have minimal defatting activity and a neutral pH; examples include Dove, Tone, Alpha Keri, Basis, Lowila, and Neutrogena. Nonsoap cleansing agents are also available, such as Aveeno and Emulave. The use of soap should be confined mainly to the intertriginous areas to avoid unnecessary defatting of other skin surfaces. Residual laundry detergent in clothes also may be irritating. Although changing detergents may help, adding a second rinse cycle to ensure the removal of soap from clothing is often more beneficial. Many patients with atopic dermatitis have hand dermatitis. Irritant contact with solvents, soaps, and detergents is probably a major factor. Patients with this problem should avoid jobs that require exposure to these irritants as well as dust, dirt, and heat. A nonaqueous cleansing method may be helpful for atopic patients with irritant hand dermatitis who need to wash frequently and are not able to apply emollients after every washing.

Sweating, whether thermal, emotional, or gustatory, may cause itching. Atopic patients should modify their ac-tivities and surroundings to minimize sweating. They should work and sleep in comfortable surroundings at a fairly constant temperature (68 to 75° F) and humidity (45 to 55 percent). Occlusive clothing may be poorly tolerated, and open weave, loose fitting garments may be preferred. Patients intolerant of woolen or stiff fabrics may find relief from cotton or cotton blend clothing.

Allergens

Aeroallergens and foods are often inciting factors in this disorder. It is important to attempt to correlate positive skin testing or RAST testing with the patient's history of environmental factors that exacerbate the dermatitis. The patient should avoid exposure to allergens when there are positive test results and a high degree of suspicion that the allergens precipitate dermatitis. Blanket restrictions are unjustified. Occasionally air cleansing with an electrostatic air purifier can help reduce aeroallergen exposure at home or in the workplace.

Dietary management of atopic dermatitis has continued to be a controversial subject among pediatricians, allergists, immunologists, and dermatologists. The most common allergens appear to be eggs, cow's milk, soy, wheat, nuts, and fish. In patients who have undergone controlled blinded food challenges that resulted in flaring of dermatitis, it is apparent that avoidance of those foods will be beneficial. Care must be taken to avoid malnutrition when restrictive diets are used. The role of bottle feeding versus breast feeding in the development of atopic dermatitis continues to be unclear; however, some believe that breast feeding may delay the onset of dermatitis if practiced for at least the first 3 months of life.

Infections

Secondary bacterial, fungal, or viral infections may occur in atopic dermatitis. The majority of infections are caused by *Staphylococcus aureus*, and these infections may cause recurrent flares of dermatitis. Staphylococcal infection should be assumed when there are acute weeping dermatitis, crusted impetiginized lesions, and small superficial pustules. Careful culturing for bacterial organisms and determination of their antibiotic sensitivity facilitate systemic treatment with the proper antibiotic.

Herpes simplex may cause extensive local or widespread infection. Topical or systemic therapy with acyclovir is indicated in such severe herpes infections.

Older children and adults may have tinea pedis superimposed upon foot dermatitis. Therefore, when standard topical therapy for foot dermatitis (see p 31) fails, scales from the feet should be collected for fungus wet mount examination and culture. Appropriate treatment is given when these tests yield positive results.

Emotional Stress

Anger, frustration, and anxiety are commonly experienced by patients with atopic dermatitis and often exacerbate the disorder. The added dimension of family hostility, rejection, and guilt can damage the family structure. During the first visit the health care team should reassure the patient and his family that such feelings and emotions are common in situations involving chronic disease. In addition patients and their families become frustrated and hostile and often press for quick "cures." This attitude can be softened by spending considerable time discussing the chronicity of the disease, exacerbating factors, and management measures. Patients and families should be offered strategies for coping with the disease that include an increased knowledge base and an understanding of therapies. Knowing that the disease can be controlled and that the majority of patients improve with age is often reassuring. Recent research has suggested a variety of new therapeutic approaches, and patients need to be given current information to avoid a sense of hopelessness.

THERAPY OF CHRONIC DISEASE

Topical Therapy

Hydration

Hydration is the key to good therapy but often is difficult to achieve because patients with atopic dermatitis have a decreased capacity to retain water in the stratum corneum. The skin is not dry because it lacks grease or oil but because it lacks water. The primary means for correcting dryness is to add water to the skin and then apply a hydrophobic occlusive substance to retain the absorbed water. This can be accomplished by either soaking the affected area or bathing for 15 to 20 minutes in tepid water. The patient leaving the bath should remove excess water by patting with a soft towel and immediately apply a water-in-oil or fatty hydrophobic base (Aquaphor, Eucerin, Crisco, white petrolatum). Use of petrolatum or Crisco without initial hydration is not effective, since it does not hydrate the skin but only prevents further transepidermal water loss. Bathing followed by the application of lubricants should be done at least daily and preferably twice daily for optimal hydration. The addition of colloid substances, such as oatmeal (Aveeno) or starch, to the bath water is soothing for some patients. Bath oils are not recommended because they give the patient a false sense of lubrication and make the bathtub very slippery. In addition, emollients—agents that hydrate the skin, such as Eucerin, Aquaphor, Lubriderm, Vaseline Dermatology Lotion, Moisturel, and Curel—should be applied as often as desired, but usage at least three or four times per day should be encouraged.

Keratin softening agents may facilitate hydration by promoting the removal of scales and crusts, especially in patients who have severe ichthyosis vulgaris as well as atopic dermatitis. Such agents include urea containing creams (Aquacare, 2 percent urea; Aquacare/HP, 10 percent urea; Calmurid, 10 percent urea; Carmol, 10 and 20 percent urea) and lactic acid preparations (Lacticare, Lac-Hydrin). These agents, however, can be irritating to open lesions and therefore may need to be withheld during an acute exacerbation of the disease.

Tar Preparations

Tars and extracts of crude coal tar have been used for their anti-inflammatory properties for years and are recommended to reduce the topical use of corticosteroids in the long term maintenance of atopic dermatitis. Coal tar products have been developed that mask the unpleasant odor, color, and staining properties of crude coal tar, making them more acceptable. Five percent LCD (Liquor carbonis detergens) in a cream base such as Aquaphor has been found to have acceptable cosmetic properties. Tar gel products (Estar Gel and Psorigel) represent a formulation of crude coal tar that is commercially available and cosmetically acceptable; however, they contain alcohol and may cause burning and irritation on acutely inflamed, eczematous skin. Tar gels are best applied under an emollient because of their drying properties. Side effects associated with tars include folliculitis, photosensitization, and contact dermatitis.

Corticosteroids

Topical corticosteroid therapy is frequently needed in the therapy of acute exacerbations of atopic dermatitis. The patient must understand how and when to use such steroid preparations. Corticosteroids possess anti-inflammatory, antipruritic, and vasoconstrictive activity when used topically. Fluorinated or esterified corticosteroids are more potent on a milligram to milligram basis than nonfluorinated and nonesterified compounds.

The choice of agents varies according to the location and extent of the lesions. As a general rule, the lowest potency corticosteroid that is effective should be used. To improve compliance, the patient's preference for a cream or ointment should be considered. Although they spread more easily, creams are less effective and may produce increased drying in some patients. Ointments are more occlusive; thus they provide better delivery of the medication and prevent water loss from the skin. Nevertheless in some cases this occlusion may result in increased pruritus or folliculitis. In this situation or in humid environments creams may be better tolerated than ointments. Sprays and lotions are best used on the scalp or other hairy areas. Steroids should be applied topically immediately after baths or soaks to take advantage of increased penetration through hydrated skin. Steroids should be applied topically no more than twice daily because more frequent application does not improve efficacy and can dramatically increase the cost.

Inadequate prescription size is a frequent problem when treating patients with widespread or frequently flaring dermatitis. Patients become frustrated at both the expense and inconvenience of refilling prescriptions for 15 and 30 gm tubes. Upon request pharmacists can provide frequently used topical preparations in half pound or pound quantities at lower cost.

Hydrocortisone ointment or cream can be used for dermatitis in infants and young children and for dermatitis of the face and intertriginous areas in adults. Patients must be repeatedly warned not to use stronger or topically applied corticosteroids on the thin skinned areas of the face, neck, axilla, and groin. Hydrocortisone 1 percent is relatively safe for daily long term use. Short, 1 to 4 week courses of topical treatment with medium potency steroids such as 0.1 percent triamcinolone or 0.025 percent fluocinolone used one to two times daily are safe and effective for flares of atopic dermatitis. Adverse effects of topical steroid treatment include skin atrophy, depigmentation, acneiform eruptions, and rarely systemic effects.

Ultraviolet Light

Ultraviolet light (UVB or PUVA) therapy may be a useful adjunctive modality in the treatment of chronic recalcitrant atopic dermatitis. Under professional supervision UVB can be effective. It requires three to four treatments per week. Patients who are not fair complexioned and who do not experience photoexacerbations of eczema should be encouraged to avail themselves of moderate amounts of natural sunlight. However, they should be warned not to sunburn and to avoid hot or humid conditions, which may actually induce more pruritus. Home sunlamp treatment is generally not recommended because of the danger of overexposure. Photochemotherapy with oral psoralen therapy followed by UVA (PUVA) is available in some dermatology departments and may be helpful in patients with severe disease. PUVA is reserved for patients with more recalcitrant disease because of the expense and the slow response rate.

The acute side effect of UVB or PUVA is sunburn. Both may increase the risk of skin cancer. Phototherapy is relatively contraindicated in patients with fair skin and is absolutely contraindicated in patients with any photoexacerbated dermatosis such as lupus erythematosus, polymorphous light eruption, photoallergic dermatosis, or photoexacerbated atopic dermatitis.

Systemic Therapy

Antibiotics

Systemic antibiotic therapy is often necessary, because atopic dermatitis is characterized by a chronic low grade inflammatory process that often is secondarily infected. *Staphylococcus aureus* causes the majority of these infections and is often penicillin resistant. Erythromycin is the first choice of therapy because of potential penicillin allergy in these patients. Many patients with atopic dermatitis also have asthma and therefore may be taking a theophylline preparation. Since erythromycin slows theophylline metabolism, erythromycin if used in these patients must be administered while following theophylline blood levels and appropriately adjusting the drug dosage. Erythromycin resistant organisms occasionally account for a poor therapeutic response and necessitate the use of dicloxacillin or clindamycin. Extended treatment ranging from 14 to 28 days is indicated with acute flares; short term therapy is often inadequate in this population. Long term maintenance therapy may be indicated in patients who repeatedly develop infections. Topical antibiotic therapy cannot be recommended, and antibacterial cleansers may worsen the condition by irritating the very sensitive skin of these patients.

Antipruritics

Pruritus is one of the most common and often least tolerated symptoms of atopic dermatitis. Systemic antihistamine treatment and antianxiety drugs may offer some symptomatic relief.

Antihistamines probably reduce scratching, mainly through tranquilizing and sedative effects. Hydroxyzine, diphenhydramine, chlorpheniramine, and promethazine are reasonable choices and should be used on a regular basis for optimal results. Increased awareness of the strong antihistamine H_1 binding affinity of the tricyclic antidepressants has led to the use of these compounds in some patients. Doxepin or amitriptyline may be given as a single 75 mg dose with the evening meal. Other patients may note more effective relief of symptoms by taking the drug in 25 mg doses three times daily. If nighttime scratching is severe and continues in spite of this, use of a sedative to offer temporary relief and allow adequate rest is appropriate. The effects of scratching can be minimized by cutting nails and using cotton gloves at night.

The topical use of antihistamines and local anesthetics should be avoided because of their adverse effects. These drugs can cause cutaneous hypersensitivity reactions. Sensitization may prevent future systemic use of these drugs and related compounds (i.e., sulfonamides, thiazides, and orally administered hypoglycemic drugs).

Corticosteroids

Some patients or parents view the oral use of steroids as a "quick cure" and find them much easier to use than hydration and topical therapy; however, they should be avoided in a chronic nonlife-threatening disorder such as atopic dermatitis. Although there may be dramatic improvement with their use, the rebound following their discontinuation is equally dramatic. The side effects of long term systemic steroid use are both unpleasant and dangerous. Unpleasant effects include acne, easy bruising, Cushingoid appearance, altered personality, sodium retention, and edema. Dangerous side effects include poor wound healing, stunted growth in children, exacerbations of diabetes mellitus and hypertension, necrosis of the femoral head, osteoporosis and fractures, and an impaired response to infections.

When a short term course of oral steroid therapy is given, it is important to taper the dosage as it is discontinued. Intensified skin care should also be instituted during the taper to suppress flaring of the dermatitis.

THERAPY OF ACUTE FLARES

It is preferable to treat acute flares at home, but hospitalization may be necessary to break the cycle of chronic inflammation. It is also helpful when family interactions become strained by hostility, sleeplessness, and irritability or when patients and physicians alike are discouraged by the failure of outpatient modalities. Frequently 5 to 10 days of vigorous inpatient skin care can result in a dramatic clearing of the dermatitis. The hospital stay may also provide time for allergy skin testing or for food challenges as well as the establishment of an effective outpatient therapy program. Hospitalization also offers the option of providing the patient with 5 to 7 days of intravenous antibiotic therapy when indicated.

During an acute flare the number of 15 to 20 minute soaking baths is increased to four or five per day to provide additional hydration and to suppress pruritus. Baths also increase the penetration of topically applied medication up to 10-fold if the medicine is applied immediately after the bath. The patient may be placed in wet wraps after baths to further accentuate hydration and medicinal penetration. Bedtime wet wraps are most practical. If only the arms and legs need to be wrapped, elasticized gauze followed by ACE bandages can be used. For total body occlusion double cotton pajamas can be used. One pair of pajamas is wetted, wrung out so as to be damp but not soaking wet, and placed on the patient. The second pair of pajamas is worn dry over the wet pair. To effect even greater occlusion, a plastic sauna suit is used instead of the dry pajamas. For wrapping the hands and feet, socks can be used in the same manner as pajamas. Baths and wraps may be needed for 3 to 7 days. The patient may require additional blankets or increased room heat during this time to prevent chilling. Baths and compresses are also effective in removing crusts and reducing exudation. Burow's 1:40 solution (one packet of Domeboro powder per quart) provides astringent and antibacterial effects for localized weeping lesions. This solution should be used for only 2 to 3 days because it is extremely drying and may predispose the skin to increased itching and cracking.

The treatment of acute hand and foot dermatitis includes soaking and occlusion as well as special topical treatment. The affected areas are first soaked in a tar solution (Balnetar) for 15 to 20 minutes followed by applications of Estar Gel, Vioform cream, and a high potency corticosteroid. The use of all these topical preparations in combination has been much more effective in recalcitrant cases than single preparation use or other combinations. Remember, however, that each patient requires individual therapy and what works for one may not work for another.

GRANULOMA ANNULARE

HOWARD N. ROBINSON, M.D.

Granuloma annulare (GA) is a dermal or subcutaneous granulomatous disease, which histologically shows foci of necrobiosis with a reactive histiocytic infiltrate. The etiology is unknown; however, there is speculation that the disease may be the result of a delayed type of hypersensitivity reaction. As clinicians we can readily discern the erythematous annular granulomatous plaques usually found on the distal extremities in children and less frequently the generalized papular lesions that tend to form annular groups in adults. The latter disorder, referred to as disseminated granuloma annulare (DGA), can be resistant to all therapeutic modalities and runs its own course, sometimes lasting decades before remitting.

TREATMENT

Localized Granuloma Annulare

The therapies that exist for the treatment of GA are many, but their efficacy must be thoroughly questioned because the disease has a periodicity that can mimic the course of drug therapy.

In children in whom the lesions are usually asymptomatic and isolated on one or two extremities, such as the dorsum of the foot or hand, a prudent treatment is no treatment at all. The granulomas usually disappear within 6 to 12 months and are more a concern of the parent than of the patient. Occasionally one encounters isolated cases of tenderness at the areas of granuloma formation, and intralesional steroid injections of 0.1 to 0.2 cc of a 5 mg per cubic centimeter concentration of triamcinolone acetonide suspension may be helpful.

For the nontender, cosmetically bothersome, superficial granulomas I prefer twice daily applications of betamethasone dipropionate ointment (Diprolene) or flurandrenolide tape (Cordran tape)—12 hours on, 12 hours off—for 2 to 3 weeks. There are now three potency tiers of fluorinated steroids that are effective topically. The higher two potencies, such as betamethasone dipropionate and clobetasol propionate (Temovate), are increasingly effective with twice daily applications. There are restrictions on the use of clobetasol propionate owing to its potential for systemic absorption and suppression of the adrenal axis. Clobetasol propionate can only be used twice daily for 2 weeks with a rest interval of 2 weeks and then a continuing cycle as necessary. I have used clobetasol propionate with good results in patients who were resistant to lower potency topical fluorinated steroid therapy.

Side effects such as epidermal and dermal atrophy, striae, adrenal suppression, and other effects seen with oral systemic steroid therapy are possible with prolonged use of any of the fluorinated topical steroid preparations.

Disseminated Granuloma Annulare

The rarer subset of GA cases are of the disseminated (DGA) form and tend to affect adults in their fifth and sixth decades. The DGA form can be quite disfiguring, producing intense anxiety in the afflicted individual. DGA is usually otherwise asymptomatic. However, there are cases in which the lesions have been extremely pruritic and tender, and one reported case involved fascial and tendon planes with subsequent deformity of the patient's hands. DGA deserves the clinician's efforts in an attempt at inducing an earlier remission than in the natural course of the disease, which could be 30 years.

The following sections describe therapeutic modalities that show some promise in the treatment of DGA.

Isotretinoin

There is one case report that describes a patient treated with isotretinoin (Accutane) 40 mg twice daily for 1 month and then once daily for 3 months with resolution of the majority of the lesions. A 6-month follow-up revealed no new lesions. Isotretinoin has recently been reported in one case to be effective also in the treatment of cutaneous sarcoidosis. Further studies are needed to determine the efficacy of isotretinoin and its derivatives for the treatment of cutaneous granulomas.

The major side effects are the same as those in treating patients with cystic acne: severe teratogenicty, elevations in the cholesterol and triglyceride levels, mucous membrane dryness, and photosensitivity. A baseline chemistry panel including fasting triglyceride and cholesterol levels and liver function tests is necessary along with monthly determinations of fasting triglyceride and cholesterol levels.

Niacinamide

One case has been reported in which oral niacinamide therapy, 500 mg three times daily, induced a remission of DGA in 6 to 12 months; there was no mention of follow-up. I have since treated two patients with oral doses of niacinamide with a similar dose schedule. In both patients there was a 50 percent remission of the lesions with subsequent return of lesions at the 3-month follow-up.

Side effects—a gastrointestinal flulike syndrome and rarely hepatotoxicity—have been reported with oral dosages of 3 to 6 g per day.

Sulfone

There have been several reports of patients treated with dapsone with dosages of 50 to 100 mg per day for 6 to 10 weeks with a significant remission of lesions. However, relapses have been documented in the majority of patients on discontinuation of therapy. One child with DGA received 50 mg per day of dapsone for 6 weeks and achieved a complete remission (including a 6-month follow-up).

Dapsone therapy requires monitoring of the complete blood count, differential, platelet level, liver function, and methemoglobin level. A screen for glucose-6-phosphate dehydrogenase (G6PD) is necessary because patients who are G6PD deficient are susceptible to hemolysis.

Potassium Iodide

In one study four patients with DGA received oral doses of potassium iodide (SSKI), starting with 3 drops three times a day with meals and increasing to 1 ml per day, which is equivalent to 900 mg per day, for 12 weeks. Two patients had marked improvement with no exacerbation after discontinuation of therapy, in one patient the disease partially cleared, and one patient did not finish the study.

One other case of DGA treatment with 900 mg per day of SSKI resulted in resolution after 6 months and recurrence 10 months later. In addition this patient became profoundly hypothyroid. Potassium iodide can cause an iodide goiter with or without hypothyroidism when an underlying thyroid disease such as Graves' disease or Hashimoto's thyroiditis is present. Therefore, baseline thyroid function studies, including T_3, T_4, TSH, and antithyroid antibody levels, should be done. The thyroid function test results should be followed intermittently during therapy.

I have treated three patients with SSKI with up to 900 mg per day for 3 months, with extensive clearing in one patient and only partial clearing in two patients. All patients developed recurrences within 3 months after ending therapy; however, two of the patients had improved by 50 percent.

Side effects other than hypothyroidism include nausea, gastric irritation, headaches, acute urticaria, angioneurotic edema, eosinophilia, arthralgia, acneiform eruption, and rarely an iododerma type of eruption.

Alkylating Agents

There are several reports of severe DGA treated with low dose chlorambucil (Leukeran) therapy, ranging from 2 mg two to three times daily for 3 to 10 months, with significant improvement.

There is one report of combination therapy with melphalan (Alkeran) and prednisone in a patient with granuloma annulare and a plasma cell dyscrasia. The patient received 10 mg of melphalan and 60 mg of prednisone for 1 week, with cycles repeated every 6 weeks for 17 months with resolution of skin lesions.

Careful screening of the complete blood cell count, platelet count, and liver and kidney function is necessary. Peripheral blood cell and platelet counts should be done weekly throughout therapy. Chlorambucil and melphalan are very toxic alkylating drugs that have been shown to cause irreversible bone marrow suppression, neutropenia, thrombocytopenia, chromatid and chromosomal damage, sterility in both sexes, gastritis (melphalan), and induction of malignant disease, such as leukemia. These drugs are known to be teratogenic. In view of the overwhelming side effects these drugs should be used only as a last resort in an informed patient.

Scarification

It has been demonstrated that manipulation via cryotherapy, surgical biopsy, or injection of a placebo solution can induce regression of an isolated lesion of GA, and rarely multiple lesions. I have on occasion performed a biopsy of a GA lesion in a child and noted rapid resolution of the lesion.

A technique known as scarification has been employed for resolution of persistent GA lesions. One uses either a 19 gauge injection needle tip or a number 11 scalpel blade to gently graze the granuloma surface and induce capillary bleeding. In my experience this technique seems to work on the manipulated lesion but rarely induces resolution of distant granulomas. In all patients in whom I have used this technique the lesions returned within 2 to 3 months.

Systemic Corticosteroid Therapy

Corticosteroids are being used systemically to treat resistant cases of GA but rarely induce long standing remission. The dosage usually cannot be tapered without exacerbation of lesions, leading to side effects such as hirsutism, cushingoid features, hypertension, elevation in the serum glucose level, easy bruisability, cataract formation, and osteoporosis. This form of therapy is a no win situation, which encourages patient dependence and insures problems in the future.

Other Therapies

Other therapies for the treatment of GA have included grenz irradiation, cryotherapy, antimalarial drugs, oral doses of vitamin E, saline intralesional injections, gold injections, sulfanilamide, bismuth, arsenic, antihistamines, and calciferol. These therapies are currently not considered to be effective in the treatment of GA.

I would like to emphasize that GA is usually asymptomatic, remits spontaneously, and is merely a nuisance disease. In its DGA form it is usually only of cosmetic concern, and therapy should be judiciously administered so as not to do more harm than the disease itself.

GRANULOMA FACIALE

ROBERT M. TAYLOR, M.D.

Granuloma faciale is a peculiar inflammatory condition of the skin of unknown origin and paradoxic histologic features: acute vasculitis with eosinophils admixed with a chronic infiltrate of lymphocytes and histiocytes. Clinically papules, nodules, and plaques are present, commonly on the face but occasionally elsewhere, which appear pink to orange-brown to red-purple. Follicular openings are prominent, and occasional telangectasias course over the lesional surface. Patients are generally middle aged caucasian adults with a male predominance. The disease is particularly indolent, with very few spontaneous remissions recorded.

Therapeutics in granuloma faciale are as much an enigma as the etiopathogenesis of the disorder. Many treatments have been attempted for granuloma faciale, but none has consistently produced acceptable results. I have had limited success with topical and intralesional corticosteroid therapy, cryotherapy, and surgery. I have not utilized PUVA (oral or topical doses of psoralens with UVA) or medications such as oral dapsone treatment.

With the advent of potent topical treatment with steroids such as clobetasol proprionate (Temovate) and betamethasone diproprionate (Diprolene), topical therapy with or without occlusion is a reasonable first line therapeutic approach to granuloma faciale. In one patient twice daily applications to facial lesions under occlusion for 14 to 21 days resulted in resolution. As long as the medication is kept on lesional skin, steroid atrophy of the surrounding skin is not a major concern. Nonetheless the patient is informed of the atrophogenic side effects of the product and is told to discontinue its use once the lesion(s) flattens or if no change is noted by the fourteenth day.

Intralesional steroid therapy using an initial 2.5 to 5.0 mg per cubic centimeter concentration (triamcinolone hexacetonide, Artistospan; or triamcinolone acetonide, Kenalog) and a 30 gauge needle is occasionally successful. The amount of steroid injected is dependent on the size of the lesion. When possible, the injection should be carried out in an arclike spray pattern rather than a depot manner. Triamcinolone injection can lead to atrophy of skin, and I have found that in addition to the amount injected,

the method of injection is important in minimizing this side effect. If two consecutive intralesional injections of triamcinolone (2.5 to 5.0 mg per cubic centimeter) 30 days apart do not effect a response (i.e., a decrease in the size and intensity of the lesion), I generally do not pursue this line of therapy further. Depending on its size, injection of more than 10 mg of triamcinolone into any given lesion over the duration of treatment is not recommended (there is a high risk of cutaneous steroid atrophy).

Cryotherapy has been used with some success, although like topical and intralesional steroid therapy, it does not produce consistent results. With a rapid delivery cryogenic system like the CRY-AC, a thorough liquid nitrogen freeze of the lesion can be achieved, including a 1 mm rim of normal tissue. In the first session a 15 to 20 second sustained freeze with thawing is carried out. If a response is seen in the lesion, I repeat with the same duration of freezing-thawing in 1 month. If blistering occurs without response, my choices are twofold: discontinue treatment or attempt one more treatment, if the patient is willing, with a 30-second freeze-thaw cycle. If no blistering occurs with or without response, I increase the freezing time another 15 to 20 seconds each session until blistering occurs or a 60-second freeze-thaw cycle has been reached. Prudence and a knowledge of the facial anatomy dictate where freezing can be attempted. For example, I do not freeze over the zygomatic arch, since in that region cutaneous nerves run in a superficial plane.

Surgery is a possibility for small lesions, but in general lesions of granuloma faciale are larger. Also recurrence is not unheard of after surgical removal.

Two additional modalities that I have not personally used but that merit mention are topical psoralen therapy with UVA (PUVA) and oral dapsone therapy. In one reported case PUVA treatment over a 9- to 10-week period at a total dosage of 24 joules resulted in clearing of a granuloma faciale nodule. In another instance dapsone, begun at a dosage of 100 mg per day in a patient with granuloma faciale, resulted in resolution of the lesion within 6 months. The latter therapy carries the risk of hemolytic anemia, and appropriate testing of hematologic parameters before and during treatment is important. In addition, a pretreatment glucose-6-phosphate dehydrogenase (G6PD) level must be obtained in order to identify G6PD deficient patients in whom hemolysis would be exaggerated if they were given dapsone.

PALMOPLANTAR PUSTULOSIS

BARBARA L. BRAUNSTEIN-WILSON, M.D.

Palmoplantar pustulosis (PPP) is a chronic recalcitrant eruption in which recurrent crops of deep seated, pruritic or tender, sterile pustules or vesicopustules develop on the palms and soles. The eruption may extend onto the dorsal surfaces of the hands and feet. The pustules, which sometimes coalesce to form lakes of pus, eventually rupture and dry up, only to be followed by similar bouts.

In most instances the cause of PPP is unknown. In many cases the eruption may be a localized form of pustular psoriasis. These patients may have evidence of psoriasis elsewhere on the body, such as the scalp or extensor extremities. In other patients PPP may be found in a "bacterid" form, a pustular eruption of the palms and soles caused by a focus of bacterial infection elsewhere in the body. Such infections include infected ulcers, sinusitis, tonsillitis, periapical abscesses, and otitis media. In such cases, when the focus of infection is eradicated, the pustular eruption resolves.

A probable variant of PPP known as acrodermatitis perstans continua is a pustular eruption that usually involves one or more distal digits and is exacerbated by infection and trauma. Scarring and destruction of the nails and digits can occur in this disorder.

APPROACH TO THE PATIENT

Other causes of pustular eruptions of the palms and soles, such as secondarily infected dyshidrotic eczema or an inflammatory dermatophyte infection, should be ruled out with appropriate bacterial and fungal cultures and a potassium hydroxide examination of a pustule and treated accordingly.

The physician should search for historical or physical evidence of a distant focus of infection that could be responsible for a "bacterid." Appropriate treatment of the underlying infection should result in clearing of the "bacterid" on the palms and soles. If no focus of infection is found, a therapeutic trial of oral doses of a broad spectrum antibiotic such as erythromycin or cephalosporin may be given in an attempt to eradicate an occult infection.

If the foregoing measures are unrewarding, one is left with a diagnosis of idiopathic PPP.

TOPICAL THERAPY

There is no cure for chronic PPP. Topical therapy is usually tried initially. However, although this is frequently helpful adjunctive therapy, in most cases it is not sufficient to control the disease. Various systemic therapies are available and may lead to remissions, but recurrences are the rule upon cessation of therapy.

If the skin is oozing and weeping, wet compresses using aluminum acetate or silver nitrate solution three times daily for 30 minutes help to dry up the skin and decrease the likelihood of secondary infection. Oral doses of antibiotics should be administered if there is evidence of secondary bacterial infection.

Topical therapy using tars and corticosteroids are sometimes helpful in decreasing pruritus and inflammation as well as pustulation. The patient should be instructed to soak the hands and feet several times daily in a basin of water to which several capfuls of tar oil such as Balnetar or Doak tar oil have been added. Immediately following the soaks, a topical tar or corticosteroid preparation should be applied. Hydration of the skin prior to the topical application of such preparations enhances the penetration of medications through the skin and thereby inceases their efficacy.

Keratolytic agents such as 5 to 10 percent salicylic acid or 10 to 20 percent urea may be added to therapeutic drugs to enhance their penetration through the thick palmoplantar skin.

Many different types of tar preparations can be used. Tar gels such as Estar gel and Psorigel are cosmetically acceptable, but these products may cause stinging on contact with broken skin because they usually contain alcohol. Also the gels, although more pleasant to use, tend to be less effective than cruder, less refined tar preparations compounded by the pharmacist. Examples of some tar preparations that can be compounded include 2 to 4 percent crude coal tar or 5 to 10 percent liquor carbonis detergens in an emollient base, such as Aquaphor ointment or Eucerin cream. Tars can be applied one to several times a day. Disadvantages of tar therapy include an unpleasant odor and staining of the clothes.

When topical corticosteroid therapy is used to treat PPP, a high potency drug is usually required. The new, very potent corticosteroids, Temovate and Diprolene, are most likely to be effective. Plastic wrap occlusion may be used to increase penetration of the steroid through the skin. The steroid should be applied to the affected skin one to three times daily. The patient should be made aware that long-term use of potent topical steroid preparations may cause irreversible atrophy of the skin, especially on the thinner skin of the dorsal hands and feet.

If topical steroid therapy is ineffective and if the eruption is fairly localized, intralesional therapy with triamcinolone acetonide suspension can be given using a 30-gauge needle and a tuberculin syringe. A maximum of about 10 mg of triamcinolone should be administered at one injection and repeated every few months. A significant disadvantage in this approach is the pain associated with the injections. Some clinicians advise diluting the corticosteroid with equal parts of lidocaine, but the lidocaine itself causes significant pain on injection. A Dermojet rather than a syringe may be used to inject the steroids and usually causes less pain.

Anthralin cream is occasionally useful in the treatment of PPP. This is available in various concentrations and is applied once daily for 20 to 40 minutes. Contact with uninvolved skin should be avoided to decrease the likelihood of irritation. Staining of clothes is a major disadvantage of anthralin therapy.

PHOTOCHEMOTHERAPY

Photochemotherapy with oral doses of psoralen and longwave ultraviolet A exposure (PUVA) is probably the most effective treatment available for PPP and is my preferred approach if the foregoing measures have failed and a PUVA unit is available. Pregnancy and lupus erythematosus are contraindications to this form of therapy. Prior to therapy an antinuclear antibody determination and an ophthalmologic examination should be done. During therapy the ophthalmologic examination should be repeated yearly. Proper eye protection must be worn to prevent ocular damage.*

Patients are treated wth PUVA three to four times weekly and are instructed to ingest 0.6 mg per kilogram of the original crystalline form of 8-methoxypsoralen 2 hours prior to the light exposure. Only the palms and soles are exposed to the ultraviolet A (UVA) light.

The starting dose of UVA can be determined by adding 0.5 J per square centimeter to the skin type (Table 1). For example, the starting dose of UVA for a patient with skin type II would be 2.5 J per square centimeter. The UVA dose is increased by 1 J per square centimeter at each treatment if no phototoxic erythema is present. When a dose of 10 J per square centimeter is attained, the dose is lowered by 0.5 J per square centimeter at each treatment. When adequate clearance has been achieved, usually a dose of about 20 J per square centimeter, the frequency of treatment can be reduced gradually. Patients usually can be maintained with one treatment every 1 to 2 weeks. Please note that if the new oral liquid capsules of 8-methoxypsoralen are prescribed, the dosage should be reduced to 0.3 to 0.4 mg per kilogram. The dose of UVA should be halved and administered at 1 hour rather than 2 hours after ingestion of the 8-methoxypsoralen. The new liquid 8-methoxypsoralen should be taken on an empty stomach.

The disadvantages of oral PUVA therapy are nausea and pruritus secondary to the psoralen as well as phototoxic erythema. Long-term side effects include ocular damage if adequate protection is not used, an increased incidence of skin cancer, and accelerated aging of the skin.

Topical psoralen therapy and UVA also constitute effective therapy for PPP. Although this method greatly decreases the likelihood of systemic side effects, there is a much higher incidence of severe localized phototoxic erythema.

TABLE 1 Skin Type Versus PUVA Dose

Skin Type	History	PUVA Dose
I	Always burns, never tans	1.5 J/cm²
II	Always burns, sometimes tans	2.5 J/cm²
III	Sometimes burns, always tans	3.5 J/cm²
IV	Never burns, always tans	4.5 J/cm²
V	Brown skin (Chinese, Mexican, American Indian)	5.5 J/cm²
VI	Black skin	6.5 J/cm²

Adapted from Morrison WL. Phototherapy and photochemotherapy of skin disease. West Haven, CT: Praeger Publishers, 1983.

TABLE 2 Contraindications to Methotrexate

Renal disease
Liver disease
Pregnancy
Severe anemia, leukopenia, thrombocytopenia
Peptic ulcer disease
Alcohol consumption
Active infectious diseases
Patient unreliability

METHOTREXATE

Methotrexate is frequently beneficial in the treatment or PPP and is indicated for severe disabling recalcitrant disease, especially if PUVA therapy is unsuccessful, contraindicated, or unavailable. There are many relative contraindications to methotrexate therapy (Table 2).

Relatively low dosages of methotrexate are used (7.5 to 25 mg) and may be administered as a once weekly dose or divided into three doses 12 hours apart.

There are many adverse reactions to methotrexate, the most common of which are nausea, vomiting, malaise, and leukopenia. Methotrexate can cause hepatic fibrosis or cirrhosis. Prior to therapy a liver biopsy should be performed and repeated periodically during therapy. The patient should undergo periodic laboratory evaluation of the hematologic, hepatic, and renal systems during therapy.

SYSTEMIC STEROID THERAPY

Oral or intramuscular treatment with corticosteroids, although very effective in clearing PPP, should be avoided if possible. The pustular eruption recurs soon after discontinuation of the steroids, and therefore long-term steroid therapy with its severe side effects would be required to control the disease. A short course of prednisone may be given to the patient with a true "bacterid" to speed resolution of the pustules while the responsible focus of infection is being eradicated. On rare occasions low dose prednisone therapy is required on a long-term basis to control the disease.

ETRETINATE

Only recently available in the United States, etretinate appears to be effective therapy for PPP. Remissions can be achieved, but therapy must be continued to avoid relapse. Some of the more common side effects of etretinate include dryness of the skin and mucous membranes, hair loss, and teratogenicity.

DAPSONE

Dapsone occasionally has been found to be useful for the treatment of PPP. The same dosage schedule and monitoring recommended for dermatitis herpetiformis are used for PPP (see chapter on *Dermatitis Herpetiformis*).

* Details about eye protection can be found in the Article by Farber EM et al. Current status of oral PUVA therapy. J Am Acad Dermatol 1982; 6:851–855.

SUBCORNEAL PUSTULAR DERMATOSIS

ROSEMARIE WATSON, M.D.

In 1956 Sneddon and Wilkinson described a chronic benign relapsing pustular eruption that occurs most frequently in women over 40 years of age. The histologic features of this disorder prompted use of the term "subcorneal pustular dermatosis." Although there has been considerable controversy in the literature since then as to whether some of these patients have variants of pustular psoriasis, the characteristic features of this syndrome warrant its place as a distinct entity in the dermatologic literature.

The primary lesion is a vesicle-pustule. When fully formed, a flaccid sterile pustule 1 to 10 mm in diameter is seen, often on an erythematous base. The pustules may be isolated or grouped, often with a tendency for bizarre circinate or serpiginous patterns to develop. Successive waves of pustules pass across previously affected areas. Sites of predilection include the groin, axillas, and submammary regions and the flexor aspects of the limbs. Pruritus is not a prominent feature, and the general health is usually unaffected unless the disease is extensive. Several reports of associated paraproteinemias, notably IgA and IgG, have been described in this disorder. The clinical course is benign, but the patient may have several relapses over many years (average, 5 to 8 years). The typical histologic appearance is a subcorneal pustule filled with polymorphonuclear leukocytes with little disturbance of the underlying epidermis. The differential diagnosis includes impetigo contagiosa, pemphigus foliaceus, pustular psoriasis, dermatitis herpetiformis, and the glucagonoma syndrome. Hematoxylin and eosin staining and immunofluorescence studies differentiate the majority.

TREATMENT

The therapeutic approach depends on the extent and duration of the disease. In localized lesions compresses with Burow's solution followed by topical applications of steroids shorten the pustular phase. Surprisingly, systemic steroid therapy is not effective in this disorder. Because the lesions initially resemble impetigo contagiosa both clinically and histologically, it is wise to initiate a 10-day course of systemic antibiotic therapy e.g., erythromycin, 250 mg four times daily.

The drug of choice for the treatment of subcorneal pustular dermatosis is dapsone (4,4-diaminodiphenylsulfone, DDS, Avlosulfon). Dapsone generally produces clinical remission in 1 to 4 weeks. The response is slower than in dermatitis herpetiformis, and the majority of patients obtain partial if not complete relief. Indeed, so impressed are Sneddon and Wilkinson by the response to dapsone that they have suggested that the absence of a response to this drug may indicate an alternative diagnosis such as pustular psoriasis. Sulfapyridine, a drug thought to be somewhat less effective, is preferred by some

physicians for the treatment of children and older individuals. It is a satisfactory alternative for patients who are unable to tolerate dapsone. Should dapsone or sulfapyridine be ineffective or should the patient be unable to tolerate these drugs, there are isolated reports of a beneficial response to PUVA phototherapy and the retinoids.

Dapsone

Mechanism of Action

Dapsone exerts its effect in infectious diseases by inhibiting para-aminobenzoic acid use by bacteria. However, the mechanism of action in subcorneal pustular dermatosis is unknown. It appears to exert its effect by suppression of polymorphonuclear leukocyte activity. Recent evidence suggests that it may block the capacity of leukocytes to respond to a chemotactic stimulus. The drug is also known to interfere with complement activity, and it may stabilize lysosomal membranes.

Pharmacology and Dosimetry

Dapsone is slowly but nearly completely absorbed in the gut, with a peak plasma concentration at 1 to 3 hours. It is detected in small amounts in the body for 8 to 12 days or longer. The drug is distributed in all tissues and fluids but is found in highest concentrations in skin, muscle, kidney, and liver. The drug is acetylated in the liver and is excreted primarily by the kidneys.

Dapsone is available in 25 and 100 mg tablets. Before starting this drug, a routine CBC, blood chemistries, and a glucose-6-phosphate dehydrogenase (G6PD) level are mandatory (Table 1). A healthy individual with a normal CBC can tolerate a starting dosage of 100 mg daily with increments of 50 mg every 1 to 2 weeks until remission occurs. Most patients are maintained on 100 to 150 mg of dapsone, but an occasional patient may require higher dosages, e.g., 200 to 300 mg. The risk of toxicity is higher at dosages over 150 mg daily. Once a remission is achieved, the dosage should be reduced gradually, i.e., 25 mg weekly. The maintenance dosage should be the lowest dosage tolerated without relapse. In some patients the drug is eventually discontinued, whereas others require continuous therapy to prevent relapse.

A lower starting dosage of 25 to 50 mg daily is recommended in both children and older individuals. Caution is also recommended in patients with cardiac disease and G6PD deficiency.

TABLE 1 Laboratory Tests to be Done Prior To Initiation of Dapsone or Sulfapyridine Therapy

CBC with differential white count
Blood urea nitrogen, creatinine, bilirubin,
  transaminases, and alkaline phosphatase levels
Urinalysis
Glucose-6-phosphate dehydrogenase level
Methemoglobin level

Sulfapyridine

Children and older individuals seem to tolerate sulfapyridine better than dapsone. Once the recommended baseline laboratory values are available (see Table 1), the recommended dosage is 2 to 4 g given in divided doses after an initial test dose of 500 mg. Once a remission is achieved, the dosage can be tapered to maintenance therapy, which is approximately 1.5 g daily. Close laboratory monitoring is also important with use of this drug, because the side effects are similar to those of dapsone. The toxicity of this drug is increased in slow acetylators. Pyribenzamine, 500 mg twice daily, potentiates the therapeutic effect of sulfapyridine in dermatitis herpetiformis, allowing for a lower maintenance dosage and fewer side effects.

LABORATORY MONITORING

Baseline laboratory tests required before the initiation of sulfapyridine or dapsone therapy are summarized in Table 1. Frequent monitoring is required to minimize the severity of potential side effects of these drugs. During the initial period of therapy, a CBC and differential white count should be obtained weekly. Once a stable dosage is achieved, a CBC should be repeated every 2 weeks for several weeks, then monthly for several months, and then once every 3 months. However, if at any time an increase in dosage is required, frequent monitoring is resumed until this dosage is again stabilized. A chemistry profile, which includes measurements of renal and hepatic function, need not be repeated as frequently as the CBC. It may be done every 2 to 3 weeks during initial therapy. Like the CBC, it eventually needs to be done only every 3 months. A urinalysis is particularly important for patients taking sulfapyridine. This should be done after the first week of therapy and at less frequent intervals thereafter. Eventually it may be required only every 3 months. After a pretreatment determination, the G6PD test need not be repeated.

ADVERSE SIDE EFFECTS

Dapsone and sulfapyridine have similar side effects. The most severe side effects occur in the first 3 months of therapy. However, exceptions to this rule are not uncommon; thus close monitoring of the patient is always necessary. It has been said that a patient who is allergic to dapsone may safely take sulfapyridine and vice versa. Although many clinicians have observed this to be true, there are reports of cross reactivity. Thus, if the patient has had a severe reaction to one of these two drugs, extreme caution should be taken in using the other agent. The side effects of these drugs are summarized in Table 2. Minor side effects are common; these include nausea, vomiting, headache, weakness, dizziness, fatigue, and nervousness. These findings were noted in 38 percent of the patients taking sulfapyridine and in 20 percent of those taking dapsone in one study. It is understandable that these minor side effects can interfere with compliance. Experience has shown that a switch from dapsone to sulfa-

TABLE 2   Adverse Effects of Dapsone and Sulfapyridine

Red blood cell: hemolytic anemia, methemoglobinemia

White blood cell: leukopenia, agranulocytosis

Gastrointestinal manifestations: anorexia, nausea, vomiting, hepatitis, cholestatic jaundice

Sulfone hypersensitivity syndrome

Skin manifestations: morbilliform rash, erythema multiforme, erythema nodosum, fixed drug eruption, urticaria, exfoliative dermatitis, toxic epidermal necrolysis

Neurologic manifestations: peripheral neuropathy, psychosis, headache, dizziness, blurred vision, insomnia

Renal manifestations: crystalluria, nephrotic syndrome, renal papillary necrosis

Miscellaneous: fever, infectious mononucleosis-like syndrome

pyridine or vice versa can result in resolution of these symptoms.

Hemolysis

Hemolysis can be expected in all patients taking therapeutic doses of dapsone or sulfapyridine. The sulfones are strong oxidizers and thus shorten the red cell half-life by approximately 50 percent. Hemolysis is markedly exaggerated in patients with G6PD deficiency whose red blood cells are more susceptible to damage by oxidants. G6PD deficiency is seen predominantly in blacks (15 percent) as a heterozygous trait and rarely in Caucasians as a more serious homozygous trait. The most severe hemolysis is seen in Caucasians with homozygous G6PD deficiency. Italians, Greeks, and Sephardic Jews have an increased frequency of deficiency of this enzyme.

Despite the variability from patient to patient, most normal individuals tolerate 100 mg per day with very little hemolysis, and G6PD deficient patients tolerate 50 mg per day well. At a level of 150 mg per day, all patients demonstrate some hemolysis. One can expect a 25 percent reduction in the hematocrit level in patients taking 300 mg per day. In patients with G6PD deficiency, if significant hemolysis is going to occur, it does so early in therapy. However, in normal individuals the hemolysis and the fall in the hematocrit level may not occur for 3 to 4 weeks after therapy is initiated. The elderly and the young are most susceptible to the hemolytic effect of these drugs. If hemolysis is severe, acute tubular necrosis may result. In general, however, after an initial fall the hematocrit value subsequently rises and levels off at a point somewhat below its original value. Patients are generally not symptomatic unless there is underlying cardiac disease, when exacerbation of angina may occur.

Methemoglobinemia

Dapsone and sulfapyridine reduce the oxygen carrying capacity of the blood by formation of methemoglobin.

Methemoglobin is detected in most patients early in the course of treatment. Clinical cyanosis becomes apparent when 15 percent of the total hemoglobin is methemoglobin. Most patients who demonstrate cyanosis are asymptomatic. Symptoms such as dyspnea, dizziness, headache, and confusion occur as the methemoglobin level increases to 30 to 40 percent. Once levels of 60 percent are reached, coma is likely. Peak methemoglobin levels usually occur by the second week of therapy. Patients with cardiac insufficiency are at risk of becoming symptomatic from this side effect. Methemoglobinemia responds partially to daily ascorbic acid ingestion (200 mg). Intravenous methylene blue therapy is an emergency treatment for methemoglobinemia.

Agranulocytosis

Agranulocytosis is a serious side effect with these drugs because it is potentially lethal. It is generally seen within the first 3 to 12 weeks of treatment. Leukopenia is said to occur in 5 percent of the patients taking sulfapyridine. The patient should be instructed to report fever, pharyngitis, or other evidence of infection to his physician; a prompt determination of the CBC and differential count is required. Frequent and regular monitoring of the CBC allows early detection of this side effect.

HYPERSENSITIVITY PHENOMENA

Cutaneous Manifestations

Some 10 percent of the patients taking sulfapyridine and dapsone develop a cutaneous eruption (see Table 2). A syndrome similar to the Dilantin hypersensitivity syndrome has also been described, primarily in patients with leprosy, 3 to 6 weeks after the initiation of therapy. The features include a rash, hepatitis, leukopenia, lymphadenopathy, and lymphocytosis with atypical lymphocytes resembling those in an infectious mononucleosis syndrome.

Peripheral Neuropathy

Peripheral neuropathy is being increasingly reported in association with dapsone therapy. The neuropathy is usually motor but can be sensory. It is generally seen after prolonged high-dose therapy, but there have been reports of its occurrence at dosages as low as 200 mg daily given for 7 weeks. The neuropathy is reversible when the dosage is decreased.

Nephrotoxicity

Nephrotoxicity is more likely to occur with sulfapyridine and is caused by precipitation of the drug in the kidney. These patients must be monitored intermittently for crystalluria to avoid renal damage. Increased fluid intake is recommended with sulfapyridine therapy. The nephrotic syndrome and renal papillary necrosis have been reported in patients taking dapsone.

CONCLUSION

Although the list of side effects of dapsone and sulfapyridine is impressive, the clinician should not be deterred. Frequent laboratory monitoring reduces the potential severity of the side effects. The majority of patients with subcorneal pustular dermatosis have an excellent response to these drugs, with partial or complete remission. Other therapeutic modalities such as PUVA therapy and the retinoids should be kept in reserve for patients who cannot tolerate or do not respond to the sulfones or sulfapyridine.

SWEET'S SYNDROME

DAVID B. VASILY, M.D.

Acute febrile neutrophilic dermatosis (AFND) was first recognized as a distinct syndrome by R.D. Sweet in England in 1964. Subsequently numerous reports of AFND, atypical variants, and new systemic disease associations have appeared.

AFND occurs predominantly in middle aged women 1 to 3 weeks after a flulike prodrome or an upper respiratory infection. The striking characteristic cutaneous lesions of this neutrophilic dermatosis erupt in asymmetric crops somewhat in a photodistribution over the face, nuchal area, arms, and upper trunk over a period of a few weeks to months.The individual lesions are typically tender, violaceous, edematous plaques with a papular or mammillated surface. The lesions rapidly expand centrifugally. Resolution with only postinflammatory pigmentation and no scarring is characteristic, although acquired cutis laxa at lesional sites has been reported.

Atypical AFND morphologic variants include lesions suggestive of cutaneous vasculitis, bacterial cellulitis, erythema nodosum, erythema multiforme, or early pyoderma gangrenosum. Vesiculobullous lesions and rarely solitary lesions have been reported. In addition to cutaneous lesions, patients are often acutely ill with severe prostration, polyarthralgias, and myalgias.

Spiking temperatures to 40° C (104° F), episcleritis or conjuctivitis, and frank joint effusions can occur. These symptoms and signs are accompanied in most cases by a marked neutrophilic leukocytosis in the 10,000 to 30,000 per cubic millimeter range (without immature forms), an elevated erythrocyte sedimentation rate (up to 150 mm per hour) and rarely proteinuria or other urinary sediment abnormalities. Relatively normal or low total white blood counts and anemia in association with vesicular, bullous, or mucous membrane AFND lesions may be markers for underlying hematologic malignant disease such as acute myeloid leukemia. Associations with lymphoma, myeloma, testicular, ovarian, and metastatic adenocarcinoma, ulcerative colitis, subacute cutaneous lupus erythematosus, Sjögren's syndrome, rheumatoid arthritis, postmyocardial infarction syndrome, and toxoplasmosis also have been reported. Despite these different systemic disease associations, the histopathologic features of AFND remain strikingly constant, consisting of a dense perivascular neutrophilic infiltrate without fibrin deposition with occasional septal pannicular involvement.

TREATMENT

Treatment of this hypersensitivity disorder, which characteristically fails to respond to antibiotics, has been and remains the systemic administration of corticosteroids.

A number of therapeutic alternatives, including indomethacin, potassium iodide, colchicine, dapsone, chloroquine, and clofazamine, have been employed with variable success.

Potassium Iodide

Of the therapeutic alternatives, potassium iodide has been used most frequently. In one series of six patients, oral treatment with potassium iodide (900 mg per day for 2 weeks) produced rapid resolution of the lesions without scarring. In another study three patients treated with potassium iodide failed to respond. In addition, the author has seen a case of AFND in a 62-year-old female receiving potassium iodide for refractory pneumonia.

If one decides to use potassium iodide, it is important to prescribe a milligram dosage and not simply recommend "5 drops three times daily", since solution concentration and drop size can vary greatly. Iodides can cause acute allergic reactions, including urticaria-angioedema (in addition to serum sickness-like reactions), worsening of cutaneous vasculitis, periarteritis nodosa, and thrombotic thrombocytopenic purpura. Gastric intolerance, including nausea, vomiting, epigastric pain, and occasionally severe diarrhea, is seen. Symptoms of upper respiratory infection, such as sinus headache, coryza, tonsillitis, or pharyngitis can occur, creating confusion with a prodrome of another episode of AFND. Development of iododerma with acneiform lesions, and more rarely eruptive vegetative lesions similar to bromoderma, can rarely occur. Thus the usage of iodides offers an inconsistent and unsatisfactory therapeutic alternative in AFND, with positive results reported by only one group of authors.

Colchicine

Colchicine has been used in divided dosages of 1.0 to 1.5 mg per day to treat AFND, with responses reported in 2 to 5 days in five patients. In one case report colchicine was given in conjunction with systemic steroid therapy and was believed to have produced a steroid sparing effect.

Colchicine is generally well tolerated in the dosage range reported to be effective in AFND, although some patients complain of gastrointestinal cramping and soft stools. Since AFND can be associated with hematologic malignant disease (e.g., preleukemia, acute leukemia, acute myeloid leukemia, acute myelomonocytic leukemia, hairy cell leukemia, chronic lymphocytic leukemia, or chronic myeloid leukemia) and since colchicine can rarely produce hematologic toxicity (e.g., agranulocytosis, aplastic anemia, or thrombocytopenia), it may be prudent to avoid colchicine in the patient with atypical vesiculobullous or mucosal lesions and in those with relatively low white blood counts or anemia. With long term usage colchicine is also capable of inducing chromosomal abnormalities and theoretically could create difficulty in interpreting bone marrow chromosome abnormalities, which can be an early marker for AFND associated with

Sweet's Syndrome / **41**

hematologic malignant disease. Colchicine must be used with great caution in women of child bearing age and should be avoided in pregnancy, since it is a confirmed teratogen in animal studies.

A few cases of AFND have responded to dapsone and indomethacin, but treatment failures have also been reported, and the role, if any, of these drugs in treating this disease remains to be confirmed.

Steroid Therapy

Although all the aforementioned drugs offer therapeutic alternatives to systemic corticosteroid therapy, it is clear that steroid therapy is the treatment of choice for AFND. Administration of steroids in the author's opinion requires more patient education and more compulsive clinical and laboratory monitoring than any other drug prescribed by dermatologists because of the high incidence of drug induced side effects and patient anxiety over taking "steroids."

Prior to initiating systemic steroid therapy it is important to identify risk factors (Table 1), including the potential for drug interactions, contraindications, and medical problems possibly aggravated by steroids. This is best accomplished by creating a check list that can be used as a baseline and for follow-up examinations for the patient taking steroids.

Additionally, steroid side effects should be detailed for the patient. The daily dosage schedule should be clearly written out and given to the patient, who is encouraged to inform the doctor of any steroid intolerance, including relatively common complaints of insomnia, mood changes, hyperhidrosis, and increased appetite, and warned to call immediately should any symptoms or signs of glucose intolerance develop.

A clinical history emphasizing any family and personal history of diabetes, tuberculosis, or hypertension is taken. A physical examination (including baseline weight and blood pressure) is performed. Baseline laboratory data including CBC and fasting SMA-12 and electrolyte levels are also recommended. Follow-up glucose electrolyte determinations are advisable in selected cases.

Therapy for the severely ill patient with AFND is initiated in the hospital with methylprednisolone sodium succinate (Solu-Medrol), 60 to 100 mg per day in two divided doses (every 12 hours). The response is dramatic, with

TABLE 1 Steroid Risk Factors

Drug interactions

  Diphenylhydantoin: reduced steroid effect
  Phenobarbital: reduced steroid effect
  Rifampin: reduced steroid effect
  Estrogen: enhanced steroid effect
  Oral doses of antidiabetic drugs: reduced efficacy of
    hypoglycemic agent
  Diuretics: steroid aggravation of potassium loss due to direct
    intrarenal kaliuric effect and antianabolic tissue effect
  Nonsteroidal anti-inflammatory drugs: synergistic ulcerogenic
    effect on gastric mucosa

Potential steroid aggravated diseases

  Hypertension (especially with proteinuria)
  Diabetes mellitus
  Peptic ulcer
  Tuberculosis
  Peptic ulcer disease
  Glaucoma

marked lessening of symptoms within 12 hours. Most cases of AFND, however, can be managed on an outpatient basis with oral steroid therapy in the form of prednisone, 40 to 60 mg per day in divided dosages for 1 to 3 days and then as a single morning dose, tapering by 5 mg every 3 to 5 days. Disease flare-ups, seen in about 30 percent of the patients, can be managed by doubling the morning prednisone dosage and resuming the tapering. Subsequent exacerbations are best managed, in the author's experience, with an 8 to 10 day course of oral doses of prednisone, 40 to 60 mg per day.

After administration and cessation of systemic corticosteroid therapy in dosages equivalent to those of prednisone, 20 to 30 mg per day, for 4 weeks or longer, it is prudent to advise the patient to carry a card in his wallet or to wear a bracelet detailing his steroid history for 1 year after cessation of therapy so that steroid cover can be provided in cases of severe stress such as major trauma or surgery. Although documented cases of addisonian crisis after steroid withdrawal are rare, it is advisable to inform the patient to report any symptoms of postural hypotension, easy fatigability, mental depression, or severe prostration during mild illnesses such as the common cold. A short ACTH stimulation test in this setting can document hypothalamic-pituitary axis suppression and the need for replacement steroid therapy.

SARCOIDOSIS

JEFFREY P. CALLEN, M.D.

Sarcoidosis is a multisystem granulomatous disorder of unknown etiology that most commonly affects the lymph nodes, lungs, skin, eyes, and reticuloendothelial system. Multiple manifestations of sarcoidosis can be present, but in this section we will discuss the therapy of only the cutaneous, pulmonary, metabolic, and ophthalmologic manifestations.

Cutaneous manifestations of sarcoidosis can be "specific" or "nonspecific." This separation of the cutaneous disease refers to the histopathologic characterization of the skin lesions. "Specific" lesions are histopathologically represented by the noncaseating granuloma, whereas the "nonspecific" lesion is usually a reactive dermatosis, most commonly erythema nodosum.

An acute self-limited process characterized by erythema nodosum and bilateral hilar lymphadenopathy, anterior uveitis, and arthritis is a common presentation of sarcoidosis. This syndrome, known as Lofgren's syndrome, is a process that in over 90 percent of the cases does not progress to chronic sarcoidosis. Thus, no treatment beyond symptomatic relief is necessary.

Cutaneous lesions, which are histopathologically represented by the noncaseating granuloma, are not necessarily diagnostic of sarcoidosis. The noncaseating granuloma can occur with other disorders. However, the lesions seen in sarcoidosis are generally clinically manifested by papules, plaques, or nodules. The papules can appear on any surface of the body and are fleshcolored, violaceous, erythematous, or hyperpigmented. Occasionally the papular lesions can become annular as they enlarge and then can clinically resemble granuloma annulare. When these small papular lesions resolve, scarring is uncommon, but pigmentary changes may occur.

Another form of cutaneous sarcoidosis is represented by persistent psoriasiform plaques. These may occur as violaceous plaques on the face with telangiectasias and resolve with scarring ("lupus pernio of Besnier"). On other surfaces sarcoid plaques with prominent telangiectasias have been termed "angiolupoid sarcoidosis." Lesions that occur surrounding the nostrils or mouth may be part of a complex of sarcoidosis involving the upper respiratory tract (SURT). SURT has been associated frequently with chronic pulmonary disease, uveitis, and bone lesions. Nodular lesions can also occur. An unusual variant of nodular lesions is a subcutaneous lesion known as "Darier-Roussy sarcoidosis." Other skin lesions that can be representative of sarcoidosis include lesions within scars, ulcerative plaques, exfoliative erythroderma, scarring alopecia, and ichthyosiform lesions. Thus many varied cutaneous lesions can be found on histopathologic examination to be represented by the noncaseating sarcoidal granuloma.

Attempts to correlate cutaneous involvement with systemic disease have led to varied results. I find that in a dermatologic practice the only clear-cut correlation is that of erythema nodosum with acute, benign, self-limited systemic sarcoidosis. Most patients (but not all) with plaques around the nostrils who have SURT and patients with lupus pernio tend to have sarcoidal parenchymal lung involvement. However, with the remaining lesions a correlation with organ involvement and severity of disease is not possible. It is important therapeutically to take into consideration the presence or absence of and type of systemic involvement.

Pulmonary disease probably occurs in all patients with sarcoidosis if extensively searched for. Changes in T and B cells can be found in the bronchial washings. Patients with normal chest roentgenographic findings may have parenchymal sarcoidal granulomas revealed on transbronchial biopsy. However, the lung lesions become clinically important only if gas exchange is affected. Therefore, all patients should undergo pulmonary function testing, including diffusion studies. There is an imperfect correlation of pulmonary function test results with the results of chest roentgenography and the prognosis can be predicted by combining these bits of information. Furthermore, the pulmonary disease may be classified by roentgenographic findings as grade 0 (no changes), grade I (hilar adenopathy), grade II (hilar adenopathy and parenychmal disease), or grade III (interstitial fibrosis without adenopathy).

Ophthalmologic involvement occurs in at least 20 percent of patients and has a myriad of manifestations. The most common finding is acute or chronic anterior uveitis. If left untreated, this involvement can result in blindness. Another important feature of eye disease is the correlation of retinal involvement of posterior uveitis with disease in the central nervous system.

Many other manifestations can occur in sarcoidosis. Hypercalcemia can be a significant problem, resulting in death or renal calculi if left untreated. Sarcoidal granulomas can infiltrate any organ or tissue. Central nervous system disease and cardiac disease may be life threatening, whereas hepatic, splenic, adrenal, or testicular infiltration may be functionally unimportant.

DIAGNOSIS AND DIFFERENTIAL DIAGNOSIS

Sarcoidosis is a diagnosis of exclusion. It can be suspected in the setting of compatible clinical, roentgenographic, and laboratory test abnormalities. Histopathologic findings, although helpful in ruling out some disorders, are likewise not diagnostic. However, the presence of noncaseating granulomas in multiple tissues, when infections and other causes of granulomatous inflammation are ruled out, is confirmatory.

Cutaneous disease most closely resembles a foreign body granuloma. Thus it is most important that appropriate testing, including polarized microscopy, be used to rule out this disorder. Other abnormalities such as a positive Kveim test or an elevated serum angiotensin-1 converting enzyme (SACE) level may also be helpful in the diagnosis of a suspected case.

EVALUATION

Therapy must be based on the findings of a thorough evaluation. The indications for certain therapies, in particular, systemic corticosteroid therapy, are based on the organ system involved and the severity of disease. Thus in all patients, in addition to a complete history and physical examination, the tests listed in Table 1 should be carried out. Those that are necessary for therapeutic decisions are listed separately. The SACE level is included among these, because it may be useful in following the response to therapy. However, an abnormal SACE level is not an indication for therapy.

PATIENT MANAGEMENT

Therapy for the patient with sarcoidosis must be individualized and is based on symptoms or system involvement. Few generalizations can be made that would apply to all patients with sarcoidosis. However, in general, two observations are possible: in most patients acute sarcoidosis resolves spontaneously, and chronic sarcoidosis may be mild or may be progressive.

Acute cutaneous sarcoidosis, represented by erythema nodosum, bilateral hilar lymphadenopathy, anterior uveitis, or arthritis, resolves spontaneously in 95 percent of the patients. Symptomatic therapy with mild nonsteroidal anti-inflammatory drugs may be used for arthritis or erythema nodosum. Indomethacin, 25 mg three to four times daily, is usually effective. Uveitis is treated topically with corticosteroid drops or intraocular injections. Systemic corticosteroid therapy is rarely necessary for acute sarcoidosis.

Cutaneous lesions in chronic sarcoidosis tend to be persistent and can lead to scarring. Lesions of lupus pernio and angiolupoid sarcoidosis should be treated more aggressively than papular lesions. Rarely has topical corticosteroid therapy been effective in an outpatient setting for my patients. Perhaps some of the newer more potent drugs like clobetasol will be more effective. The problem lies in expense, fewer applications than the number recommended, and poor penetration of the drug. The need for

the drug is in the dermis, but epidermal atrophy may limit the use of the more potent drugs.

The intralesional administration of corticosteroids can be helpful in disease control. I use triamcinolone acetonide, 3 to 4 mg per milliliter, and inject minute amounts into the involved dermal lesions. This is repeated every 3 to 4 weeks until resolution occurs. In patients with persistent skin lesions, I then add oral doses of hydroxychloroquine sulfate given in a dosage of 200 to 400 mg per day, depending on the patient's weight. In open clinical trials I have observed a positive response in 75 percent of the patients, and in 50 percent there has been total control of the lesions. The dosage is then reduced to the lowest tolerable level needed for control of the disease. However, I have observed the development of systemic disease in patients taking hydroxychloroquine.

When these drugs fail, one needs to decide whether systemic corticosteroid therapy or an immunosuppressive-cytotoxic drug is necessary. Disfiguring skin lesions are included in most lists as a relative indication for systemic corticosteroid therapy. If the patient has any other indication, this drug should be used. I prefer oral doses of prednisone and for skin lesions begin with a dosage of 20 mg on alternate days. The dosage can be raised or lowered depending upon the response. Immunosuppressive-cytotoxic drugs include chlorambucil (2 to 4 mg per day orally) or oral or intramuscular doses of methotrexate (7.5 to 25 mg per week). Anecdotal reports of success have been published for both these drugs, but I have not had the need to use them in any of my patients. Lastly, oral treatment with isotretinoin has been used successfully in an occasional patient. I have not had the opportunity or the need to use this drug.

Systemic manifestations of sarcoidosis should be managed by an experienced specialist. However, often the patient with systemic disease has cutaneous disease also; thus a knowledge of systemic disease therapy is of importance for the dermatologist. The mainstay of treatment continues to be the use of systemically administered corticosteroids. Table 2 lists the current indications for corticosteroids.

TABLE 1   Evaluation of the Patient with Sarcoidosis

Tests necessary for therapeutic decisions

Cutaneous examination
Ophthalmologic examination
Calcium levels (serum and urine)
Electrocardiogram
Chest film
Pulmonary function studies (including diffusion studies)
Bone films
Serum angiotensin-1 converting enzyme level

Tests in standard evaluation (these do not alter therapy)

Protein electrophoresis
Liver function tests
Skin tests (delayed type hypersensitivity)

TABLE 2   Indications for Systemic Corticosteroid Therapy in Sarcoidosis

Absolute indications

Intrinsic ocular disease
Neuropsychiatric sarcoidosis
Cardiac involvement with functional impairment or severe conduction defects
Hypercalcemia
Hypersplenism
Severe pulmonary disease with progressive functional disability

Relative indications

Disfiguring cutaneous lesions
Mild pulmonary disease
Bone or joint disease
Mucosal lesions
Persistent lymphadenopathy
Fever

There is still some controversy relating to the role of corticosteroids in pulmonary sarcoidosis. A classic well controlled study in the 1970s failed to demonstrate benefits from corticosteroids on the long term pulmonary function in the patient with sarcoid. However, several subsequent studies have demonstrated possible benefits, such as lack of progressive deterioration of pulmonary function test results. There is still a need for a long term, well controlled study of this problem. When corticosteroids are given for pulmonary disease, the recommended oral dosage of prednisone is at least 40 mg daily (or equivalent). Although alternate day corticosteroid therapy is safer, it also appears to lack the benefits possibly seen with daily corticosteroid therapy. Immunosuppressive and antimalarial drugs have also been used, with mixed results.

About one third of my patients with cutaneous sarcoidosis have ocular disease. This is managed with an experienced ophthalmologist. The medication usually used is a corticosteroid, which may be given by topical eyedrop, local injection, or oral administration. One potential complication is my therapy of the skin lesions with Plaquenil (hydroxychloroquine), which possibly has ophthalmic toxicity. This has not been a problem in my patients. Ocular sarcoid and antimalarial retinopathies have differing pathogenetic mechanisms and different clinical manifestations; they generally can be distinguished and managed appropriately.

PYODERMA GANGRENOSUM

THOMAS T. PROVOST, M.D.

Pyoderma gangrenosum is an uncommon, highly destructive, inflammatory skin disease characterized by single or multiple skin ulcerations, which can occur at any age. These skin ulcers generally arise as painful purplish papulonodules, which subsequently develop into pustules. The pustule breaks down and extends centrifugally over a period of a few days to weeks, producing a large necrotic ulceration (5 to 10 cm in diameter) characterized by a distinctive raised, purplish, undermined border. Surrounding this border is a halo of erythema. The ulcers are generally very painful and deep, extending through the subcutaneous tissue. The ulcers have a boggy necrotic base and may discharge a purulent or hemorrhagic exudate. Pressure on the purplish border may release pus into the ulcer or through tiny sinus tracks. The base of the ulcer is generally covered with necrotic debris and may be studded with small abscesses. Irregular granulation is commonly seen. Healing generally occurs spontaneously, producing a thin atrophic, generally cribriform scar.

These lesions can occur anywhere on the body but most commonly the abdomen and legs. Pathergy (cutaneous trauma, e.g., venisection site, producing a new lesion) is seen in approximately 20 percent of the patients.

The etiology of pyoderma gangrenosum is unknown, although recent data indicate that vasculitis (perhaps immune complex mediated) may play a pathologic role. Research during the past 50 years has established beyond doubt that the lesions are not induced by an infectious disease process.

Immunologic abnormalities have been variably described. These consist of cutaneous anergy in response to a battery of skin tests (suggesting a defect in recall or a secondary immune mediated response) and inability to be sensitized by dinitrochlorobenzene (suggesting an inability to mount a primary immune response). Other studies have demonstrated defects in lymphokine production. Abnormalities in leukocyte phagocytosis, random migration, and chemotaxis have also been described, and in one isolated report defects in monocyte chemotaxis and phagocytosis were observed.

The histopathologic features are nondiagnostic. Biopsy specimens from the ulcers generally demonstrate edema, neutrophilic infiltrates, thrombosis of small and medium sized vessels, together with hemorrhage and necrosis. Recently investigators have subjected the periphery of the lesions to biopsy examination, and some have described fibrinoid necrosis with leukocytoclasis. Other investigators have demonstrated the deposition of immunoreactants (IgM, C_3, and fibrin) in the papillary and dermal blood vessels on the periphery of pyoderma gangrenosum lesions.

Pyoderma gangrenosum has been associated with ulcerative colitis, Crohn's disease, seropositive and seronegative rheumatoid arthritis, chronic active hepatitis, and a variety of hematologic disorders, including paraproteinemia, myeloma, and leukemia. It must be emphasized that in this author's experience most cases of pyoderma gangrenosum have occurred without an associated systemic disease. The original description reported that approximately 80 percent of the patients with pyoderma gangrenosum had ulcerative colitis. Indeed subsequent reports have indicated that 30 to 60 percent of the patients with pyoderma gangrenosum have underlying ulcerative colitis. There seems to be a gross correlation between activity of the ulcer and bowel disease activity. In general, the symptoms of ulcerative colitis precede pyoderma gangrenosum, although pyoderma gangrenosum can exist in the presence of subclinical ulcerative colitis. Other studies indicate that 2 to 5 percent of the patients with ulcerative colitis subsequently develop pyoderma gangrenosum.

In addition to its association with ulcerative colitis, pyoderma gangrenosum has been associated with Crohn's disease. One study indicated that 20 percent of the patients with pyoderma gangrenosum had Crohn's disease. Only 1.2 percent of the patients with Crohn's disease have been shown to develop pyoderma gangrenosum.

Other studies have shown that pyoderma gangrenosum is found in association with rheumatoid arthritis. One study indicated that as many as 47 percent of the cases of pyoderma gangrenosum were associated with rheumatoid arthritis.

It seems likely that these data regarding the prevalence of pyoderma gangrenosum in association with systemic disease reflect the screening bias of the referral patient population. Thus, rheumatologists see pyoderma gangrenosum in association with arthritis, gastroenterologists see it in association with chronic granulomatous disease of the bowel, and dermatologists frequently see pyoderma gangrenosum in the absence of associated systemic disease.

The differential diagnosis of pyoderma gangrenosum involves fungal infection, especially North American blastomycosis, bromoderma, atypical Mycobacterium infections, cutaneous amebiasis, malignant disease, ichthyma gangrenosum, and cutaneous vasculitis with infarction (Wegener's granulomatosis and cutaneous polyarteritis nodosa).

Because of personal experience, I recommend that all patients with pyoderma gangrenosum have a biopsy of the margin of the ulcer. The ulcer biopsy specimen should be submitted for routine pathologic examination, direct immunofluorescence examination, and *Mycobacterium*, bacterial, and fungal cultures. In addition, the patient should have a barium enema and a sigmoidoscopic examination.

TOPICAL THERAPY

The treatment of pyoderma gangrenosum must be directed at the associated disease as well as the cutaneous ulcers. The cutaneous ulcers are characteristically very painful. Therefore, topical treatment should be undertaken with the judicious use of analgesics (e.g., meperidine, 50 mg orally or intramuscularly every 6 hours). The ulcers are debrided employing aluminum subacetate, saline, or acetic acid (0.25 percent) solutions. These soaks are applied for 1 hour three to four times a day. In addition, if the patient is hospitalized or if outpatient whirlpool therapy can be provided, once or twice daily whirlpool therapy has been shown to be effective. Following the soaks or whirlpool therapy, the lesions are treated with polysporin ointment and covered with a gauze pad or telfa. As an alternative, silver sulfadiazine (Silvadene) may be applied. However, many patients complain that the Silvadene cream burns. On occasion, especially when the ulcer is exuding much material, a Vigilon dressing has been found to be effective in alleviating the pain. This dressing, however, should not be left in place for more than 18 to 24 hours because bacteria can rapidly multiply under it.

On occasion we have found that small ulcerations may respond rapidly to the intralesional subcutaneous injection of triamcinolone (10 to 20 mg per cubic centimeter). These injections are made at the periphery through the erythematous halo into the ulcer. The patient is given an analgesic 30 minutes to 1 hour before these injections. Following the healing of these lesions we have found that local support in the form of an Ace bandage or a Jobst stocking is an important adjuvant to the therapy, reducing edema and protecting the very thin scar.

Multiple lesions of large pyoderma gangrenosum lesions demand intensive systemic therapy. In our hands, the most effective systemic therapy is oral doses of prednisone, 60 to 100 mg daily. Such steroid doses generally result in rapid disappearance of the pain and surrounding erythema.

Because of the large defects produced by the ulcers, healing is slow; therefore grafting (full thickness) is often considered. We have found that once the patient has taken high doses of corticosteroids for 2 to 3 weeks and the pain and erythema have disappear from the lesions, one can safely graft the lesions without fear of inducing additional lesions (pathergy). Some plastic surgeons have found that a xenograft (pig skin) applied to the graft site results in exuberant granulation tissue and that subsequent full thickness autologous grafts have a much better take.

Other investigators have found that pulse methylprednisolone therapy (1.0 g in 150 ml of dextrose in water infused over a 1 hour period for 5 days) provides a dramatic therapeutic effect on pyoderma gangrenosum ulcers. Subsequently the patient is maintained on alternate day corticosteroid therapy (60 mg on alternate days). The course of pulse therapy is repeated at 3 to 4 week intervals if necessary. It is important to note that large doses of methylprednisolone produce changes in sodium, potassium, and calcium fluxes across the myocardium, and the patients appear to be at risk for cardiac arrythmias. Therefore, special caution should be exercised regarding the electrolyte status in patients receiving pulse methylprednisolone therapy.

In addition to steroids, which are the mainstay of treatment in pyoderma gangrenosum, dapsone, 50 to 100 mg daily, has been found to be effective in treating some patients. Prior to treating the patient with dapsone, it is important to carry out a glucose-6-phosphate-dehydrogenase determination. Sulfapyridine (2 to 4 g per day) has also been employed to treat the lesions of pyoderma gangrenosum. Because of the tendency of sulfapyridine to result in crystalluria, it is important that the patient drink copious amounts of water while taking this drug. Weekly blood counts should be obtained for at least the first 4 weeks of sulfapyridine and dapsone therapy in order to detect the presence of hemolytic anemia and, potentially, sulf- and methemoglobinemia.

Immunosuppressive drugs (azathioprine, 100 to 150 mg daily, and cyclophosphamide, 100 to 150 mg daily or 1 to 2 mg per kilogram) have also been effectively employed in treating pyoderma gangrenosum. Both these drugs can produce bone marrow suppression, and azathioprine on occasion can produce hepatitis and interstitial lung disease. Furthermore, cyclophosphamide metabolic products can produce hemorrhagic cystitis with subsequent scarring and contracture of the bladder. Thus, copius quantities of water must be taken by the patient in order to avoid this complication.

Finally, recent evidence indicates that clofazimine (Lamprene), 100 mg three times a day, is effective in treating pyoderma gangrenosum. I have not personally employed this drug in the treatment of pyoderma gangrenosum. The action of clofazimine in the treatment of this disease is unknown. Clofazimine enhances phagocytosis and the intracellular killing of bacteria by neutrophils and macrophages. Unfortunately this drug produces a reddish discoloration and xerosis of the skin.

The course of pyoderma gangrenosum is variable. The disease process, although explosive and dramatic in onset, may rapidly respond to therapy, remaining quiescent for months or years before exacerbating again. When associated with a systemic disease, pyoderma gangrenosum may parallel the systemic disease activity. In patients with pyoderma gangrenosum unassociated with a systemic disease, especially those responding to treatment, the prognosis is good, but there may be considerable scarring and disfigurement.

BULLOUS DISEASES

ERYTHEMA MULTIFORME

JOHN A. KAZMIEROWSKI, M.D.
KIRK D. WUEPPER, M.D.

Erythema multiforme (EM) is an acute self-limited inflammatory disorder of the skin and mucous membranes, with characteristic histopathologic changes, a tendency to recur, and sometimes a distinctive clinical appearance. A sizable body of evidence indicates that EM is a hypersensitivity disorder occurring in response to any one of a variety of precipitating factors, including drugs, neoplasms, and infections (especially herpes simplex and *Mycoplasma*). Both circulating immune complexes and sensitized lymphocytes have been implicated in the pathogenesis of EM.

A wide spectrum of manifestations are included in the clinical presentation of EM, and these may involve the skin alone, mucous membranes alone, or both skin and mucous membranes. Some patients present with a relatively mild disorder (EM minor) consisting of a few focally located erythematous skin lesions and mucosal inflammation. Others have severe mucocutaneous disease (EM major or Stevens-Johnson syndrome), with systemic symptoms as well as numerous inflammatory bullous and erythematous lesions on both mucosal and cutaneous surfaces. In some cases the nasal mucosa, urethra, vagina, trachea, and esophagus are involved in addition to the lips, oropharynx, and conjuctiva. The most common skin lesion is the iris or target lesion, which consists of a central violaceous or erythematous region surrounded by an erythematous and edematous ring. The necrotic areas sometimes evolve into hemorrhagic bullae. The clinical course of EM is variable, ranging from a mild acute syndrome lasting about 10 to 14 days to a severe disorder which lasts several weeks and in rare cases can be fatal.

THERAPY

The therapy of EM must take into account the clinical presentation of the patient and the severity of the disease. Although a precipitating cause cannot always be identified in cases of EM, when it can be treated or stopped, this should be done as soon as possible. Often, in mild disease with a known cause, no more therapy than removal of the initiating factor is necessary. Therefore, obvious mycoplasmal infections should be treated with erythromycin, offending drugs withdrawn, or neoplasms aggressively treated with appropriate chemotherapy or radiotherapy when these specific etiologies can be identified. In cases of EM associated with herpes simplex, prompt topical treatment of the initiating infection with antiviral drugs (e.g., acyclovir, 5 percent ointment applied 5 to 7 times per day) is recommended, but there are no specific data to suggest that this substantially alters the final course of the associated EM. Recurrent erythema multiforme associated with herpes simplex infection has been successfully treated by employing oral doses of acyclovir (200 mg five times per day for 7 to 10 days).

Oral acyclovir treatment also has been recommended prophylactically (200 mg three to five times per day) to treat frequent herpes simplex infections. This dosage should be given for no more than 4 to 6 months.

Some controversy exists about the treatment of patients with severe disease, but the literature seems to favor the use of systemic corticosteroid treatment. We use high dose corticosteroid therapy for severe disease, beginning with a single oral daily dose of 60 to 80 mg of prednisone or its equivalent, slowly tapering this dose over 2 to 4 weeks. Patients who are unable to take medications orally because of mucosal involvement can be treated with daily intravenous doses of corticosteroid preparations of similar potency and switched to an oral regimen once resolution of oral erosion begins. Intramuscular repository corticosteroid preparations are not recommended; they give the physician little control over situations in which dosage changes may be indicated, and they often do not provide a high enough steroid dose. Such side effects as fluid retention, gastrointestinal discomfort, psychiatric disturbances, muscle weakness and wasting, osteoporosis, glaucoma, and glucose intolerance must be kept in mind when treating patients with high dose corticosteroid regimens. Usually an initial favorable response can be seen after 3 to 5 days of corticosteroid therapy, but severe necrotic lesions may take weeks to resolve.

Although most patients do not require hospitalization, those with severe mucocutaneous involvement may need careful monitoring of the fluid and electrolyte balance and aggressive local care of lesions that can be provided only in a hospital setting. Occasionally secondary bacterial infection or septicemia may complicate EM, and this should be promptly and vigorously treated.

Antihistamine and antipruritic drugs may be used to treat itching in mild cases but have no effect on the long term course of the disease. Hydroxyzine hydrochloride, 25 to 50 mg orally every 6 to 8 hours, or Periactin, 4 mg orally every 6 to 8 hours may be helpful. Well established necrotic cutaneous lesions often are painful rather than itchy and are not helped by this therapy. Care must be taken to avoid the marked sedation caused by these drugs in some patients.

Local measures for cutaneous lesions are often not very effective, but bullous lesions should be treated with cleansing solutions and soaks (Burow's solution every 3 to 4 hours until drying occurs) to avoid secondary bacterial infection. If this is suspected, cultures should be taken and appropriate antibiotics started.

Oral lesions are frequently quite painful and require an aggressive treatment regimen, since secondary bacterial infection of severely damaged oral mucosa can readily occur. Hydrogen peroxide diluted 1:1 with water can be used regularly to remove necrotic material. Anesthetic drugs such as diphenhydramine elixir diluted 1:1 with water or viscous lidocaine, can help to control pain, especially when taken before meals. Bacterial superinfection should be treated with penicillin or erythromycin for 7 to 10 days, and candidal infection should be treated with nystatin, clotrimazole troches, or oral doses of ketoconazole, 200 mg per day, for 10 to 14 days.

Ophthalmic lesions require careful observation, and an ophthalmology consultation is indicated, since cicatrix formation can occur. Eye irrigation and wet compresses are sometimes indicated in severe cases, but usually topical instillation of corticosteroids is sufficient. Antibiotics are indicated when secondary infection occurs.

As already noted, there is some controversy concerning the use of corticosteroids in EM, but we believe that they are indicated early in the disease in most patients. Rarely, in patients with uncontrollable recurrent EM that is unresponsive to high dose corticosteroid therapy, we have added azathioprine, 100 mg per day, to the oral corticosteroid regimen, and results have been favorable. Caution is recommended in the long term use of corticosteroid therapy in patients with recurrent disease, especially disease associated with herpes infections. We have seen a marked increase in the frequency of herpes infection and associated EM in some patients taking corticosteroids regularly; only after the steroids were discontinued could both disorders be adequately controlled. In most patients with EM, however, short courses of corticosteroids are an important part of the therapeutic regimen.

TOXIC EPIDERMAL NECROLYSIS

SHARON R. HYMES, M.D.

The development of toxic epidermal necrolysis (TEN) is a potentially devastating medical emergency. This relatively rare syndrome is characterized by distinctive and widespread cutaneous involvement. As it evolves, many other organ systems can be affected, producing complex medical management problems. Anticipation of these problems enables the clinician to better manage the complications as they occur.

When a known precipitin initiates an acute onset of TEN, there is little difficulty with diagnosis. In contrast, some patients have a more insidious onset. Burning, itching, or skin tenderness may accompany headaches, fever, and nausea. Lethargy, malaise, and arthralgias are also common. Early cutaneous manifestations may include macular erythema, a morbilliform rash, or even annular lesions that progressively become confluent. Areas of affected skin may develop large flaccid bullae, which slough with minor trauma, resulting in widespread epidermal loss. The extension of epidermal separation with minimal trauma (Nikolsky's sign) is a nonspecific yet characteristic clinical feature. Mucous membrane involvement is also a prominent feature, and in severe cases nail matix damage creates nail dystrophy and loss. Mortality incidences of 30 to 50 percent are reported.

TEN on occasion may be confused with other dermatologic conditions. The staphylococcal scalded skin syndrome (SSSS) may present with clinically similar features but because of its significantly different etiology requires different treatment. Although SSSS is more common in the pediatric age group, age alone is not a reliable means of distinguishing it from TEN. The level of cutaneous split, determined histopathologically, is different in TEN and SSSS and accurately distinguishes these two entities. Because definitive permanent pathologic sections may take 24 to 48 hours to process, frozen sections of the blister roof or exfoliated skin may be used to immediately confirm the clinical impression. If available, this method can determine the level of epidermal split within hours. A Tzanck preparation of the denuded skin base may also be useful. Clinical impression along with immediate laboratory confirmation allows prompt initiation of treatment.

TREATMENT

Identification of the precipitating cause should, if possible, precede the initiation of specific therapy. Drug reactions remain the most commonly associated factor. Common offending drugs are antibiotics, anticonvulsants, nonsteroidal anti-inflammatory drugs, and allopurinol, but virtually any drug may be associated with TEN. Multiple drug regimens may make it difficult to incriminate a specific drug, in which case all medications should be discontinued if possible. If replacement therapy is indicated, efforts should be made to do so with chemically unrelated medication. Viral, bacterial, and fungal infections also have been associated with TEN and should be diagnosed and treated. Less common causes include neoplasms, vaccinations, and radiotherapy. In some cases the etiology cannot be identified.

The treatment of TEN with corticosteroids remains controversial. When deciding whether to treat with steroids, I consider the possible etiology of the condition, the duration of the TEN at the time of consultation, and any associated medical problems the patient might have. In most patients with TEN and a noninfectious etiology, I use high dose corticosteroid therapy early in the course. In adults the dose may range from 100 to 200 mg of prednisone or its parenteral equivalent, depending on body size and disease severity. If therapy is started late in the disease when extensive exfoliation has already developed, the risk of local bacterial superinfection, sepsis, and impaired wound healing may outweigh any potential benefit. The steroid dose is tapered when active disease extension has stopped.

Supportive therapy remains the mainstay of treatment. Patients are best managed using protective isolation in a burn unit setting if this is available. Frequent assessment of vital signs, daily weight measurement, accurate intake and output measurements, and regular monitoring of chemistry and hematology values are essentials of good management. In most patients intravenous access is needed for fluid and electrolyte replacement. Unstable patients may require central venous pressure monitoring for adequate assessment of volume status. Because of the danger of catheter induced sepsis, the strictest sterile techniques in line placement must be employed. A baseline chest x-ray view is useful for serial comparison if pulmonary problems should arise. Culturing denuded skin every 3 to 4 days makes possible both quantification and identification of potentially dangerous organisms. The patient's room temperature must be strictly controlled to compensate for the loss of epidermal barrier protection. Turning frames that allow easy nursing access with minimal trauma are also very helpful.

It is important that nurses who care for patients with TEN be educated about the fundamentals of the disease. Although these patients functionally have second degree body burns, some aspects of their care differ significantly from that of burn patients. Although the extent of a burn injury is usually known upon admission, the exfoliative process in the skin of a patient with TEN continues to evolve over time. Trauma to even mildly erythematous skin may cause further sloughing, leaving more dermis at risk of infection. Vigorous debridement by scrubbing is done in some burn patients but is unnecessary in patients with TEN. Localized debridement may be accomplished with wet sterile saline soaks alone or in combination with hexachlorophene or Burow's solution. As the epidermis becomes loose and nonviable, sterile debridement with forceps and scissors is effective. Hydrotherapy is also useful in some patients.

Once the epidermis is denuded, bacterial infection and sepsis are significant causes of death, but the topical use of antibacterial drugs may decrease the risk of infection by providing an antimicrobial barrier. Sterile soaks followed by the application of 1 percent silver sulfadiazine (Silvadene) may be used every 12 to 24 hours without a dressing. The application is painless and the incidence of allergy is low. In addition, it protects the skin from drying and contamination and reduces pain. The complications of silver sulfadiazine usage include reversible leukopenia and obscuring of the skin lesions, hindering evaluation. On occasion the drug is difficult to remove without disturbing the surrounding skin. Mafenide acetate, 10 percent cream (Sulfamylon), has been used to treat TEN, but it is usually painful when applied, inhibits epithelialization, and sometimes produces metabolic acidosis. Silver nitrate, 0.5 percent solution, has also been tried, but it obscures the skin with tissue staining and has been reported to cause electrolyte imbalance and methemoglobinemia.

In selected patients biosynthetic dressings may be successfully employed. Hydrogel formulations of water and polyethylene oxide (e.g., Vigilon) absorb wound odor and bacteria, conform to body configuration, and reduce evaporative water and protein losses. These dressings may be refrigerated for 1 hour before use to maximally relieve pain. Skin substitutes (e.g., Biobrane) may also be useful in some patients. When used on a clean based area, these dressings reduce pain and may encourage epithelial regrowth. Their lack of specific antibacterial activity may be a relative disadvantage. If infection does not intervene, skin substitutes remain in place until regrowth is complete. Once these areas are well epithelialized, bland emollients are sufficient for topical care. Systemic doses of antibiotics are added only if there is a definite source of infection. In such cases attempts are made to identify and determine specific antibiotic sensitivity.

Mucous membrane involvement contributes significantly to the morbidity of TEN. Eye involvement ultimately may culminate in keratitis, ulceration, and blindness as well with entropion, ectropion, or trichiasis. Ophthalmologic guidance should be obtained early in the course of the disease. Involvement of the mouth and lips not only is painful but also interferes with nutrition. Despite the potential complications, supplemental alimentation, either centrally or with a feeding tube, may be necessary to maintain a positive nitrogen balance. Methodical oral hygiene using foam swabs and a dilute solution of hydrogen peroxide every 2 hours allows gentle manual debridement of necrotic tissue. Frequent saline mouthwashes are also useful, as is viscous Xylocaine for pain. The mucosal involvement may extend down the gastrointestinal tract, and the subsequent sloughing of this mucosa increases the risk of bleeding and stricture formation. Since patients with TEN are already potentially at high risk for gastric bleeding from stress and high doses of corticosteroids, oral doses of antacids or H2 blocking agents are advisable. The examination of stools for occult blood should be routine in these patients. Rectal ulcerations may be treated topically with steroids and sitz baths if tolerated. Rectal strictures may become a chronic problem.

Involvement of the respiratory mucosa must be anticipated, and results in bronchitis and tracheitis. Pneumonia potentially can be caused by ciliary motility abnormalities, aspiration, or atelectasis. Every patient should be encouraged to breathe deeply and cough frequently to prevent atelectasis. In cooperative patients incentive spirometry may be helpful. Intermittent positive pressure breathing and nasotracheal suctioning are unnecessarily traumatic and should not be used unless infection is already present. Patients with pulmonary infiltrates need frequent monitoring of arterial blood gas levels, since ventilatory assistance may become necessary in severe cases.

Involvement of the genitourinary system with vaginal and urethral ulceration is often prominent. Again topical steroid therapy may be helpful. Acute tubular necrosis with subsequent renal failure sometimes occurs in association with sepsis, fluid imbalance, or glomerulonephritis. Appropriate supportive measures must be taken in such cases.

Some of the other systemic manifestations of TEN may be severe but are rather nonspecific. Hepatitis as well as leukocytosis and leukopenia may occur. Disseminated intravascular coagulation is a very serious but fortunately rare complication. Altered mental status associated with metabolic abnormalities, steroids, and burn unit confinement is not uncommonly noted. In the clinical setting of hemorrhage, fever, sepsis, and fluid imbalance, these complications may become major problems.

The management of these critically ill patients is necessarily a team effort, especially if it is to be successful. Patients with severe TEN require intensive support throughout the acute phases of the disease, and this support must continue through the chronic problems that may remain after its resolution.

STAPHYLOCOCCAL SCALDED SKIN SYNDROME

ALFRED T. LANE, M.D.

Staphylococcal scalded skin syndrome (SSSS) presents as a distinct clinical condition associated with production of a specific epidermal toxin (epidermal necrolysin, exfoliatin) by a *Staphylococcus aureus* infection. The most severe form, generalized exfoliative disease, presents with the abrupt appearance of diffuse, erythematous, tender skin, which progresses to wrinkling, flaccid bullae, and epidermal separation in sheets. The generalized scarlatiniform eruptions present with the abrupt appearance of diffuse erythematous skin, which does not exfoliate. Bullous impetigo, the mildest form, presents with flaccid bullae and erosions. SSSS most commonly occurs in children under 5 years of age and has its highest mortality when it occurs in the neonatal period. Confirmation of the diagnosis depends on the characteristic cutaneous eruptions associated with culture of epidermolytic toxin producing phage group 2 staphylococci. In addition, the diagnosis of the exfoliative form in adults requires a skin biopsy showing intraepidermal cleavage at the level of the stratum granulosum.

THERAPY IN THE NEONATE

The functionally deficient immune response of the neonate allows systemic spread of localized infection. Therefore the therapy of neonatally acquired cutaneous infections must be aggressive and closely supervised. The infant with bullous impetigo should be evaluated initially for signs of neonatal sepsis, such as vomiting, diarrhea, fever, poor feeding, lethargy, and infrequent urination. If uncertainty exists regarding the diagnosis, fluid from one of the vesicles should be Gram stained and cultured. In the nonseptic appearing infant, therapy should commence with oral antistaphylococcal antibiotic therapy (Table 1). Local

TABLE 1 Antibiotic Therapy of Staphylococcal Scalded Skin Syndrome*

Neonate	
Oral	Dicloxacillin sodium, 12.5 to 25 mg/kg/day, in four divided doses
Parenteral	Methicillin sodium, 50 to 150 mg/kg/day; exact dosage and frequency are dependent on the age of the neonate
Child or adult	
Oral	Dicloxacillin, 12.5 to 25 mg/kg/day, in four divided doses up to a maximum of 1 g/day
Parenteral	Methicillin, 100 to 150 mg/kg/day, in four divided doses up to a maximum of 4 g/day

* Another penicillinase resistant penicillin, cephalosporin, or erythromycin may be substituted, depending on the sensitivity of the organism and any history of drug allergies.

care should include warm baths to remove the crusting. The recently circumcised male or the infant with a surgical wound should be closely observed for signs of cellulitis at the surgical site. Once therapy is started, follow-up by daily examinations or daily telephone contact with the parents should be carried out until the lesions begin to resolve. Marked improvement should be noted within 2 days.

The neonate with a generalized scarlatiniform eruption, with or without exfoliation, should be hospitalized and treated aggressively. After culture specimens are obtained from the conjunctiva, pharynx, rectum, and blood, antibiotic therapy is started at the appropriate parenteral dose (see Table 1). Because of possible excessive transcutaneous fluid loss, the fluid and electrolyte balance must be closely observed by strict measurement of oral and intravenous fluid intake as well as urinary excretion. Serum electrolyte levels are determined daily. Urinary output, easily calculated by the weight difference between dry and wet diapers, should be maintained above a minimum of 30 ml per kilogram per day. Frequently applications of emollients, such as Keri lotion or Vaseline Dermatology Formula lotion, are recommended to prevent fissuring and cracking of eroded skin. Topical steroid or topical antibiotic therapy is not indicated. Gentle handling and soft bedding are necessary to protect the fragile, tender, erythematous skin. Strict isolation of the affected infant is necessary in order to prevent spread of the pathogenic organism. Culture confirmation requires several days but therapy should not be delayed pending culture results.

THERAPY IN THE INFANT OR CHILD

The older infant or child with SSSS does not have a high mortality risk but still suffers significant morbidity. The possibility of developing sepsis from localized bullous lesions is greatly decreased. Frequently the flaccid bullae are not seen by the examining physician because they are ruptured by normal activity. Residual erosions with a collarette of scale remain as secondary changes of a previous bulla. Early oral antibiotic therapy, moist compresses to remove the crust, and observation for other infected contacts are the only therapy needed.

The older infant and child with generalized exfoliative disease usually has a prodrome of purulent conjunctivitis or rhinorrhea. Subsequently malaise, fever, and irritability develop associated with facial erythema, tenderness, bullae, and erosions. Characteristically new lesions extend onto the trunk with sparing of the extremities. The infant or child with severe involvement requires hospitalization for close observation and frequent topical care. Multiple sites—nasopharynx, skin, conjunctiva, and rectum—should be cultured in order to identify the infecting organism. Early parenteral or oral therapy with antibiotics should be instituted (see Table 1). Aspirin or acetaminophen reduces the associated fever and pain. Warm, soft compresses, followed immediately by emollients, help to keep the involved area clean and more comfortable. The less severely affected child can be treated at home with oral doses of antibiotics and the frequent topical application of emollients.

THERAPY IN THE ADULT

Exfoliative SSSS is unusual in the adult and may be difficult to distinguish from toxic epidermal necrolysis with secondary infection (see chapter on *Toxic Epidermal Necrolysis*). Therapy for the adult and neonate may be similar in that both may involve underlying immune deficiency. Early intervention with frozen section skin biopsy is indicated to identify SSSS in the adult. Once cultures are obtained, intravenous antibiotic therapy is indicated. Topical skin care includes the frequent application of moisturizing emollients in addition to avoiding trauma to the skin. Because the epidermal separation is more superficial than with toxic epidermal necrolysis, silver sulfadiazine cream is not necessary. Bullous impetigo in the adult can be treated with oral doses of antibiotics and warm water compresses to remove the crust.

Although resolution of SSSS may occur as a result of toxin neutralizing antibodies, early aggressive antibiotic therapy is recommended. With a decreased number of viable organisms, less toxin is produced and the patient has fewer organisms to transmit to others. For the adult or neonate with SSSS, the potential for staphylococcal sepsis is decreased with systemic antibiotic therapy. Oral therapy can be substituted for parenteral therapy once the patient has shown significant improvement. Antibiotic therapy can usually be stopped after 7 to 14 days. Steroids, topical or systemic, are not indicated for SSSS and should not be used.

PEMPHIGUS

GRANT J. ANHALT, M.D.

There are several different clinical syndromes, all of which are called pemphigus, and all of which share common features. These syndromes are pemphigus vulgaris, pemphigus foliaceus, pemphigus vegetans, pemphigus erythematosus, and endemic Brazilian pemphigus foliaceus (fogo selvagem). Specifically these syndromes present with blisters and erosions of the skin or mucous membranes, loss of normal cell–cell adhesion in the epidermis with the development of intraepidermal acantholytic blisters, and the presence of autoantibodies of the IgG class that bind to a cell surface protein of the epidermis. It is certain that these autoantibodies cause the cellular injury in the epidermis. Both in vitro and in vivo systems have been developed to study the mechanisms by which the autoantibodies induce acantholysis. There is still debate about these mechanisms, and it has not been possible so far to develop any specific way of significantly altering acantholysis in vivo when the autoantibodies are present. This means that all current therapies ultimately succeed by reducing autoantibody production rather than by affecting the events that occur after antibody binding in the skin. For this reason the efficacious therapy of pemphigus requires treatment of the bone marrow primarily, and the skin itself only secondarily.

Prior to the development of corticosteroids the disease was considered uniformly fatal, and if a patient survived the illness, the diagnosis was in doubt. Mortality is now uncommon, but morbidity from drug therapy of the disease remains a major problem and it can be severe. In general, pemphigus vulgaris is a serious disorder and requires aggressive therapy. Pemphigus vegetans is likely a variant of pemphigus vulgaris. Pemphigus foliaceus (including fogo selvagem and pemphigus erythematosus) is a more benign and more indolent disease and can be treated much less aggressively.

PEMPHIGUS VULGARIS

The diagnosis of pemphigus vulgaris is established by obtaining a histologic specimen showing suprabasilar intraepidermal acantholysis, direct immunofluorescence showing IgG (and often C3) bound to the cell surfaces of perilesional skin or mucosa, and demonstration of pemphigus antibodies in the serum by indirect immunofluorescence. If one excludes sampling and laboratory error, in my experience all patients with pemphigus have these three diagnostic features. Therefore, if any of these features is absent, the diagnosis or the laboratory results should be questioned.

Virtually all patients with pemphigus vulgaris develop painful oral erosions prior to developing cutaneous lesions. These patients are frequently misdiagnosed as having oral aphthae or other more common diseases and are treated with topical therapy or oral corticosteroid therapy. The possibility of oral pemphigus usually is entertained when the lesions persist or recur when the oral steroid dosage is decreased or when the patient develops cutaneous lesions. It has been my impression that patients with limited oral disease respond to therapy more quickly than those who have developed extensive lesions, but this may be due to variations in the aggressiveness of the disease itself.

Acute pemphigus requires early systemic drug treatment. A favorable response to treatment is demonstrated initially by halting formation of new lesions, the disappearance of the Nikolsky sign, and finally by re-epithelialization of existing lesions. I use serum pemphigus antibody titers initially as a diagnostic tool and occasionally to help evaluate the patient's status. It is generally not helpful to carry out numerous antibody determinations when treating acute disease, for one should never treat a titer. The response of the acute disease to treatment is determined by the clinical status of the patient, and in the majority of patients, as the disease improves clinically, the antibody titers gradually fall. I do find the titers helpful in management under certain circumstances. Specifically, if a patient is under good control on a stable dose of medication and develops a minor flare of the disease, if the antibody titer remains low, I feel more confident about not altering treatment. If the antibody titer is rising, however, it may be an indication that medication changes are required.

Systemic Therapy

Corticosteroids are the drugs of first choice in all patients with pemphigus vulgaris. It previously was popular to use a regimen with an initial dosage of prednisone of 80 mg per day. If satisfactory control of the disease was not observed in about 1 week, the dosage was doubled to 160 mg per day. If necessary, after 1 week the dosage was doubled again. With this regimen patients often were exposed to dosages of prednisone in the range of 200 to 400 mg per day. In my experience the potential for life threatening complications such as sepsis increases dramatically whenever the dose exceeds 2 mg per kilogram per day; consequently I never use this regimen.

Most patients can be controlled with prednisone, 1.0 to 2.0 mg per kilogram per day in divided doses. Subsequently this may be consolidated into a single daily dose and then tapered. The tapering may be relatively rapid at first (5 to 10 mg per week) but should proceed more slowly as the dosage reaches 40 mg per day. Once this dosage is achieved, an alternate day regimen should be started. This can be done by tapering the dosage administered on every other day until the values are 40 mg and 0 mg on alternate days. The alternate day high dosage then can be tapered. The disease is apt to develop flares of activity during this period, and treatment of such relapses must be individualized. Some patients can be maintained for decades on low doses of prednisone, and alternate day therapy reduces the well known side effects of steroids dramatically.

One must be careful about possible variability of generic preparations of prednisone. If a patient is not demonstrating a uniform response to oral prednisone therapy, it may be advisable to prescribe Deltasone rather than generic prednisone to eliminate variations in bioavailability of the drug. Prednisone is the corticosteroid used most frequently in the United States for pemphigus, but in other countries oral triamcinolone therapy is used because it is believed that there are fewer long term complications with this particular formulation. I have had no experience with this drug and cannot comment on this point.

Corticosteroid "pulse therapy" has also been used in certain patients. In this regimen 1 g of methylpredniso-lone is given daily in an intravenous infusion lasting 3 hours on 5 consecutive days. This is reported to provide rapid healing of lesions. I have not used this treatment because of the risk of sepsis, sudden death due to arrhythmias in elderly or debilitated patients, and possible aseptic necrosis of the femoral heads. I find that almost all patients can be controlled with lower doses of corticosteroids used in combination with immunosuppressive drugs.

I have found it necessary to use immunosuppressive drugs in addition to prednisone in about half the cases of pemphigus vulgaris that I have treated. Immunosuppressive drugs used in the treatment of pemphigus include cyclophosphamide (Cytoxan), azathioprine (Imuran), and methotrexate. They are listed here in order of their effectiveness (in my own experience). Immunosuppressive drugs are usually started when the prednisone tapering has begun. During initial therapy with large doses of prednisone, the addition of these drugs may produce profound immunosuppression with hazardous consequences.

I have found Cytoxan to be the most efficacious immunosuppressive drug. It has a greater effect in reducing immunoglobulin synthesis than does azathioprine or methotrexate, and I have found the side effects to be reasonably predictable. Cytoxan is given in a single dose of 1 to 2 mg per kilogram daily. The major side effects are bone marrow suppression, hemorrhagic cystitis, bladder fibrosis, sterility, and an increased risk of malignant disease. Marrow suppression is expected with the use of Cytoxan, and frequently one does not observe a clinical effect until the leukocyte count has decreased. It is important to remember, however, that the effect on the white cell count is masked by high doses of prednisone, that elderly patients are more sensitive to the drug than younger patients, and that the drug appears to kill hematopoietic stem cells, so that the longer a patient is treated with the drug, the lower the dose that is required. The risk of hemorrhagic cystitis and bladder fibrosis can be reduced by insisting on an oral fluid intake of 2 liters per day. The most serious potential side effects involve malignant change. The risk that such treatment will result in the emergence of a bladder carcinoma or other malignant tumor is not known exactly, but the possibility of this effect makes one reluctant to use this drug in a young patient.

Azathioprine, an alternative immunosuppressive drug, is preferred by some physicians. It is also administered in a dosage of 1 to 2 mg per kilogram daily and can be used if cyclophosphamide does not produce satisfactory results or if urinary tract complications develop. The side effects encountered with azathioprine are compared with those of Cytoxan in the chapter on *Bullous Pemphigoid* and are not reiterated here (Table 1). Like Cytoxan, the use of azathioprine has the potential for allowing the emer-

TABLE 1 Summary of Relative Effects and Side Effects of Immunosuppressive Drugs Employed in the Treatment of Bullous Pemphigoid

	Cyclophosphamide	Azathioprine
Effects		
Lymphopenia	++	+
Mitostatic effect	+	++
Depression of primary immune response	++	++
Depression of secondary immune response	++	+
Anti-inflammatory effects	+	++
Depression of cell mediated immunity	++	+
Side effects		
Bone marrow suppression	+	+
Hepatic damage	−	+
Teratogenesis	+	+
Gastrointestinal intolerance	+	−
Infection	+	+
Hair loss	++	−
Azoospermia	++	−
Anovulation	++	−
Oral ulcers	−	−
Cystitis	++	−

gence of malignant disease, and it should be used judiciously.

Methotrexate initially was used more extensively because most dermatologists were more familiar with this drug than with either Cytoxan or Imuran, but it is not as effective as these other drugs.

The intramuscular administration of gold sodium thiomalate has also been used for both pemphigus vulgaris and pemphigus foliaceus. The mechanisms by which it works are unknown. The treatment regimen is similar to that for rheumatoid arthritis. A test dose of 5 or 10 mg is given, followed by 25 mg 1 week later. After that, 50 mg is given at 1 to 4 week intervals; a therapeutic effect usually is expected after a total dosage of 500 mg has been achieved. A complete blood count, urinalysis, and examination of the urine sediment must be done prior to each injection.

The possible side effects include a persistent and troublesome lichenoid dermatitis, acute nephritis, thrombocytopenia, and neutropenia. Nephritis usually is detected early only by an abnormal urinary sediment, often by the appearance of microscopic hematuria. Proteinuria and the nephrotic syndrome may progress even if the drug is discontinued, and rarely glomerulonephritis may occur. The probability of side effects requiring discontinuation of the drug is about one in four.

Reports in the literature indicate that chrysotherapy is of benefit in some patients, but the exact value of this treatment is unclear. I have not been convinced that it is efficacious in pemphigus vulgaris, and two of my patients have developed sudden and significant complications. One patient developed allergic pneumonitis requiring admission to intensive care for a prolonged period; a second patient developed acute nephritis and proteinuria in excess of 4 g per day that persisted for 6 months. I have not had any experience as yet with oral gold therapy, but considering the unimpressive therapeutic effects of intramuscular gold therapy, I doubt that it will be more helpful.

Plasmapheresis also has been reported to be of benefit in the disease, and there is a rational basis for its use. It is proven that the IgG autoantibodies produce the cutaneous lesions; therefore removing large amounts of IgG from the circulation should decrease the autoantibody titer and control the disease. In brief, the treatment does just that, but there are substantive problems with this treatment modality. First, removal of the circulating antibody is expensive and requires multiple high volume exchanges to adequately affect the titers. Often six to 10 exchanges (about 3 liters per exchange) are required to produce healing of lesions. In our institution the first exchange costs $1000 and subsequent exchanges cost $600 each. Second, the effect of the plasmapheresis is very temporary. Because this only removes the end product (IgG), autoantibody production continues and actually can be stimulated by the procedure. Unless there is concomitant immunosuppression, there can be a rebound flare when the exchanges are discontinued. For these reasons plasmapheresis should be used only occasionally, when it is necessary to reduce antibody levels quickly while waiting for systemic drug therapy to become effective.

Additional Therapeutic Measures

During the acute phase frequent cultures and appropriate antibiotic therapy should be employed to reduce bacterial colonization. When extensive cutaneous erosions are present, topical treatment with Domeboro compresses three times daily followed by the application of silver sulfadiazine cream (Silvadene) also helps reduce colonization of the wounds and provides some pain relief. Recently I have used semipermeable dressings (Vigilon) on weeping erosions of acute pemphigus vulgaris with surprisingly good results. The dressing provided excellent pain relief, reduced serum exudation from the lesions, and allowed temporary re-epithelialization of the wound to occur. The benefits of these dressings are temporary, for as long as the disease is active, the regenerated epithelium will peel away with every dressing change. Therefore the use of these dressings is limited to the very acute phase of the disease and provides some relief for the patient while waiting for systemic drug therapy to become effective.

It has been stated that intralesional injections of Kenalog (10 mg per milliliter) promote healing of localized lesions, especially oral lesions that may persist despite overall improvement. I have found them not to be of much benefit. Topical steroid treatment can provide limited benefit in pemphigus vulgaris. Twice daily applications of Lidex gel can help reduce the crusting of scalp lesions and benefit oral lesions to a limited extent.

PEMPHIGUS FOLIACEUS

By light microscopy pemphigus foliaceus differs from pemphigus vulgaris in that the intraepidermal blister formation is very superficial, occurring just below the stratum corneum. Clinically it can also be differentiated. Oral lesions are rarely observed, and hyperkeratotic and crusted lesions are prominent. Fogo selvagem is an epidemic form of pemphigus foliaceus that occurs mainly in central Brazil.

In general the options available for the treatment of pemphigus foliaceus are similar to those used in pemphigus vulgaris, but one is much less aggressive with drug therapy because the disease has a better prognosis than pemphigus vulgaris. Most patients can be controlled with a combination of very low oral doses of corticosteroids and potent topical steroid therapy. The use of immunosuppressive drugs is rarely required, but in the rare severe case that requires a second drug, the choice of drugs and their usefulness are similar to that outlined for pemphigus vulgaris.

DRUG INDUCED PEMPHIGUS

Cases of pemphigus have been reported to occur during treatment with several different drugs. Most commonly a clinical disease resembling pemphigus foliaceus occurs during treatment with d-penicillamine and captopril. It is important to recognize that not all patients with drug induced pemphigus have demonstrable evidence of autoantibody production. The skin biopsy shows acantholysis, but direct immunofluorescence shows only complement components in the epidermal intercellular spaces, and indirect immunofluorescence examination for circulating antibodies will be negative. In these cases it is likely that the acantholysis is due to a direct action of the drug on the epidermis. In support of this theory it has been shown that penicillamine and captopril can produce acantholysis in organ cultures of skin without the addition of human antibodies. In these cases in which autoantibody production is not demonstrable, the disease resolves over a period of 6 to 8 weeks after withdrawal of the drug. It is not necessary to treat these patients with systemic steroid therapy or other drugs, although topical application of a potent steroid such as Topicort (desoximetasone, 0.25 percent) helps reduce crusting and discomfort in the lesions.

There are cases in which patients treated with these drugs do develop autoantibodies, both present in the perilesional epidermis and circulating in the serum. The relationship of drug treatment to the development of true autoimmunity in these patients is a challenging question for investigators. These patients appear to have true pemphigus and must be treated as if they have idiopathic pemphigus foliaceus.

CICATRICIAL PEMPHIGOID

DOUGLAS A. JABS, M.D.
GRANT J. ANHALT, M.D.

Cicatricial pemphigoid, also known as benign mucous membrane pemphigoid or ocular cicatricial pemphigoid, is a chronic inflammatory disease primarily affecting the mucous membranes. The pathogenesis of this disease is presumed to be related to autoantibodies directed against an antigen of the basement membrane zone of mucous membranes and skin. These autoantibodies are thought to bind to the basement membrane zone, activate complement, and incite an inflammatory response leading to damage and scarring of involved mucous membranes.

The majority of patients affected are over 60 years of age, but younger patients, 40 to 50 years of age, are known to us. The conjunctiva, oropharynx, and nasopharynx are the areas most frequently involved, the skin being involved much less commonly. Other involved areas include the genitalia, larynx, esophagus, and rectal mucosa (Table 1). A spectrum of disease exists wherein a patient may have exclusively conjunctival disease with no other mucous membrane involvement or involvement of other mucous membranes without conjunctival disease or a mixture of both. Skin involvement is variable.

The natural history of cicatricial pemphigoid is dismal, with only one sustained spontaneous remission reported in the four largest series totaling 174 untreated patients. Blindness is the most serious consequence, developing in one third of the patients with conjunctival involvement followed for an average of 6 years. The end stage of conjunctival involvement is ankyloblepharon with complete obliteration of the conjunctival fornices, total cornification of the conjunctival mucous membrane, and a vascularized blind cornea. Less common problems include esophageal, laryngeal, or rectal strictures.

Despite the apparently similar pathogeneses of cicatricial pemphigoid and bullous pemphigoid, the clinical presentations are different. Bulla formation is rarely seen in the conjunctiva in cicatricial pemphigoid; the clinical presentation is that of conjunctival scarring. Ulcers and erosions are commonly seen in the oropharynx and nasopharynx. Patients often present with complaints of ocular irritation, epistaxis, or recurrent oral ulcers. Trauma, particularly surgical trauma, such as intraocular surgery, is sometimes the precipitating event in conjunctival disease.

At our institution all patients suspected of having cicatricial pemphigoid are evaluated jointly by an ophthalmologist and a dermatologist. A detailed history is taken, with particular attention paid to previous diseases or topical medication usage that may produce a disease that mimics cicatricial pemphigoid (Table 2). Other important medical conditions include hematologic or malignant diseases precluding the use of immunosuppressive drugs, diabetes, active peptic ulcer disease, tuberculosis, or other infections.

It is frequently not appreciated that the net result of ocular surface disease of many diverse causes can be a scarring condition similar to that of cicatricial pemphigoid. For example, severe conjunctival inflammation due to previous episodes of erythema multiforme, toxic epidermal necrolysis, and alkali burns can cause sufficient disruption of the normal surface epithelium and tear film so that chronic and progressive cicatrizing conjunctivitis can ensue. It is also important to recognize that certain topically applied medications, when used for many years, can produce toxic effects on the conjunctival epithelium. This insult to the ocular surface also can produce a chronic disease that is difficult to distinguish from idiopathic cicatricial pemphigoid. Such cases of drug induced pseudoemphigoid of the eye are well known to ophthalmologists, and this possibility must be excluded.

Patients should receive both a complete ophthalmologic examination and a dermatologic examination. The clinical hallmark of the disease in the conjunctiva is the formation of symblepharons, which are adhesions between the bulbar and palpebral conjunctiva formed by conjunctival shrinkage. Ophthalmologic examination of active pemphigoid often discloses subconjunctival erythema and may also disclose fine grayish white subconjunctival fibrosis. Examination of other mucous membranes may disclose erosions or ulcers, and occasionally cutaneous bullae may be present.

Biopsy of involved mucous membranes is then performed. When ocular involvement is present, our preference is to have the ophthalmologist perform a conjunctival biopsy. However, biopsy of the involved oropharynx or skin may be equally useful. Biopsy specimens are submitted both for routine histologic processing and for direct immunofluorescence studies. Routine histologic studies may reveal inflammation of the subepithelial structures, fibrosis, and cornification of previously noncornified epithe-

---

TABLE 1   Cutaneous and Mucous Membrane Involvement in Cicatricial Pemphigoid

Site	Frequency (%)
Conjunctiva	80
Mouth	70
Pharynx	39
Nose	37
Skin	24
Genitalia	22
Larynx	19
Esophagus	9

TABLE 2   Diseases That May Mimic Cicatricial Pemphigoid

Erythema multiforme
Toxic epidermal necrolysis
Alkali burns
Drug induced pseudopemphigoid of conjunctiva
   (from topical application of ocular medications)
      Ecothiophate iodine (phospholine)
      Pilocarpine
      Epinephrine compounds
      Idoxuridine

lium; electron microscopy may show destruction of the basement membrane zone.

Immunofluorescence studies are used to detect deposition of either immunoglobulins (primarily IgG) or the third component of complement in the basement membrane zone of the tissue. These studies are particularly helpful in distinguishing active cicatricial pemphigoid from conditions that may mimic it (pseudopemphigoid). In addition, blood is drawn for indirect immunofluorescence studies to look for circulating autoantibodies to the basement membrane zone. In contradistinction to bullous pemphigoid, in which circulating autoantibodies may be demonstrated in two thirds of the patients, circulating autoantibodies are uncommon in cicatricial pemphigoid.

Antibodies in the blood are usually detected only in patients who have active disease and mucous membrane involvement in addition to ocular disease. It is rare to detect circulating antibodies in patients with only ocular disease; hence the need for conjunctival biopsy for confirmation of the diagnosis. However, when the biopsy findings are equivocal, the diagnosis of cicatricial pemphigoid occasionally may be made on the basis of finding circulating autoantibodies.

In addition, a variety of baseline laboratory studies are performed prior to therapy, including a complete blood count, platelet count, differential white blood count, urinalysis, serum chemistries, and chest x-ray examination.

THERAPY

Various forms of therapy have been used, often with limited success. These have included the topical application of corticosteroids, high oral doses of corticosteroids, dapsone (diaminodiphenylsulfone), and immunosuppressive drugs. Topical corticosteroid therapy is ineffective. Systemic corticosteroid therapy may suppress the disease inflammation, but high dosages (1 mg per kilogram per day) are needed, and the disease activity often recurs with even minimal dosage reduction. The side effects of systemic doses of corticosteroids preclude their usage at this dosage level for prolonged periods. Diaminodiphenylsulfone (dapsone), in a dosage of 100 mg per day, has also been reported to suppress disease activity. However, in our experience dapsone exerts only minimal control of the disease process, and ocular pemphigoid has always recurred when the diaminodiphenylsulfone was discontinued.

The most successful form of therapy to date appears to be the use of immunosuppressive drugs, either alone or in combination with systemic corticosteroid therapy. Cyclophosphamide (Cytoxan), at a dosage of 1 to 2 mg per kilogram per day, appears to be highly effective for controlling the disease activity. Azathioprine (Imuran) appears to be less effective than cyclophosphamide in suppressing the activity of the disease, but may be used to maintain a remission once attained. Therefore, our prefer-

ence has been to use cyclophosphamide, 1 mg per kilogram per day, and prednisone, 1 mg per kilogram per day, as initial therapy for cicatricial pemphigoid. Should there be a contraindication to the use of prednisone, this drug may be omitted, but control of the disease will be slower. Patients are treated with this regimen for 1 month, and the disease activity is reevaluated clinically. Should the disease continue to be active with this treatment, the dosage of cyclophosphamide is increased in 25 mg increments monthly as tolerated. The goal of therapy is complete suppression of the active inflammation in the conjunctiva and the erosive disease in the other mucous membranes.

After 1 month of the initial regimen, the systemic corticosteroid dosage is tapered. We generally taper rapidly to 40 mg of prednisone every morning and then to 40 mg every other morning over 1 month. Subsequently the every other day corticosteroid dosages are tapered and discontinued over 1 to 2 months. Once the disease is quiescent, cyclophosphamide is continued for 1 year. Therefore a total course of cyclophosphamide therapy of 18 months is usually required. This form of therapy holds the promise of a sustained remission without further drug therapy, and it is our practice to taper the dosage and discontinue the cyclophosphamide after the disease has been in remission for 1 year.

The side effects of cyclophosphamide include alopecia, leukopenia, anemia, thrombocytopenia, hemorrhagic cystitis, and possibly an increased chance of malignant disease. The most common side effect is leukopenia, and patients must be monitored closely. We insist that all patients being treated with this form of therapy also have an internist, oncologist, or rheumatologist familiar with this drug and willing to participate actively in following its usage. Patients are initially monitored weekly with a complete blood count, differential, platelet count, and urinalysis. After 3 months, if the dosages of medications are stable, patients are checked every 2 weeks and later every month. The lower acceptable limit for the white blood count while immunosuppressive drugs are being given is 3,000 cells per cubic millimeter, with at least 1,500 granulocytes per cubic millimeter. Should the white count fall below 3,000 cells per cubic millimeter, the cyclophosphamide is temporarily discontinued and reinstituted at a slightly lower dosage.

The importance of concomitant adjunctive therapy by the ophthalmologist must be stressed. In this disease trichiasis is eventually present in all cases, and without adequate ablation of the lashes that constantly abrade the cornea, continued conjunctival irritation, corneal abrasion, and the potential for devastating corneal ulcerations will be present. Such complications can occur even though there is adequate medical control of the underlying disease. Aggressive removal of lashes by cryotherapy and adequate lubrication of the eye are essential.

BULLOUS PEMPHIGOID

HARISH P. PATEL, M.D.

Bullous pemphigoid is an autoimmune, inflammatory, subepidermal, blistering disease of the elderly. The blister formation in bullous pemphigoid occurs at the dermal-epidermal junction of the skin, and the individual blisters are characterized as being tense. In contradistinction to pemphigus vulgaris, the application of pressure to the blister or shearing force to the normal appearing skin does not produce extension of the existing blister or denuding of the skin.

These blisters arise in the axillary and inguinal regions and are characterized generally by the presence of significant surrounding erythema. This is a relatively benign, transient disease with low mortality, even in patients with untreated bullous pemphigoid. These patients, however, can develop widespread denuding of the skin accompanied by exudation and secondary infection.

Direct immunofluorescence examination of the skin of patients with bullous pemphigoid invariably demonstrates a linear deposition of IgG or the third component of complement along the dermal-epidermal junction of perilesional skin. In addition, other immunoglobulins are found together with both early and late components of the complement sequence—properdin, properdin factor B, and beta-1H globulin. The immunoreactants are localized to the lamina lucida of the dermal-epidermal junction of the skin. Approximately 75 to 80 percent of the patients with bullous pemphigoid demonstrate serum antibodies reactive against an antigen in the lamina lucida of the skin.

Recent in vitro studies reported by Gammon et al have shown that cryostat sections of human skin incubated in the presence of bullous pemphigoid serum, neutrophils, and a fresh source of complement bind pemphigoid antibodies and fix complement along the dermal-epidermal junction. Neutrophils are attracted to the dermal-epidermal junction and release their lysosomal enzymes, producing subepidermal separation of the epidermis from the dermis. This blister formation is similar, if not identical, to the blister formation of bullous pemphigoid.

Additional in vivo studies carried out in the rabbit cornea have also demonstrated the pathogenic role of bullous pemphigoid antibodies. The intraocular injection of the bullous pemphigoid sera results in deposition of human IgG and complement along the basement membrane zone separating the rabbit cornea from the stroma. Polymorphonuclear leukocytes attach to the epithelial-stromal junction, and a subepithelial blister identical to that seen in bullous pemphigoid occurs.

Clinical studies have also demonstrated that the bullous pemphigoid disease process almost always occurs in the presence of IgG or C3 deposition along the skin basement membrane zone. Furthermore, with successful treatment of the clinical disease, the pemphigoid antibody disappears from both the serum and the skin of the affected patient. With relapse of clinical disease activity there is a reappearance of the bullous pemphigoid antibody in the serum and the appearance of linear C3 basement membrane zone deposits.

These findings strongly suggest a cause and effect relationship between the bullous pemphigoid antibody and the bullous pemphigoid disease process. These studies also strongly support the hypothesis that the bullous pemphigoid antibody mediates the development of the characteristic blistering skin disease, at least in part, by the activation of the complement sequence. The aforementioned clinical and laboratory studies form the rationale for our therapeutic regimen, which is designed not only to eradicate the clinical disease but also to eliminate the bullous pemphigoid antibody.

The majority of the patients with bullous pemphigoid go into complete clinical remission following successful therapy. In addition, the bullous pemphigoid antibody disappears from the serum and, finally, from the skin of these patients. Once the pemphigoid antibody disappears from both the skin and the serum, all therapy can be gradually tapered completely. The majority of the patients with bullous pemphigoid need treatment for 4 to 6 months. Most remain in complete serologic and clinical remission, off all therapy. Recurrences are seen in approximately 15 to 20 percent of the patients.

TOPICAL THERAPY

Isolated bullous pemphigoid, generally localized to the lower extremities, may respond to saline or aluminum subacetate wet dressings and the frequent topical application of a potent fluorinated steroid (e.g., triamcinolone, 0.1 percent four to six times per day).

SYSTEMIC THERAPY

The mainstay of therapy for bullous pemphigoid is the parenteral administration of steroids. Forty to 60 mg of prednisone daily is generally an adequate oral dosage for the treatment of the majority of the patients with bullous pemphigoid. With this dosage of corticosteroids, the individual pemphigoid blisters generally heal within a 2 to 3 week period, and new blister formation ceases within approximately 3 weeks.

Immunosuppressants (azathioprine, 100 mg per day, and cyclophosphamide, 100 mg per day) alone or in combination with steroids may be used to suppress the blistering disease.

Prior to the institution of immunosuppressive or steroid therapy, a careful review of the patient's history is conducted to evaluate for a history of duodenal ulcer, diabetes, or exposure to tuberculosis. In addition to a routine CBC and differential counts and urinalysis, a chest roentgenogram is obtained. If evidence of tuberculosis is found, an infectious disease consultation is obtained. Generally, if there is a history of tuberculosis, the patient is treated with isoniazid, 300 mg per day, as long as he is receiving steroid or immunosuppressive therapy.

The immunosuppressive drugs are generally detoxified in the liver and the kidney; the function of these organs is evaluated by appropriate blood chemistry tests prior to the initiation of immunosuppressive therapy. In addition, potential bone marrow toxicity is monitored weekly with a complete blood count, including a platelet estimate during the first month of therapy and every 2 weeks thereafter (Table 1).

Clinically the combination of these drugs is thought to result in an additive therapeutic effect minimizing side effects of both the steroids and the immunosuppressive drug.

Azathioprine, 100 to 150 mg per day, appears to be an especially effective drug to be employed together with corticosteroids in the treatment of bullous pemphigoid. The combination of these drugs, i.e., prednisone, 20 to 30 mg per day, and azathioprine, 100 to 150 mg per day, is given until the patient ceases to demonstrate new blister formation and previous blisters heal. Following the disappearance of the bullous pemphigoid antibody from the serum, the presence of bullous pemphigoid antibody in the skin is determined by direct immunofluorescence examination of a skin biopsy specimen. If the bullous pemphigoid antibody is not detected, all therapy is gradually tapered completely. (Prednisone is completely tapered at a rate of 2.5 mg per week. Then azathioprine is tapered over a 1 to 2 month period after the steroids have been discontinued.) The patients are then examined for disease recurrence, clinically and serologically, every 3 to 4 months.

Dapsone (diaminodiphenylsulfone) alone, 100 mg per day, or in combination with steroids has been noted by some investigators to be of benefit in the treatment of bullous pemphigoid and its variant, benign mucous membrane pemphigoid. This, however, must be confirmed; its value in these two conditions appears to be marginal.

Before employing diaminodiphenylsulfone, a glucose-6-phosphate determination should be done with the patient's red blood cells. Older red blood cells, normally deficient in glucose-6-phosphate, hemolyze in the presence of diaminodiphenylsulfone. The presence of a deficiency in all red blood cells during sulfone therapy results in pronounced hemolytic anemia. Methemoglobinemia and sulfhemoglobinemia are also infrequent

TABLE 1 Summary of Relative Effects and Side Effects of Immunosuppressive Drugs Employed in the Treatment of Bullous Pemphigoid

	Cyclophosphamide	Azathioprine
Effects		
Lymphopenia	++	+
Mitostatic effect	+	++
Depression of primary immune response	++	++
Depression of secondary immune response	++	+
Anti-inflammatory effects	+	++
Depression of cell mediated immunity	++	+
Side effects		
Bone marrow suppression	+	+
Hepatic damage	−	+
Teratogenesis	+	+
Gastrointestinal intolerance	+	−
Infection	+	+
Hair loss	++	−
Azoospermia	++	−
Anovulation	++	−
Oral ulcers	−	−
Cystitis	++	−

complications of sulfone therapy.

The mechanism of action of dapsone is unknown. Some evidence indicates that the sulfones interfere with the leukocyte myeloperoxidase system. Whether this mechanism is responsible for the mild anti-inflammatory effect of diaminodiphenylsulfones is unknown.

The major aim of present day therapy of bullous pemphigoid is to design therapeutic regimens that not only control the disease but also minimize the substantial morbidity and mortality potential related to the drug therapy. The combination of low doses of steroids with an immunosuppressive drug has been a successful form of treatment for this bullous disease. In addition, determination of the autoantibody disappearance in this disease has prevented needless maintenance therapy and minimized the morbidity of steroid and immunosuppressive therapy.

CHRONIC BULLOUS DERMATOSIS OF CHILDHOOD

JOHN J. ZONE, M.D.

Chronic bullous disease of childhood (CBDC) has been referred to by some as IgA linear dermatosis of childhood and may be regarded as a counterpart of IgA linear dermatosis of adults. The practical distinction between the two disorders at this time is the age of onset, although some differences do exist. CBDC is an idiopathic, self-limited, nonhereditary, blistering disease, which primarily affects children of preschool age. The course of the disease is characterized by waxing and waning of clinical activity for a period of 2 to 6 years, at which time spontaneous remission is the rule. The disorder does not persist into puberty and is seldom associated with serious systemic complications. Recent clinical and immunopathologic studies have served to differentiate CBDC from other subepidermal blistering diseases, including classic dermatitis herpetiformis of childhood, bullous pemphigoid of childhood, and childhood erythema multiforme.

Clinically CBDC is characterized by pruritus, which may vary from minimal to severe. The eruption is usually focused in flexural areas, particularly the lower trunk, thighs, and groin, but lesions also may occur in the central facial area. Grouping of lesions is common, with arcuate and annular vesicles frequently arising on an erythematous base. Primary lesions consist of tense vesicles and bullae filled with clear or occasionally hemorrhagic fluid. Some lesions may consist of erythematous plaques alone. Secondary excoriation with crusting is common. Patients are usually in good health with no associated congenital or systemic disease.

The histopathology of CBDC is not unique and may be difficult to distinguish from classic childhood dermatitis herpetiformis (granular IgA disease) and childhood bullous pemphigoid. CBDC is characterized by subepidermal bulla formation with infiltration by neutrophils or eosinophils. The histopathologic picture therefore can be readily confused with either classic dermatitis herpetiformis or childhood bullous pemphigoid.

Immunopathology has served to define more sharply the blistering diseases of childhood. Classic dermatitis herpetiformis is now confirmed immunopathologically by the presence of granular IgA deposition in dermal papillary tips in biopsy specimens of perilesional skin. Childhood bullous pemphigoid is characterized by the linear deposition of IgG and complement components in a tubular fashion along the basement membrane. Pemphigus vulgaris characteristically demonstrates intercellular deposition of IgG within the epidermis. Although initial reports showed no immunopathologic changes, most authorities agree that testing with monospecific antibodies reveals linear IgA deposition along the basement membrane in the majority of cases of chronic bullous disease of childhood. This finding is of sufficient value to warrant a repeat biopsy of fresh perilesional tissue if the initial specimen is negative and routine histopathologic study reveals a subepidermal blistering disorder.

Some cases of subepidermal blistering disease in children may show, in addition to linear IgA deposition, a similar, less distinct deposition of IgG along the basement membrane. Such patients have been said to show a clinical picture leaning toward that of bullous pemphigoid. From a therapeutic standpoint they are best treated in the same manner as in CBDC with linear IgA alone, although supplemental systemic therapy with steroids is more likely to be necessary. Indirect immunofluorescence may reveal circulating IgA antibasement membrane antibody in less than 50 percent of the cases of CBDC. However, the association of this antibody with disease activity is presently unknown and basing therapeutic decisions on such antibody levels is of questionable clinical value.

Childhood dermatitis herpetiformis is characterized by granular IgA deposition in dermal papillary tips and is associated with gluten sensitivity, as is the case in adult dermatitis herpetiformis. However, CBDC, unlike granular IgA dermatitis herpetiformis, does not appear to be regularly associated with gluten sensitive enteropathy. Clinical malabsorption is not a significant finding in CBDC. Small bowel biopsy findings have been reported to be normal in the small number of children with known linear IgA CBDC who have undergone this procedure. To confirm the lack of this association, it would be necessary to perform larger numbers of small bowel biopsies in children with CBDC. There does appear to be a significant association of CBDC with the HLA B8 haplotype, although no familial aggregation of cases has been reported.

Linear IgA disease in adults is defined as a subepidermal blistering disease with basement membrane deposition of IgA as the predominant immunoglobulin. Clinically patients with adult linear IgA disease are heterogeneous. Approximately half the patients have the same clinical findings as in classic dermatitis herpetiformis, the remainder having clinical findings resembling those of bullous pemphigoid. The association of adult linear IgA disease with the HLA B8 haplotype and gluten sensitive enteropathy appears to be less frequent than for classic dermatitis herpetiformis, if present at all. Lawley and co-workers found no association between adult linear IgA disease and either HLA B8 or gluten sensitive enteropathy, whereas Leonard et al found that these associations were present but weaker for linear IgA disease than for granular IgA disease. From a therapeutic standpoint, most authorities currently regard linear IgA disease in adults as a nongluten sensitive disease, although results of trials of gluten free diet therapy in such cases are lacking.

Adult linear IgA disease does have a significant association with cicatrizing conjunctivitis that is not reported in CBDC.

TREATMENT

Therapeutic Alternatives

Sulfapyridine and dapsone are considered to be the drugs of choice in the therapy of both CBDC and linear

IgA disease in adults. Systemic supplementation with steroids may be necessary in both disorders. Mild cases may be managed with antihistamines and potent fluorinated topical steroid therapy on occasion. Topical steroid application, however, generally is inadequate to control lesions, although it may provide relief of occasional lesions that develop in otherwise adequately controlled patients. This approach allows patients to treat lesions without increasing dosages of sulfapyridine, dapsone, or systemic steroid therapy.

At this time gluten free diet therapy is not recommended for patients with CBDC, since a significant association with gluten sensitivity has not been established. Likewise gluten restriction has not been recommended in linear IgA disease in adults. However, the author has seen a single case of classic linear IgA disease in which gluten sensitive enteropathy was diagnosed and eventual improvement was accomplished with gluten free diet therapy. In general, however, most authorities agree that a basis for treating linear IgA disease in adults with gluten free diet therapy has not yet been established.

Linear IgA disease in adults has been reported to respond to oral doses of colchicine in one case. One might also consider medications that have been reported to be successful in classic dermatitis herpetiformis. These include nicotinic acid, sodium chromolyn, and cholestyramine. However, there is no reported experience with medications in linear IgA disease in adults or CBDC, and such treatments should be considered as a last resort only if the preferred therapeutic approach has not been successful.

Preferred Approach

The majority of cases of CBDC respond to either sulfapyridine or dapsone therapy. It is the author's opinion that the side effects of sulfapyridine are less significant than those of dapsone, and that initial therapy with sulfapyridine is preferred. Sulfapyridine is given in an initial dosage of approximately 70 mg per kilogram per day in divided doses. Sulfapyridine does not produce significant hemolytic anemia, peripheral neuropathy, or psychosis, as have been reported with dapsone. Patients with allergic reactions to dapsone may take sulfapyridine, and vice versa. Patients taking sulfapyridine are subject to the known complications and side effects of therapy with other sulfa drugs, including nephrolithiasis.

If symptoms are initially partially controlled by sulfapyridine, the dosage is increased to allow nearly complete control of lesions. However, sulfapyridine may not completely control symptoms at any dosage level, and in such cases therapy with dapsone is necessary. Initial dapsone dosages of 1 to 2 mg per kilogram per day are given. If there is minimal or no improvement, the dosage is increased at weekly intervals until the symptoms are adequately controlled. The dosages of sulfapyridine and dapsone should never exceed 100 mg per kilogram per day and 3 to 4 mg per kilogram per day, respectively. In the author's experience dapsone or sulfapyridine is usually adequate for control, and systemic therapy with steroids is usually not necessary.

The clinical management of the therapeutic response to dapsone or sulfapyridine should stress maintenance with the smallest dosage necessary to control the disease. Occasional new lesions (one to two per week) are to be expected with an optimal dapsone dosage and are not an indication for altering the dosage. Spontaneous remission does occur, and such remissions become obvious if the suppressive dosage is minimized to allow occasional new lesions to develop. For pediatric use, sulfapyridine and dapsone tablets may be crushed and incorporated into a flavored syrup.

Side effects from dapsone can be significant and may limit therapy. These include hemolysis, which is particularly severe in patients with glucose-6-phosphate dehydrogenase deficiency, methemoglobinemia, toxic hepatitis, cholestatic jaundice, psychosis, and either motor or sensory peripheral neuropathy. Hypoalbuminemia may occur after chronic use. Carcinogenicity of dapsone has been reported in mice and rats but has not been documented in humans. Experience suggests that dapsone is safe for use in children and does not have any significant effect on growth and development. (The side effects of dapsone are discussed in further detail in the article on dermatitis herpetiformis.)

An infectious mononucleosis syndrome with fever and lymphadenopathy occurs rarely with dapsone therapy but may be severe. Death from agranulocytosis and aplastic anemia associated with the use of dapsone has been reported. Idiosyncratic cutaneous reactions that demand discontinuation of the drug include exfoliative dermatitis, erythema multiforme, erythema nodosum, and urticaria.

Severe side effects or complications from dapsone or sulfapyridine therapy are best managed by discontinuing the drug and treating with the alternative.

Recommendations for follow-up of patients taking dapsone include the following:

1. A baseline complete blood count and liver function tests should be carried out. Glucose-6-phosphate dehydrogenase levels should be determined prior to initiating therapy in Asians, blacks, and those of southern Mediterranean descent.

2. The complete blood count should be checked weekly for the first month, monthly for the next 5 months, and semiannually thereafter.

3. The chemistry profile should be checked at 6 months and then annually to monitor for possible hepatotoxicity, changes in renal function, and hypoalbuminemia.

4. Patients should be made aware of potential hemolytic anemia and a blue-gray skin discoloration associated with methemoglobulinemia in order to avoid undue alarm on the part of the patient or other physicians treating the patient.

In cases that are difficult to control it may be necessary to use corticosteroids (prednisone) in conjunction with either dapsone or sulfapyridine. The initial dosage of prednisone should be 1 mg per kilogram per day, and the dosage may be increased weekly to a level necessary to control symptoms. Such therapy should be reserved for severe cases that are incompletely responsive to dapsone or sulfapyridine, since the complications of long term systemic steroid therapy in children may be significant. However, if systemic steroid therapy is necessary, the effect on growth is likely to be minimized, since most children develop remission of CBDC before puberty.

Linear IgA disease in adults can be controlled by dapsone or sulfapyridine in about 75 percent of the cases. The remaining 25 percent require supplemental systemic prednisone therapy, as discussed for CBDC. Once again, in linear IgA disease in adults, it is recommended that the dapsone or sulfapyridine dosage be titrated to the minimal dosage required to suppress symptoms.

Since patients with adult linear IgA disease are known to have a significant incidence of cicatrizing conjunctivitis, it is advised that all such patients undergo careful eye examinations. If cicatrizing conjunctivitis is found, the patient should be followed closely in conjunction with an ophthalmologist.

Pros and Cons of Treatment

Rare patients with mild disease may elect not to undergo treatment. There seems to be little harm in this, except for discomfort and possibly an increased risk of secondary infection. However, in the majority of cases therapy is advisable to halt progression of lesions, severe pruritus, and secondary infection.

HERPES GESTATIONIS

ROBERT E. JORDON, M.D.

Herpes gestationis is an uncommon, intensely pruritic vesiculobullous disease of pregnancy and the immediate postpartum period. Although herpes gestationis may be more common than the reported incidence, the disease process is thought to occur about once in every 10,000 deliveries. The onset usually occurs in the second trimester of pregnancy, but well documented cases in the first trimester and the immediate postpartum period have also been reported. Herpes gestationis is usually self-limited, but with subsequent pregnancies bullous lesions may occur earlier and may be more severe. Estrogen or progesterone containing medications are contraindicated, as these may initiate an episode of the disease process. A high frequency of occurrence of the HLA alloantigens DR3 and DR4 suggesting a genetic predisposition has recently beeen demonstrated. The etiology remains unknown.

The clinical presentation of herpes gestationis varies. Erythematous and urticaria-like lesions, vesicles (often in an annular configuration), and large tense bullae may be clinically apparent. The abdomen, extremities, and flexural areas are common sites of involvement, but the palms, soles, chest, back, and face may also be involved. The blistering process and accompanying pruritus may be mild or severe. Although transient urticarial and vesicular lesions have been documented in some infants born of affected mothers, most infants are not affected. An increased mortality in infants born of affected mothers, however, has been documented. A relationship between disease severity and fetal complications has also been reported.

The histopathologic features of herpes gestationis are thought to be somewhat characteristic. Like other lesions of the pemphigoid group, bullous lesions are subepidermal. Necrosis of the tips of the basal cells is thought to be a histologic hallmark, but the same phenomenon may be seen in selected cases of bullous pemphigoid. By electron microscopy the earliest change appears to be vacuolar degeneration of the endoplasmic reticulum in the basal cells with destruction of plasma membranes.

Immunopathologically the hallmark of herpes gestationis is heavy deposition of C3 along the basement membrane zone of perilesional skin, often in absence of IgG. A variety of other complement components, particularly those of the alternative pathway, have also been noted at the basement membrane zone in herpes gestationis skin. Unlike bullous pemphigoid, antibasement membrane zone antibodies are detectable by indirect immunofluorescence in only 10 to 20 percent of these patients. Almost all these patients, however, have a C3 fixing factor (herpes gestationis factor), which circulates in the serum. This factor has been shown to be an avid complement fixing IgG autoantibody, which is present in low levels, thus escaping detection by routine indirect immunofluorescence methods. The immunopathogenesis of this disease process, then, is thought to be similar to that of bullous pemphigoid. Because of the similarities to bullous pemphigoid, some investigators have suggested that the term herpes gestationis be changed to pemphigoid gestationis.

TREATMENT

Treatment of herpes gestationis should not be designed to entirely suppress the disease process. Instead therapy should be directed toward suppressing the appearance of new lesions and relieving the intense pruritus. The design of therapy should also depend on the extent of the disease.

In moderate to severe cases prednisone, 20 to 40 mg per day, is often adequate to suppress new blister formation and relieve symptoms. Once new blister formation has been suppressed, the prednisone dosage may be decreased just enough to maintain control and relieve symptoms. Alternate day therapy might be more appropriate and should be attempted at this point. Immunosuppressive drugs such as azathioprine obviously are contraindicated unless used in non-nursing mothers in the postpartum period. If the disease flares in the immediate postpartum period, prednisone, 20 to 40 mg per day, should be reinstituted. A higher dosage may be instituted at this time if necessary.

Topical steroid treatment is also helpful in cases of herpes gestationis, particularly in mild cases. This should be used rather than systemic therapy in mild cases. Fluorinated corticosteroid preparations, such as triamcinolone cream, 0.1 percent, should be applied to affected areas three or four times daily. These preparations may be used with or without tap water wet dressings. As symptoms subside, applications may be decreased every few days, with the eventual topical use of less potent steroid preparations, such as hydrocortisone. Wet dressings with Burow's solution also may be used for moist weeping lesions. These should be applied for 15 to 20 minutes two to three times daily to help relieve discomfort and dry the affected areas. If pruritus is severe, Benadryl may be given orally, although other antihistamines are usually contraindicated during pregnancy.

The systemic use of corticosteroid therapy during pregnancy has been the subject of some controversy. Some studies suggest that there is increased fetal mortality in patients who receive high dose systemic corticosteroid therapy during pregnancy. In studies of patients with severe asthma who require corticosteroid therapy during pregnancy, however, an increased fetal risk does not appear to be present. Physicians, however, should use these drugs cautiously during pregnancy. Therapy in herpes gestationis needs to be designed for the control of symptoms rather than cure.

EPIDERMOLYSIS BULLOSA ACQUISITA

WRIGHT CAUGHMAN, M.D.

Whenever one assesses any therapeutic modality for any disease, valid conclusions regarding the outcome, be they positive or negative, are totally dependent upon a proper diagnosis. Although the criteria for diagnosis are well established for many disorders, those for some, such as epidermolysis bullosa acquisita (EBA), are still evolving. Although EBA has been described as a distinct entity for over 80 years, it is only over approximately the past 15 years that criteria have been more clearly defined. Moreover, although we now know much more about the pathophysiology of EBA, many questions remain. With the help of several diagnostic procedures, the diagnosis now can be made with a fair degree of confidence. Our focus in this article is primarily on therapeutic modalities, but it is essential that we review both the spectrum of clinical presentations and the diagnostic techniques available so that all clinicians who approach the question of "how" to treat this disorder can feel an appropriate level of confidence about "what" they are treating.

What we know about EBA as a clinical entity influences our approach to any patient with the disease. EBA is an acquired immunobullous blistering skin disorder that, although rare, may be more common than previously thought. Blisters and skin fragility are most frequently evident over joints and are frequently induced by mild trauma. Because of the relatively deep plane of blister formation, atrophic scarring and milia are common. Dystrophic nail changes and cicatricial alopecia may be evident as well as scarring involving the nasal, oral, ocular, and esophageal mucosa. The disease traditionally is viewed as a noninflammatory disorder, but patients may present with generalized inflammatory bullous pemphigoid-like lesions. Thus there is a spectrum of clinical presentations, and the clinical picture in any given patient may or may not change over time. In one patient extensive noninflammatory skin fragility and scarring may predominate; in another pruritic inflammatory blistering may be the cardinal feature; and in another occasional traumatic blisters may amount to no more than a sporadic nuisance. Thus, the severity and the character of the disease may vary both within and among patients followed over time, and both these parameters naturally influence therapeutic decisions.

With such diverse clinical presentations, it is easy to understand why more common diagnoses such as bullous pemphigoid, dermatitis herpetiformis, and porphyria cutanea tarda are often ruled out, even repeatedly in the same patient, before a diagnosis of EBA is seriously entertained. Indeed until recent years the diagnosis of EBA was essentially one of exclusion. There are now, however, specific tests—indirect immunofluorescence on salt-split normal human skin and immunoblotting—that can confirm the diagnosis. Both the indirect immunofluorescence and the immunoblotting tests rely upon the fact that ap-

proximately 50 percent of the patients with EBA have in their serum an antibody that binds specifically to a basement membrane zone component known as the EBA antigen. Aside from determining that the blistering disorder is subepidermal, histopathologic study of EBA may provide less specific information concerning the diagnosis than immunofluorescence studies. Indeed, on a histologic basis, EBA may be considered the great mimicker among bullous diseases, because it may reveal a picture totally compatible with dermatitis herpetiformis, linear IgA disease, bullous pemphigoid, cicatricial pemphigoid, or even porphyria cutanea tarda. Direct immunofluorescence studies distinguish porphyria cutanea tarda and dermatitis herpetiformis from EBA, and if IgA in a linear pattern is not seen, linear IgA disease may be ruled out as well. However, a pattern of linear IgG and C3 along the basement membrane zone by direct immunofluorescence and a circulating anti-basement membrane zone antibody on indirect immunofluorescence are common features of both bullous pemphigoid and EBA and less frequently of cicatricial pemphigoid. However, if the normal human skin specimen used as substrate for indirect immunofluorescence is first soaked in a 1.0 M sodium chloride solution, a microscopically detectable split occurs between the epidermis and dermis. By using this salt-spilt skin, bullous pemphigoid and EBA sera can be distinguished by their binding patterns—bullous pemphigoid sera showing binding along the roof or epidermal side of the split and EBA sera showing binding along the base or dermal side of the split. This differential binding pattern in salt-split skin is a consequence of the ultrastructural locations of the basement membrane zone antigens to which these autoantibodies are directed and also reflects the differences seen on the second test, immunoblotting. Bullous pemphigoid sera bind to a 220 kd protein, and EBA sera bind to a protein with subunit molecular weights of 290 and 145 kd. Thus although bullous pemphigoid and EBA can be strikingly similar if not indistinguishable clinically, histologically, and even by routine immunofluorescence studies, they can be distinguished by the location and nature of the proteins to which autoantibodies are directed.

Thus, coupling these immunohistologic and immunobiochemical studies with previously established features, we see that the criteria and clues for the diagnosis of EBA currently can be summarized as follows:

1. Clinical lesions of dystrophic epidermolysis bullosa with increased skin fragility, trauma induced blisters, and atrophic scarring and milia over extensor surfaces, or generalized bullae occurring over inflammatory bases with pruritus.
2. Histologically, subepidermal blister formation that may be cell poor and reminiscent of porphyria cutanea tarda, or cell rich and indistinguishable from either bullous pemphigoid, cicatricial pemphigoid, dermatitis herpetiformis, or linear IgA disease.
3. By electron microscopy, a sublamina densa split with dense amorphous deposits in the papillary dermis.
4. By direct immunofluorescence, linear IgG and C3 along the dermal-epidermal basement membrane zone.

5. By indirect immunofluorescence, circulating anti-basement membrane zone IgG antibody that binds to the dermal side of salt-split normal human skin.

6. By immunoelectron microscopy, in vivo bound and circulating anti-basement membrane zone antibodies located just below the lamina densa.

7. By immunoblotting, circulating anti-basement membrane zone antibodies directed against a unique basement membrane zone polypeptide with subunit molecular weights of 290 and 145 kd.

Thus the clinical criteria for the diagnosis of EBA remain somewhat contradictory, in that it can appear as both a noninflammatory mechanobullous disorder and an inflammatory immunobullous disorder. On the other hand, the criteria at the immunohistologic and immunobiochemical level are distinctive. However, these distinctive immunologic criteria are not all-encompassing, because there remains a large subset of patients (more than 40 percent) who by clinical, direct immunofluorescence, and electron microscopic studies have a mechano-immunobullous disorder consistent with EBA, but who have no detectable circulating anti-basement membrane zone antibody that can be used to confirm the diagnosis. There is an even smaller subset (less than 5 percent) who have clinical, histologic, and electron microscopic features consistent with a diagnosis of EBA, but who exhibit no abnormalities on immunofluorescence studies.

Another feature of EBA that is inconsistently observed is its association with numerous other autoimmune and lymphoreticular disorders—including inflammatory bowel disease, systemic lupus erythematosus, rheumatoid arthritis, diabetes mellitus, thyroiditis, cryoglobulinemia, lymphoma, and leukemia. Indeed it is in these patients that one can be paradoxically somewhat more optimistic about therapy, in that successful management of the associated disorder often is accompanied by a remission of the skin disease.

THERAPY

If one has taken the pains to establish a diagnosis of EBA as confidently as is practically possible, what then can be done therapeutically? Three arenas of therapy should be considered: systemic therapy, topical management, and consultative support. The obvious first question to be addressed is whether any trials of systemic therapy are indicated. This decision is one that requires a thorough understanding of the risks and benefits of the therapeutic options, the likelihood of favorable responses, and a careful assessment of the patient's need and appropriateness for therapy. This question should be addressed not only before any systemic therapy is entertained but also when contemplating changes in the therapeutic regimen that inherently involve changes in the risk-benefit ratio. Such decisions require thorough patient education and participation in the decision making process, with particular attention to the patient's assessment of daily activity compromise caused by the disease.

If the decision is made that systemic therapy is indicated, the character of the clinical situation and histologic findings aid the physician in choosing among the alternatives. Basically EBA that presents with inflammatory pruritic lesions and is similar clinically and histologically to other acute immunobullous diseases such as bullous pemphigoid and dermatitis herpetiformis shows some response to most drugs employed to treat these more common entities. Specifically one should employ systemic doses of corticosteroids or therapy with sulfones first. Initially prednisone at a dosage of at least 1 mg per kilogram per day, and often as much as 2 mg per kilogram per day, is required before a response, if any, can be seen. Unlike the situation in bullous pemphigoid and dermatitis herpetiformis, responses are not complete, with a total cessation of new lesions; rather the response should be judged in terms of the frequency of new lesions and the symptomatic amelioration of pruritus, if present. The steroid dosage should be tapered as expeditiously as possible with conversion to alternate day therapy an early goal of management. Skin fragility improves only in relation to fragility that occurs as a consequence of inflammation. Since EBA is a chronic disorder, commitment to corticosteroid therapy makes the long term risks of therapy significant. Although a cataloguing of those risks is unnecessary, the physician must be aware that the benefits, if any, may be minimal. EBA is traditionally considered a relatively steroid resistant disease. Thus one may tend to push the steroid dosage to the point of significant side effects without obtaining a significant response. When a significant inflammatory component is present, corticosteroids may be useful. Also, because inflammatory flares sometimes occur in some patients, briefer periods (3 to 6 weeks) of high dose steroid therapy may prove beneficial. High dose maintenance therapy should be avoided.

It is our experience that sulfones, in the form of dapsone primarily, also can be helpful in the inflammatory forms of EBA, either as the sole therapeutic drug or as an adjunct and steroid sparing drug in patients requiring prednisone as well. When it is properly monitored, the benefits of dapsone can far outweigh both the inherent risks of the therapy and the long term side effects of the moderate (0.5 mg per kilogram per day) to high dosage corticosteroid therapy that these patients may require.

Before dapsone therapy is instituted, a complete blood count, liver and renal function tests, and the glucose-6-phosphate dehydrogenase level should be checked. A patient with glucose-6-phosphate dehydrogenase deficiency may experience life threatening hemolysis if sulfones are administered. All patients taking dapsone experience some degree of hemolysis—a decrease of up to 2 g of hemoglobin initially but averaging about a 1 g decrease over time. This drop in hemoglobin is accompanied by an increase in the reticulocyte count and Heinz body formation. The hemolysis is tolerated by most patients but must be considered a potential risk in older patients and in those with anemia or cardiovascular disease.

Another pharmacologic effect of dapsone is methemoglobinemia, an effect that usually is dose dependent, rarely exceeding 12 to 15 percent of the hemoglobin level. Patients should be informed of the gray-blue cyanosis that is often seen during dapsone therapy as a consequence of methemoglobenemia. An extremely rare but potentially lethal idiosyncratic response to dapsone is agranulocytosis, which usually occurs, if at all, during the first 3 to 4 months of therapy. Thus the complete blood count should be monitored weekly or biweekly during the first 4 months and every 3 to 4 months thereafter.

If responses are seen in the form of decreases in inflammation and pruritus, the dosage should be reduced to a minimal level that remains effective. The initial dosage should be 100 mg per day, but one should not conclude that there has been a failure to respond until dosages of up to 400 mg per day have been tried for at least 2 to 3 weeks. The response is not as immediate or as complete as in dermatitis herpetiformis, but almost all patients with EBA inflammatory lesions have shown at least partial improvement with dapsone therapy. As with corticosteroids, however, dapsone has afforded no benefit in those with skin fragility problems occurring in the absence of inflammation. Side effects seen at higher dosages include headache, nausea, anorexia, fatigue, and abdominal pain. Some of these symptoms may be attributable to methemoglobinemia, but they also can be seen in patients taking dapsone without significant methemoglobin formation.

The second tier of systemic therapeutic options involves immunosuppressive and cytotoxic drugs. Although azathioprine (Imuran) and cyclophosphamide (Cytoxan) have traditionally been the mainstays of adjunctive and steroid sparing immunosuppressive therapy in the treatment of pemphigus and bullous pemphigoid, the results to date in our patients with EBA have been uniformly unimpressive. There is perhaps a key to both the heterogeneity of the laboratory findings in EBA patients and the essential pathogenesis of this disease in this failure of azathioprine and cyclophosphamide to effect a beneficial response. Both drugs are believed to exert a primary immunosuppressive effect on humoral rather than cellular immune events. Thus autoimmune disorders in which autoantibodies play a critical role in the pathogenesis, such as pemphigus and bullous pemphigoid, are more likely to exhibit a positive response to these drugs.

The role of circulating autoantibodies in the pathogenesis of EBA remains unclear, although in in vitro tests these antibodies are capable of fixing complement and promoting neutrophil attachment to the dermal-epidermal basement membrane zone. Nevertheless inflammatory and noninflammatory forms of EBA exist in which no circulating or even in vivo bound anti-basement membrane zone antibodies can be detected. Thus the primary immunologic events may be cellular and not autoantibody dependent. These cellular immune events may remain relatively unresponsive to azathioprine and cyclophosphamide. In some patients autoantibodies may occur as an epiphenomenon rather than as a pathogenetic event, and thus they are not seen in all patients with EBA.

Further support, albeit extremely limited, for a cellular rather than a humoral immunologic pathogenesis in EBA is provided by our experience with cyclosporine A in one patient. Cyclosporine A, an immunosuppressive drug, is widely used in organ transplantation therapy. Its primary immunosuppressive effect is exerted at the cellular level through alteration of T cell capacity to produce or respond to interleukin 2, an essential lymphokine in T cell activation and function. It is not a cytotoxic drug and does not cause leukopenia. Recently researchers have been studying the efficacy of cyclosporine A in experimental and clinical autoimmune disease and have encountered some significant responses, even in some diseases that have an apparent humoral immune component. However, cyclosporine A is not a panacea for autoimmune diseases and is not without significant toxic effects, the most serious of which are nephrotoxicity and hypertension. In one patient with chronic EBA and extensive inflammatory lesions who was responsive only to high dose corticosteroid and dapsone therapy, significant improvement (to the point of being nearly lesion free) was noted even at dosages as low as 0.5 mg per kilogram per day. Although therapy was suspended because of hypertension and nephrotoxic side effects, the favorable response was observed following short term reinstitution of therapy and thus provides encouraging results for pursuing this therapeutic alternative in other patients with EBA. However, it must be stressed that the use of cyclosporine A in autoimmune skin disease should be considered entirely experimental at this point. Nevertheless it is a drug with significant promise for both systemic and possibly topical therapeutic use.

Forms of EBA that are exclusively more classic in clinical manifestations (that is, noninflammatory, trauma induced blistering with increased skin fragility, atrophic scarring, and milia formation) are in our experience less amenable to therapeutic intervention. Fortunately many of these patients have disease that is limited in extent, such that, given the risks of the options discussed, systemic therapy is usually not warranted. The only systemic therapy that has been employed in these patients with any regularity is vitamin E at dosages of up to 1600 IU per day divided over four doses. Although there are reports of the efficacy of this modality in EBA, we have not been impressed that vitamin E therapy results in any dramatic decrease in blister formation or skin fragility, but no controlled trials have been performed. In patients with extensive noninflammatory EBA, there are currently no rational alternatives that have shown any significant benefit. However, if all cases of EBA are indeed immunobullous in pathogenesis, it may be that immune modulators such as cyclosporine A may prove to be useful, but recommendations concerning their appropriateness await further study.

As for topical management, efforts should be made to keep intact blisters sterile and erosions clean. Most patients with EBA report that both pain or pruritus and extension of the blister are aborted by draining the blisters with sterile precautions soon after their formation. Patients with extensive erosions and delayed healing have found nonadhesive water based gel dressings such as Vigilon or Second Skin to be soothing and protective. High and mid range topical steroid therapy may be useful for occasional and limited inflammatory lesions that "break through" maintenance systemic therapy. As always, patients with open skin lesions who are taking immunosuppressive drugs should be informed of the risks of both localized and systemic infection, and appropriate antibiotics should be given when indicated.

Obviously patients soon become aware of the activities that are most likely to lead to blister formation and learn to avoid these when possible. In the noninflammatory forms of EBA, avoidance of trauma is perhaps the best therapy currently offered. Unfortunately, when skin fragility is extreme, even the mildest of friction or trauma can lead to lesions and thus cannot be avoided. In some situations changes in vocation may be necessary, and the physician must be willing to pursue and cooperate with the appropriate support services to accomplish such changes. Other consultative services are often required in the management of EBA. Mucosal inflammation and scarring may require assessment and therapy by an otolaryngologist and an ophthalmologist, and their contributions in regard to management can be extremely helpful.

Finally, the management of EBA requires of both the physician and the patient a willingness to accept frustration and often only limited success. As should be apparent, the process of properly diagnosing EBA requires diligence and an awareness of the pitfalls that may arise. Furthermore, since there is currently no totally successful therapy, patients can be expected to become disenchanted with the physician's skills, and the physician may learn to resent a patient's failure to improve. Such situations can be minimized and possibly avoided if the physician is both supportive and honest with the patient from the outset and encourages the patient's input in management decisions. It is to be hoped that as more is learned about the pathophysiology of this disorder, more therapeutic alternatives will come to light and be of greater benefit than those currently available.

DERMATITIS HERPETIFORMIS

RUSSELL P. HALL III, M.D.

Dermatitis herpetiformis (DH) is a chronic, extremely pruritic papulovesicular disease, which generally begins in the second to fourth decade. Although periods of clinical remission occur, the disease should be considered to be lifelong and requires long-term therapy. DH is characterized clinically by very pruritic papules and vesicles, which occur in groups on extensor surfaces (elbows, knees, buttocks) and the scalp. Biopsy of an early lesion reveals a subepidermal blister with collections of neutrophils at the dermal papillary tips (papillary microabscesses). Although this histologic picture is characteristic of DH, a similar pattern can be seen in some patients with bullous pemphigoid and in those with the bullous eruption of systemic lupus erythematosus. In addition, biopsy of older vesicles or bullae in DH most often does not show the characteristic papillary microabscesses. Direct immunofluorescence of normal appearing perilesional skin reveals either granular deposits of IgA (85 percent of the patients) or a linear band of IgA at the dermal-epidermal junction (15 percent of the patients). Although the clinical and histologic presentation is, in general, identical in patients with either granular or linear deposits of IgA, the pattern of the cutaneous IgA deposits is important in planning therapy for patients with DH.

In patients with DH and granular IgA deposits there is a high prevalence of the histocompatibility antigens HLA B8 and DR3 and an associated asymptomatic gluten sensitive enteropathy. In addition, the skin disease in these patients often responds to a gluten free diet (to be discussed). By contrast, DH patients with linear IgA deposits have a normal prevalence of HLA antigens B8 and DR3 and do not appear to have associated gluten sensitive enteropathy, and there is no evidence suggesting that a gluten free diet is effective in treating the skin disease. It has been proposed that the name dermatitis herpetiformis be reserved for the disease in patients with granular IgA deposits and that those with linear IgA deposits be designated as having "linear IgA dermatosis."

THERAPY

The cornerstone of effective therapy for both DH and linear IgA dermatosis is establishment of the correct diagnosis. There should be appropriate clinical and histologic presentations and granular or linear IgA deposits should be evident on direct immunoflorescence. Most false negative results in immunofluorescence tests are a result of obtaining lesional skin for direct immunofluorescence examination. If the normal appearing perilesional skin does not reveal IgA deposits in a patient thought to have DH, direct immunofluorescence should be repeated using fresh tissue (without "transport media"), multiple sections being evaluated for IgA deposits. The clinical

response to therapy with dapsone is not a useful criterion for the diagnosis of DH owing to the numerous other conditions that also respond to dapsone.

Dapsone (diaminodiphenylsulfone) is the drug of choice for both DH patients with granular IgA deposits and those with linear IgA dermatosis. Most patients respond quickly to dapsone, noting a marked decrease in the pruritus and a lack of new lesion formation within 12 to 48 hours after starting dapsone therapy. Although some patients with linear IgA dermatosis require systemic corticosteroid therapy and dapsone to control the disease, in my experience all these patients have responded to dapsone therapy alone.

Dapsone, however, does have serious adverse hematologic effects that necessitate careful pretreatment evaluation and close follow-up. Dapsone causes dose related hemolysis, which can be severe in patients with glucose-6-phosphate dehydrogenase (G6PD) deficiency. G6PD deficiency occurs most frequently in blacks, Asians, and those of Southern Mediterranean descent, and in these individuals the G6PD level should be determined before therapy is begun. All individuals who take dapsone have a degree of hemolysis that results in a decreased hemoglobin level. This hemolysis is minimal at 25 to 50 mg of dapsone per day but can result in up to a 2 g reduction in hemoglobin at dosages of 150 to 200 mg per day. In patients who are not iron, folate, or vitamin B_{12} deficient, a compensatory reticulocytosis occurs and the hemoglobin rises nearly to pretreatment levels. Patients with cardiac or pulmonary disease should be evaluated carefully to determine that they will not be compromised by the expected drop in hemoglobin that occurs with dapsone therapy.

Methemoglobinemia also occurs during dapsone therapy in a dose related fashion. This can result in a slate blue discoloration in some patients but is generally well tolerated at the levels seen during dapsone therapy (12 percent methemoglobin or less). The patient needs to be made aware of this side effect and carry a card detailing his medications in order to avoid confusion during any possible medical emergency. Other symptoms of methemoglobinemia can include weakness, tachycardia, nausea, headache, and abdominal pain, but usually do not develop at methemoglobin levels lower than 20 percent. In patients with severe cardiopulmonary disease the effect of relatively low levels of methemoglobinemia may be more severe.

The other side effects of dapsone are either idiosyncratic or allergic and are listed in Table 1. For the most part these side effects disappear on discontinuation of the drug. Agranulocytosis has been reported in patients taking dapsone. This is a rare complication and has always occurred within the first 3 to 4 months of therapy. When agranulocytosis is recognized promptly, it appears to be reversible on withdrawal of the dapsone. Finally, although dapsone has been classified as a "weak carcinogen" in rats, evidence of carcinogenicity does not exist in humans.

The pretreatment evaluation prior to dapsone therapy should include a history and physical examination, a complete blood count with a differential, liver and renal function tests, urinalysis, and, when indicated, a G6PD level.

TABLE 1 Adverse Reactions to Dapsone

Hemolysis
Methemoglobinemia
Headache
Gastric irritation
Anorexia
Hepatitis, infectious mononucleosis-like
Cholestatic jaundice
Morbilliform eruption
Erythema nodosum
Erythema multiforme
Toxic epidermal necrolysis
Psychosis
Leukopenia
Agranulocytosis
Hypoalbuminemia
Peripheral neuropathy (most commonly
    motor)

After this complete pretreatment evaluation, patients with DH or linear IgA dermatosis should be begun on 50 to 100 mg of dapsone per day. The long half-life of dapsone allows most patients to take a single daily dose. A complete blood count with a differential should be done weekly for the first 4 to 6 weeks, then biweekly for an additional 2 to 3 months, and finally at 8 to 12 week intervals while dapsone therapy is continued. This frequent follow-up allows for the potential early detection of agranulocytosis before serious morbidity occurs and for close monitoring of the hemolysis and resultant anemia that occur with dapsone. Liver and renal function should be assessed every 4 to 6 months. Patients also should be tested for distal motor weakness or sensory deficits on follow-up visits. Most patients respond within 24 to 48 hours after the institution of dapsone therapy with a marked decrease in itching and the cessation of new lesion formation. After 1 to 2 weeks the dosage of dapsone should be adjusted to the minimal dosage required to control the patient's symptoms by changing the daily dosage by 25 to 50 mg every 1 to 2 weeks.

Most patients' symptoms can be controlled with 100 to 150 mg of dapsone per day. Patients and physicians, however, should be aware that some lesions may still occur (two to three lesions every 1 to 2 weeks) at this dosage and that this normal variation in disease activity should not lead to an increase in the dapsone dosage. When a patient experiences long periods without any active skin disease, I recommend that the dosage of dapsone be decreased slowly in order to re-establish the minimal amount needed to control symptoms. It should be emphasized to the patient that dapsone is an effective drug that is well tolerated by most patients but that it has potentially severe side effects. It is important to discuss these side effects carefully with the patient and to explain that many are directly dose related. In this way the hazards of self-medication are emphasized as is the need for close and frequent follow-up care.

Patients who are unable to tolerate dapsone can be given sulfapyridine at initial oral doses of 500 mg twice daily. Although the side effects of sulfapyridine are less severe, the drug is also less effective. Sulfapyridine cannot be taken by patients who are allergic to sulfa drugs

and must be taken with adequate fluid intake and close monitoring of renal function because renal calculi can occur. The dosage of sulfapyridine can be increased to 3 to 4 g per day, if needed, to control blistering; however, frequently even this dosage level is insufficient to control the disease.

In general, patients who are thought to be allergic to sulfapyridine can safely take dapsone and vice versa. Rare cases of cross reactivity have been reported, however, and such patients should be followed carefully when initiating therapy. Likewise the history of an allergic reaction to sulfa drugs is not thought to be an absolute contraindication to dapsone therapy, but these patients also should be observed closely for potential adverse effects.

A number of other drugs have been reported to be useful in DH. These include pyridoxine, cholestyramine, colchicine, nicotinic acid, and oral doses of antihistamines. In my experience these drugs have proven to be only minimally effective in most cases of DH. Topical steroid therapy, although not effective in controlling the eruption, occasionally is helpful in decreasing the symptoms associated with the sporadic lesions of DH that occur during therapy and perhaps may help in healing these lesions.

Since DH often affects women of child-bearing age, the question of the use of dapsone during pregnancy frequently is raised. There is little information documenting the safety of dapsone during pregnancy. It is my policy to discuss the issue with the patient at the time of the initial diagnosis and to suggest that she adhere to a gluten free diet during pregnancy (see next paragraph), which ideally should be started 6 to 12 months prior to the pregnancy. If this is not possible, the patient should be advised regarding the lack of data regarding the possible teratogenicity of dapsone. If the patient desires treatment, I favor low dose sulfapyridine (500 to 1,000 mg per day) or low dose dapsone (25 to 75 mg per day) therapy. The patient should be advised to take the minimal dose required to allow her to tolerate her symptoms. The patient's other physicians, including the pediatrician, should also be advised of the use of dapsone or sulfapyridine during the pregnancy. Finally the patient should be advised that dapsone is secreted in breast milk and can cause hemolytic anemia in the newborn and that she therefore should avoid breast feeding.

As mentioned previously, patients with DH and granular IgA deposits have an associated gluten sensitive enteropathy. This association has led to trials of a gluten free diet for control of the skin disease. It has been found by a number of investigators that patients with DH and granular IgA deposits who strictly adhere to a gluten free diet can decrease the dapsone requirement by 50 to 75 percent or more after 9 to 16 months with the diet. However, there is no evidence suggesting that a gluten free diet is of any value in the patient with linear IgA deposits (linear IgA dermatosis). The gluten free diet requires the total avoidance of all wheat containing foods for as long as 9 to 16 months before any substantial benefit to the patient can be noted. The patient should also be aware that as many as 25 to 30 percent of the cases of DH do not appear to respond to the gluten free diet and that it is currently not possible to predict who will respond to gluten restriction. It also appears that total gluten restriction is necessary for maximal benefit, even to the extent of avoiding the small amount of wheat additives found in some ice cream, sauces, and other foods. I advise my patients not to begin diets that eliminate only 50 to 75 percent of wheat protein, for in all probability this will offer little benefit. The complexity of this diet necessitates consultation with a dietitian who has been educated by dermatologists regarding DH as well as a well motivated patient. Patients should be made aware of resources available from the National Celiac-Sprue Society (5 Jeffrey Road, Wayland, MA 01778), which can help in planning and executing the gluten free diet.

MALIGNANCIES

BASAL CELL AND SQUAMOUS CELL CARCINOMA

JOHN W. SKOUGE, M.D.
THEODORE A. TROMOVITCH, M.D.

BASAL CELL CARCINOMA

Basal cell carcinoma (BCC) is the most common cancer that affects man. It is estimated that there are over 500,000 newly diagnosed cases per year in the United States.

The etiology of BCC is multifactorial. Causes include hereditary factors, radiation exposure, and certain types of skin injury. In the majority of cases BCC is associated with a long history of exposure to ultraviolet light, most often in the form of sun exposure, in a patient with a hereditarily predetermined susceptibility. Skin that always burns and never tans is at the highest risk for the development of BCC, whereas black skin only rarely develops the cancer. People with skin types in between are at intermediate risk. There are, however, certain families that seem to demonstrate a predisposition despite skin color. Certain specific hereditary diseases carry a very high risk. These include nevoid basal cell carcinoma syndrome and xeroderma pigmentosum.

Before discussing our preferred methods for treating BCC, we must consider several factors that have marked effects on recurrence incidences – tumor type, size, and location. The advantages and disadvantages of the various treatment modalities must be understood so that the most appropriate one will be chosen.

Type

There are three major types of BCC – nodular, superficial and sclerosing.

1. Nodular BCC, the most common type, presents as the classic pearl colored, telangiectatic or ulcerated nodule. The tumor evolves as a slowly enlarging, opalescent mass at whose margins small subclinical finger-like extensions develop. Nodular BCC occurs predominantly on the face and neck.
2. Superficial BCC presents as a slow growing, erythematous, and scaling plaque, most commonly on the trunk. Only at a late stage of development does a deeper vertical growth phase develop. Some lesions may be mistaken for psoriasis.
3. Sclerosing BCC accounts for less than 2 percent of the cases of BCC. It presents as a firm scarlike patch and may have a slightly elevated, pearly border. This form of BCC is characterized histologically by small thin strands of basaloid cells with a rich surrounding stroma of scarlike tissue. Ulceration occurs late and thus the diagnosis is often delayed. Because of the associated stroma, the tumor edges most often blend into the surrounding skin, making margin determinations extraordinarily difficult. This type of BCC may invade widely and deeply and has the capacity to invade tissues such as cartilage, bone, muscle, and nerve. It most commonly occurs on the face but can occur elsewhere.

Size

The size of the tumor affects its curability irrespective of the treatment modality employed. As nodular BCCs increase in size, the histologic pattern often changes. The deeper component may develop small, deeply invasive strands. The lateral margins develop large subclinical extensions. In lesions of small size (less than 2 cm) these extensions measure 3 to 5 mm. Tumors that are larger than 2 cm in diameter have been shown to develop subclinical extensions that measure 10 mm or more. Sclerosing BCCs often prove to be two to three times the clinical diameter of the tumor.

Location

There are certain high risk sites on the face that consistently show higher incidences of recurrence. These high risk areas include the periauricular, periorbital, and perinasal areas as well as the lateral forehead and, in women, the scalp.

Cure incidences for primary tumors in low risk areas, using any of a variety of standard therapies (curettage and desiccation, excision, radiation, and cryosurgery) range between 90 and 95 percent. This is in sharp contrast to the high risk areas where, utilizing the same modalities, cure rates for even small primary BCCs may be 80 percent or lower.

Treatment

The standard methods available to treat BCC include curettage and electrodesiccation, scalpel excision with or without primary closure, cryosurgery, radiation, and Mohs micrographic surgery.

The choice of modality usually depends upon the training and experience of the practitioner, but each technique has advantages and disadvantages. These points should be considered along with tumor type, size, and location when planning therapy.

Curettage and Desiccation

This method works by taking advantage of the textural difference between the soft friable tumor and the firm surrounding dermis. Use of the curette permits preferential removal of tumor with little destruction of surrounding normal skin. When used in conjunction with desiccation, which adds a small additional margin, and when the whole process is performed three times, excellent cure rates can be obtained. When this textural difference is no longer present, curettage and desiccation must be abandoned.

An example of this situation is when the curette drops through the dermis and into the subcutaneous tissue. Since fat and tumor are both soft and friable, the differential upon which the technique is dependent is lost. Another example is in the context of sclerosing or recurrent BCC when the tumor mass and surrounding tissue have similar fibrous textures. Again the textural difference is not present, and curettage and desiccation are no longer effective.

Experience with this modality is critical, as was seen in a recent study that showed markedly different rates of cure when curettage and desiccation were performed by experienced practitioners as compared with that performed by residents in training. Advantages of curettage and desiccation include the small amount of time needed to perform the procedure and the excellent rate of cure. The disadvantages include the long healing time and the resultant white, sometimes atrophic or hypertrophic scar. In the patient with a dark or ruddy complexion, this may yield an unacceptable cosmetic result.

Surgical Excision

Surgical excision requires estimation of the margins by eye and palpation. We know that this is generally possible for small tumors, but because of long subclinical extensions, it is difficult in large tumors.

Excision by scalpel results in an incidence of cure approximately equivalent to that with curettage and desiccation. The procedure itself is standard and requires no comment here. There are several advantages that this mode of therapy has over the others. Because the skin edges are approximated with sutures, healing time is much less and the resultant scars are, with some exceptions, superior. There are also some disadvantages. This type of surgery requires a moderate amount of training, especially when entering the realm of flap and graft repairs. Equipment and instrument needs are generally greater and a greater knowledge of sterile technique is required.

Radiation Therapy

Radiation therapy is an excellent modality. Good results require a therapist who understands skin cancer and the effects of radiation on the skin. Treatments must be given in small doses spread over many sessions if the acute consequences of ulceration and radiation burn are to be avoided.

The benefits of treatment by this modality are several. Because treatments are painless, it is frequently preferable in very ill or debilitated patients who will not tolerate a surgical procedure. When it is performed properly, there is often little distortion of tissue, so important in certain parts of the face, i.e., the nose, ears, and eyelids. The modality has several limitations. Margins are again determined by eye and palpation and accuracy may be limited in some tumors.

Recognition of the long term sequelae caused by ionizing radiation is important. Radiation changes generally result in dry mucosal surfaces and scars, which are often superior in quality early but which get worse as the years go by. This is in contrast to surgical scars, which generally improve over time. Other long term radiation changes include poikiloderma, ulceration, and cutaneous carcinoma.

Cryosurgery

Cryosurgery using liquid nitrogen is a relatively noninvasive procedure in the treatment of BCC. Except in the most experienced hands, the incidence of cure is not as good as with other modalities. Advantages are its noninvasiveness and the relatively short treatment time. Disadvantages include the long recovery period, with the patient having to deal with an oozing weeping wound. Wounds may heal satisfactorily, but generally white depressed scars result. Freeze injury to cartilage may result in substantial retraction defects in the treatment of lesions of the nose and ear.

Mohs Micrographic Surgery

Mohs surgery is a precise, multistaged, microscopically controlled method for treating BCC, squamous cell carcinoma, and other cutaneous tumors. The main disadvantage is that it requires specialty training, and there are therefore a limited number of surgeons available in remote areas who are qualified to use this method. Because tumors are meticulously traced out microscopically, the incidence of cure is in the 99.5 percent range for primary BCCs (even in high risk areas) and in the 96 to 98 percent range for recurrent BCCs. Cure rates are slightly lower for squamous cell carcinoma.

Preferred Method

It is clear that a number of factors come into play in deciding which modality to employ, depending on the type of basal cell carcinoma.

Primary Basal Cell Carcinoma. For small (less than 2 cm), nodular, and superficial BCCs in low risk areas, we generally use curettage and electrodesiccation or excision and primary closure. We believe that the cosmetic result is most often superior with sutured closure. Because scalpel excision is limited from the standpoint of margin determination, we generally combine the benefits of the foregoing two procedures by first curetting in order to better define the limits of gross tumor, following this with excision with the appropriate margin.

Special consideration must be made in reference to the other categories of BCC. Curettage and desiccation are clearly not appropriate in the treatment of sclerosing BCC. Because of this limitation and the fact that margins are so poorly defined, generally we treat these by Mohs surgery. The same is true for nodular BCCs larger than 2 cm, since subclinical extensions make margin determination extremely difficult. If this modality is not available, wide excision or radiation with a wide portal is a reasonable alternative.

We generally refer elderly patients with BCCs on cosmetically critical structures (ears, nose, eyelid) for radiation therapy, for these are patients in whom concern for long term sequelae is minimal. Radiation is also recommended for tumors in patients who are for whatever reason unable to undergo surgery. We may also use it for palliation in large destructive tumors for which surgery is impossible.

Recurrent Basal Cell Carcinoma. In general, once a BCC has recurred, the incidence of cure drops from 90 to 95 percent for primary BCCs to the 40 to 60 percent level for recurrent tumors. The factors that account for this dramatic decline have been alluded to in the discussion of primary BCCs. Scar tissue that occurs with healing obscures tumor edges and often makes estimation of margins impossible. Tumor recurrence at the deep margin is hindered in upward growth by scar tissue or surgical covering such that a recurrence may not be detected until late. Often recurrent tumors change their histologic pattern and become more invasive.

For recurrent BCC we recommend Mohs surgery because of the good prognosis for cure. When this modality is not readily available, wide excision or radiation may be substituted in an attempt to clear margins of tumor, recognizing that the chances of recurrence will be great.

SQUAMOUS CELL CARCINOMA OF THE SKIN

In determining the proper therapeutic modality to use in the treatment of squamous cell carcinoma (SCC) of the skin, there are a few factors that must be considered.

One must determine whether SCC has arisen within an actinic keratosis, in conjunction with a scar, or de novo, as this affects the incidence of metastasis. The risk of metastasis is low, when an SCC arises within an actinic keratosis. The incidence is estimated to be as low as 0.1 percent. Those that arise within a scar have an intermediate rate of metastasis, whereas de novo SCC metastasizes in as many as 40 percent or more of the cases.

Size and location are also important considerations. Small SCCs (less than 2 cm) rarely metastasize. SCCs located on the head and neck metastasize less often than those on the upper extremity, which metastasize less often than those on the lower extremity.

Preferred Treatment

For small SCCs of actinic etiology, we recommend curettage and desiccation or excision and primary closure. Considering the extremely low risk of metastasis, this is a reasonable approach. For larger SCCs (larger than 2 cm) and for tumors that have arisen in scar tisssue or are on the trunk and extremities, we use Mohs surgery. Otherwise wide excision is recommended. Primary closure is performed when possible, and split thickness grafts are used for larger defects to avoid hiding deep recurrences.

Recurrences are of major concern because of the high overall incidence of metastasis in recurrent SCC.

ACTINIC KERATOSIS AND KERATOACANTHOMA

STUART J. SALASCHE, Col. M.C., U.S.A.

ACTINIC KERATOSIS

Actinic keratoses are scaly erythematous papules or plaques that appear on the sun damaged skin of predisposed persons. At highest risk are those who have fair skin and light colored eyes and are of Celtic origin. The number and severity of lesions depend on the anatomic subsite and the amount and duration of excessive ultraviolet exposure. Lesions of the scalp and dorsal hands and wrists tend to be thicker and more discrete than those occurring elsewhere and may be termed hypertrophic actinic keratoses. There is a small but definite risk of malignant degeneration and subsequent metastatic potential in neglected lesions.

Therapy

Therapy is directed against this low malignant potential and at the unsightly cosmetic appearance of the lesions. Therapy should be individualized, depending on the number and extent of the lesions, the condition of the surrounding skin, the anatomic subsite, and the general condition of the patient. Since some of the therapeutic modalities cause discomfort and temporary unsightliness, it is well to consider whether the patient has any impending socially important events or has the ability to care for himself or herself.

After assessing the lesion(s) and these variables, it is best to outline a therapeutic plan that includes the sequential and continuing use of a combination of the available therapeutic techniques. I advise the patient that although therapy may cure all apparent lesions, new lesions caused by prior sun damage may be expected to continue to appear for a while. No matter which mode of therapy I choose, all patients are instructed how to limit further sun exposure and are advised strongly to use a sun screen whenever they go outside. The therapeutic choices available for definitive therapy are cryotherapy with liquid nitrogen, topical 5-fluorouracil therapy, curettage and electrodesiccation, surgical excision, and dermabrasion.

The preferred therapeutic modality for individual discrete lesions is cryotherapy, with liquid nitrogen as the cryogen. This is the most popular agent of choice because of its effectiveness, ease of application, and availability. Cryotherapy is also a noninvasive approach that does not require anesthesia because the pain is only mild, yet tolerable.

Liquid nitrogen is effective in treating individual lesions, with treatment of as many lesions as the patient can tolerate in one sitting as the goal. It can be applied with either a commercially available spray device or a cotton-tipped applicator. With either mode of delivery the key is to apply the liquid nitrogen directly to the center of the lesion until frosting occurs. The length of time the cryogen is applied is an aspect of the art one develops with experience. Thinner lesions on frail elderly women with atrophic surrounding skin obviously require less cryogen than thicker lesions on younger sturdier skin. I prefer a thin directed spray applied in short bursts to maintain frosting for several seconds, trying not to stray beyond the border of the keratosis into the normal skin for more than a millimeter or so. I attempt to keep the lesion frosted for about 3 to 5 seconds, and then I wait for a comparable or slightly longer thaw time before repeating the process. The freeze time and number of freeze-thaw cycles depend on the thickness of the lesion and its response upon visual inspection to the cryogen.

The keratosis and surrounding area become erythematous and edematous within minutes, certainly by the time the patient leaves the office. These effects persist for 24 to 48 hours. If the cryotherapy has been vigorous, a blister or bulla may develop. The blister splits the skin at the derma-epidermal junction and, if troublesome, may be punctured with a sterile needle and deflated. Otherwise a necrotic crust forms within days and sloughs within a week or two, depending on the thickness of the lesion. No specific wound care or dressing is required and the patient may bathe or shampoo as usual. The sequence of events should be reviewed beforehand so that the patient may arrange his social schedule accordingly.

During cryotherapy the patient remains in a lying or supported sitting position. This avoids head injury if a vasovagal response occurs. I proceed in an orderly systematic fashion so that on each visit I routinely examine all exposed areas. I use a small thermos-like container with a blunted needle tip to deliver the spray. The cannister is lightweight and can be held easily in one hand.

My usual routine is to visually inspect and digitally examine an area while almost simultaneously spraying the newly discovered lesions with the spray device being held in the other hand. Newly erupting, small lesions are often better felt than they are seen. Having to look away frequently to dip a cotton tipped applicator would break my concentration. Using a heavy spray machine would make this routine too long and cumbersome. A hypertrophic actinic keratosis may require multiple freezings at 1 to 2 week intervals. I ask the patient to return every 3 to 6 months for a full examination. Complications are extremely uncommon with this cryotherapy and, when they do occur, are usually due to overzealous spraying, which may cause dermal scarring or epidermal dyspigmentation.

Topical chemotherapy with 5-fluorouracil is the treatment of choice for multiple or extensive actinic keratoses. It is a remarkable treatment modality in that normal skin is unaffected, whereas solar keratoses and clinically unapparent lesions are unmasked ("lit up") and removed during therapy. This unmasking of incipient lesions is a therapeutic bonus. Be forewarned, though, that topical therapy with 5-fluorouracil may result in superficial but inadequate therapy of other forms of cutaneous tumors, such as basal cell carcinoma and squamous cell carcinoma, which results in more biologically active recurrences of these tumors when they resurface at a later date. It is therefore imperative that a thorough skin examination, with appropriate biopsies and treatment, be accomplished before instituting topical chemotherapy 5-fluorouracil. Because successful therapy with 5-fluorouracil depends on patient compliance, I render rather specific instructions and counseling. It must be made clear that some discomfort in the form of tenderness and pain and an unsightly appearance are inherent in effective treatment. It is also important to show the patient time-course photographs (available from Roche Laboratories, Nutley, NJ 07110) of similarly affected patients.

Although 5-fluorouracil is available in 1, 2, and 5 percent solutions and creams, I use the 5 percent cream almost exclusively. Treatment is required for approximately 2 weeks for lesions on the face, 4 weeks for those on the neck, 4 to 6 weeks for those on the limbs and chest, and about 6 weeks or more for those on the hands, arms, and scalp. I instruct my patients to wash and dry the area to be treated, to apply the cream twice daily, and to expect lesions on the face to "light up" in about 3 to 5 days and within a few days later elsewhere. This reaction includes erythema, mild tenderness, and scaling. I also tell them that seemingly unaffected areas may respond to the treatment.

With continued therapy, erosions, shallow ulcerations, and weeping occur as well as increasing gradations of pain and tenderness. When the situation becomes too uncomfortable, the patient usually stops therapy just shy of the proposed regimen. If the inflammatory reaction is particularly brisk, it may be prudent to reduce the concentration of 5-fluorouracil to 2 percent, to reduce the applications to once a day or every other day, or even temporarily to interrupt therapy. Once medication is discontinued, cold tap water compresses followed by topical application of a nonfluorinated steroid cream three or four times a day speed recovery. Severe or vesiculating inflammatory responses early in the treatment course may be due to allergic contact dermatitis to the 5-fluorouracil. It is best to see patients at weekly intervals to provide support and to ensure that all is going well.

Two to 3 weeks after completion of the course of 5-fluorouracil the skin takes on a healthy, smooth, keratosis free appearance. Larger, thicker, recalcitrant keratoses may then be treated with liquid nitrogen. It is extremely important in this post-treatment period that the patient use a sunscreen with a high sun protection factor to protect the vulnerable "new" skin. Developing good sunscreen habits in this phase helps give the patient a longer lasting keratosis free period. The 5-fluorouracil chemotherapy may be repeated every 2 to 3 years as required.

An alternative, although more invasive, method of therapy is superficial dermabrasion of the face (involving the scalp if applicable). In this modality the skin is planed into the papillary dermis with subsequent regeneration of a keratosis free epidermis and papillary dermis. The procedure not only treats the actinic damage but gives the face a rejuvenated appearance and adds a degree of prophylaxis against the development of new keratoses.

Thicker solitary lesions may be surgically excised or treated by curettage and electrodesiccation. These adjunctive procedures play only a minor role in the treatment of actinic keratosis.

KERATOACANTHOMA

Keratoacanthomas are pseudomalignant tumors. They exhibit a characteristic clinical morphology and course and a tendency for spontaneous resolution. The typical solitary keratoacanthoma appears initially as a firm, red, round papule, which grows rapidly over a period of 4 to 6 weeks to attain its final size of 1 to 2 cm. In its "mature" form it is a skin colored, dome shaped lesion, which has been likened to a volcano having smooth slopes and a central keratin filled crater. The majority of lesions spontaneously resolve within 4 to 8 months. Despite this spontaneous resolution, keratoacanthomas can be destructive as they evolve, leaving disfiguring atrophic scars. Rapidly growing lesions, attaining a size of 2 cm or greater, are referred to as "giant" keratoacanthomas and can also be aggressive and destructive. Rarely multiple keratoacanthomas may occur as a consequence of either a hereditary condition or an immunosuppressed state or in conjunction with Torre's syndrome.

Therapy

As with actinic keratoses, the clinician has many therapeutic modalities from which to choose. These include awaiting spontaneous resolution or providing surgical excision, curettage and electrodesiccation, cryotherapy, radiation, and intralesional injection with either steroids or cytotoxic drugs. The clinician's primary obligation in reference to keratoacanthoma is to make a proper diagnosis. This is usually not difficult when it is based on an accurate history and clinical morphology. The primary differential diagnosis is with squamous cell carcinoma. If reasonable doubt exists, I perform either excisional biopsy or full thickness central incisional biopsy.

Keratoacanthomas have no malignant potiential, but they can be locally destructive and cosmetically unacceptable. Anatomic location is important; involvement of functional or cosmetic structures such as the nose and lip or proximity to the eye lids is an absolute indication for immediate therapy. I choose to await spontaneous resolution only if the lesion is already showing signs of involution. Healing is usually foretold by loss of the central keratotic plug, which is followed by flattening of the tumor walls and obliteration of the central crater.

I have found intralesional 5-fluorouracil therapy to be more efficacious than intralesional injection with triamcinolone acetonide (10 mg per cubic centimeter). In my experience the incidence of cure and the cosmetic results with electrodesiccation and curettage and with cryotherapy with liquid nitrogen have not been as good as with the treatment modalities to be outlined.

If the clinical diagnosis is reasonably assured, my initial treatment of choice is intralesional injection with 5-fluorouracil. This is a relatively inexpensive noninvasive form of therapy with a high incidence of cure. A commercially available 10 cc vial (50 mg per milliliter) is divided into 1 cc aliquots and drawn into tuberculin syringes. With a 1 inch, 30 gauge needle approximately 0.3 ml is injected into the tumor wall tangentially toward the base. Injection is continued slowly until the site blanches. This process is continued circumferentially at three or four sites until the whole lesion is injected. The remaining syringes to be used may be labeled, dated, and stored in the refrigerator for up to 1 month. Injections are repeated at weekly intervals.

Resolution begins after the first or second injection and a total of three or four weekly injections are required. Involution usually appears as "soupy" purulent degeneration of the tumor. Final healing is seen as a flat, slightly hypopigmented, soft scar. If substantial healing has not occurred by the fourth injection or if increased or continued growth occurs during this time, I perform an excisional or incisional biopsy of the lesion. Injections are usually painless or only slightly uncomfortable. If considerable discomfort arises, the area may be anesthetized using 1 percent lidocaine with epinephrine. This anesthetized state may have the added benefit of keeping intralesional 5-fluorouracil at the site longer. Since squamous cell carcinomas do not respond well to intralesional 5-fluorouracil therapy, use of these guidelines probably would not jeopardize the patient's health.

Radiation therapy is a useful adjunct for treating aggressive, destructive, or giant keratoacanthomas. In these cases there is usually a question of the differential diagnosis with squamous cell carcinoma, and it is imperative that a cancericidal dose be given. Our usual program is to give 20 fractionated treatments over 4 weeks up to a total tumor dose of 4,000 to 5,000 rads. During the course of therapy the tumor becomes erythematous and weepy and develops a black surfaced eschar. Resolution is normally total and the cosmetic result excellent.

BOWEN'S DISEASE

DONALD E. CLEMONS, Col. M.C., U.S.A.

Bowen's disease, a form of squamous cell carcinoma in situ, may arise on both sun exposed and nonsun exposed skin. Because of the propensity of Bowen's disease to involve the outer root sheath of the hair follicle but to spare the acrosyringium, the choice of therapy depends a great deal on the anatomic site involved. Adequate surgical excision to the depth of the subcutaneous tissue and close histologic examination of the surgical margins constitute the preferred therapy for Bowen's disease. In critical areas such as the periorbital region, Mohs surgery, if available, should be employed for its tissue sparing effect. Alternatively electrodesiccation and curettage may be considered for areas with predominant vellus hair growth if care is taken to curette past the suspected level of involvement. Cryosurgery with liquid nitrogen utilizing thermocouples to ensure adequate depth of freezing may also be employed, and in older or debilitated patients radiation therapy may be advantageous.

Five percent 5-fluorouracil cream is the treatment of choice for Bowen's disease of the glans penis (erythroplasia of Queyrat, considered to be a separate entity from Bowen's disease but mentioned here for therapy only). Because of the possibility of tumor extension occurring deeply along hair follicles, 5-fluorouracil should be used only on nonhairbearing skin or mucosa, except for selected cases. Application of 5-fluorouracil twice daily for 6 to 8 weeks should ensure adequate treatment.

If any form of therapy other than surgical excision with evaluation of margins is utilized, post-treatment biopsies should be performed to document cure of disease. Once Bowen's disease evolves into an invasive squamous cell carcinoma, management should be directed at the treatment of a squamous cell carcinoma as detailed on page 73.

The relation of Bowen's disease to internal malignant disease remains controversial. However, it is reasonable to evaluate patients for internal malignant disease if Bowen's disease lesions are on nonsun exposed skin or on the anogenital region in women.

KAPOSI'S SARCOMA

ANTOINETTE F. HOOD, M.D.

Kaposi's sarcoma (KS) is a multifocal vascular neoplasm that affects the skin, lymph nodes, and viscera. Histologically the tumors are composed of variable mixtures of spindle cells and irregular vascular spaces lined by endothelial cells, extravasated erythrocytes, hemosiderin laden macrophages, lymphocytes, and plasma cells. Recent immunohistochemical studies provide strong evidence of the vascular endothelial cell histogenesis of the tumor.

Kaposi's sarcoma occurs in several distinctively different populations of patients. The clinical appearance of the disease, natural progression, and treatment vary from population to population. Table 1 compares the clinical subtypes of KS.

CLASSIC KAPOSI'S SARCOMA

The classic form of KS is rare and accounts for less than 1 percent of the cases of malignant disease in the United States today. It affects older individuals, usually men, often of Mediterranean or eastern European Jewish lineage. Lesions first appear insidiously on the distal lower extremities as red, violaceous, or brown macules and patches, which gradually progress to papules, plaques, and nodules. Over many years there may be extensive involvement of one or, more commonly, both legs; lymphedema may be a prominent feature. Ulceration and secondary infection are common recurrent complications. Lesions are often limited to the skin. Spread to internal organs has been reported in 10 to 70 percent of the patients, but when that occurs, it does so late in the course of the disease. The extracutaneous organ most commonly involved is the bowel; other organs frequently involved are the spleen, adrenal glands, pericardium, lymph nodes, liver, lungs, and bone. Only 20 percent of the patients with classic KS die as a direct result of the tumor, and those deaths are usually due to gastrointestinal or pulmonary involvement.

Many patients develop secondary malignant disease, particularly lymphomas, which carry approximately the same incidence of mortality as KS itself. Other neoplasms associated with KS include Hodgkin's disease, multiple myeloma, and carcinoma.

The studies recommended for evaluation of disease involvement are given in Table 2. Adequately staging a patient with KS is important for management purposes, especially if chemotherapeutic drugs are being considered as part of therapy.

Treatment of classic Kaposi's sarcoma is directed toward eliminating the tumor burden and managing complications. KS is quite radiosensitive, and treatment in the early localized stage consists of irradiation. This may be in the form of spot therapy for individual lesions or limited field or extended field radiotherapy. The total dosage ranges from 1,200 to 3,000 rads and is usually administered in fractionated doses over a 4 week period. However, a single dose of 800 rads may cause complete remission of KS. Cobalt-60 and electron beam therapy have also been used successfully. Other modalities including surgery, laser therapy and cryotherapy with liquid nitrogen have met with limited success but might be considered if radiotherapy cannot be utilized.

Reducing lymphedema often results in improved limb function and diminished discomfort. The use of well fitted Jobst stockings should be required in all KS patients with lower limb involvement. Culture and prompt treatment of crusted fissures or ulcers is very important, since these areas of barrier breakdown may serve as a source of recurrent localized infection, cellulitis, or sepsis. Using synthetic semipermeable dressings such as Vigilon on ulcers may hasten healing and reduce pain.

Extensive incapacitating cutaneous disease, visceral involvement, or relapses after radiotherapy require systemic chemotherapy. This has been administered as a single drug (vincristine, vinblastine, actinomycin D, nitrosoureas, bleomycin, doxorubicin) or as a combination of drugs (vincristine and actinomycin D, nitrosoureas and bleomycin, or doxorubicin and DTIC). Remission has been reported in more than 80 percent of the patients treated with chemotherapy.

TABLE 1 Comparison of Clinical Manifestations in Kaposi's Sarcoma

	Age (Years)	Male:Female Ratio	Location of Cutaneous Lesions	Lymphadenopathy; Visceral Involvement	Course
Classic KS	50–70	15:1	Lower extremities	Uncommon; late in course of disease	Indolent growth and slow progression
African KS					
Adults	25–44	17:1	Lower extremities	Uncommon	Locally aggressive
Children	1–10	3:1	Rare	Common	Progressive and fatal
KS associated with iatrogenic immunosuppression	27–60	2:1	Lower extremities, occasionally generalized	Uncommon	May remain localized but often is progressive and fatal
KS in acquired immunodeficiency syndrome (AIDS)	25–50	20:1	Upper extremities, trunk, head, and neck	Common	May remain stable or may rapidly progress

TABLE 2 Diagnostic Evaluation of Patient with Kaposi's Sarcoma

1. Biopsy of representative skin lesions; photograph prior to initiating therapy
2. Physical examination; stool guaiac test
3. CBC, chemistry profile, and chest x-ray examination
4. CT scan of abdomen and pelvis
5. Biopsy of palpable or enlarged nodes
6. Endoscopy, colonoscopy, and gastrointestinal contrast studies
7. Bronchoscopy if chest x-ray findings are abnormal
8. Bone scan if alkaline phosphatase level is elevated

AFRICAN KAPOSI'S SARCOMA

Kaposi's sarcoma is a frequent tumor in equatorial Africa, accounting for 9 to 11 percent of all cases of malignant disease in some areas. In Africa the disease is sharply localized in Zaire, Tanzania, Uganda, and Kenya. Four clinically distinctive forms of the disease have been described in Africa:

1. A locally aggressive form of the disease occurs in young adults, most commonly in the fourth and fifth decades. Patients with this form of KS usually develop tumors on the lower extremity that are exophytic and infiltrate deeply, often invading underlying bone.

2. A childhood lymphadenopathic form of KS occurs in the first and second decades and, unlike all other subclassifications of Kaposi's sarcoma, affects females more commonly than males. Skin findings are usually absent. The disease is rapidly progressive and the mortality high.

3. The classic disease is also reported in Africa.

4. There is an increasing number of patients with acquired immunodeficiency syndrome (AIDS) associated KS, including homosexuals, hetersexuals, prostitutes, and children born to high risk, human immunodeficiency virus (HIV) infected women.

Treatment of locally aggressive and lymphadenopathic KS requires systemic chemotherapy. Drugs that have been used include the vinca alkaloids (vincristine, vinblastine) and the vinca alkaloids in combination with actinomycin D or DTIC.

KS ASSOCIATED WITH IMMUNOSUPPRESSION

Patients who are iatrogenically immunocompromised by medication are at increased risk for the development of Kaposi's sarcoma. KS has been observed in patients being treated for lupus erythematosus, dermatomyositis, and multiple myeloma and in organ transplant recipients. Although this tumor may occur in patients who are receiving only systemic corticosteroid therapy, KS occurs more commonly in patients who are taking azathioprine in addition to corticosteroids. This variant of Kaposi's sarcoma is typically diagnosed 9 to 16 months after the initiation of immunosuppressive therapy.

The lesions may occur anywhere, but are commonly seen on the upper and lower extremities. The disease may remain stable and localized, progress slowly, or become rampantly progressive and disseminate to visceral organs.

Complete regression may occur when the immunosuppressive treatment is discontinued. When lesions do not clear or if immunosuppression cannot be stopped, local irradiation or systemic chemotherapy may be required for control of the disease.

Personal note: When examining chronically immunosuppressed individuals, there should be a high index of suspicion for KS, and appropriate diagnostic biopsy specimens should be obtained even of innocuous appearing lesions.

KS ASSOCIATED WITH ACQUIRED IMMUNODEFICIENCY SYNDROME

Epidemic Kaposi's sarcoma occurring in homosexual males was one of the earliest reported manifestations of the acquired immunodeficiency syndrome (AIDS). Because of the unusually high incidence of Kaposi's sarcoma in patients with acquired immunodeficiency syndrome, this neoplasm is now considered a major criterion for the diagnosis of AIDS. Physicians are required by law to report to their state communicable disease registry the names of patients less than 60 years old with a biopsy confirmed diagnosis of KS. Kaposi's sarcoma has been reported as the initial manifestation of AIDS in approximately 30 percent of the cases. Although KS is seen most frequently in homosexual men, the neoplasm has been described in all groups at risk for the development of AIDS, including intravenous drug abusers, children, and hemophiliacs. Kaposi's sarcoma is seen most frequently in patients with AIDS from New York and California, in white individuals, and in homosexuals. Although the prognosis for AIDS patients with KS alone is better than for those with KS and opportunistic infections or opportunistic infections without KS, the incidence of mortality is still approximately 41 percent with overall survival said to be 18 months.

This variant of KS initially presents with a single or, more frequently, multiple red to violaceous macules, papules, or nodules on the skin or mucosal surfaces. Unique morphologic findings include oval or linear lesions, a peripheral halo of yellow discoloration, and a distribution on the trunk along skin lines (pityriasis rosea-like). As the lesions become larger, they appear darker red or red-violet and may form raised plaques or tumor nodules. In contrast to the acral distribution of classic KS and the aggressive, local African form of KS, this subtype often appears on the head, especially in a pre- and postauricular location, and on the trunk, genitalia, and oral mucosal surfaces, especially the hard palate. Histologically Kaposi's sarcoma lesions from patients with AIDS cannot be distinguished from those of the other variants of KS.

Although typically more fulminant than other forms of KS, in some patients the disease may remain localized and stable for many months or may be very slowly progressive. Visceral involvement is common and has been reported in 98 percent of the cases in one autopsy series.

The poor prognosis in patients with AIDS related KS is less related to tumor load than to diminished functional capacity of the patient's T and B cell populations. The exact association between the human immunodeficiency virus (HIV) and epidemic KS is not understood. There is actually a direct relationship between antibody titers and prognosis for both the tumor and opportunistic infection; patients with elevated HIV titers apparently have a better prognosis than those with lower titers.

Although opportunistic infections are the major cause of death in all patients with AIDS, the development of widespread Kaposi's sarcoma contributes significantly to the morbidity of these patients and justifies attempts at therapy. Treatment of KS associated with AIDS is difficult because the disease is often widespread and less amenable to radiation and the administration of chemotherapy may result in significant immunosuppression that subjects the patient to an increased risk of opportunistic infections or progression of HIV infection.

Radiation therapy is often effective for the palliation of lesions. Doses between 1,800 and 3,000 rads are effective in reducing the size of tumor nodules. This form of therapy is useful for treating large erosive lesions, areas of extensive lymphedema, or painful lesions of the feet. The argon laser, which emits a blue-green visible light, has been reported to have practical albeit limited applications in the treatment of small lesions. It may be a valuable adjunctive palliative therapy effective in patients with slowly progressive or widely dispersed lesions that cannot be treated with more conventional modes of therapy.

Systemic chemotherapeutic drugs that have been found to be effective and useful include vinblastine, vincristine, etoposide (VP-16), and the combination of doxorubicin, bleomycin, and vinblastine or alternating vincristine and vinblastine. Intralesional administration of the vinca alkaloids has also been reported to be effective without producing the systemic immunosuppression associated with systemic chemotherapeutics. These drugs (either vinblastine or vincristine) are injected intralesionally at a dose of 0.1 to 0.2 mg per cubic centimeter every 2 to 3 weeks with a limit of 2 cc per session.

Interferons, which combine antitumor, immunomodulatory, and antiviral properties, would seem to be ideally suited for the treatment of AIDS related KS. Recent studies indicate that interferon alfa-2a given at high dose can induce the regression of Kaposi's sarcoma. Furthermore, patients whose tumors respond to interferon treatment also show both a lower incidence of opportunistic infection and a longer survival than nonresponders. Patients who demonstrate relative preservation of immune function at the onset of the administration of interferon have a significantly higher incidence of response than patients with altered immune function. Studies are currently underway to assess this drug's capacity to inhibit the HIV in patients with AIDS.

Thus effective treatment of Kaposi's sarcoma requires a thorough evaluation of the patient to determine the extent of involvement and selection of a therapy appropriate for the subtype of disease, age and immunologic status of the patient, and degree of involvement. Patients with Kaposi's sarcoma benefit most from a team approach to treatment that coordinates the talents and efforts of the dermatologist, internist, radiation therapist, and oncologist.

MYCOSIS FUNGOIDES AND THE SÉZARY SYNDROME

STANFORD I. LAMBERG, M.D.

Mycosis fungoides (MF), with its leukemic variant, the Sézary syndrome (SS), is a lymphoma of thymus derived helper lymphocytes. MF and SS are malignant lymphomas and not "reactive" or inflammatory disorders, as evidenced by the findings that cells from patients with MF form cell lines in vitro; that the infiltrating cells have abnormal DNA content and show irregular clonal rearrangements in genes for cell surface receptors, alterations not present in benign disorders; and that the disease follows a course that often leads to death.

CLINICAL MANIFESTATIONS

Males are affected twice as often as females and races are affected equally. The average age of onset is 55, although cases in young adults do occur. Occupational exposure to heavy manufacturing or chemicals is associated with an increased risk of MF, but most patients recall no such exposure. Family members of patients appear to have a higher than expected frequency of other leukemias or lymphomas, but less than 10 instances of families with more than one case of MF have been reported.

Most cases of MF begin with clinically suggestive and pathologically diagnostic lesions. However, about 20 percent have a premycotic clinical phase that either resembles a common benign disorder, such as psoriasis or atopic eczema, or appears with one of several highly suggestive patterns, including poikiloderma atrophicans vasculare, alopecia mucinosa, and large plaque parapsoriasis. The individual lesion characteristic of MF is a thickened, reddish brown, annular or serpiginous plaque. The first lesions appear most commonly on the lower part of the trunk. Most patients with MF or SS have pruritus; itching is especially severe is SS. Patients with SS have widespread erythroderma with atypical lymphocytes composing more than 10 percent of the total of lymphocytes. With progression of MF, thick nodules and tumors, which may ulcerate, appear on the skin, enlarged lymph nodes occur, and involvement of deeper viscera and blood becomes apparent. Extracutaneous dissemination, which most commonly involves the lungs, liver, and spleen, is found at autopsy in three-fourths of those who die with MF and in all with SS. Evidence of extracutaneous disease is less apparent during life because the malignant infiltrate tends to be microfocal without interfering with organ function. Sepsis, often following ulceration of tumors or chemotherapy, is the most common immediate cause of death.

In one form of T cell leukemia, patients have cutaneous lesions resembling those of MF, but also frequently have hypercalcemia, lytic bone lesions, and early lymphadenopathy. This form is more aggressive than the usual case of MF. It has been found mostly in patients from certain areas, especially Japan, the Caribbean, and the southeastern United States. A human type C retrovirus has been associated with this lymphoma.

PROGNOSTIC FACTORS AND STAGING

We have examined more than 20 factors for their prognostic significance, including clinical, pathologic, serologic, and occupational variables, and found that only the extent of skin involvement (T) and the numbers of clinically involved lymph node sites (N) were independently correlated with survival. However, histologically proven extracutaneous lymphoma in blood (B) or viscera (M), generally seen only in advanced disease, indicates further shortening of survival (for definitions, see Table 1). When the T and N variables are combined, the disease can be grouped into four clinical stages that have significantly different incidences of survival. Patients in stage TN_1 (less than 10 percent skin involvement with papules, eczematous patches, or plaques and 0 to 1 enlarged lymph node site) have an actuarially corrected 5 year survival incidence of 83 percent. Survival falls to 64 percent in stage TN_2 (less than 10 percent skin involvement with more than 1 enlarged lymph node site or more than 10 percent skin involvement and 0 to 1 enlarged lymph node site), to 50 percent in stage TN_3 (more than 10 percent skin involvement with more than 1 enlarged lymph node site or 3 or more tumors) and to 35 percent in stage TN_4 (erythroderma). This staging classification also can be used to assign patients to treatment.

WORK-UP

After a skin biopsy diagnosis of MF is confirmed, map the extent of the skin lesions for the medical record and record the numbers of sites of clinically enlarged peripheral lymph nodes. Obtain routine blood counts and chemical test results to establish a baseline and to identify coexisting disorders. Peripheral lymphocytes should be examined by an experienced hematologist. Chest roentgenograms rarely show evidence of intrathoracic lymphoma at the time of first diagnosis. However, involvement frequently develops later in the course.

Liver and bone marrow biopsy specimens rarely are positive in the absence of lymphadenopathy or peripheral blood or lymph node involvement. Consequently these biopsies are recommended only for patients with advanced disease if the information is important for verifying the cause of visceral enlargement, or dysfunction, or for following the response to treatment. Abnormalities of liver function tests alone are unreliable indicators of hepatic involvement, because infiltration, when present, generally is focal and microscopic and does not interfere with function. Although lactic acid dehydrogenase isoenzymes and immunoglobulin E serum levels are elevated in about 10 percent of the patients with MF and SS, their significance is unclear. On rare occasions renal failure has been

TABLE 1 TNM Classification of Mycosis Fungoides

Class	Description
T: Skin *	
T_0	Clinically or histopathologically suspicious lesions
T_1	Eczematous patches, papules, or plaques covering less than 10% of the skin surface
T_2	Eczematous patches, papules, or plaques covering 10% or more of the skin surface
T_3	Tumors, one or more (three or more according to the MFCG)
T_4	Generalized erythroderma
N: Peripheral lymph nodes†	
a. Clinical	
N_{0-8}	The number of sites of palpable peripheral lymph nodes
b. Pathologic	
If available, involvement should be indicated (dermatopathic lymphadenitis, foci of atypical cells, partial or full effacement)	
B: Peripheral blood	
B_0	Atypical circulating cells not present or less than 5%
B_1	Atypical circulating cells present in 5% or more (the actual numbers per 100 lymphocytes recorded), total WBC, and total lymphocyte counts
M: Visceral organs	
M_0	No involvement of visceral organs
M_1	Visceral involvement (must have confirmation of disease; organ involved should be specified)

* Skin biopsy of T_{1-4} must be diagnostic of MF. When characteristics of more than one T exist, all are recorded and the highest is used for staging, for example, $T_{4(3)}$.
† Cervical (left + right = 2), epitrochlear (1), submandibular (1). Total possible = 8. According to the clinical scheme, information about LN disease is not needed for staging or selection of therapy (see discussion).

associated with MF and SS as well as with other malignant lymphomas.

Lymphangiography is not a useful staging procedure because of the high frequency of false positive results. The place for abdominal computer assisted tomography and ultrasonography has not been established but is probably minor.

Sufficient information is available from clinical evaluation of peripheral lymph nodes for staging purposes, but knowledge of pathologic involvement of the lymph nodes may be desired for further prognostication. However, interpretation of lymph nodes is difficult, and nonspecific changes, so-called dermatopathic lymphadenitis, are found in nearly all lymph node biopsy specimens in stages TN_1 and TN_2.

TREATMENT

The optimal therapy for patients with MF and SS has not yet been established. However, preliminary results

from a randomized trial at the National Cancer Institute (NCI) appears to confirm numerous nonrandomized reports of improved survival and even cures in patients treated aggressively while still in an early stage of disease. On the other side, and not too surprisingly, late stage patients in the NCI study did more poorly with more aggressive treatment. In treatment studies using data from the Mycosis Fungoides Cooperative Group, patients in stages TN_1 and TN_2 treated with electron beam therapy alone achieved a higher incidence of remission and remained in remission for a longer period of time than those treated with topical nitrogen mustard therapy alone. Furthermore, the chances of inducing remissions and remaining in remission were lower for patients in stage TN_2 compared to those in stage TN_1 regardless of the treatment modality. The likelihood of remission was further lowered in stage TN_3.

Separate series of stage TN_1 and TN_2 patients treated with total skin electron beam therapy report 3 year disease free survivals of 30 to 40 percent compared to about

15 percent in those treated with topical nitrogen mustard therapy. With a 5 year follow-up there appeared to be little further fall-off in the electron beam treated groups, whereas the incidence of disease free survival with nitrogen mustard fell further to 9 percent at 5 years. Although the incidence of cure appears to be higher with electron beam therapy than with topical nitrogen mustard therapy, electron beam radiation has potentially significant short term and long term complications that must be considered when helping the patient make a choice; side effects are detailed in the individual treatment sections that follow.

Numerous systemic therapy protocols have been tried in late stage patients and patients with visceral involvement, but present modes of treatment have not been curative.

The development of optimal schedules for present therapies and investigation of new forms of therapy are improved when patients with MF are entered into continuing treatment protocols whenever possible. (Information about studies in progress can be obtained by calling the Cancer Information Service, National Cancer Institute, Bethesda, MD. 1-800-4CANCER.)

Treatment Plan by Stage

Stage TN₁

Therapy is generally limited to the skin with either electron beam radiation or topical nitrogen mustard therapy. The combination of electron beam therapy followed by long term topical therapy with nitrogen mustard appears no more effective than electron beam therapy alone. Topical carmustine therapy (BCNU) is generally used in patients who have failed to respond to both modalities or who have become allergic to nitrogen mustard. Studies to evaluate the role of additive systemic chemotherapy during this stage are in progress at several centers.

Stage TN₂

An effective treatment rationale must consider the larger MF mass in the skin and the greater likelihood of recurrence after treatment. Therefore, the addition of systemic chemotherapy to either total skin electron beam or topical nitrogen mustard therapy may be appropriate.

Stage TN₃

Electron beam radiation, often supplemented with orthovoltage radiation to thick tumors, is generally more effective in patients with tumors or extensive plaques and adenopathy than is topical nitrogen mustard therapy, but nitrogen mustard may be used, perhaps supplemented with orthovoltage radiation to tumor areas. Patients generally are given systemic chemotherapy as well.

Stage TN₄

The primary treatment in the erythrodermic Sézary syndrome is systemic, since all patients in this group have visceral disease. Presently most systemic regimens consist of cytotoxic drugs, but other measures are being evaluated (see section on experimental measures).

General Measures

Pruritus is a common, sometimes overwhelming problem. Moderate relief may be gained by the systemic use of antihistamines, such as hydroxyzine, 25 mg orally every 4 hours as needed, and topically applied emollients, such as Eucerin, or topical therapy with corticosteroids, such as beta-methasone, fluocinonide, or triamcinolone, in either cream or ointment form applied as needed or overnight under plastic wrap occlusion.

Phototherapy (PUVA)

Longwave ultraviolet light treatment combined with psoralen (PUVA) suppresses early thin lesions, and claims of cures in patients with early disease have been made. However, I believe that the long term cure of patients with histologically proven MF is unlikely with PUVA alone, and that at least some of the patients said to have been cured have had the large plaque form of parapsoriasis, which often does respond and may clear with PUVA. Furthermore, I believe that PUVA treatments may suppress or "hide" activity and prevent prompt initiation of more effective and potentially curative therapy.

Particular Measures

Electron Beam Radiotherapy

MF is radiosensitive and nearly all patients respond to electron beam radiation, at least temporarily. Electron beam radiation has a distinct advantage over orthovoltage radiation; the penetration of electrons, being particles, can be controlled to reach depths as shallow as a few millimeters, whereas orthovoltage wave form radiation passes deeply into tissues. Thus, a large surface dose can be given with electron beam therapy without deep tissue injury or bone marrow suppression. Therapy generally is fractionated over 6 to 10 weeks to a total of about 3,000 to 3,600 rads. All portions of the body must be treated; a higher incidence of recurrence has been found in patients who elected scalp shielding to prevent hair loss. There does not appear to be any additional benefit in adding topical nitrogen mustard therapy after completion of electron beam therapy.

The advantages are as follows: (1) Disease free 5 year cure incidence of 30 to 40 percent are seen in early disease. (2) The course of treatment is a single 2 month period. (3) There is no visceral toxicity. (4) Most large cities now have at least one medical center capable of providing electron beam radiotherapy.

The disadvantages are as follows: (1) Treatment sessions are rigorous, requiring long periods of standing in prescribed positions, which is difficult for the older patient. (2) Acute side effects include skin edema, erythema, and fissuring. These usually subside in the month following therapy. (3) Late side effects include pigmentation, hair loss, nail loss, and "dry" skin. Hair, nails, and sweat gland function usually return in 3 to 6 months. (4) Treatment is costly, $5,000 to $10,000, although insurance generally covers most or all of the expenses. (5) Other skin cancers have appeared in a few patients following electron beam therapy.

Topical Chemotherapy

Topical Mechlorethamine Therapy (Nitrogen Mustard, Mustargen). Mechlorethamine, a nitrogen mustard, is an alkylating agent used topically in MF for more than 20 years. The majority of patients with early disease respond to the drug and long term "cures" are claimed, although sustained remissions probably require continued use of the drug.

The advantages are as follows: (1)Nitrogen mustard is easy to apply topically. (2) It is nonirritating, although patients often mention excessive "dryness." (3) The treatment can be used easily by older patients. (4) There is no associated hair, nail, or eccrine sweat loss. (5) No bone marrow suppression or other systemic toxicity develops.

The disadvantages are as follows: (1) Long term disease free cures are unlikely. (2) Up to 40 percent of the patients develop contact allergy. (3)Treatments must be given daily or nearly so for up to several years. (4) The medication costs about $4 a day. (5) Other skin cancers have appeared in a few patients following nitrogen mustard therapy.

Instructions: The patient should be instructed to pry off the metal cap of a 10 mg vial of nitrogen mustard with pliers and mix the contents just before use in 1 to 2 oz of distilled water, purchased from a grocery or drug store by the gallon. The painting is most conveniently done at bedtime, generally following a shower but after the skin is dry. A 2 inch nylon paint brush is convenient and minimizes hand irritation. Most of the solution is applied from head to toe, but the intertriginous areas are spared and painted last with the residual solution, which is diluted with extra water to reduce irritation. A teaspoonful of glycerin may be added to the solution to ease residual dryness, especially during the winter. If dryness is excessive, the patient may apply an emollient, such as Eucerin, on arising. Treatment is used daily until complete clearing occurs, which takes 6 months to 2 years. After complete clearing the frequency may be reduced to every other day or less, but the patient should be warned that the treatment must continue for several years or even indefinitely. Unfortunately allergic reactions to the drug develop in up to 40 percent of the patients after long term use. Desensitization can be accomplished in about half the patients who develop allergy by graded increases of diluted nitrogen mustard, generally performed by dermatologists with prior experience with the drug.

Topical Carmustine Therapy. Topical carmustine (BCNU) therapy appears to be an effective alternative to nitrogen mustard. Allergic reactions are uncommon, but local irritation and persistent telangiectasis may develop, and because the drug is absorbed, reversible bone marrow depression may develop.

Instructions: The pharmacist dissolves a 100 mg vial of BCNU powder in 50 ml of 95 percent or absolute ethyl alcohol. This is the stock solution and is refrigerated by the patient. For treatment, 5 ml of the stock is added to about 60 ml of distilled water; this solution is applied once daily to the entire body, as with nitrogen mustard. The solution may be further diluted when used in the intertriginous areas to minimize irritation. Treatment should continue for 6 to 8 weeks, depending on the degree of irritation. Steroid cream may be used topically if excessive irritation develops. After a 6 week rest period, the course may be repeated. If the response is incomplete, the concentration may be doubled (10 ml of stock per 60 ml of water) for another 6 to 8 weeks. During rest periods residual lesions may be treated with the full strength alcohol stock solution, up to twice daily for up to 6 weeks not exceeding 70 mg (35 ml of stock) per week.

Complete blood counts, including platelet counts, should be obtained every 2 to 4 weeks during and for 6 weeks after BCNU applications. The cycle of treatment may be repeated as necessary to suppress visible lesions.

Systemic Chemotherapy

Single drug chemotherapies with which documented complete remissions have occurred include methotrexate, systemic nitrogen mustard therapy, bleomycin, cyclophosphamide, chlorambucil, doxorubicin, and VP-16. Combination chemotherapies used most frequently include methotrexate, cyclophosphamide, and prednisone; cyclophosphamide, vincristine, and prednisone (CVP); mechlorethamine, vincristine, procarbazine, and prednisone (MOPP); cyclophosphamide, vincristine, and prednisone with or without bleomycin (COP or COP-Bleo); Ara-C and doxorubicin; and chlorambucil and prednisone. Additional drugs being studied for effectiveness in MF include L-asparaginase, cis-platinum, cyclosporine A, 2' deoxycoformycin (Pentostatin), dibromodulcitol, hexamethylmelamine, hydroxyurea-cytosine arabinoside, ICRF-159, gallium nitrate, methyl-GAG, N-methylformamide, thiotepa, vinblastine, VM-26, and VP-16.

An attenuated CHOP protocol given after electron beam radiation used by the Mycosis Fungoides Cooperative Group consists of the following: On day 1, cyclophosphamide (500 mg per square meter intravenously); doxorubicin (40 mg per square meter intravenously); vincristine (1.4 mg per square meter intravenously); and on days 1 to 5, prednisone (60 mg per square meter orally), repeated every 21 days for a maximum of six courses.

Experimental Measures

Other attempts to control late stage or recurrent MF and SS include combinations of total skin electron beam and topical or systemic chemotherapy, or total lymphoid or total body irradiation. In addition to cytotoxic chemotherapy with the single and combination regimens just listed, other current programs are evaluating serotherapy with antithymocyte globulin, human interferon (alpha, beta, and gamma), and monoclonal antibodies directed against T lymphocytes or against malignant T cell surface markers, leukapheresis for removal of circulating atypical Sézary cells, local hyperthermia, and extracorporeal phototherapy.

MALIGNANT MELANOMA

DAVID E. ELDER, M.B., Ch.B., B. Med. Sc., F.R.C.P.A.

The management of malignant melanoma is primarily surgical. Surgery directed at the primary tumor may range from simple excision biopsy to formal "wide" excision of a piece of skin the size of a tennis ball. An area of controversy relates to the exact margin width that produces an optimal balance between a low level of local recurrence, acceptable morbidity, and survival. Also controversial is the indication for elective nodal surgery in stage 1 melanomas. In our view, however, a survival benefit has not been convincingly demonstrated for this procedure.

There is no effective therapy for metastatic melanoma, and surgery, although presumably effective in preventing the continuing accumulation of metastases from primary tumors, is not capable of eliminating micrometastases that may already be established at the time of diagnosis. However, incidence of survival in patients with melanoma has improved from only 12.5 percent in the first quarter of the century to over 80 percent today. Since there has been no dramatic advance in the surgical strategy employed, the improved survival is no doubt due to earlier diagnosis. Any physician who manages patients with melanoma must have a clear idea of the criteria for the diagnosis of early melanoma. Further, common and dysplastic nevi have been associated with an increased risk of developing melanoma. Thus, strategies available today to reduce the mortality from melanoma include public education in the recognition of early melanomas and the identification of individuals at high risk of developing melanoma so that they can be screened and followed.

COMMON ACQUIRED NEVI

Common acquired melanocytic nevi are small (usually less than 4 to 6 mm), symmetrical, uniformly pigmented benign tumors. Only a few of the vast numbers of nevi in the normal population ultimately give rise to melanoma. Furthermore, many melanomas arise de novo in clinically normal skin. Thus, it is inappropriate to excise nevi with the aim of preventing melanoma by eliminating potential precursor lesions. Indications for excision include the following:

1. Cosmetic indications and patient preferences. In this situation only, shave excision may be acceptable. A specimen must always be submitted for pathologic examination, and the patient should be advised that an additional excision may be required if there is atypia. The dermatologist should be alert for nuances of pathologic descriptions that might indicate that the lesion is not an ordinary nevus; he should discuss these with the pathologist and have a low threshold for re-excision.

2. Atypical morphology suggesting the possibility of melanoma. In this and the following situation, an excision biopsy should be done with a request for margin evaluation if indicated.

3. A history of growth or any other change in an adult patient. Nevi in children may be observed to undergo normal evolutionary changes, but each such lesion must be evaluated carefully on its own merits. Especially in patients at high risk for melanoma (see later discussion), any lesion that the patient convincingly states has changed should be excised or followed, preferably with photographic documentation.

DYSPLASTIC NEVI

Dysplastic nevi are broader than most nevi (usually 4 mm or more), are entirely or mostly flat (though side-lighting reveals them to be slightly raised) with some variegation of shades of tan and brown, and have an irregular, "hazy," indefinite edge. In these attributes dysplastic nevi to some extent resemble plaques of "early" radial growth phase melanoma, but the melanomas are large (7 mm and usually much larger), more variegated with blue-black hues, and more irregular.

Dysplastic nevi, like common nevi, are potential precursors of melanoma. Their potential for transformation, though greater than that of common nevi, is still very low. It has been estimated that it would be necessary to excise hundreds of dysplastic nevi to prevent the development of one melanoma. Thus, there is no indication for prophylactic excision.

More important than their very low potential precursor risk is the role of dysplastic nevi as markers of risk for melanoma. Dysplastic nevi are found in 5 to 8 percent of "normal" populations and in 30 to 50 percent of patients with melanoma. On the average, patients with dysplastic nevi are about 10 times more likely to develop melanoma than a normal person. However, the large pool of patients with dysplastic nevi (perhaps 10 million in the United States alone) is heterogeneous with respect to this risk. The most important added risk factor is a family or personal history of melanoma. For example, patients with dysplastic nevi and a family history of melanoma in two or more relatives, or with a personal history of melanoma, may be as much as 400 times more likely to develop (another) melanoma than the general population. There is some evidence that the number and size of the nevi are also related to risk. Thus, an individual with only one or two dysplastic nevi and no history of melanoma may be at little or no risk, whereas the risk for members of hereditary melanoma families approaches 100 percent over their lifetimes.

The principle of management of dysplastic nevi is to detect a melanoma, should it occur in a given patient, in its early, always curable, stage. The means to facilitate this early diagnosis include patient education in the diagnosis of early melanoma and physician screening in a series of periodic follow-up examinations. The patient should be given brochures depicting early lesions of melanoma and describing a method of monthly self-examination. Suitable publications are available from the Skin Cancer Foundation, the American Cancer Society, and the National Cancer Institute. Photography is done in selected cases to permit detection of new lesions when they are small.

The management of dysplastic nevi should be individualized according to the patient's imputed risk of developing a melanoma and the "difficulty" of follow-up (Table 1). Patients with few abnormal nevi may be at lower risk, and they are also easier to educate and follow than individuals who are covered with large variegated nevi. Even an expert may have difficulty distinguishing dysplastic nevi and melanomas in the latter, fortunately uncommon, group of patients. At the low risk and "easy to follow" end of the spectrum, photography may be unnecessary. A patient who has only a few small dysplastic nevi on his skin probably can be left to observe his own skin at occasional intervals. A phenotypically similar patient who has, in addition to a few dysplastic nevi, a family or personal history of melanoma is putatively "high risk" but is still "easy to follow." This individual should be followed for life, but the photographic documentation need not be extensive. At the other end of the spectrum, patients who have a melanoma history and are covered with (often highly variable and atypical) dysplastic nevi should be followed for life, and their skin should be carefully documented with segmental photographs and closeup views.

Although a case can be made for more frequent follow-up in high risk subsets of dysplastic nevus cases, it is the opinion of this author that few, if any, patients require follow-up more than once a year provided nevi are stable (showed no interval changes at the last examination) and the patient knows that he should return if changes occur. After the initial work-up, patients are seen 6 months later and then annually if the lesions are stable. Excisions are recommended in the following circumstances: for diagnosis at an initial visit, to rule out melanoma in "atypical" lesions, for any nevus that has shown change of any kind, and for lesions that are in locations where they are difficult to follow, especially the scalp. In these cases the threshold for excision is lower than in locations such as the face where the lesion is constantly in the patient's view.

MALIGNANT MELANOMA

Diagnosis and Staging

Accurate diagnosis is the cornerstone of rational management. Not only must benign simulants of melanoma be recognized clinically and histologically, but so must unusual forms of melanoma that may resemble benign lesions. Further, accurate staging and microstaging of melanomas are essential. Staging is primarily a clinical exercise that determines the extent of the disease (Table 2). Most patients (80 percent) present in stage I. For these patients, a set of so-called "microstaging" attributes can divide the cases into three or more groups with low (less than 5 percent), intermediate (less than 20 percent), and high risks of recurrence, metastasis, or death. Current practice recommends different types of management for these groups, but the principles of therapy are the same, namely, complete extirpation of local areas of disease ("wide" local excision) and careful follow-up directed at regional nodes, skin, and visceral organs.

TABLE 2 Staging of Melanoma

Stage I   Tumor confined to a node drainage region

    A. Localized to a single cutaneous site
    B. Satellites within 5 cm of primary site
    C. In-transit metastases beyond 5 cm but still regional

Stage II   Tumor in regional lymph nodes

    A. Less than 20% of nodes involved
    B. More than 20% involved

Stage III   Tumor beyond a node drainage region

    A. Nonregional cutaneous metastases
    B. Visceral metastases
      i. "Solitary"
      ii. Disseminated

TABLE 1 Management of Dysplastic Nevus

Group	Definition	Management Photos	Follow-Up
Low risk	No personal history of malignant melanoma No family history of malignant melanoma	Overviews	Every 12 months for 5 years; educate in self-examination
High risk, easy or hard to follow	Personal or family history of malignant melanoma	Overviews laterals, ± close-ups	Every 12 months of life and more often if nevi are changing; educate
Easy to follow and low risk	Few lesions, slight clinical atypia	Optional	At least two vists for education; optional follow-up
Hard to follow, low or high risk	Many lesions, marked clinical atypia	Overviews, laterals, close-ups	Every 12 months for life and more often if changing; educate

The majority of melanomas present in clinical stage 1, localized without satellites or in-transit metastases. By definition, the regional lymph nodes are "clinically negative." Although these patients, as a group, enjoy much longer survival (more than 80 percent for 7 years) than stage II (less than 30 percent) or stage III cases (less than 10 percent), their survival is heterogeneous. There are subsets of stage I melanoma in which survival is essentially 100 percent and other subsets whose survival percentage is little better than if they had presented with lung metastases (though their survival duration is longer). These subsets are defined by microstaging, using microscopic and some clinical criteria to define a prognostic model that "predicts" survival for groups of stage I patients.

The attributes used in microstaging are summarized in Table 3. Most important are the "phase" of tumor progression (radial or vertical growth phase), thickness, level of invasion, mitosis rate, and lesion location. The phase of tumor progression in melanoma is under investigation by our group at the University of Pennsylvania as a prognostic attribute. Patients with melanomas in the histologically defined phase of radial growth, when the clinical lesion is a plaque that expands outward along the radii of a disk or a circle and histologically there is no tumorigenic growth in the dermis, have enjoyed a 7 year survival incidence of 100 percent. Melanomas thinner than Breslow's 0.76 mm are associated with a similar 97 percent survival and Clark level II melanomas with 98 percent survival. Those few "thin" or level II melanomas that have metastasized have all had a small focus of "vertical growth," a qualitatively new phase in the natural history of a melanoma when a clone of cells appears to acquire the property of tumorigenicity and presents clinically as an initially small (but expanding) nodule within the antecedent radial growth phase plaque.

For clinical management a relatively simple model gives adequate stratification. Indeed treatment can be based on thickness alone, defining a low risk group of patients with tumors thinner than 0.76 mm, an intermediate risk group with a thickness between 1.5 and 3.99 mm, and a high risk group with a thickness of more than 4 mm. The precision of the prognostication can be refined by using multiple attributes. One relatively simple model is presented in Table 4.

TABLE 3 Prognostic Attributes Used in Microstaging of Stage I Melanoma

Microscopic	Clinical
Phase of tumor progression*	Lesion location
Thickness	Sex*
Level of invasion	Age*
Mitosis rate	?Immune status*
Microscopic satellites	
Ulceration	
Lymphocytic infiltrate*	

* Controversial or unconfirmed.

Therapy of Melanoma

The detailed management of stage III melanoma is beyond the scope of this review. In general, the therapy for disseminated stage III melanoma consists of systemic modalities such as traditional chemotherapy or investigational immunotherapy. Stage III disease confined to the skin is usually managed surgically, and patients may survive for relatively long periods with occasional excision of new dermal deposits. Isolated perfusion with chemotherapeutic drugs is effective in palliating (and, perhaps, curing) disease confined in a single limb. Uncommonly patients present with apparently isolated visceral metastases amenable to surgical intervention. Surgery is inappropriate, however, for the more common presentations with multiple metastases. In the remainder of this section the indications and rationales for local and nodal therapy of clinical stage I and II melanoma will be discussed. Details of techniques can be found in standard surgical and dermatologic texts.

Local Therapy

The rationale for traditional "wide" local excision is to ensure complete extirpation of the tumor (together with any nearby satellites) at the local site. The aim is to prevent any local recurrences that might be due to continued growth of residual tumor. Most melanomas grow in a contiguous fashion (without satellites) and are circumscribed rather than highly infiltrative. Thus, most specimens from re-excisions after a complete excision biopsy do not contain any residual lesion at all. Satellites and in-transit metastases, if they occur, are most likely to be seen in thick tumors (larger than 2 mm) and are most likely to be close to rather than distant from the tumor. Thus, the optimal margin width would be a function of the probability of micrometastases at various distances from the primary sites of tumors stratified by thickness. Unfortunately such data are not available. It is known, however, that formal wide level excision is effective in preventing all but a few local recurrences. At the same time, paradoxically, the extent of resection has not been related to the most important outcome parameter—survival. These facts suggest the following:

1. The traditional 5 cm wide excision is excessive therapy for almost all melanomas.

2. Margin widths can be quite narrow for thin melanomas in which the probability of satellites approaches zero.

3. Melanomas larger than about 1.5 to 2 mm in thickness, with a finite probability of satellites, should be excised with somewhat greater margins in order to prevent local recurrence but without the expectation that the extent of this therapy will influence survival.

4. A randomized trial of various margin widths is needed to assess the relationships among thickness, margin widths, and survival. Such a trial is under way at present.

TABLE 4 Prognostic Categories for Stage I Melanoma

Low risk	EITHER	tumor in radial growth phase only	
	OR	thickness <0.76 mm*	
	OR	level II	
Intermediate risk	Vertical growth phase present		AND
	EITHER	thickness <1.5 mm †	
	OR	thickness 1.5–3.99 mm	
		AND located on a limb	
		OR mitosis rate <6 per sq mm	
High risk	Vertical growth phase present		AND
	EITHER	thickness >3.99 mm	
	OR	thickness 1.5–3.99 mm AND mitosis rate >6 per sq mm	
	OR	thickness 1.5–3.99 mm AND not located on a limb	

* 0.85 mm and † 1.70 mm may be equally or more appropriate cutoff points.

For the present, our management plan for stage I primary melanoma is based simply on the risk status of the primary tumor (Table 4). The plan is shown in Table 5. Margins should be adjusted when there is a nearby vital structure. In these circumstances it is especially important that the pathologic examination include a careful assessment of the margins. In desmoplastic and neurotropic melanomas infiltration may extend well beyond the gross tumor, and margins therefore should be carefully examined for nerve involvement.

Nodal Therapy

The regional lymph nodes are the commonest site of initial treatment failure, and lymph node metastases are often the harbingers of visceral metastases. It is generally agreed that clinical stage II melanomas should be treated by excision of the nodal tumor in a "therapeutic" node dissection. Although the prognosis remains poor, dissection of tumor bearing nodes at least prevents many instances of bulky symptomatic tumor development in the node basin.

For clinical stage I melanomas the management is controversial. In intermediate and high risk subsets, the incidence of positive nodes at "elective" node dissection is greater than 20 percent. The same patients, if the elective dissection had not been done, would probably have presented later with palpable tumor. It can be argued that elective dissection, done in 100 percent of these patients, might be lifesaving if the disease in 20 percent of the cases were confined at presentation to the nodes only, and if dissemination from the nodes to the viscera might have occurred in the interval between excision of the primary lesion and the patient's later presentation with clinical

nodal disease. This approach would then result in "unnecessary" dissections, with attendant morbidity and expense, in 80 percent of the cases. An alternative theoretical viewpoint argues that lymph node metastases are not commonly the locus of dissemination to the viscera, but serve as markers of risk for visceral disease. Thus, lung metastases in patients with positive nodes are derived from the primary tumor prior to its extirpation. In this view, node dissection should not be done electively but should be held in reserve for the 20 percent of the patients who present with pathologic nodes in follow-up examination.

This problem cannot be resolved by theoretical debate. The test of the hypothesis that elective dissection is associated with longer survival depends on the direct observation of survival incidences in a clinical data base. Unfortunately the available data are conflicting. Several retrospective series have shown apparent benefit in patients with melanomas in the thickness range of 1.5 to 3.99 mm. Patients with thinner tumors do not often develop metastases, and presumably those with thick tumors who develop visceral metastases already had disseminated disease at presentation. Other retrospective series, our own included, and two randomized trials involving limb melanomas have shown no benefit from elective node dissection, provided the patients are followed closely and "therapeutic" node dissection is done promptly if nodes become palpable. Pending the results of a continuing randomized trial, we have therefore concluded that there is no compelling indication for elective dissection.

Follow-Up

Particularly if an elective node dissection is not done, close follow-up is essential. The examinations should be directed toward inspection and palpation of the scar and its region and palpation of regional nodes, with a general physical examination including the abdomen. Equally important, since patients with melanoma are at risk of developing a second primary, is a complete skin examination. Preferably the skin should be documented photographically at the first appointment, and any new melanocytic lesions thereafter should be excised. Most of the patients in our data base who have developed multiple primaries

TABLE 5 Margin Widths for Melanomas by Thickness

Risk Group*	Margin Width (Radius,cm)
Low risk	≤1
Intermediate risk	1-2
High risk	2-3

* See Table 4.

TABLE 6 Follow-up Schedule for Melanoma

Risk Group	Schedule	Investigations
Low risk	Every 6 months, 2 years Every 12 months, 8 years*	Photography at first visit Physical examination Skin examination, educate* CXR,[†] blood studies
Intermediate risk	Every 3 months, 2 years Every 6 months, 3 years Every 12 months, 5 years*	Photography at first visit Physical examination Skin examination, educate* CXR,[†] blood studies
High risk	Every 3 months, 3 years Every 6 months, 2 years Every 12 months, 5 years*	Photography at first visit Physical examination Skin examination, educate* CXR,[†] blood studies

* For patients with dysplastic nevi, skin follow-up is continued for life, and family screening is recommended. All patients should be educated about the diagnosis of early melanoma and method of self-examination.
[†] CXR–chest radiograph

also have dysplastic nevi, which are seen in 50 percent of all cases and in over 90 percent of patients with multiple primaries. These individuals should have skin follow-up examinations for life, and their families should be screened and followed if necessary (see foregoing discussion). At each follow-up examination for melanoma, we order a chest radiograph, a blood screen, and a chemistry profile. We do not order CT scans, isotope scans, or magnetic resonance imaging (MRI) scans unless there is a specific indication. Our follow-up schedule is summarized in Table 6.

CUTANEOUS HISTIOCYTOSIS

William H. Zinkham, M.D.

The appearance of a skin rash may be the first manifestation of a histiocytic disorder. Although this book emphasizes the treatment of dermatologic disease, additional objectives of this presentation are to review the perplexing and often confusing terminology applied to the histiocytoses, their clinical signs and symptoms, and the importance of early diagnosis and long-term evaluation. The justification for this approach is based on two considerations. First, the frequency of occurrence of the idiopathic histiocytoses is sufficiently low that the physician may never encounter one of these patients. And second, most of the drugs with proven efficacy are chemotherapeutic agents. Therefore, their selection and the schedule of administration require the availability of an experienced chemotherapist.

TERMINOLOGY

Idiopathic forms of histiocytosis are associated with abnormal proliferation of histiocytes in one or more organs. In some patients there is a single benign lesion that resolves spontaneously, whereas in others there is widespread disease with a high mortality. The etiologic factor remains elusive, although a variety of disorders of known etiology may exhibit a similar histologic picture, e.g., infections due to viruses (rubella, cytomegalic inclusion disease, and herpes), bacteria (*Brucella,* atypical mycobacteria), fungi (histoplasmosis), parasites (leishmaniasis), host immune defense abnormalities (Chédiak-Higashi syndrome and chronic granulomatous disease), and certain malignant diseases (monocytic leukemia and histiocytic medullary reticulosis). The natural history of the idiopathic histiocytic disorders and the histologic findings are extremely variable. Consequently there is no universally acceptable classification, even though the literature is replete with efforts to devise one.

In 1953 Lichtenstein noted that the compulsion of many clinicians to devise their own system of terminology had created a body of literature that was "fast becoming a veritable Babel as a consequence." To circumvent this problem he coined the term "histiocytosis X" to encompass disorders previously designated as Letterer-Siwe disease, reticuloendotheliosis, eosinophilic granuloma, and Hand-Schüller-Christian disease. Several years later Lieberman proposed another classification—unifocal eosinophilic granuloma signifying solitary lesions, and multifocal eosinophilic granuloma designating patients with multiple sites of involvement. The most recent classification that has been developed is based on the finding that the Langerhans' cell is the predominant type of cell in most of the nonmalignant types of histiocytic disorders. Therefore, one can anticipate that in the future the terms previously used will be replaced by the following: Langerhans' cell histiocytoses for Letterer-Siwe disease, Hand-Schüller-Christian disease, and eosinophilic granuloma and non-Langerhans' cell histiocytoses for the malignant histiocytoses, virus-induced hemophagocytic syndromes, and familial forms of histiocytoses.

CLINICAL PRESENTATION

Cutaneous involvement is frequent in the idiopathic histiocytic disorders, but seldom is the skin the only site of disease. To date approximately 20 patients with disease confined to the skin have been reported. A rash usually appears during the first 2 years of life and in some may be present at birth. The male:female ratio is approximately 2:1 and most of the patients are white. Characteristically the lesions appear as erythematous papules, which may at times exhibit a greasy yellow crust. In some patients petechial lesions are present. Sites of predilection include the scalp, postauricular regions, auditory canal, axillary and inguinal areas, and occasionally the thorax and abdomen. Frequently there is a superimposed bacterial infection. The seborrhea-like character of the rash frequently results in a delay in diagnosis.

The majority of the patients with cutaneous histiocytosis have disease in one or more other tissues, including the liver, spleen, lung, bone, lymph nodes, teeth, paronychial regions, and the hypothalamic-pituitary axis. Important signs and symptoms of extracutaneous disease are defects of the skull, intractable otitis media, loss of teeth, chronic ulcerations of the palate, gums, and vulva, pain in the pelvic or long bones, enlargement of the liver or spleen, adenopthy, diabetes insipidus, hypothyroidism, growth failure, dyspnea, and anemia. Any patient being treated for seborrheic dermatitis who develops any of these complications should undergo a skin biopsy.

MANAGEMENT OF THE PATIENT

In many respects the guidelines for the management of patients with histiocytosis resemble those developed for patients with malignant tumors: diagnosis, staging, and therapy. First and foremost is a prompt and precise tissue diagnosis. Since cutaneous involvement is a frequent occurrence, the dermatologist may be the first to establish the diagnosis, for which a detailed history, physical examination, and skin biopsy are essential.

The skin biopsy should be performed in a site free of crusting, infection, or ulceration. Usually there is a dense infiltrate of pale staining, mature histiocytes in the upper and mid-dermis, with scattered inflammatory cells and eosinophils. The epidermis may be atrophic and in some areas replaced by a histiocytic infiltrate. If the results of the first biopsy are equivocal, a second biopsy should be carried out.

In 1979 Nezelof noted that idiopathic histiocytosis is fundamentally a proliferation of Langerhans' cells. Electron-microscopic examination of these cells reveals the presence of rod-shaped or racquet-shaped bodies, the so-called Birbeck granules. These granules are the hallmark of Langerhans' cells and are usually present in the skin of patients with cutaneous histiocytosis as well as in other affected tissues. The density of these cells in the biopsy specimen is quite variable, so that many sections have to be made to demonstrate their presence. Other identifying features of the Langerhans' cells include their reactivity with anti-T6 antibody and anti-HLA-DR antibodies. Most of the cells also react with anti-S100 protein antibody. However, the S100 antibody also reacts with other types of cells, including melanocytes and neural cells, so it is not a specific marker for Langerhans' cells. Thus, electron-microscopic examination of the biopsy specimen, together with immunopatholgic techniques, may be necessary to confirm the diagnosis. In this respect it is important to note that the antibodies to the T6 antigen react with Langerhans' cells but not with monocytes or macrophages, thereby enabling one to differentiate between normal proliferation of macrophages or monocytes and the overgrowth of histiocytic elements that one sees in the idiopathic histiocytoses.

Once the presence of cutaneous histiocytosis has been established, studies should be initiated to determine the extent of the disease (staging). Histiocytosis can involve many different tissues. Since pure cutaneous histiocytosis is a rare disorder, the patient with biopsy-proven histiocytosis of the skin frequently has lesions in other areas. Furthermore, the extent of the disease and its effect on organ function have prognostic significance. In general, the greater the number of tissues or systems affected, the poorer the prognosis. Other important prognostic indicators are functional abnormalities of the liver (hyperbilirubinemia, hypoalbuminemia), lung (dyspnea, reduced pO_2), and bone marrow (leukopenia, thrombocytopenia, or anemia). A search for disease in extracutaneous sites has to be carried out before one can develop an appropriate therapeutic program.

THERAPY

The treatment of the cutaneous forms of histiocytosis depends on whether skin involvement is associated with disease in other areas. In cases of "pure" cutaneous histiocytosis, a variety of therapeutic modalities have been applied. Because of marked variations in the natural history of the disease and the occurrence of spontaneous remissions, the therapeutic effectiveness of any single drug or group of drugs is difficult to evaluate. In one report of 11 cases, 3 patients received local radiation therapy, 5 were given systemic corticosteroid treatment, 1 responded to vinblastine, and 4 had spontaneous remissions. Disease did not recur in the skin or other organs during a follow-up period of 1 to 8 years. Since relapses may occur as long as 5 to 10 years following remissions, it is possible that the duration of follow-up was insufficient to gauge the success of therapy.

In two of our patients with "pure" cutaneous histiocytosis, oral treatment with prednisone was ineffective. Dramatic resolution of the lesions occurred following four once-weekly injections of vincristine, 2.0 mg per square meter. One patient subsequently relapsed and responded to oral doses of Cytoxan, 2.5 mg per kg per day, which were continued for 1 year.

The effectiveness of vinca alkaloids and other chemotherapeutic drugs has been established by their capacity to control disease in patients with involvement of the skin and extracutaneous sites. A variety of drugs has been used, including vinblastine, vincrisine, 6-mercaptopurine, methotrexate, cyclophosphamide, chlorambucil, procarbazine, and daunomycin. Either singly or in combination, these drugs may be effective. Because of their short- and long-term toxic effects, they should be administered by someone familiar with their side effects.

Recently a 20-year-old man with recurrent and crippling disease received an allogeneic bone marrow transplant. Obviously this type of therapy should be reserved for patients who have a severely crippling or life-threatening form of the disease. Another form of therapy currently being evaluated is a thymic extract. Early observations suggest that it may be effective in controlling the disease in patients with multisystem involvement.

Longitudinal observations of the patient are essential to determine whether the disease has affected organs other than the skin. For example, the subject with presumed "pure" cutaneous histiocytosis who suddenly develops polyuria and polydipsia may have histiocytic involvement of the hypothalamic-pituitary axis. In this situation immediate radiation therapy of the suprasellar and sellar regions is indicated. In general, radiotherapy should not be used in the patient with solitary skin involvement.

MUCOUS MEMBRANE DISEASES

RECURRENT APHTHOUS STOMATITIS

ROY S. ROGERS III, M.D.

Recurrent aphthous stomatitis is not a disease *sui generis* but rather a mucosal manifestation of a variety of conditions characterized by aphthous ulcers of the mucosa. Thus, underlying conditions may be identified in approximately 30 percent of the patients (Table 1). In assessing a patient with recurrent aphthous stomatitis, it is incumbent upon the clinician to exclude underlying conditions. Unfortunately, in 70 percent of the patients the disease remains idiopathic. This represents a challenge to clinical investigation.

BEHÇET'S SYNDROME

Behçet's syndrome is characterized by recurrent oral ulcers, recurrent genital ulcers, and recurrent ocular inflammation. This condition is discussed in more detail elsewhere in the book.

FORMES FRUSTES OF BEHÇET'S SYNDROME: SEVERE APHTHOSIS

Some patients suffer recurrent oral ulcers with occasional genital ulcerations of an aphthous nature. Few of them develop the full blown Behçet syndrome, although the disease activity may be intense and more continuous than intermittent. Likewise some patients with aphthous ulcers limited to the oral mucosa have severe and frequent episodes, sometimes even continuous disease activity with new lesions developing as old ones heal. These patients do not respond to the usual therapeutic approaches and may require aggressive therapy.

Among the therapeutic alternatives are dapsone, colchicine, thalidomide and other nonsteroidal anti-inflammatory drugs. Dapsone may act on the function of the polymorphonuclear leukocyte or monocyte. The treatment course would be similar to that used to treat dermatitis herpetiformis (see chapter on *Dermatitis Herpetiformis*). Colchicine is an anti-inflammatory drug that perturbs spindle function and may act on polymorphonuclear leukocytes or migrating inflammatory cells or the release of prostaglandins. The dosage is 0.6 mg daily for 1 week, twice daily for the second week, and then three times daily until a remission is achieved. The dose is tapered to the lowest dose that maintains a remission. Cholchicine is a toxic drug, particularly to the gastrointestinal tract, causing such side effects as nausea, vomiting, diarrhea, and abdominal pain. Both dapsone and colchicine should ameliorate the disease activity in 6 to 12 weeks. If a beneficial effect is noted, long-term administration, as for dermatitis herpetiformis or gout, may be considered. If no therapeutic benefit is noted in 6 to 12 weeks, the trial may be abandoned.

Thalidomide is a potentially highly toxic drug that appears to possess anti-inflammatory activity. Teratogenicity and peripheral neuropathy are two of its major potential complications. Some patients with severe aphthosis have responded to doses of 100 to 200 mg per day. Use of thalidomide in women of child bearing age requires very careful discussion and consideration. Other nonsteroidal anti-inflammatory drugs such as indomethacin may be tried.

Some patients require intermittent systemic prednisone therapy. For long-standing severe episodes, doses in the range of 1 mg per kg per day are necessary to abort the disease activity and induce a remission. This regimen would be tapered over a 3 to 6 week period and discontinued. For shorter, less severe episodes, a 2 to 3 week course of systemic corticosteroid therapy, starting with doses of 0.5 to 0.75 mg per kg per day, may be effective. Systemic corticosteroid use should remain intermittent,

TABLE 1 Conditions Associated with Recurrent Aphthous Stomatitis

Condition	% of Population
Behçet's syndrome	1
Severe aphthosis	2
Menstrually related disorder	2
Inflammatory bowel disease	1
Gluten sensitive enteropathy	2
Hematinic deficiencies	22
Idiopathic disorder	70
	100

treating disabling and severe episodes as necessary.

None of these therapeutic approaches induces a long-term remission. Therefore, the clinician must be cautious and observe the patient for side effects of long-term drug administration.

MENSTRUALLY RELATED APHTHOUS STOMATITIS

Some women describe a flare of lesions in the premenstual phase of the menstrual cycle. These patients respond to the oral administration of estrogen dominated contraceptives such as Ovulen. A period of 3 to 6 months may be necessary to note the beneficial effect of the anovulatory drug. The mechanism of action is obscure, although estrogen promotes mucosal hyperkeratosis, which may protect against trauma.

INFLAMMATORY BOWEL DISEASE

Crohn's disease and ulcerative colitis are associated with recurrent aphthous stomatitis. Indeed oral aphthous ulcers may presage a flare of the bowel disease. The aphthous stomatitis tends to improve with improvement of the underlying condition.

GLUTEN SENSITIVE ENTEROPATHY

Patients with gluten sensitivity often are afflicted with recurrent aphthous stomatitis. As the bowel disease improves with gluten restriction, so do the oral aphthous ulcers. Some patients with no evidence of gluten sensitive enteropathy note a marked diminution of aphthous ulcer activity with a gluten free diet.

HEMATINIC DEFICIENCIES

According to some investigators, as many as one in five patients with oral aphthous ulcers have a deficiency of vitamin B_{12}, folate, or iron, or a combination of two or three of these hematinic drugs. Replacement of the deficiency yields a remission or marked decrease in disease activity in the majority of patients. This process takes 1 to 3 months. Vitamin B_{12} deficiency should be confirmed by appropriate testing. Doses are standard replacement doses. Our studies indicate that our patient population is as likely to be deficient as the British populations studied.

ZINC DEFICIENCY

We have not confirmed a zinc deficient subpopulation among sufferers of recurrent aphthous stomatitis.

IDIOPATHIC RECURRENT APHTHOUS STOMATITIS

The majority of patients who suffer from recurrent aphthous ulcerations have few episodes of short duration. The etiology remains obscure. Symptomatic therapy includes viscous lidocaine suspension to anesthetize the mucosa. This may be used before meals and at bedtime. Topical application of local anesthetics such as Diclone may be used throughout the day to alleviate pain. Proprietary, over-the-counter preparations such as Cank-Aid are also helpful in alleviating symptoms. A warm saline mouthwash (1 teaspoon salt to 1 pint water) may be salutary.

In view of the putative immunologic mechanism involved in the pathogenesis of recurrent aphthous stomatitis, the topical application of corticosteroids may ameliorate or abort early lesions. Potent fluorinated corticosteroids in ointment, cream, or gel bases are applied to early lesions every 1 to 2 hours while the patient is awake. Once the ulcer is fully developed, topical application of corticosteroids should be discontinued, as they may retard wound healing. Symptomatic measures are then used.

Some episodes are aborted by topical application of caustics such as silver nitrate. These medicaments provide pain relief and convert the lesion to a burn wound.

Topical or systemic doses of antibiotics may provide benefit in individual episodes. For the herpetiform variant of recurrent aphthous stomatitis, tetracycline may be administered. Double blind studies have failed to demonstrate efficacy but a trial is recommended.

COMMENTS

Spontaneous long-term remission may be anticipated in the majority of patients with the minor and herpetiform variants. Major aphthous ulcers tend to be a more chronic problem. Most therapeutic trials are characterized by a study population that is heterogeneous and not divided into the aforementioned subsets. Therefore, studies are difficult to perform and interpret. Nonetheless numerous double blind studies have been conducted, and the majority have failed to demonstrate efficacy of various therapeutic trials. This points out the need for the clinician to evaluate the patient with recurrent aphthous stomatitis with respect to classification into one of the subsets.

In treating recurrent aphthous stomatitis, therapeutic nihilism is not appropriate as long as it is tempered with the cautious use of the numerous therapeutic measures just described.

DISEASES OF CUTANEOUS APPENDAGES

ALOPECIA AREATA

RONALD J. SWEREN, M.D.

Alopecia areata is a nonscarring alopecia of unknown etiology that classically begins as one or more well defined, discrete patches of hair loss on the scalp. Although it is usually asymptomatic, patients occasionally describe "paresthesias" in areas of involvement. The clinical course is unpredictable, with periods of regrowth and recurrence often without regard to therapy. Disease activity may be described as active (continuing hair loss) or stable. Progression of hair loss with coalescence of patches results in alopecia totalis, the loss of all or most of the scalp hair. Alopecia universalis is the loss of all or most of the body hair.

The diagnosis usually can be made clinically. Physical examination reveals sharply circumscribed patches of complete hair loss (usually) with an otherwise normal appearing scalp. Exclamation point hairs are said to be diagnostic; these are short broken hairs that are tapered much like an "exclamation point," usually present at the periphery of the lesion. Associated nail findings may include splitting of the nail plate, onycholysis, and pitting. Biopsy of the scalp is not usually necessary but when done, reveals a perifollicular round cell infiltrate. Uncommonly hair loss may be rapid, with complete loss in a few weeks or months. Rarely patches of hair loss may be incomplete, making the diagnosis of alopecia areata more difficult.

A poor prognosis has been associated with an early age of onset, disease of longer than 1 year's duration, rapid progression, and "ophiasis"—a band of alopecia extending from the postauricular scalp on one side to the other side.

TREATMENT

The evaluation of various modalities of therapy remains difficult because of the capricious nature of this disease. My approach to the patient with alopecia areata depends on several factors—the activity and extent of disease, the age of the patient, and the concerns of the patient, both real and imagined (Table 1).

I usually begin with topical corticosteroid therapy with Diprolene or Temorate, either the cream or the ointment, which is applied to the involved areas once or twice a day. Follow-up examination is usually recommended in 4 to 6 weeks. If any hair regrowth is noted, therapy is continued. A lack of response or continued hair loss indicates a need for additional or alternate therapy.

Intralesional corticosteroid therapy (triamcinolone, 3 to 10 mg per milliliter) has been shown to be useful in individuals with a few localized patches of alopecia. Multiple injections may preclude its use in individuals with numerous patches or in children, but it may be especially useful for treating cosmetically important areas such as the eyebrows. Unfortunately hair regrowth is not permanent and repeated injections may be necessary to maintain regrowth. The most significant complication is localized atrophy at the site of involvement (Table 2).

Systemic corticosteroid therapy should be reserved for the few individuals with rapidly aggressive hair loss. Side effects of chronic use are obvious. Again, hair regrowth may be transient, with hair loss recurring as the dosage of medication is tapered.

Minoxidil is a potent antihypertensive drug that, when applied topically, has been shown to induce hair regrowth in both androgenetic alopecia and alopecia areata. Its mechanism of action remains unknown, although both immune modulation and vasodilation have been proposed as mechanisms of action. The topical use of minoxidil (Rogaine) remains unapproved by the FDA, although its approval is anticipated. Patients are given a 2 or 3 percent solution of minoxidil to apply to involved areas twice a day (for the formula see Table 3). Unfortunately minoxi-

TABLE 1 My Approach to the Patient with Alopecia Areata

Localized disease
   Topical corticosteroid therapy
   Intralesional corticosteroid therapy (except in children)
   Topical minoxidil therapy
   Short contact anthralin therapy

Numerous patches or alopecia totalis-universalis
   Same as above
   Limited intralesional corticosteroid therapy for eyebrows
   Consider 4 to 6 week course of prednisone early in disease (especially if rapid loss) after appropriate discussion with patient, PUVA

TABLE 2   Complications of Therapy

Topical corticosteroid therapy:	Atrophy, systemic absorption
Intralesional corticosteroid therapy:	Atrophy, systemic absorption, central retinal artery thrombosis (frontal scalp)
Systemic corticosteroid therapy:	Fluid retention, increased appetite, mood elevation or depression, fat redistribution, acne, cataracts, increased infections
Anthralin:	Irritant dermatitis
Minoxidil:	Irritant dermatitis, folliculitis, allergic contact dermatitis
PUVA:	Phototoxicity ("sunburn"), pruritus, nausea, skin cancer

dil has been found to be effective in only 30 to 40 percent of the patients studied.

This application of irritants to the scalp to promote hair regrowth, the most popular of which is anthralin, has regained renewed interest. Drithocreme or Lasan cream (concentrations of 0.1 to 1 percent) is applied to involved areas of the scalp for increasing lengths of time using the short contact anthralin therapy (SCAT) protocol used for the treatment of psoriasis. Therapy is continued until mild erythema is attained and then continued until hair regrowth is noted or lack of progress is documented. It is unclear whether the reaction caused by anthralin represents an irritant or true allergic contact dermatitis. Nonetheless investigators have hypothesized that the production of an inflammatory response allows for the generation of suppressor T cells and immunoregulation. True allergic contact dermatitis may be induced with any of the following:

TABLE 3   Formula for 3 Percent Minoxidil (to make 50 ml)

1.5 minoxidil
30% propylene glycol (must have 10% propylene glycol for every 1% minoxidil)
Vehicle N qs ad 50 ml
Let sit for 3 days
Filter three times
Vehicle N qs ad 50 ml (to replace volume lost by filtering)
SIG: apply twice daily

dinitrochlorobenzene, squaric acid dibutylester, and diphencyprone. Recently dinitrochlorobenzene has been shown by the Ames test to be mutagenic, which should limit its clinical usefulness.

Patients with alopecia totalis or universalis may be treated with photochemotherapy or PUVA (psoralens and UVA). Immune modulation is suspected as the mechanism of action. Treatment protocols have included topical psoralen therapy and local UVA, oral doses of psoralens and local UVA, and oral psoralen therapy and whole body UVA. Unfortunately hair regrowth makes it more difficult for light to penetrate to the scalp, making it a less effective therapy once a response is noted.

Other therapies currently under investigation include inosiplex, transfer factor, and cyclosporine. Their clinical use must await more extensive, controlled studies.

Hair pieces and wigs cannot be dismissed in the treatment of patients with alopecia areata. For some individuals this is a markedly severe psychosocial disease. Therapy may be frustrating to both patient and clinician. Time must be spent with these patients to answer all questions as honestly as possible while reassuring them that many individuals do experience hair regrowth. When necessary, counseling should be encouraged. Most important, patients should be given the address of the local or national chapter of the Alopecia Areata Foundation, so that they can benefit from an excellent "peer" support group (National Alopecia Areata Foundation, P.O. Box 5027, Mill Valley, CA 94941).

NAIL DISORDERS

LAWRENCE A. NORTON, M.D.

Treatable disorders of the nails include infections, tumors, trauma, and dermatologic diseases. Systemic and topical drug reactions, including reactions to cosmetics and occupational diseases, are not included here because their treatment consists merely of recognizing and avoiding the causative agent.

The nail is a unit or organ that consists of the nail plate, nail folds, nail matrix, nail bed, and hyponychium. Any or all parts of the unit may be affected by disease, and the choice of treatment depends on the part affected.

INFECTIONS

The most common nail infections are fungal. The term onychomycosis refers to infection of the nail with dermatophytes, nondermatophytes, or *Candida*. It is helpful to classify these infections by the route of invasion taken by the responsible organism. *Candida albicans* does not invade the nail plate except in the special disorder of mucocutaneous candidiasis found in immunodeficient patients. This organism is found, however, in the nail folds in paronychia and frequently in onycholysis. Dermatophytes and nondermatophytic fungi may enter the nail unit distally (distal subungual onychomycosis), superficially (superficial white onychomycosis), or proximally via the proximal nail fold (proximal subungual onychomycosis).

Superficial invasion of the nail plate, which occurs only on the toenails, is easily recognized as a chalky white to yellow-white discoloration of the surface of the nail plate. The organism, which is usually *T. mentagrophytes* or a nondermatophyte, can be eliminated by mechanical scraping of the white material with a scalpel blade. Scraping should be followed by the topical application of clotrimazole, 1 percent, miconazole, 2 percent, econazole, 1 percent, ketoconazole, 2 percent, or haloprogin, 1 percent, in cream or lotion form for 2 to 3 weeks.

In distal subungual and proximal subungual onychomycosis, the responsible organism should be identified by microscopic examination and culture because topical treatment of these infections is almost universally unsuccessful and several conditions, including psoriasis, eczema, lichen planus, contact dermatitis, and traumatic nail injuries, may mimic onychomycosis. If culture proof of a susceptible organism (i.e., a dermatophyte) is not achieved, biopsy of the nail bed with periodic acid–Schiff staining of the specimen may demonstrate fungi.

Once the diagnosis has been established, the treatment of choice is griseofulvin in an adequate dosage until the nails are clear by gross and microscopic examination. The mechanism of action of griseofulvin is not completely proven, but evidence suggests that this fungistatic drug works by inhibiting production of cytoplasmic microtubules, which in turn affect synthesis of the hyphal cell walls. The duration of treatment varies with the degree of involvement, but is usually 5 to 6 months for the fingernails and 8 to 12 months for the toenails. The prospect of cure is much better on the upper than on the lower extremities, and the patient should be advised of the length and expense of treatment required.

The most common side effect is headache, but gastrointestinal distress, fatigue, and photosensitivity may occur. Bone marrow suppression and leukopenia are extremely rare, but blood surveys (at 1- to 3-month intervals) are advisable during prolonged courses of therapy. Griseofulvin interacts with some other drugs, most notably warfarin and barbiturates, requiring adjustment in dosage. Cross reaction with known penicillin allergy has not been reported.

The decision to treat must take into account the fact that reinfection may occur after treatment. If only one or two digits are involved, the duration of treatment can be significantly shortened by initial surgical or chemical avulsion of the involved nails prior to griseofulvin administration. The dosage of griseofulvin is 500 mg of the microsize form twice a day or 250 mg of the ultramicrosize polyethylene glycol products twice a day. The patient should be examined at 1- to 2-month intervals to see whether areas of nail plate involvement are progressing distally consistent with the expected rate of nail growth. If not, the dose should be doubled and monthly follow-up continued. Resistance of dermatophytes to griseofulvin has been reported but is rare; failure of treatment is more likely to be due to patient noncompliance.

If a patient cannot tolerate griseofulvin because of side effects or drug interactions, or if the organism is resistant, an alternative approach is to remove the involved nails either surgically or chemically by the Farber and South technique, using 40 percent urea paste. This paste is formulated by mixing 40 percent urea, 20 percent anhydrous lanolin, 5 percent white wax, and 35 percent white petrolatum. The paste is applied to the nail plate after protecting surrounding skin and left on under an occlusive dressing for 7 to 10 days. After this the nail plate may be removed easily. Alternative chemicals for nonsurgical removal are 50 percent potassium iodide or a mixture of 20 percent urea with 10 percent salicylic acid. The chemical removal is followed by topical application of one of the previously mentioned antifungal drugs until a new nail has grown. The incidence of success with this approach has been disappointing.

A final treatment possibility is the new drug ketoconazole, which is not yet approved for use in onychomycosis by the FDA. In extreme cases of fingernail involvement, treatment with this drug may be justified, provided the patient is well aware of the potential side effects of hepatotoxicity, endocrine effects, neuromuscular complaints, and cutaneous eruptions. Its mechanism of action is to inhibit ergosterol synthesis, which is necessary for normal cell membrane permeability in fungi. The dosage is 200 mg per day for the same period as that required for griseofulvin therapy. The patient should be educated regarding symptoms of toxicity and should be monitored with liver function tests.

In many cases, particularly when only the toenails are involved, no treatment may be the best choice in terms of risk-benefit.

Acute paronychia, a bacterial infection of the nail folds, usually follows trauma. *Staphylococcus* and *streptococcus* are the most common causative organisms. Treatment consists of warm soaks for 15 minutes three times a day with systemic antibiotic therapy. Drainage present should be cultured for sensitivity studies. I prescribe erythromycin, 250 mg four times daily, unless sensitivities indicate the need for a more specific drug. Surgical drainage is rarely needed.

Chronic paronychia lasting weeks or months is generally caused by occupational exposure to moisture (e.g., in waitresses, bartenders, beauticians), by chemical irritation, or by foreign bodies (e.g., metal filings, hair, steel wool). Emphasis should be placed on dryness, avoidance of soaks and occlusive dressings, and thorough drying after washing. When available, a hair dryer is a helpful instrument for achieving dryness in the nail folds.

In most such infections *Candida* or a mixture of *Candida* and bacteria is discovered on culture. Four percent thymol in absolute alcohol, applied topically three times a day, helps to maintain dryness, and this is usually combined with clotrimazole, miconazole, econazole, or ketoconazole topically. If cultures show predominantly bacterial growth, an antibiotic such as bacitracin, neomycin, or gentamicin should be used topically.

Onycholysis, or separation of the nail plate from the nail bed, has multiple causes. The differential diagnosis includes psoriasis, allergic contact dermatitis, dermatophyte infection, photoallergy, and thyroid disease. The rapidity of onset, the number of digits involved, and accompanying skin and nail changes, as well as the drug history, help to distinguish these conditions. Onycholysis usually involves just one or two digits. It is idiopathic in origin but usually occurs in females, involves fingernails only, and like paronychia, may be associated with moisture exposure, trauma, and occupation. The treatment consists of clipping the involved nails back to the most proximal portion of separation, which is marked by a pink transverse band. Since scrapings generally reveal yeast and cultures isolate *Candida*, dryness should be emphasized and an antiyeast drug such as nystatin, amphotericin B, miconazole, or clotrimazole, applied topically. Repeat trimmings may be necessary at monthly intervals until the lysis is resolved. Extreme cases may require nail avulsion for cure.

Bacteria have already been incriminated as playing a role in paronychia. They seldom involve the nail plate per se, except in the cases of green nails produced by *Pseudomonas aeruginosa*. The recommended treatment consists of cutting back the nails and the topical application of colistin sulfate otic suspension, 1 percent silver sulfadiazine cream, or gentamicin, 0.1 percent cream.

The most common viral problem involving nails is warts. Those involving nail grooves or the nail bed are probably the most difficult to eradicate. Treatment resistance is compounded if the patient is a chronic nail biter or if he has hand eczema with fissuring of the digits.

If the warts are multiple and large, I usually initiate treatment with either plain Zonas tape occlusion or 40 percent salicylic acid plaster covered with plain tape. This measure usually softens the warts, reduces their size, and may even eliminate them. In children it allows time for establishing rapport and building confidence. The involved fingers are kept occluded for 6 days each week. If this treatment fails or is only partially effective, remaining wart tissue may be removed by curettage and desiccation under local anesthesia without epinephrine, by topical di- or trichloroacetic acid application, or by cryotherapy. In addition, the patient may be instructed to use 16.7 percent lactic acid and 16.7 percent salicylic acid in flexible collodion at home.

The treatment that I now find to be most effective is intralesional injection of bleomycin sulfate followed immediately by cryotherapy. The patient should be informed that this use of the drug is not yet FDA approved, and the local side effects of necrosis and pain should be explained. Bleomycin is a glycopeptide antibiotic that inhibits mitosis and DNA synthesis. It is believed that epidermal microsomal enzymes act synergistically with the drug to produce DNA chain breakage in the virus. The intralesional injection consists of 0.1 to 0.2 ml of a 0.01 percent solution of bleomycin, with or without prior local anesthesia. This is followed by a 10- to 15-second application of liquid nitrogen. The wart turns black in 4 to 5 days and can be dissected away in 10 days. Since Raynaud's phenomenon has been reported with higher dosages of this drug, I never inject more than one wart on a single digit at a time and never treat a wart more than twice by this technique. Contraindications to bleomycin treatment should include collagen vascular disease, impaired circulation, a long-standing wart without biopsy, and pregnancy.

A second viral infection that may involve the nail folds is herpes simplex (herpetic whitlow). Recognition is the important issue here, and surgery, which can make the condition worse, is to be avoided. If, on the basis of the history, it appears to be a primary infection, following culture of the virus acyclovir, 200 mg given orally five times a day for 10 days, may reduce the pain and shorten the illness.

TUMORS

Tumors involving the nail unit may be divided into benign, premalignant, and malignant types. The most common benign tumors of the nail are warts (already discussed under infections), mucous (myxoid mucoid) cysts, pyogenic granulomas, and fibromas.

Mucous Cysts

A mucous cyst is a localized smooth swelling of the dorsum of the digit between the distal interphalangeal joint and the proximal nail fold. The nail plate usually displays a depressed longitudinal groove distal to the tumor. In a high percentage of cases there is evidence of osteoarthritis in the distal joint. The tumor may also be subungual in the nail bed or matrix. Some cysts connect with the distal joint space and some do not. If the patient is asymptomatic, frequent puncture of the cyst with a sterile needle expressing the viscid material may eventually eliminate the cyst.

Intralesional injection of triamcinolone acetonide, 5 mg per milliliter, or betamethasone sodium phosphate and betamethasone acetate, 3 mg per milliliter, in a volume of 0.1 ml to 0.2 ml at 3-week intervals may be curative. More resistant cases require destruction with curettage and desiccation, cryotherapy with a 15- to 20-second application and 60 second thaw time, or, finally, wide excision and grafting or a rotation flap. Caution should be taken to avoid matrix injury whenever possible. When the cyst is located in the distal portion of the proximal nail fold, simple excision of the nail fold, including the cyst, allowing for healing by secondary intention, may be very satisfactory.

Pyogenic Granulomas

Pyogenic granulomas develop as a result of injury, most commonly from pulling a hang nail or secondary to an ingrown nail. They are easily destroyed by curettage and desiccation, but a biopsy specimen should be taken prior to electrodesiccation because early malignant disease may mimic the lesion.

Periungual Fibromas

Periungual fibromas (Koenen's tumors) are significant as markers of tuberous sclerosis, but may exist without the disease. Neurofibromas, acquired digital fibrokeratomas, and other benign fibrous tumors also may occur in this location. They can be locally excised or destroyed by electrosurgery. When they are sizable and involve the lateral folds, the patient should be advised that temporary or permanent damage to the sensory nerve is a possible complication.

Keratoacanthoma of the nail bed behaves differently from the same tumor elsewhere and is difficult to recognize because of its subungual location. As elsewhere, it grows rapidly and because of its location produces early bone erosion. The tumor is less likely to resolve than keratoacanthomas elsewhere, or else pain compels the patient to be treated before that event occurs.

All subungual tumors should be studied by diagnostic radiography. Following that, the nail should be avulsed and the lesion subjected to biopsy followed by local destruction. In cases of multiple mutilating subungual tumors, systemic treatment with methotrexate or intralesional 5-fluorouracil or bleomycin therapy should be considered. Histologic differentiation from squamous cell cancer may be difficult, but the latter grows slowly and invades bone late.

Bowen's Disease

Bowen's disease of the nail bed is being reported more frequently and probably represents the horizontal growth phase of squamous cell cancer. Because electrosurgery and topical 5-fluorouracil therapy have both resulted in a disappointing number of recurrences, my choice of treatment for both Bowen's disease and frank squamous cell cancer is Mohs microscopically controlled surgery. This affords maximal preservation of function. Amputation seems too radical for a tumor that is known to metastasize late, and x-ray therapy also is less desirable.

Melanoma

Melanoma of the nail bed has undergone extensive study in the past 5 years. The biologic behavior of this tumor is different from that of melanoma of the skin and is more similar to that of mucous membrane melanoma. Because of certain distinct histologic features, the most common form of melanoma in this area is referred to as acral lentiginous melanoma.

The most important aspect of treatment, and unfortunately the most difficult, is early diagnosis. Recent series show that the chances for survival depends much more on the level of invasion at the time of diagnosis than on treatment. To trace this dilemma back to its origin, the starting point is the pigmented nail band. With the exception of the extremely rare amelanotic melanomas, some form of pigmentation is present when this tumor begins to form. This may be masked by infection or a traumatic injury. Once pigmentation is recognized, hematoma must be ruled out, along with benign melanocytic hyperplasia, atypical melanocytic hyperplasia, pigmented nevus, or acral lentiginous melanoma. Table 1 lists a differential diagnosis of benign pigmentation of the nail bed. The significance of pigmentation is far more serious if these conditions are ruled out. Its presence in a Caucasian, an onset after the age of 40 years, and involvement of the big toe or thumb greatly increase the likelihood of malignant disease. Biopsy requires good visualization of the matrix after formation of a flap in the proximal nail fold and avulsion of the nail followed by removal of all the apparent source of pigmentation. If pigmentation persists following a benign biopsy, the burden of proof is on the physician to show that the remaining source of pigmentation is benign. Biologically melanoma of the nail bed has a

TABLE 1   Benign Causes of Hyperpigmentation of the Nail Bed

Cancer chemotherapy
X-ray therapy
Trauma
Heavy metal exposure
Normal in high percentage of blacks and some Orientals
Peutz-Jeghers syndrome
Laugier's syndrome
Cushing's syndrome (postsurgical)
Pigmented nevi
Idiopathic benign melanocytic hyperplasia
Hematoma
Antimalarial drugs
Chlorpromazine

horizontal growth phase followed by a vertical growth phase. Although superficial spreading melanoma and lentigo maligna melanoma have been reported in this area, the overwhelming majority of tumors are the acral lentiginous variety. This is recognizable by giant melanocytes with large dendrites in the basal layer, absence of pagetoid cells, and other histologic features.

The treatment is amputation of the digit. Recent series show no increase in survival with more radical amputation or node resections. If nodal involvement or other distant metastases are present at the time of diagnosis, chemotherapy or immunotherapy must be considered. Table 2 summarizes the treatment approaches to nail tumors.

TRAUMA

The most common traumatic injury to the nail is subungual hematoma. When the injury is acute and painful, instant relief may be obtained by touching a red hot, opened paperclip to the nail plate until it is penetrated, releasing the underlying blood. Chronic asymptomatic accumulation of blood under the nail is particularly common in people who engage in tennis, basketball, and running. Normally this accumulation progresses outward with outward growth of the nail plate. Sometimes, however, the hematoma does not migrate and biopsy is required after 3 to 4 months to rule out melanin as the source of pigment.

Another common traumatic entity of the nail is the self-induced deformity of habit tic. This condition is characterized by horizontal ridges over the central portion of the nail plates, which are usually depressed; the cuticles and proximal nail folds appear irritated and the lunulae are enlarged. This deformity is almost always bilateral on the thumb nails, but other nails may be involved. The patient grinds the second, third, and fourth nail plate into the proximal nail plate or proximal nail fold as a neurotic habit. Tactful explanation to the patient and the topical application of steroid cream covered with Blenderm tape over the involved area often succeed in breaking the habit.

Split nails vary from a fine line extending longitudi-nally the length of the nail plate, with a wedge of subungual hyperkeratotic material at the distal end, to complete lengthwise separation of the nail plate into two sections. The cause is usually a traumatic injury. The source of the defect is in the nail matrix. The degree of defect and the degree to which the patent is bothered by catching the nail on objects determine whether surgical correction is advisable. If elected, this treatment requires exploration of the matrix, excision of visible scar tissue, and careful realignment of the matrix after undermining.

Ingrown toenails result from improperly-fitting shoes, nail picking, or orthopaedic deformities that place unusual stress on the normal nail plate–soft tissue relationship. The nail plate undermines the skin, and a foreign body reaction occurs. The choice of treatment depends on the severity of the condition. In an early ingrown toenail, there is swelling and redness of the distal lateral nail fold. The nail should be cut straight across and the distal corner of the nail plate wedged with cotton to keep it from impinging on the nail fold. The patient can be taught to replace the cotton until a normal distal edge of nail plate is established. In more advanced cases there is more pronounced swelling of the lateral nail fold, granulation tissue, and drainage. The patient has usually cut the nail plate back into the corner, and lateral to that there is a buried spike of nail. This spike should be excised under local anesthesia and the granulation either excised or cauterized with silver nitrate. Postsurgical treatment consists of warm water soaks twice a day followed by topical antibiotic therapy. Long-standing ingrown nails with marked distortion of the end of the toe and a deeply embedded nail may require systemic antibiotic therapy and soaks initially to clear up infection prior to surgical correction. The treatment of choice is then to permanently narrow the nail by excising the lateral portion of the matrix on the involved side. This requires an incision into the proximal nail fold to obtain good visualization of the entire proximal horn of the matrix. Following excision, the incision is sutured, excess granulation tissue removed, and a nonadherent dressing applied.

An alternative method is chemical destruction of the lateral matrix with 89 percent phenol (Otto Boll method)

TABLE 2 Therapy of Nail Tumors

Therapy	Kinds of Tumor
Local destructive techniques or injection (office procedure)	Warts, fibromas, neuro-fibromas, fibrokeratomas, pyogenic granulomas, mucous cysts, keratoacanthomas
Sterile operating room surgery	Exostoses (local excision), osteochondromas, enchondromas, glomus tumors, giant cell tumors of the tendon sheath, melanoma (amputation)
Mohs microscopically directed surgery	Bowen's disease, squamous cell cancer, basal cell cancer

applied for 2 minutes, followed by neutralization with alcohol. The surrounding skin should be protected with petrolateum when applying the phenol. Another technique for eliminating the lateral matrix is use of the carbon-dioxide laser. Those familiar with this instrument note the advantages of a bloodless field and less postoperative pain.

DERMATOLOGIC DISEASES

Both psoriasis and lichen planus may cause extensive nail unit changes, and to some extent, these changes can be lessened by treatment. The classic signs of psoriasis of the nail are pitting of the nail plate, onycholysis, subungual hyperkeratosis, and accumulation of a serum-like material under the plate (oil spot sign). Evidence of psoriasis is usually present elsewhere on the skin and scalp. If not, scrapings and cultures and sometimes biopsy are needed to rule out fungal infection.

Treatment of more generalized psoriasis may help the nails secondarily (see chapter on *Psoriasis*).

Direct treatment of the nails may be attempted with triamcinolone acetonide, 0.5 percent cream, fluocinolone acetonide, 0.2 percent cream, clobetasol propionate, 0.05 percent cream or ointment, or betamethasone dipropionate, 0.05 percent cream or ointment, two times a day with Saran Wrap or Blenderm tape occlusion at night. This should be applied to the nail folds and nail plate. An alternative to occlusion is to mix the steroid cream with 10 percent benzoyl peroxide gel or tretinoin, 0.025 percent gel. A greater concentration of steroid can be delivered to the matrix by direct intradermal injection with a 26 gauge needle. Triamcinolone acetonide, 5 mg per milliliter, or betamethasone sodium phosphate or betamethasone acetate, 3 mg per milliliter, is injected in doses of 0.2 to 0.4 ml per nail. Some patients respond to short contact therapy with 1 percent anthralin paste applied for one-half hour daily. The topical application of 5-fluorouracil cream has been reported to help, but results in my practice have been disappointing.

With the ready accessibility of hand and foot ultraviolet light boxes for psoralen-plus-light therapy (PUVA), this

TABLE 3 Treatment for Psoriasis of Nails

0.5% triamcinolone acetonide topically with occlusion

0.5% triamcinolone acetonide topically with 10% benzoyl peroxide—or with 0.025% tretinoin gel

Intralesional injection of triamcinolone acetonide, 5 mg/ml

Topical application of 5-fluorouracil

Anthralin paste, 0.1 to 0.5%

PUVA

X-ray therapy

modality may well be the best approach, particularly if the patient is already receiving therapy for generalized psoriasis. Recent studies indicate that the nail plate prevents a significant percentage of light from penetrating. Therefore, the dosage has to be higher than for similar involvement of adjacent skin (see chapter on *Psoriasis*). The same can be said for superficial x-ray therapy. Table 3 summarizes the treatment approaches to nail psoriasis.

Lichen planus produces dystrophic changes in the nail, most commonly displayed as longitudinal ridging and grooving, thinning of the nail plate, ground-glass opaqueness of the nail plate, pterygium formation, and visible papules sometimes on the nail folds or nail bed. The first three treatments listed for psoriasis are appropriate. The disease process may be severe (bullous lichen planus), with the possible sequela of total nail destruction. In these cases prednisone in systemic doses of 50 to 60 mg per day may be justified for limited periods of time, tapering as the inflammation subsides.

Brittle nails are the equivalent of xerosis in the skin. The normal nail contains 18 percent water by weight. If the content falls below 16 percent, brittle nails result. Water penetrates the nail plate well, but keeping it in the nail is the problem. I have patients soak their nails for 15 minutes and then apply Complex 15 phospholipid moisturizer cream or Lac-Hydrin, 12 percent ammonium lactate lotion.

HIDRADENITIS SUPPURATIVA

JOHN W. SKOUGE, M.D.
THOMAS T. PROVOST, M.D.

Hidradenitis suppurativa is a chronic inflammatory disease of the apocrine sweat glands. It is characterized by "attacks" of tender erythematous abscesses occurring in the axillary and anogenital areas and on the areolae of the breasts. These abscesses slowly enlarge and may perforate the overlying skin, discharging purulent material. If they are not treated, sinus tracks form. These "attacks" may be isolated or may occur simultaneously in multiple apocrine areas and are recurrent. With each recurrence more and more fibrosis and sinus tract formation occur. At worst, large, tender, erythematous, boggy masses with multiple sinus tracks discharging seropurulent material occur in the axillary and anogenital areas.

The initial episode may or may not be associated with a prior local skin condition such as folliculitis or a primary irritant. Hidradenitis suppurativa can be aggravated by obesity and in some cases is associated with acne lesions in other areas of the body. There does not appear to be any familial history or an association with underlying systemic diseases.

TREATMENT

Optimal treatment occurs when the disease is quickly diagnosed in its beginning stage. At that stage, characterized by small, tender, inflammatory pustules in the apocrine regions, systemic antibiotic therapy is the treatment of choice. Although the hidradenitis suppurativa disease process is not produced by a bacterial infection, bacterial contamination of the lesions is common. Therefore, appropriate cultures and sensitivity determinations for both aerobic and anaerobic organisms should be obtained, and these findings should determine the antibiotic employed. Generally in our experience this usually involves the use of tetracycline or a tetracycline derivative (minocycline). Tetracycline, 1.0 to 1.5 g per day, should be employed as the initial treatment for 2 to 4 weeks. At the end of that time, depending on the initial response, the disease process should be reevaluated; if the patient has improved, the tetracycline dosage should be reduced to 500 mg daily. If there is still increased activity, reculturing is done and the antibiotics altered depending on the bacterial sensitivity data.

Other antibiotics that have been employed in the treatment of this phase of hidradenitis suppurativa include erythromycin, penicillin, dicloxacillin, ampicillin, and the cephalosporins. The duration of this antibiotic therapy is empiric, but in the initial episode we usually treat for approximately 3 to 6 months. At the end of that time if there is no evidence of disease activity, we completely taper the antibiotics. Often, however, there is evidence of residual disease activity and we are forced to continue the tetracycline (0.5 g per day) or its equivalent indefinitely. Periodically reculturing is done.

Persistent localized lesions may respond to the local injection of triamcinolone (5 to 10 mg per milliliter). If necessary, these injections may be repeated every 2 to 3 weeks for about 6 weeks. It must be stressed that rapid diagnosis and aggressive initial therapy in this stage of development of hidradenitis suppurativa offer the best chance for a cure.

Complications of this type of therapy are generally minimal. However, with high doses of tetracycline (more than 1.0 g per day) one frequently encounters gastrointestinal upset and on unusual occasions phototoxicity and yeast vaginitis. All can be appropriately handled by alterations in the drug therapy.

Topical antibiotic therapy is advocated by many. We, however, have not found this to be helpful in the treatment of the hidradenitis per se, but these topical preparations are useful as antiperspirants. We advocate topical therapy with erythromycin or clindamycin (Cleocin) to be applied to the area twice a day. Shaving of the axillary hair and use of depilatories are indicated.

During the acute phases in which there are numerous abscesses, many patients obtain symptomatic relief by the application of warm compresses (saline or aluminum subacetate) for half an hour at a time, three to four times a day.

Systemic Steroid Therapy

On unusual occasions in which there are multiple abscesses in the apocrine areas and there has been an initial failure to respond to high dose antibiotic therapy, we prescribe a 2 to 3 week course of prednisone, beginning with 30 to 40 mg daily for 1 week, then 20 mg daily for 1 week, and then 10 mg daily for 1 week before completely tapering. This type of therapy coupled with oral tetracycline therapy is effective in gaining control of the disease process. However, if there is a good deal of scar formation, such aggressive therapy will fail.

Hormone Therapy

On unusual occasions when hidradenitis suppurativa in a woman has failed to respond to conventional antibiotic and anti-inflammatory drugs, oral estrogen therapy is considered. The mechanism of putative therapeutic action is the suppression of the androgen responsive apocrine glands. However, it must be emphasized that there are no data to support this hypothesis.

We have employed Enovid E birth control pills to treat several recalcitrant patients. (This therapy has been continued for 4 to 6 months.) This has been usually a desperation form of therapy used after all else has failed. Unfortunately it is not uniformly successful. Because of the increased thromboembolic complications of high doses of estrogens, we use this form of therapy for no more than 1 year.

Surgical Treatment

Early surgical intervention, in conjunction with medical therapy, is often helpful in the control of early hidradenitis suppurativa. Individual abscesses can be incised and drained under local anesthesia, providing rapid relief. This should be followed with appropriate antibiotics as determined by culture. Intervention at this time may prevent some of the scarring and sinus tract formation that characterize this disease in its later stages.

The sinus tracts that form in this disease process are nearly always superficial, involving only the dermis and subcutis. Again, under local anesthesia, these tracts can be safely unroofed. The extent of the tract is determined by placing a blunt tipped probe into the tract until it can go no farther. The overlying roof then can be removed, using the probe as a guide to the depth and extent. This tissue can be excised with electrocautery, heat cautery, or with a steel blade. The base of the tract need not be desiccated, and the wounds may be allowed to close by secondary intention.

Localized areas of severely involved tissue can be excised and closed primarily. This may provide long-term relief, but because other apocrine gland containing tissue remains behind, recurrences can be expected. Definitive treatment, as recommended for severe disease or disease not responsive to medical management, involves excision of the entire area of skin that contains the affected apocrine glands as well as the diseased tissue affected by sinus tract formation and fibrosis.

For axillary disease a transverse primary closure, as described by Pollock, Vernelli, and Ryan (Plast Reconstr Surg 1972; 31:307-311), can be performed even in the patient with apparently infected, draining sinuses. This procedure permits early mobilization and minimal hospitalization. Various other types of closure have been described for use after axillary vault excision. These include triangular, rhombic, and Z-plasty procedures. Split thickness skin grafting techniques as well as secondary intention healing have also been described.

For extensive perineal disease, wide excision of all involved tissues remains the only definitive treatment. Such procedures may leave a more extensive wound than would secondary intention healing. Secondary intention healing, although necessitating a long recovery period, has provided good results. Split thickness skin graft repairs and various regional flaps have also been described for the repair of wounds in this area.

It is important to remember that squamous cell carcinoma may arise in conjunction with the chronic draining sinuses of hidradenitis suppurativa.

ACNE

PETER E. POCHI, M.D.

Acne is a prevalent skin disorder, with a peak occurrence in the mid to late teens. However, adults are by no means immune from it, and some dermatologists' practices may actually comprise more adults than teenagers with the disease.

Although research on acne in the past two to three decades has elucidated a good deal of information about the pathogenic factors involved, two crucial matters about the disease remain elusive, namely, why it comes and why it goes. With time most cases of acne undergo complete or near complete involution, but the reason for it is a mystery. In terms of early development, susceptible pilosebaceous follicles of the face and trunk are affected, with abnormal keratinization occurring in the follicular epithelium. Again the reason for this follicle disturbance has not been adequately explained. Proliferation of anaerobic diphtheroids (*Propionibacterium acnes*) that require sebaceous lipids for subsistence is a central event in the induction of the inflammatory lesions of acne. These bacteria possess chemoattractant properties for neutrophils that initiate a series of events culminating in the expression of inflammation, both immune and nonimmune mediated. Characteristically an inflammatory lesion lasts 2 to 3 weeks, usually healing without a trace but occasionally leaving behind scars, mostly atrophic but occasionally hypertrophic.

GENERAL THERAPEUTIC APPROACH AND BASIS OF MANAGEMENT

From the foregoing brief summary of the etiologic events in acne, it is evident that such a multifactorial disorder would require a multifaceted therapeutic regimen. This is often desirable and necessary, although a unitarian approach may prove sufficient to control the disease, particularly mild cases or those early in their onset, or as maintenance therapy. Combination treatment may embrace the topical use of two or even three medications or the use of oral as well as topical therapy.

The decision about specific drugs or measures to use in acne depends on two broad considerations, namely, the severity of the acne and the type of acne present, i.e., whether it is predominantly inflammatory or noninflammatory. Before undertaking or recommending treatment it is important that time be taken to obtain an accurate history from the patient concerning the acne. Too often this aspect is overlooked or glossed over quickly. Important in this regard is the natural evolution of the acne and the response to prior treatments, including over the counter preparations. Women should be questioned about menstrual cycles and the presence of other possible manifestations of androgen excess, such as hirsutism or scalp hair recession or thinning. A history of drug ingestion can be important too, since certain medications such as lithium, excessive iodides, and anticonvulsants may aggravate existing acne. Even if little of the history obtained proves helpful for the overall management, the initial visit provides an important basis for a positive interaction between physician and patient. At times the patient, particularly a teenager, may seem indifferent to the physician's inquiry, but the opposite is more often the case.

After examination the disease should be explained to the patient, although the amount of time spent at this point depends on the simplicity or complexity of the problem and the physician's perception of how much of a "didactic" exercise the patient wishes to engage in. However, it is important to mention the general inutility of extrascrupulous cleansing, special diets, and the probable lack of association of the acne with the patient's sexual practices. Once a treatment plan is decided upon, the dermatologist should be sure that the following are explained to the patient: (1) Treatments by and large are suppressive rather than curative, so that therapy must be maintained, or changed if later necessary, until the condition undergoes natural involution, which it does in most cases. (2) Most treatments work by preventing the formation of new lesions rather than by healing more rapidly those lesions already present. Moreover, this preventive effect is not ordinarily observed until 3 to 6 weeks have elapsed. (3) Apropos to this, medications must be applied topically to all the affected areas rather than to individual lesions per se. (4) Trunk acne seems to be less well controlled by topical therapy than facial acne.

ANTIKERATINIZING (COMEDOLYTIC) EFFECT

Tretinoin (retinoic acid) is the most effective drug topically because of its capacity to reverse, at least in part, the abnormal follicular hyperkeratosis, the earliest known event in the formation of the acne lesion. By the same token it can help to prevent the transformation of early noninflammatory microcomedones (lesions not clinically visible) into inflammatory sequelae. Salicylic acid also has a keratolytic action, although its benefit in acne via this mechanism appears to be much less than that of tretinoin. Comedolytic assays have shown benzoyl peroxide to have a similar action, but its effect also seems to be comparatively weak.

The commonest objection patients have to the use of tretinoin is the primary irritant reaction it frequently causes. This can be lessened or even prevented by a number of measures that include waiting 20 to 30 minutes after washing before applying it; when using it at bedtime, not retiring until a half-hour has passed; using it every other day at first, rather than the recommended daily application, to allow for accommodation of the skin to its irritant effect; and at first, especially in the winter or dry climates, using the milder cream preparations. Tretinoin is available in creams (0.05 and 0.1 percent) and gels (0.01 and 0.025 percent) and in a liquid formulation (0.05 percent) (Table 1).

Another complaint patients may have about tretinoin, which is less frequent but more annoying to the patient,

TABLE 1 Tretinoin Preparations

Form	Concentration (%)
Cream	0.05
	0.1
Gel	0.01
	0.025
Liquid	0.05

is that there is a flare-up of the acne in the early weeks of treatment. In my experience this occurs to some extent in about 20 percent of the patients and at times can be quite marked. Fortunately the flare-up subsides within a few weeks or sooner, but very uncommonly the worsening may continue unabated and requires discontinuation of medication.

Oral therapy with isotretinoin, the 13-cis isomer of tretinoin, also, as one might expect, has antikeratinizing properties, but it has other antiacne actions as well. Treatment of acne with this drug is described later in this article.

ANTIMICROBIAL THERAPY

The therapy most commonly utilized for acne is antimicrobial therapy, owing in great measure to the availability of a wide variety of preparations for both topical and oral use. Implicit in the widespread use of antibacterial drugs is the recognition, mentioned earlier, that the inflammatory lesions of acne for which most patients seek a physician's attention result from the presence of *P. acnes* within acne susceptible pilosebaceous follicles. One could postulate, with reasonable certainty, that if these follicles could be depleted of these anaerobic diphtheroids, inflammatory acne could be reduced to zero, regardless of whether abnormal keratinization was affected. In actuality suppression of *P. acnes* by antimicrobial therapy, whether topical or oral, is only partially achievable, although sometimes just enough to effect marked or complete amelioration of the inflammatory lesions.

For mild to moderate cases of inflammatory acne, benzoyl peroxide and topical antibiotic therapy have attained prominence in management. Benzoyl peroxide, longest in use for acne, is available in concentrations ranging from 2.5 to 10 percent and in a variety of vehicles—lotions, creams, gels, washes, and soaps. There are at least 30 different marketed preparations that are available with or without a prescription. The majority of nonprescription products are lotions and creams. There is no evidence that prescription products are more efficacious than over the counter preparations, although it is possible that gel formulations do possess some superiority.

Benzoyl peroxide may be applied one to two times daily, again being certain that the patient applies it to the entire affected area, although it has been reported (but not confirmed) that individual lesions may heal more quickly following its use. Benzoyl peroxide possesses two advantages over topical antibiotic therapy. First, it is, in general, more effective. Second, *P. acnes* resistance does not develop, so that if a patient's acne worsens during benzoyl peroxide therapy, it is because the acne has become more active rather than because the benzoyl peroxide somehow has been rendered less effective.

There are, however, disadvantages to the use of benzoyl peroxide compared with antibiotics. First, it is almost invariably more irritating than topically applied antibiotics, even if the lowest concentration, 2.5 percent, is used. Second, sensitization may occur (rare with topical antibiotic therapy), although the precise incidence has not been clearly established. In my experience fewer than one in 100 patients develop allergic contact dermatitis in response to benzoyl peroxide. Third, the irritant effect of benzoyl peroxide may accentuate the postinflammatory hyperpigmentation seen in dark skinned persons. Last, it may bleach hair and colored fabrics.

Topical antibiotic therapy has come to occupy a prominent niche in the treatment of minimal to moderately inflamed acne. Such preparations include, in order of their introduction into the clinical practice, tetracycline, clindamycin, erythromycin, and meclocycline sulfosalicylate (Table 2). All have been shown in controlled studies to be more effective in reducing the number of inflammatory lesions than control vehicles, although as a general rule, the percentage difference in inhibition between active drug and control vehicle is less than that between the vehicle and the baseline valves. Most of these antibiotics are in liquid vehicles, although some are available as pledgets, creams, and ointments. The latter two are better tolerated and more useful in patients with sensitive skin. Although, as noted, their effectiveness over a wide range of patients is less than that of benzoyl peroxide, one advantage is that the antibiotics are virtually devoid of allergenicity. A concern in regard to their use has been the potential for the development of resistant bacterial organisms, but to date this fear does not appear to have been realized, at least not at a clinical level.

The effect of benzoyl peroxide and of topical antibiotic therapy can be enhanced by the concomitant use of tretinoin. Often this combination, i.e., the use of each one daily or more frequently, is not well tolerated. However, if tolerated, a regimen of tretinoin with topical antibacterial therapy remains the most effective way, to date, of suppressing less than severe cases of acne. Benzoyl peroxide has also been combined with erythromycin in a single gel base preparation.

Systemic antibiotic therapy has been used for decades in the treatment of acne. The three that are clearly effective in the majority of cases of inflammatory acne are

TABLE 2 Antibiotics for Acne

Topical therapy
  Clindamycin
  Erythromycin
  Meclocycline sulfosalicylate
  Tetracycline

Oral therapy
  Tetracycline
  Erythromycin
  Minocycline
  Trimethoprim-sulfamethoxazole
  Clindamycin

tetracycline, erythromycin, and minocycline (see Table 2). Also effective is clindamycin, although it is infrequently used nowadays because of the risk, albeit very small, of the development of pseudomembranous colitis. The indications for the oral use of antibiotics in acne are as follows: moderately severe to severe inflammatory acne; less severe cases of acne not adequately responsive to topical therapy; still milder cases of acne, in which the individual because of sensitive skin (atopics often) is unable to tolerate topical therapy or in which there is evidence of active scarring; and patients with predominantly truncal acne, which ordinarily does not respond satisfactorily to externally applied medications.

The oral doses of antibiotics used vary with the severity of the disease, although I tend to start with "full" dosages, viz., 1.0 g of tetracycline daily or its equivalent for other antibiotics, even if the acne is only of moderate severity. A more rapid response is achieved and is decidedly preferable if there is any evidence of the development of scarring. An exception to this starting dosage of antibiotic is minocycline, which in dosages of 200 mg per day can cause symptoms of ototoxicity. Only if the disease is severe would I start with this dosage. Tetracycline must be taken on an empty stomach and for logistic reasons can be taken in twice daily doses of 500 mg, although occasionally this amount is not tolerated by the upper gastrointestinal tract. Erythromycin is less affected by the ingestion of food and minocycline, the least.

The advantages and disadvantages of the different antibiotics vary. Gastrointestinal effects occur most frequently with erythromycin. Phototoxicity is moderate with tetracycline, minimal with minocycline, and absent with erythromycin. *Candida* vaginitis is most frequent with tetracycline, occurring in about 15 percent of the patients taking long term therapy. A special problem with minocycline is the occasional development of pigmentary changes, consisting either of small bluish tattoo-like macules on the face, often in scars, or less commonly a brownish hyperpigmentation elsewhere. These pigmentary changes are reversible on drug discontinuation.

The advantage shared by these three antibiotics is the very low incidence of allergic sensitization with their use. This is in contrast to trimethoprim-sulfamethoxazole, which is also effective for acne but with which allergic reactions are far more common.

Other antibiotics used in acne include ampicillin and the cephalosporin group of antibiotics. Controlled studies to assess their effectiveness are lacking. Ampicillin suppresses *P. acnes* weakly.

ANTI-INFLAMMATORY DRUGS

The most rapid and most predictable way of reducing the severity of inflammatory acne is the systemic use of corticosteroids in anti-inflammatory dosages, e.g., 30 to 50 mg of prednisone daily. Once the dosage is reduced to 10 to 15 mg per day, the acne begins to flare up. Obviously such treatment is replete with drawbacks, and its use is limited to patients who have periodic severe but infrequent and brief flare-ups.

The principal use of anti-inflammatory steroids is their injection into inflamed lesions to shorten their duration. I use triamcinolone acetonide suspension in a concentration of 2.5 to 10 mg per milliliter. The lower concentration is usually effective. In fact the results of one report have revealed that a concentration of 0.6 mg per milliliter is virtually as effective as higher ones. The risk of a 10 mg per milliliter concentration is the induction of atrophy, even though it almost always reverts with time.

Topical corticosteroid therapy seems to have little effect on acne, although the reason is not certain. The generally held view is that there is inadequate penetration of the steroid into the involved site. Moreover its use is thought to be contraindicated because of the weakening effect of the steroid on the follicular wall, with the possible consequent development of folliculitis ("steroid acne").

Studies with nonsteroidal anti-inflammatory drugs (e.g., naproxen, ibuprofen) have not shown an overwhelming benefit, even when administered in high dosages. However, one study showed unequivocally that the administration of high dosages of ibuprofen (2.4 g per day) enhances the antiacne effect of concomitantly administered tetracycline in a dosage of 1.0 g daily.

SEBACEOUS GLAND INHIBITION

Sebum, the secretory product of the sebaceous glands, is an integral factor in the pathogenesis of acne. A substantive reduction in the activity of these androgen sensitive glands results in a decrease in the intensity of the disease. To date no topical therapy has been discovered that will effectively suppress sebaceous activity. Systemic therapy is required, involving the use of hormonal therapy for androgen suppression.

The drug longest in use for this purpose is estrogen, whose action is to inhibit the pituitary-ovarian axis, with consequent reduction of ovarian androgen production. Some effect on the adrenal gland may occur as well. The drugs are those marketed for oral contraception. Although no controlled studies have clearly delineated the effectiveness of oral estrogen treatment, clinical experience has disclosed that this form of therapy can be beneficial. However, uncomfortably high dosages of estrogen are usually needed, i.e., more than 50 μg of ethinyl estradiol or mestranol daily, to yield a reasonable chance of success. The response is slow, requiring 2 to 4 months for clear-cut improvement to become evident. Moreover, as with virtually all other acne treatments, the effect is suppressive rather than curative, so that even if there is a good result, recurrence of the acne is the consequence of treatment discontinuance.

Another disadvantage of estrogen therapy is the problem of the concomitant use or need for oral antibiotic therapy for the acne or other medical conditions. There have been reports that antibiotics may decrease the level of the administered estrogen in the blood. As a consequence, if the estrogen is being taken for the dual purpose of acne treatment and contraception, protection against pregnancy might be reduced. The chance that such an interaction will lead to pregnancy is not known but is likely to be very low.

Another method for androgen suppression is low dose

glucocorticoid administration to decrease adrenal elaboration of androgens, particularly dehydroepiandrosterone. In many studies this androgen, either free or sulfated, has been found to be increased in women with persistent acne, even without collateral signs of androgen excess. Treatment of such patients with dexamethasone, 0.25 to 0.5 mg daily, or with prednisone, 5 to 10 mg daily, has been reported to decrease the acne. However, as with estrogen, controlled studies are still lacking so that the true benefit from low dose steroid treatment remains unestablished. What has been demonstrated, however, is that combined estrogen-glucocorticoid treatment effects a marked reduction in sebum levels and very significant acne improvement.

Spironolactone in high dosages, i.e., 100 to 200 mg daily, has a peripheral antiandrogen effect. It has been reported to be helpful in women with acne. I have found it to be effective in approximately 25 percent of the patients, the remainder showing only modest to no improvement. Common side effects from spironolactone are menstrual irregularity and fatigue, symptoms that can decrease despite continued administration of drug.

With any form of hormone therapy I generally try not to exceed 9 months of treatment but occasionally continue the therapy for up to 12 months. The occurrence of side effects in any given patient might curtail the use of whatever regimen has been selected.

ISOTRETINOIN

Introduced into clinical practice in 1982, the synthetic retinoid, isotretinoin, has proved to be superior in the treatment of acne and the drug to use in patients with severe nodulo-cystic acne in whom traditional regimens, including systemic antibiotic therapy, have failed. In fact, it is only in this class of patient that the drug has been approved for use. However, my inclination is to extend its use to the occasional patient who has less severe cystic acne or even noncystic acne but who is developing active scarring and has resisted the standard treatments. The oral dosage of isotretinoin is 0.5 to 2.0 mg per kilogram per day. The dosage that should suffice for most patients is 80 mg per day, although heavy individuals or those with predominantly truncal acne may require the higher dosages. The drug generally induces a high incidence of remission despite the severity of the disease and its previous recalcitrance to treatment.

Numerous side effects preclude the use of the drug in all forms of acne, although most of the reactions are more of a nuisance than a danger. These changes are chiefly in the skin and mucous membranes and most commonly consist of cheilitis, various types of dry skin rashes, dry eyes, minor degrees of scalp hair loss, and occasional musculoskeletal discomfort. Perhaps the most annoying side effect, insofar as the patient is concerned, is a temporary worsening of the acne, not dissimilar to that seen with tretinoin given topically, but more severe, and observed in about one-third of the patients treated with isotretinoin.

Minimal hyperostoses have been seen in spinal x-ray views in acne patients treated with conventional doses of isotretinoin. They have occurred in 10 percent of the patients, have been asymptomatic, and have not progressed on discontinuation of treatment. The most serious side effect of isotretinoin is its teratogenic potential. One study demonstrates a 25-fold increase in the development of major fetal abnormalities in women who were pregnant or became pregnant while receiving the drug. Prevention of pregnancy while the patient is taking this treatment and for 1 month afterward is an absolute necessity, with the responsibility shared by the physician and the patient.

MISCELLANEOUS FORMS OF THERAPY

Cryotherapy

In addition to intralesional injections of steroid to combat inflammation in individual lesions, the use of cryotherapy is a useful alternative, although in my experience not as effective. Liquid nitrogen or dry ice is applied to individual lesions. Even less effective is the application of ice, but this has the advantage that the patient can do it at home. No standard regimen has been developed for lesional "ice cube" treatment, but I suggest to the patient that at the first evidence of a new inflammatory lesion forming, an ice cube be applied for 5 to 10 minutes to the lesion three to four times daily for 1 to 2 days. Some patients claim benefit from this treatment.

Surgical Measures

In active disease both noninflammatory and inflammatory lesions can be decreased by minor surgical procedures. Comedones can be removed with ease and little discomfort. Open comedones can be extracted directly, but closed comedones first need to have the small poral opening enlarged by inserting and rotating the opening with a 20 gauge needle.

Inflammatory lesions may be drained if pus is evident, but care must be taken not to incise widely. If the pustular contents cannot be drained easily following simple needle puncture, the lesion is best left alone or instead injected intralesionally with steroid.

A variety of procedures are used to improve the appearance of scars that may form during the healing of inflammatory lesions. If the scars are hypertrophic (usually on shoulders, upper back, and anterior chest), they can be injected with triamcinolone acetonide suspension in concentrations ranging from 10 to 40 mg per milliliter. Hypertrophic scars, however, have the tendency to decrease slowly in size spontaneously.

Atrophic scars are permanent. A variety of techniques are available for their removal, including dermabrasion, simple excision, excision with punch grafts, and bovine collagen implants.

ACNE ROSACEA

THOMAS T. PROVOST, M.D.

Acne rosacea is a chronic inflammatory dermatosis involving the central portion of the face. It is characterized by erythema, telangiectasia, edema, papules, and pustules. The disease process can be seen at any age but tends to occur most commonly in women between the ages of 30 and 50.

The disease may begin as a prominent flush involving the malar eminences and nose. Infrequently this erythema may involve predominantly the chin and perioral area (perioral dermatitis). On unusual occasions the central portion of the forehead may also be involved. With time, pustules and papules may occur as well as telangiectasia. The skin is frequently oily and on occasion a cystic-nodular formation may occur in this area. Unlike acne vulgaris, there are no comedones. In its most severe form acne rosacea results in thickening and lobulated overgrowth of sebaceous glands and connective tissue in the nose, producing disfigurement (rhinophyma).

Ten to 15 percent of patients with acne rosacea have ocular involvement—blepharitis, conjunctivitis, iritis, keratitis, and episcleritis. The ocular lesions tend to be chronic and progressive. The relationship between the ocular and cutaneous findings of rosacea is unknown, but it is a clinical paradigm that once the cutaneous lesions of acne rosacea are controlled, the ocular lesions generally tend to regress.

The etiology of acne rosacea is unknown. In the past caffeine in the form of tea and coffee together with other hot drinks, tobacco, alcoholic beverages, and spicy foods were all thought to have a causative role. However, it now appears that these agents aggravate the pre-existing acne rosacea by producing flushing in the central portion of the face. Psychiatric factors and stress also were once thought to be causative. Their relationship to the disease process is unknown, but most likely they aggravate the condition by heightening the vascular response (i.e., increased flushing).

In recent years it has been recognized that the long-term topical application of fluorinated steroids on the face can induce a rosacea-like disease characterized by erythema, telangiectasia, and atrophy. In addition, papules and pustules can be induced by topical fluorinated steroid therapy.

The histopathologic changes in acne rosacea include the appearance of a variable number of lymphocytic inflammatory cells around the upper dermal blood vessels, telangiectasia, and edema. In the papular or nodular cystic form of acne rosacea, more intense inflammatory cell infiltrates consisting of numerous histiocytes and occasional giant cells are seen. Most of these lesions also show prominent telangiectasia and solar elastosis. Disruption of follicular epithelium results in release into the dermis of keratin and cellular debris which are thought to be responsible for the granulomatous response.

The differential diagnosis of acne rosacea includes seborrheic dermatitis, carcinoid flush, and lupus erythematosus. In general, the typical papulopustular lesions in the central portion of the face in middle aged individuals serve to differentiate this condition from those just mentioned.

TREATMENT

The cutaneous and ocular manifestations of acne rosacea are responsive to therapy. General measures employed in the treatment of these patients include avoidance of activities and foods that induce flushing of the central portion of the face. For example, saunas, steam baths, and hot tub baths should be avoided. Alcohol, caffeine, and hot spicy foods also should be restricted, if not completely avoided. Excessive sun exposure should also be avoided because of its erythrodermic capabilities. Diet restriction, however, does not seem to be a very effective form of therapy.

In addition to these general measures, I have found that most cases of acne rosacea respond to tetracycline, 500 to 1,000 mg per day. The initial course is given for 6 weeks at which time the patient is reevaluated. Generally within a 6 week period one sees a marked improvement in the acne rosacea—usually a decrease or absence of further pustule formation and a diminution in the size of the papules. The erythema, however, persists for prolonged periods of time. At the reevaluation at 6 weeks I generally begin to decrease the tetracycline dosage to 250 to 500 mg daily. The patient is subsequently reevaluated in approximately 2 months. I usually continue tetracycline therapy for at least 18 months before completely tapering. In general the maintenance dosage is 250 mg daily. Unfortunately attempts to discontinue the tetracycline have met with varied success. Within 6 months after discontinuing tetracycline a number of patients have experienced a reemergence of the disease and have needed retreatment. Thus, my experience, like that of most dermatologists, indicates that acne rosacea is a chronic, lifelong disease entailing prolonged tetracycline therapy (years).

In addition to tetracycline I generally give my patients either 0.5 or 1 percent hydrocortisone cream to be applied to the face two to three times per day during the first month of therapy. This generally produces a great deal of vasoconstriction and helps decrease the erythema, which in many women is cosmetically objectionable. The hydrocortisone is discontinued after 1 month of therapy because of the possibility of aggravating the acne rosacea or producing epidermal atrophy and telangiectasia.

If oiliness is a prominent feature, I prescribe 5 percent Benzagel, to be applied to the face at night. This generally is discontinued within the first 2 to 3 months of therapy, depending upon the clinical response.

Frequently, after the inflammatory process has been eradicated, a number of areas of telangiectasia are left that are cosmetically objectionable. These may be destroyed by employing superficial electrodesiccation. Rhinophyma may be cosmetically objectionable and may require surgical correction. This can be done by either an experienced dermatosurgeon or a plastic surgeon. The techniques used to correct this deformity include surgery, electrosurgery, and, perhaps most commonly, dermabrasion.

The ocular manifestations of acne rosacea generally clear after the institution of tetracycline therapy. However, the ocular problems may be persistent, responding only to 1 or 2 drops of Cortisporin ophthalmic solution per day. If the ocular problems persist, I refer the patient to an ophthalmologist. However, it should be re-emphasized that generally the ocular problems associated with acne rosacea resolve as the cutaneous manifestations come under control with systemic antibiotic therapy.

HIRSUTISM

WILMA F. BERGFELD, M.D.
GEOFFREY P. REDMOND, M.D.

Hirsutism in females is defined as the excessive growth of coarse pigmented terminal hair in a male hair distribution. The true incidence of hirsutism is unknown, but it appears to be more clinically prominent in females whose origins are western European countries; however it is also common in South Asian and black women. In a study of North American women, an 11 percent incidence of hirsutism was reported. The most common sites of hair growth are the extremities (84 percent), linea alba (35 percent), upper legs (20 percent), periareolar area (17 percent), lumbosacral area (16 percent), and upper pubic triangle (10 percent).

Classically two types of terminal coarse pigmented hair are clinically distinguished: asexual hair, which is independent of androgens; and sexual hair, which is dependent on androgen metabolism. Terminal hair is commonly found on the scalp, eyebrows, and to a lesser extent the forearms and legs in both sexes. At all ages asexual hair follicles appear to be only minimally influenced by hormonal (androgenic) secretions. The conversion of vellus (fine) hair to terminal coarse hair on the face, chest, shoulders, back, and abdomen requires levels of androgens similar to those found in the male or androgen sensitive hair follicles.

Hirsutism represents a large heterogenous group of disorders previously classified into four types, which now have limited relevance. Although in the past investigators have cited a 1 percent incidence of endocrine abnormalities in the hirsute family, in our experience about half the patients have excessive levels of one or more androgens. If clinical signs of virilization are present, such as oligomenorrhea, acne, alopecia, enlargement of the clitoris, deepening of the voice, an increase in body musculature, or skeletal growth, androgen excess is likely to be evident in the laboratory screening test results. Technical advances in studying hormonal secretions have revealed that 50 to 85 percent of hirsute women demonstrate some form of hyperandrogenemia. With the new radioassay techniques, the familial and idiopathic forms of hirsutism now can be investigated more thoroughly for major and minor androgen metabolism defects. These defects can be seen centrally within the endocrine organs or in the hair follicle.

All androgens and their immediate precursors are of adrenal or gonadal origin. In women the ovaries and adrenal gland contribute equally to the secretion of testosterone, the most potent androgen. Ovarian hyperandrogenemia usually results from polycystic ovaries and very rarely from masculinizing ovarian tumors. Adrenal androgen levels are elevated in late onset adrenal hyperplasia, congenital adrenal hyperplasia, Cushing's syndome, hyperprolactinemia, and acromegaly (Table 1). In most cases the reason for the exaggerated adrenal androgen secretion is unknown. The most common disorder of an-

TABLE 1 Causes of Hirsutism

Adrenal disorders
  Exaggeration of normal androgen secretion
  Hyperplasia
    Late onset adrenal hyperplasia
    Congenital adrenal hyperplasia
  Cushing's syndrome
  Tumors
    Steroid secreting
    Testosterone secreting
Ovarian disorders
  Polycystic ovaries
  Ovarian hyperthecosis
  Tumors and hyperplasia
    Luteoma of pregnancy
    Ovarian hilus cell hyperplasia
    Ovarian stromal hyperplasia
Combined disorders
  Adrenal and ovarian disorders
Other causes
  Pituitary disorders
    Hyperplasia
    Adenoma
  Exogenous neoplasms
    Carcinoid
    Choriocarcinoma
    Metastatic lung disease

drogen excess is secondary to acquired adult onset, mild adrenal hyperactivity with resulting hyperandrogenemia. A specific marker for this entity is an elevation of the dehydroepiandrosterone sulfate (DHEA-S) level. Ovarian and adrenal hyperandrogenemia usually can be differentiated by a 7 to 10 day dexamethasone suppression test.

The major adrenal androgens are androstenedione and alpha-dehydroepiandrosterone (DHEA) and the sulfated product, DHEA-sulfate (DHEA-S). Both these androgen metabolites are weak androgens. Eighty percent of the DHEA-S is secreted by the adrenal glands and 20 percent by the ovaries. Because of this difference in secretion, DHEA-S has served as an adrenal marker of androgen excess and has been the most important marker for minor adrenal hyperactivity in adult hirsute patients with acne and alopecia. In the female DHEA influences the function and metabolism of hair follicles as well as the site of peripheral metabolism of DHEA and its metabolite, androstenediol. Increased DHEA and its metabolite may adversely affect the scalp hair, producing premature shedding and thinning. Elevated levels of DHEA and its metabolites acting on skin areas other than the scalp ultimately may induce a hirsute condition. The suggested mechanism is an elevation of the androstenedione level with ultimate increased production of dihydrotestosterone. Elevated circulating testosterone levels similarly affect hair growth on both the scalp and other areas.

Previously hirsutism had been attributed to polycystic ovaries and other gynecological endocrinopathies. It has been suggested that elevations of DHEA or DHEA-S levels in rats induce cystic ovarian changes. Therefore, it is hypothesized that adrenal hyperandrogenism can induce polycystic ovarian disease in humans. This results in androgenic skin changes, such as hirsutism, acne, and alopecia, and may be associated with abnormalities of menstruation and fertility.

Hyperprolactinemia is also thought to be associated with elevations of the DHEA-S level due to action of prolactin on the adrenal cortex. Hyperprolactinemia has been reported in a variety of conditions, but the highest levels are associated with pituitary adenomas. Drugs reported to produce prolactin hypersecretion include birth control pills, cimetidine, antihypertensives, and phenothiazides.

In the past, laboratory evaluations included the 17-ketosteroid level, which was measured in the urine and might be found to be elevated in patients with hirsutism. The DHEA-S adrenal marker however, has replaced the 17-ketosteroid urine test for the detection of adrenal androgen excess.

Androstenedione and the potent androgen testosterone are produced by the ovaries. The ovaries and adrenal glands contribute comparative amounts of the circulating pool of androstenedione, approximately 50 percent of the circulating pool of androstenedione. Approximately 50 percent of the circulating androstenedione is derived from peripheral conversion of androstenedione and the remainder from the secretions of the adrenal glands and ovaries.

Approximately 70 percent of testosterone is derived from the ovaries and 30 percent from the adrenal glands and peripheral tissue. Although there is considerable individual variation in these ratios, testosterone exerts an androgenic effect on specific tissues, for example, muscle, embryonic wolffian duct, and hair follicles. Therefore, both androstenedione and testosterone are characterized by dual secretion from the ovaries and the adrenal glands. In females with menstrual abnormalities the source of the androgen excess is likely to be ovarian, whereas in those with normal menstruation the source of androgen excess is likely to be the adrenal glands.

DRUG INDUCED HIRSUTISM

Drugs that have been noted to induce a hirsute condition include testosterone, danazol (Danocrine), adrenocorticotropic harmone/(ACTH), metyrapone, phenothiazide, anabolic steroids, and acetazolamide (Diamox). Other drugs that have also been noted to induce localized or generalized hirsutism include cyclosporin, phenytoin (Dilantin), diazoxide (Dyazide), minoxidil, high doses of glucocorticoids, hexachlorobenzene, penicillamine, and psoralens (Table 2). Some of these drugs may induce hair growth in areas where androgens do not, such as between the eyebrows, on the forehead, and on the upper anterior cheek area.

ANDROGEN EXCESS SYNDROME

Androgen overproduction syndromes have been noted to produce hirsutism and virilizing change. For clinical purposes these disorders including excessive androgen production are classified as being of ovarian, adrenal, and

TABLE 2 Hirsutism Secondary to Drugs

Androgenic	Nonandrogenic
Testosterone	Cyclosporin
Danazol	Dilantin
ACTH	Diazoxide
Metyrapone	Minoxidil
Anabolic steroids	Chlorobenzene
Progestins	Penicillamine
	Psoralens

mixed origin. Hyperthecosis or polycystic hyperplasia of the ovaries, polycystic ovaries, and hilus cell hyperplasia in ovarian tumors (such as arrhenoblastoma and hilus cell, adrenal rest, granular cell, and Brenner tumors) induce hirsutism.

Similarly the adrenal gland may demonstrate minimal or major areas of hyperplasia, which may be present in Cushing's syndrome, congenital adrenal hyperplasia, and late onset adrenal hyperactivity. Other adrenal tumors that induce virilization include carcinomas or adenomas.

The local effects of androgens on hair follicles can be present without marked elevations of serum or urine androgen levels. Androstenedione and 5-alpha-dihydrotestosterone actively stimulate amino acid uptake and protein synthesis in intact human hair follicles. Although levels of testosterone are lower in women than in men, DHEA and androstenediol appear to play a significant role in hair growth. In women the serum DHEA level is 400 times greater than in males. The female hair follicle has 100 times more androstenediol and 10 times more DHEA than that in males. Studies of human hair follicles reveal that DHEA and 5-alpha-androstenediol alter hair growth. In the female it appears that hirsutism is most commonly induced by increased serum DHEA-S levels and altered metabolism of DHEA within the hair follicle with occasional increases in androstenedione (Fig. 1).

LABORATORY EVALUATION OF PATIENTS WITH HIRSUTISM

Because hormonal abnormalities induce widespread effects, an extensive history and a complete physical examination, including observations of all body surfaces and a complete physical examination, including observations of all body surfaces for contour changes as well as hair type and distribution, are necessary. Patients with rapidly progressive or severe manifestations of virilization or changes in menstruation require the most extensive laboratory investigation. Disorders such as Cushing's disease and congenital adrenal hyperplasia usually are detected in the history and physical examination, but they may be subtle and be detected only by laboratory tests.

Patients who are not obviously diagnosed are those with long-standing hirsutism with or without menstrual abnormalities and who probably constitute the majority of those seen for this problem. Again, those with menstrual abnormalities usually have ovarian androgen abnor-

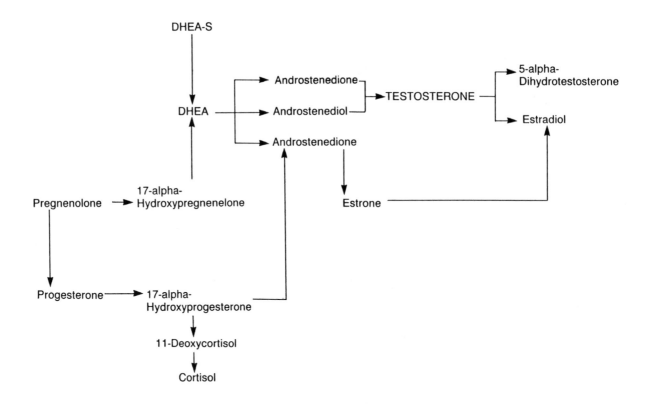

Figure 1 Important androgen pathways

malities. Only a few patients have serious systemic disease or tumors that are life-threatening. In these cases initial tests should include a minimal screen of adrenal, ovarian, and pituitary function (Table 3).

The basic endocrine survey for hirsute individuals should include the following tests: total and free testosterone, androstenedione, DHEA-S, and prolactin. If the free testosterone test is not available, the sex binding globulin ratio or the ratio of testosterone to testosterone-estradiol

TABLE 3 Basic Hirsutism Work-Up

Ovarian androgen excess
    Total testosterone
    Free testosterone
    Androstenedione*

Adrenal androgen excess
    DHEA-S
    Androstenedione*
    17-Hydroxyprogesterone*†
    Compound S (11-deoxycortisol)*†
    Cortisol*†

Pituitary
    Prolactin

* Advanced studies.
† Urinary adrenal steroids.

binding globulin protein gives an indirect measure of the free testosterone. Elevated prolactin levels can be seen in patients with minor adrenal hyperactivity and polycystic ovarian disease. Occasionally patients taking cimetidine, phenothiazines, antihypertensive drugs, and other drugs demonstrate elevated prolactin levels, which suggest the presence of a pituitary adenoma. The DHEA-S marker of adrenal androgen hypersecretion is usually elevated in patients with hirsutism. Blood levels of androstenedione, which is secreted in equal amounts by the ovaries and the adrenal glands, should be determined 10 to 15 days after menses for the best interpretation of androgen excess.

The interpretation of laboratory results is important. For example, in the patient who has an elevated DHEA-S level, the probable cause of hirsutism is adrenal androgen hypersecretion, whereas elevated free testosterone and normal DHEA-S levels often indicate ovarian androgens. However, even in this situation the source may be the adrenals. More elaborate studies of adrenal function should include free cortisol, urinary adrenal steroids, 17-hydroxyprogesterone, and compound S (11-deoxycortisol) levels. The 17-hydroxyprogesterone and compound S levels are elevated if the patient has congenital adrenal hyperplasia, Cushing's syndrome, or an adrenal tumor. Cortisol levels are elevated only in Cushing's disease.

Specialized dexamethasone suppression tests can be

used to further evaluate the presence or absence of adrenal tumor. These tests vary from institution to institution and vary in their interpretation. An endocrinologist should be called upon to do this evaluation.

At the present time there is no adequate laboratory test or tissue examination for the measurement of hair follicle androgen production, rates, or metabolism. The use of 5-alpha-diol, androstenediol glucuronide (a follicular androgen) has not proved helpful in our experience.

In our recent review of 191 females with signs of androgen excess, we were unble to identify specific androgen profiles with specific clinical signs. The patterns of androgen levels were similar in all three conditions of hirsutism, alopecia, and acne.

Frequently with increased age, especially in the perimenopausal female, a fall in the estrogen level may also affect hair growth. After menopause, ovarian androgen production falls, but androgen production is occasionally excessive. Clinically it appears that androgen secretion and action on the hair follicle increase with menopause.

TREATMENT OF HIRSUTISM

The endocrine factors that contribute to hirsutism are controllable, but usually are not curable except in rare surgically treatable cases of Cushing's disease, prolactinoma, or adrenal secreting tumors of the ovary or adrenal glands.

Hyperandrogenemia without the presence of a tumor can be treated with a variety of drugs. If adrenal suppression is needed to convert minor or major adrenal androgen hypersecretion, low bedtime doses of glucocorticoids can be employed. For example, prednisone (5 mg at night) or low doses of dexamethasone (0.125 to 0.375 mg) are preferred. Close patient monitoring is essential to avoid potentially serious adverse affects. Recently spironolactone (Aldactone), an antihypertensive drug with antiandrogenic activity, has been used in doses of 100 to 200 mg per day with notable suppression of elevated testosterone levels and subsequent gradual reduction of the hirsute condition. Spironolactone works at two sites: the steroid producing cell to inhibit androgen biosynthesis, and the androgen receptor sites on the hair follicle or other target organs. By binding with cytosol receptors, androgen action is antagonized.

Cyclic estrogen therapy has been used for both adrenal and ovarian hypersecretion, but it is most efficacious in the treatment of ovarian androgen excess. Great care should be taken in the selection of contraceptives for oral treatment. Norgestrel and levonorgestrel should be avoided, since they appear to have some androgenic activity (Table 4).

In European and other countries, cyproterone acetate, a potent antiandrogen-progesterone, has been found to suppress terminal hair growth and has been used successfully in the treatment of hirsutism, acne vulgaris, and seborrhea. Its mechanism of action is twofold: pituitary-gonadal axis suppression combined with interference with androgen binding on the target cell receptors, similar to the spironolactones. The recommended dosage is 50 to 100 mg per day on days 5 to 14 in the menstrual cycle. Ethinyl estradiol, usually 0.05 mg, is given on days 5 to 26. The expected duration of therapy in all cases of systemic treatments of hirsutism is at least 2 years (Table 4). Topical antiandrogen therapy has not proved successful in a limited unreported study.

Cosmetic management of hirsutism has specific advantages and disadvantages. Specific management includes epilation, shaving, electrolysis, waxing, and the use of depilatory creams.

Epilation basiclally involves plucking individual hairs from the hairy area and may induce skin irritation and acne lesions. Prevention of these secondary events can be accomplished by the topical use of aseptic detergents, soaps, and antibiotics. If the skin is irritated, a low potency corticosteroid is sometimes helpful in reducing skin redness. Epilation should not be used near the eyes.

Shaving is the easiest, cleanest, and cheapest way of removing hair but is psychologically unacceptable to most women. Hair growth after shaving is not increased nor is the hair fiber thickened. Shaving of the extremities is a common practice and psychologically acceptable.

Electrolysis is probably the only permanent method of removing hair. However, it may induce focal scars at the site of removal. Also, with this therapy, minor acneform eruptions have been noted and should be treated as acne with topically applied antibiotic solutions and drying agents. Patients undergoing electrolysis should be aware of the possibility of contracting infectious hepatitis from the needles. It is also advisable to avoid electrolysis if the patient has active herpes simplex. Electrolysis is less successful when disorders involving androgen excess are inducing the continued appearance of hair. Time and expense may be saved if electrolysis is deferred until hormonal therapy has slowed the appearance of new hair. Waxing preparations are melted to produce a pliable material that can be applied easily to the skin surface. When this wax hardens, it is quickly removed or ripped off and the hair follicles are mechanically epilated. However, this induces focal skin irritation and occasionally folliculitis. One disadvantage of waxing is that the hairs have to be at least 1 mm in length before they can be gripped by the wax and epilated. This problem can be minimized by waxing different areas at different times and bleaching any obvious hair until it is long enough to be waxed again. The procedure is quite effective for the upper lip. Intervals between treatment range from 2 to 6 weeks.

Depilatory creams contain calcium thioglycolate,

TABLE 4 Treatment of Hirsutism

Adrenal
  Dexamethasone suppression (0.125–0.375 mg/day h.s.)
  Spironolactone (100–200 mg/day)

Ovarian
  Cyclic estrogens
  Demulen
  Ortho-Novum
  Ovcon

which acts by reducing the disulfide bonds of the hair fiber, resulting in a soft hair, which is easily wiped off. These creams are applied to the skin for specific periods of time and are also classified as to use on certain body areas. These specifications reflect the concentrations of calcium thioglycolate in the product.

It is mandatory that patch testing be done prior to the use of a depilatory cream. A 24 hour patch test should be applied to the anterior aspect of the wrist. If mild skin irritation is induced, this can be easily treated with a topical application of corticosteroid. If severe irritation is induced at the patch test site, the depilatory product should not be used as treatment. The main disadvantages of depilatory creams are that they are expensive and application must be repeated.

RHEUMATOLOGIC AND IMMUNOLOGIC DISEASES

CHRONIC URTICARIA

MARTIN D. VALENTINE, M.D.

When a thoughtful medical evaluation of a patient in whom hives have been recurring for more than 6 weeks fails to reveal a specific cause, the condition is designated "chronic idiopathic urticaria." After systemic illness has been ruled out, the physician's role in such cases is to provide the therapeutic support that enables the patient to reduce symptoms to a manageable minimum while awaiting a spontaneous remission. Because chronic urticaria may adopt a cyclic pattern and usually regresses spontaneously, often to recur at a later date, what sometimes appears to be a therapeutic triumph may actually turn out to be the natural course of the disease. Although chronic urticaria is usually confined to the skin, mucosal and visceral symptoms occasionally occur, requiring separate therapeutic consideration, as noted later in this article.

Histamine is generally considered to be the primary mediator in most cases of chronic urticaria; thus, antihistamines taken systemically are the mainstay of therapy. Topical therapy with antihistamines or other drugs is rarely helpful, although certain general measures relating to skin care may help the patient feel more comfortable. These include avoidance of conditions that heat the skin, such as hot baths or showers and heavy bed clothing. Other items, such as chili peppers, spicy foods, and systemic ethyl alcohol also result in cutaneous vasodilation and increased susceptibility to urticaria. Clothing should be loose, comfortable, and no heavier than necessary. Skin dryness exacerbates pruritus and should be prevented with moisturizing lotions or creams.

Most H1 histamine antagonists also cause drowsiness. Some physicians believe that this is a desirable effect of a drug used for treating urticaria, but I disagree. The antihistamine that produces maximal effect in the skin with minimal sedation would be the drug of choice; several H1 antagonists are currently available, including ethanolamine derivatives, ethylenediamine derivatives, and alkylamines. Terfenadine (Seldane), an antihistamine with less sedative and anticholinergic effect than other H1 antagonists, is worth trying because of its reduced side effects. Although some patients do well with these drugs, I find hydroxyzine and cyproheptadine, and occasionally the cyproheptadine relative azatidine, generally superior to the other drugs. The phenothiazine drugs are generally avoided because of the side effects associated with this family of compounds, although one might consider their use in a patient in whom other H1 antihistamines had failed. Because of inherent differences in the pharmacology of hydroxyzine and cyproheptadine, their use is to be considered separately. Antihistamines work better when taken regularly in a prophylactic regimen; when taken after hives appear, they may relieve itching but do not reverse already visible lesions.

HYDROXYZINE

This drug is available as the pamoate (Vistaril and generic equivalents) and the hydrochloride (Atarax, Durrax, and generic equivalents). Either form may be used, both having inherently long durations of action when administered orally. The hydrochloride is available in smaller oral dosage forms, 10 mg being the smallest tablet dose available for the hydrochloride and 25 mg being the smallest capsule dose available of the pamoate. Both are available as liquids. Either form is relatively contraindicated in early pregnancy, because hydroxyzine has caused fetal abnormalities in rats when given in doses substantially above the human therapeutic range. Drowsiness may occur with hydroxyzine, although the duration of sedation with this drug seems to be far shorter than its duration of effect in the skin. Although most people tolerate 10 mg orally three to four times per day without drowsiness, some patients find this dosage to have sedative properties; for such patients an attempt may be made to give the entire day's dosage at bedtime. Some particularly sensitive patients may do well with as small a dosage as 10 mg at bedtime, although this is the exception. As a rule most patients improve with 20 to 40 mg daily, and some patients tolerate—and require—25 to 50 mg every 6 hours. Sedation is common but not universal with the higher dosages. In patients in whom hydroxyzine does not seem to be therapeutically successful, I try cyproheptadine.

CYPROHEPTADINE

In addition to being an antihistamine, this drug is also a serotonin antagonist whose nonapproved uses include prophylaxis against vascular headaches and maintenance therapy in certain patients with Cushing's syndrome. Although drowsiness is the major side effect associated with cyproheptadine, increased appetite or weight gain has also been associated with its use, and at one time it was approved for use as an appetite stimulating drug in children. In addition, I have found an occasional patient to experience otherwise unexplainable emotional depression while using this drug. It is not as inherently long acting as hydroxyzine and thus does not lend itself to single bedtime dosing. However, drowsiness does appear to be minimized if the drug is begun at a low dosage that is gradually increased. In practice, I suggest beginning with 2 mg twice a day, making incremental increases at 2- to 3-day intervals or as tolerated by the patient. After 2 mg twice daily the next dosages are 2 mg three times daily, 4 mg twice daily, and 4 mg three times daily to a maximum of 4 mg four times daily.

COMBINATION THERAPY AND H2 ANTAGONISTS

A single H1 antagonist may be insufficient in the management of patients with chronic urticaria. Although some advocate combinations of two or more H1 antagonists, I believe that other measures are more suitable. I would first consider maintaining the chosen dosage of the H1 antagonist, for example, hydroxyzine or cyproheptadine, and then adding an H2 antagonist, such a cimetidine or ranitidine. Some patients apparently respond to the combination of H1 and H2 antagonists with resolution of the urticaria. It is usually the case, however, that the patient who responds favorably to the addition of the H2 antagonist is the patient who has already responded partially to administration of the H1 antagonist. Certain patients may respond partially to the combination of H1 and H2 antagonists and still need additional therapy. Although steroid therapy may be considered for such patients, I would first consider adding ephedrine sulfate, 25 mg three to four times daily. The combination of alpha-adrenergic and B_1 and B_2 activities may be a useful adjunct in the patient with urticaria. Some authorities have favored B_2 agonists because of the inhibitory effects such drugs have on mediator release, but I believe that such selective drugs are less likely to be useful than the combination of alpha and mixed-beta effects of ephedrine.

TRICYCLIC ANTIDEPRESSANTS

It is known that drugs belonging to the tricyclic antidepressant family have great affinity for H1 receptors in certain binding assays in vitro. This has led to therapeutic trials in patients with chronic urticaria; some successes have been reported. In addition to H1 antagonism, some of the tricyclics, such as doxepin, have significant anti-H2 activity. A trial of doxepin may be warranted if a single conventional H1 antagonist is ineffectual in a patient with chronic urticaria.

CORTICOSTEROIDS

A minority of patients cannot be managed adequately even with a combination of H1 and H2 antagonists with ephedrine. In such patients it may be necessary to resort to systemic corticosteroid therapy. In cases of chronic urticaria one must keep in mind that since the condition may persist for months or even years, if steroids are employed, they may be necessary—with their attendant potential for side effects—for that period of time as well. In general, the rules for the use of steroids in urticaria are the same as they would be for asthma: one should use a drug that is short acting to avoid suppression of the pituitary-hypothalamic-adrenal axis, and should use the drug initially in a dosage sufficient to suppress symptoms completely and taper the dosage fairly rapidly until one can determine the dosage necessary to achieve satisfactory suppression of symptoms. A subgroup of the physical urticarias known as delayed pressure urticaria often responds poorly, if at all, to antihistamines and often requires steroid therapy.

The nonsteroidal anti-inflammatory drugs may have a beneficial therapeutic effect on physical urticaria and should be tried before steroids. Some clinicians believe that the nonsteroidal anti-inflammatory drugs are relatively contraindicated in chronic urticaria of the usual variety, however, and routinely advise against their use even if specific sensitivity to the drug in question is not suspected.

CUTANEOUS VASCULITIS

Cutaneous vasculitis may present as urticaria. This may be seen in the acute or chronic phase of viral hepatitis or other viral illnesses, and in other immunologically mediated syndromes, such as systemic lupus erythematosus, for which patients with urticaria should be screened. In both these examples the skin lesions appear to result from the local deposition of circulating immune complexes with an accompanying local inflammatory reaction, which may include the diapedesis of red blood cells into the skin, producing lesions that persist longer than 24 hours at individual sites and ecchymoses at the sites of individual lesions. This lesion is easily identified in a small punch skin biopsy specimen and also may be present in patients without any underlying systemic illness. In patients with cutaneous vasculitis an elevated erythrocyte sedimentation rate and abnormal serum complement levels are usually seen. Such patients are often unresponsive to conventional therapy for idiopathic urticaria until oral corticosteroid therapy is employed. If the cutaneous lesions are a manifestation of systemic vasculitis, consideration must be given to immunosuppressive therapy.

DRUGS NOT INDICATED

Patients with inherited or acquired deficiency of the inhibitor of C1 do not have urticaria but are susceptible to attacks of cutaneous and mucosal angioedema, which do not respond to epinephrine, antihistamines, or corticosteroids. In these syndromes, confirmed by appropriate immunochemical studies, various anabolic steroids ("impeded androgens") help prevent attacks by promoting biosynthesis of the normal C1 inhibitor protein. Such therapy is not indicated in chronic idiopathic urticaria for two reasons: benefit has not been shown in appropriately blinded and controlled clinical trials, and the anabolic steroids are hepatotoxic and may be tumorigenic.

ACUTE EXACERBATIONS

Occasionally the patient with chronic urticaria may experience an acute exacerbation requiring urgent treatment because a previously effective drug regimen has failed. Acute intervention may also be requested by a patient when urticaria involves an area that results in transient disfigurement, such as the lip or eyelid, causing embarrassment or social inability to continue normal activities. In such situations 0.3 mg (0.3 cc of a 1:1,000 solution) of aqueous epinephrine given by subcutaneous injection is often rapidly effective in reversing cutaneous lesions. Mucosal urticaria or angioedema may also require and benefit from such intervention to prevent airway compromise. Visceral urticaria can produce pain in the gut; esophageal lesions may produce pain that mimics angina but that is rapidly relieved with epinephrine.

CUTANEOUS VASCULITIS

ROBERT A. SWERLICK, M.D.
THOMAS J. LAWLEY, M.D.

In this article we limit the discussion to cutaneous necrotizing vasculitis. Also known as leukocytoclastic vasculitis, cutaneous necrotizing vasculitis is manifested most commonly by palpable purpura. The purpuric lesions usually begin on and are commonly confined to the lower extremities, but widespread involvement sometimes occurs. The typical lesion is an erythematous papule 3 to 10 mm in diameter, which progressively becomes purpuric within 12 to 48 hours after its appearance. In some instances the lesions may become pustular or necrotic. In the extremely unusual chronic form of necrotizing vasculitis, erythema elevatum diutinum, the lesions become nodular, particularly over the knees, elbows, and buttocks. In recent years chronic urticaria-like lesions have been recognized as a cutaneous manifestation of leukocytoclastic vasculitis. In some instances with leukocytoclastic vasculitis, there may be associated constitutional or organ related signs and symptoms; primarily fever, malaise, arthralgias or arthritis, gastrointestinal pain with or without associated bowel blood loss, proteinuria, and hematuria.

The diagnosis of leukocytoclastic vasculitis is confirmed by a skin biopsy. This typically demonstrates swollen damaged endothelial cells, infiltration of polymorphonuclear neutrophils in and around vessel walls, extravasated erythrocytes, nuclear dust, and fibrin deposition around involved vessels. For immuno-fluorescence testing it is best to carry out a biopsy of an early lesion less than 1 to 2 days old. Direct immunofluorescence of early lesions often reveals deposits of immunoglobulin, particularly IgM, or C3 in vessel walls.

THERAPEUTIC ALTERNATIVES

Aside from merely observing the lesions, the drugs that have been used for treatment include antihistamines, nonsteroidal anti-inflammatory drugs, oral corticosteroid therapy, dapsone, and colchicine.

PREFERRED APPROACH

The approach to therapy must take into consideration the natural history of the disease. A majority of patients have a single episode that resolves spontaneously, but perhaps up to 10 percent of the patients may have a recurrence or recurrences at intervals of months to years. A small but significant number manifest chronic disease, with recurrent crops of lesions developing as old lesions heal. In addition, the vasculitis may be associated with an underlying disorder or precipitating event or agent. Removal of the offending agent or treatment of the underlying disease may obviate the need to treat the cutaneous vasculitis. Lastly it is important to determine whether sig-

nificant tissue damage is limited to the skin or whether it also involves other vital organs.

After establishing the diagnosis, it is important to obtain a complete history, concentrating on ingestion of prescription, over the counter, or illegal drugs; preexisting symptoms suggestive of a chronic or acute disorder; or a recent infection or exposure to an infectious agent. The physical examination should be directed toward revealing conditions that predispose the patient to cutaneous vasculitis (Table 1). In the absence of specific symptoms or signs of an underlying systemic disorder, the initial laboratory evaluation should include CBC and differential counts, serum chemistry tests with liver function tests, hepatitis B surface and core antigen determinations, urinalysis, examination of three consecutive stool specimens for occult blood, erythrocyte sedimentation rate determination, and an ASO titer. Additional tests should be selected according to the findings on the history and physical examination.

The initial treatment should concentrate on removal of offending drugs or treatment of associated conditions. This is followed by symptomatic treatment. Most patients with cutaneous vasculitis have only minimal to moderate discomfort, have a disorder that is self-limited, lasting a few weeks to a few months, and do not require therapy. In some instances antihistamines such as hydroxyzine, up to 50 mg four times daily, may help alleviate discomfort and potentially retard the development of new lesions. We have never been impressed with the latter. Often patients complain of general malaise and arthralgias, which can be responsive to nonsteroidal anti-inflammatory drugs such as ibuprofen in dosages up to 400 mg four times daily.

If the cutaneous involvement is severe, early institution of oral corticosteroid therapy may be indicated. Prior to institution of steroid therapy, a more extensive serologic work-up including ANA, rheumatoid factor, anti-Ro (SS-A) antibody, CH_{50}, and cryoglobulin determinations and, if possible, an immune complex assay should be done. If these studies do not reveal an associated underlying disorder, prednisone given at an initial dosage of 60 mg daily in divided doses should be sufficient to control symptoms in patients with cutaneous disease alone. Since most patients have episodes that resolve spontaneously in 3 months or less, rapid tapering over approximately 1 month or less should be attempted after disease activity has been controlled.

Patients who develop chronic disease represent a sig-

TABLE 1 Selected Disorders Associated with Cutaneous Necrotizing Vasculitis

Drug induced reactions
Acute or subacute bacterial or viral infections
Collagen vascular disorders
Hypergammaglobulinemic purpura
Cryoglobulinemia
Ulcerative colitis
Inherited complement deficiency syndromes
Henoch-Schönlein purpura
Erythema elevatum diutinum
Idiopathic disorders

nificant therapeutic problem. They generally respond well to moderate oral doses of corticosteroids, but the disease promptly exacerbates when therapy is stopped. Since the morbidity associated with chronic oral corticosteroid therapy may be worse than that associated with vasculitis limited to the skin, the goal of therapy should be to use the minimal oral dose of prednisone at the least frequent interval. This can be done through a number of approaches. First, an attempt should be made at alternate day steroid therapy. A daily dosage that controls disease activity should be used initially. The dosage on alternate days should then be tapered 5 to 10 mg weekly while an equivalent amount is added on alternate days. For example, an individual controlled on 25 mg of prednisone daily would be switched over 3 to 4 weeks to 50 mg on alternate days. If the disease remains quiescent, the alternate day dosage is tapered slowly. If the disease flares during the attempt to change to alternate day treatment, the dosage is increased back to the level at which control was seen and a slower tapering is attempted.

Unfortunately symptoms in some patients are not controlled by a low daily dosage or alternate day steroid treatment. In these patients other drugs can be tried instead of or in conjuction with oral corticosteroid therapy. Colchicine in a dosage of 0.6 mg once to four times daily has produced variable success, but its usefulness is often limited by gastrointestinal distress, particularly diarrhea, when dosages equal or exceed 1.2 mg daily. We have found that some patients respond to the addition of dapsone in dosages up to 200 mg daily. In particular, patients with erythema elevatum diutinum respond in dramatic fashion to the initiation of dapsone therapy: within 48 hours no new lesions appear and there is rapid resolution of most preexisting lesions. Some patients with more typical cutaneous necrotizing vasculitis gradually respond over 1 week or more, allowing a decrease in the oral corticosteroid dosage.

Dapsone should be used with caution, particularly in those with cardiovascular or pulmonary compromise. In addition, individuals with G6PD deficiency may experience life threatening hemolysis if therapy is started with this drug. Although this condition is most common in blacks and individuals of Mediterranean descent, it is prudent to check all patients before starting therapy and not to use dapsone in G6PD deficient patients. Treatment should be started with a dosage of 50 to 150 mg daily. Initially patients need to be followed closely for evidence of severe hemolysis; a 2 g decrease in the hemoglobin level can be expected. We obtain CBC and differential counts and an SMA-12 evaluation every 1 to 2 weeks for 3 months to check patients taking dapsone for evidence of leukopenia or agranulocytosis. Serum chemistry levels should be determined to check for evidence of liver function abnormalities, which may be an early sign of dapsone hypersensitivity. If dapsone is tolerated, the dosage may be increased to as much as 400 mg daily before the patient is considered nonresponsive. High dosages of dapsone may be associated with significant anemia, methemoglobinemia, and fatigue, and in long-term therapy with peripheral neuropathy.

The role of immunosuppressive drugs in the treatment of vasculitis limited to the skin has not been extensively studied, and there is little evidence suggesting that their use would be prudent or effective. In a small group of patients with vasculitis limited to the skin, the use of cyclophosphamide was not helpful in controlling the disease. Given the generally benign course of chronic cutaneous vasculitis, it is difficult to justify the use of potentially life threatening immunosuppressive drugs in the absence of compelling evidence of their effectiveness.

Patients with vasculitis limited to the skin in whom chronic disease persists should be checked regularly for the development of systemic disease. In particular, regular examination of the urine sediment should be carried out, since renal involvement may start silently, without any symptoms. Other studies are dictated by symptoms and findings on the physical examination.

RELAPSING POLYCHONDRITIS

THOMAS M. ZIZIC, M.D., F.A.R.A.

Relapsing polychondritis is a relatively rare multisystem disorder with a predilection for affecting tissues that have a relatively high glycosaminoglycan content, such as cartilage, aorta, sclera, cornea, and parts of the ear. The most characteristic lesion in the disease is cartilaginous inflammation, which is polyfocal. Although 15 percent of the patients have continuous symptomatic disease, the remainder in one large series had intermittent inflammatory manifestations, with an average of five episodes over a 6-year mean period of follow-up. Hence, the name—relapsing polychondritis.

Although the disease can affect adolescents or the geriatric population, the median age at diagnosis is in the fifth decade. There is an equal sex frequency, but the frequencies of some disease manifestations appear to differ between the sexes. External ear chondritis and scleritis or episcleritis appear to be more common in men and saddle nose deformities and subglottic strictures more common in women. It is postulated that anatomic differences in cartilage mass and dimensions may account for this observation. There does not appear to be any familial predisposition, and there is no evidence of increased frequency of any of the HLA-A or B locus alloantigens in relapsing polychondritis.

Auricular chondritis is the most frequent initial manifestation (present in more than one-quarter), and it occurs in over 85 percent at some time during the course of the disease. It characteristically begins with the sudden onset of a painful, swollen, beefy red ear. The ear lobe, lacking cartilage, is always spared. The chondritis tends to be recurrent, and although succeeding attacks are less severe, many patients eventually develop soft floppy or "cauliflower" ears. In 95 percent of the patients the involvement is bilateral and, along with a history of episodes of spontaneous resolution, indicates relapsing polychondritis rather than infection or another disorder.

Nasal chondritis is also a frequent presenting manifestation and eventually occurs in three-quarters of the patients with relapsing polychondritis. It is usually of sudden onset and painful, but at times there may only be a sensation of fullness in the nasal bridge and surrounding tissues or epistaxis. Although involvement of the nasal cartilage is less likely to be recurrent than auricular chondritis, approximately half the patients with nasal chondritis develop a "saddle nose" deformity. Occasionally this occurs with little or no clinical evidence of inflammation. A saddle nose deformity occurs most frequently in younger patients, especially females.

Arthropathy is also a common initial manifestation and eventually develops in three-quarters of the patients. It is typically migratory, nonerosive, and asymmetric. Peripherally the large joints are predominantly involved, and there is a predilection for the sternoclavicular, costochondral, and sternomanubrial joints. Severe cases may be complicated by dislocation of the clavicles and ribs, or a flail chest wall secondary to lysis of costosternal cartilage.

Virtually any part of the eye can be involved in relapsing polychondritis, but in the majority of patients episcleritis or scleritis occurs. Conjunctivitis, iritis, and keratitis are common, while chorioretinitis, extraocular muscle palsies, optic neuritis, and exophthalmos occur less frequently.

Involvement of the respiratory tract may be a presenting manifestation and eventually develops in half the patients. Hoarseness and a cough may be initial symptoms, and wheezing and dyspnea may be signs of airway stenosis. When respiratory involvement occurs early in the course of relapsing polychondritis, it usually involves inflammation and swelling in the glottic, laryngeal, or subglottic soft tissues and may necessitate a tracheostomy. Like the saddle nose deformity, subglottic strictures, which eventually develop in one-quarter of the patients with relapsing polychondritis; occur most frequently in younger patients, especially females. Respiratory disease later in the course of relapsing polychondritis often is manifested by obstructive pulmonary disease secondary to tracheal or bronchial cartilage dissolution, stenosis, and collapse.

Audiovestibular damage occurs in half the patients and may be bilateral or unilateral. It may begin gradually or suddenly, and the hearing loss may be conductive or sensorineural. In addition, there may be tinnitus, vertigo, nystagmus, nausea, and vomiting. Hearing loss is seen in all age groups, but vertigo, which may be seen alone, but generally is associated with hearing loss, occurs almost exclusively in patients under the age of 50.

Cardiovascular involvement is a major cause of morbidity and mortality in relapsing polychondritis. Aneurysms or arteritis of the large vessels, including the cerebral vessels, the proximal and distal aorta, the mesenteric arteries, and the subclavian artery, may develop in patients with relapsing polychondritis. Many develop thromboses of large arteries, including the abdominal aorta, but venous thromboses are less frequent. Valvular lesions (aortic more than mitral) can occur by two mechanisms. The more common mechanism is secondary to annular dilation as a result of disintegration of the aortic root and valve ring. The less common mechanism involves changes in the architecture of the aortic cusp. Analysis of the involved valves reveals decreased amounts of hydroxyproline and glycine, which are amino acid constituents of collagen.

Cutaneous involvement in relapsing polychondritis occurs in about one-quarter of the patients. As we and others have reported, it can vary from furuncular eruptions, erythema nodosum-like lesions, cutaneous vasculitis, and pyoderma gangrenosum to neutrophilic dermatosis. The central nervous system manifestations of relapsing polychondritis have recently been appreciated, although no detailed neuropathologic study has been performed. Cranial nerve abnormalities are most frequent, but hemiplegia, cerebellar signs, and diffuse cerebral dysfunction (seizures, confusion, hallucinations, and headaches) also can occur. Although renal involvement has not been a prominent feature of relapsing polychondritis, occasionally severe glomerulonephritis may occur.

Patients with relapsing polychondritis have many nonspecific laboratory features found in chronic inflammatory diseases, such as anemia and an elevated erythrocyte sedimentation rate. Roentgenographic findings can include calcification of the pinna, nose, and trachea. Measurement of the maximal expiratory and inspiratory flow-volume loop and airway resistance can indicate the presence, location, and degree of fixation of the upper airway obstruction. This can be confirmed with radiography, computed tomography, or tracheography. Routine chest roentgenograms, as well as soft tissue views of the neck, should be made to detect narrowing of the trachea. Of course, the chest x-ray view may also reveal pneumonia or atelectasis as a result of collapsed airways or cardiomegaly, pulmonary congestion, widening of the aortic arch, and prominence of the ascending or descending aorta when cardiovascular involvement is present.

The characteristic histopathological findings on light microscopy of involved cartilage, regardless of its location, are similar: There is a loss of basophilic staining of the cartilage matrix (reflecting the loss of matrix acid mucopolysaccharides); perichondral inflammation; and eventual cartilage destruction with replacement by fibrous tissue. Deposits of IgG, IgA, and C_3 have been demonstrated at the fibrocartilage junction by direct immunofluorescence.

Although the etiology of relapsing polychondritis is unknown, vasculitis and autoimmunity appear to be important factors. Vasculitis has been documented in many patients and not only may contribute to the clinical manifestation, but when systemic may be a major cause of death from arterial thromboses or complications relating to aneurysmal disease.

Autoimmunity to type II collagen or cartilage may be important in the pathogenesis of relapsing polychondritis. The coexistence of relapsing polychondritis with other immune diseases, including systemic lupus erythematosus, rheumatoid arthritis, Hashimoto's thyroiditis, Sjögren's syndrome, and glomerulonephritis, is well known and has been reported in as many as one-quarter of the patients with relapsing polychondritis.

The main constituents of the interstitial space of cartilage are type II collagen and proteoglycans. Structurally identical collagen type II is also present in the cornea, retina, and vitreous of the eye. It has been shown that immunization against native type II collagen can induce arthritis in rats and mice, and the disease can be transferred to normal animals by either cells or the IgG fraction of the serum from arthritic animals. Moreover, in this model some animals have developed a delayed auricular chondritis similar to that in human relapsing polychondritis. There were high titers of circulating antitype II collagen as well as deposits of immunoglobulin and complement in the auricular cartilaginous lesions.

In patients studied by us, antibodies to proteoglycan were not found, but one-third of the patients had antibodies to type II collagen of the IgG or IgA subclass. The antibodies could be absorbed from the serum by rat native type II collagen, and the titers appeared to correlate with the activity and severity of the disease. A case report of transplacental transfer of relapsing polychondritis suggests that the autoantibodies present are pathogenic.

In a recent review of 112 patients with relapsing polychondritis at the Mayo Clinic, the median survival from the time of diagnosis was 9 years for men and 16 years for women. The 5 and 10 year probabilities for survival after diagnosis were 74 and 55 percent, respectively. Infection is the most common cause of death, often in association with steroid therapy or laryngotracheal involvement and strictures. Cardiovascular involvement with an underlying systemic vasculitis or large artery aneurysm dissection or rupture, acute respiratory failure due to airway collapse, and renal failure secondary to glomerulonephritis are other disease related causes of death. Anemia at the time of diagnosis is a poor prognostic sign in patients of all ages with relapsing polychondritis, and in patients who are less than 50 years old a saddle nose deformity and systemic vasculitis are poor prognostic signs.

TREATMENT

About one-quarter of the patients with relapsing polychondritis can be treated solely with nonsteroidal antiinflammatory drugs. Generally these patients have mild chondritis of the ears or nose or arthritis.

Until recently the treatment in the majority of patients has consisted of corticosteroids either for persistent disease or for more serious organ involvement with laryngotracheal symptoms, vasculitis, glomerulonephritis, or audiovestibular or neurologic disease. Corticosteroids suppress acute flares, decrease the frequency and severity of recurrences, and decrease the anemia. They appear to be anti-inflammatory and antichondrolytic. Generally prednisone, 40 to 60 mg per day, is used, although occasionally higher dosages may be required. In one study, for example, of the 13 patients with documented sensorineural hearing loss who were treated, eight improved with corticosteroid therapy. In the 75 percent of the patients with relapsing polychondritis who survive 5 years, only one-third continue to require corticosteroids, and in 90 percent of these the dosage of prednisone was tapered to 10 mg per day or less.

Sulfones are used in several dermatological diseases, and in the past decade there have been increasing reports of the use of dapsone (diaminodiphenylsulfone) in relapsing polychondritis. The mechanisms of action is thought to be related to the capacity of the drug to block the lysosomal activity of polymorphonuclear cells. Dapsone oxidizes intracellular glutathione, therefore decreasing the amount of reduced glutathione, which normally acts as a catalyst for lysosomal enzymes that damage chondrocytes. Unfortunately reduced glutathione also protects red blood cells from hemolysis, which is the major side effect of dapsone (especially in patients who are deficient in glucose-6-phosphate dehydrogenase). Other side effects include lethargy, nausea, agranulocytosis, and aplastic anemia.

Generally dosages of dapsone of 25 to 200 mg per day are recommended. In our experience disease in the majority of patients can be controlled with dosages in the lower ranges: six of eight patients required only 50 to 100 mg of dapsone per day throughout the course, and the remaining two, who required higher dosages intially, eventually were controlled with 50 or 100 mg per day. One of our patients treated with only 100 mg of dapsone had resolution of hearing loss with this therapy and has never required corticosteroids. Although dapsone eventually may become the drug of choice for relapsing polychondritis, until more experience is available it is probably most prudent to administer corticosteroids in addition to dapsone in severe disease. Once clinical manifestations have been controlled, the steroid dosage may be tapered slowly. One of our patients was tapered off both corticosteroids and dapsone and had no recurrence of the disease 5 years after discontinuation of both drugs.

About 10 percent of the patients with relapsing polychondritis require immunosuppressive or cytotoxic drug therapy. Cyclophosphamide and azathioprine have been used most frequently. Because of evidence of the role of anticollagen II immunity in relapsing polychondritis and evidence of macrophage–T cell interactions of pathogenetic importance in affected cartilage, cyclosporine A has recently been used successfully in a patient with severe tracheal cartilage damage that was progressive despite treatment with corticosteroids, dapsone, azathioprine, and cyclophosphamide.

At times complications secondary to respiratory difficulties, such as airway collapse and obstruction, can be surgically alleviated. Because patients with airway collapse may be difficult to intubate and bronchoscopy may be difficult, early tracheostomy placement is the preferred procedure. Airway narrowing due to perichondral inflammatory masses and granulation tissue can be corrected by surgical removal of the excess mass and tissue. Cardiac valvular disease and aortic aneurysm are also surgically treatable.

LUPUS ERYTHEMATOSUS

RICHARD D. SONTHEIMER, M.D.

The skin is the second most frequently affected organ in lupus erythematosus (LE), and cutaneous disease is the second most common presenting manifestation of this clinically heterogeneous autoimmune disorder. In some patients the disease process manifests itself exclusively in the form of characteristic skin lesions, whereas in others cutaneous involvement occurs in the context of a relatively mild or potentially life threatening systemic illness. In the latter circumstance certain patterns of cutaneous disease are known to correlate with certain patterns of systemic involvement. The dermatologist is therefore in a unique position to contribute significantly to the management of LE patients through both his understanding of the ways in which the cutaneous and systemic manifestations of this disorder can be related (the *principles* of management) and his special knowledge of the specific drugs that are most useful in treating LE skin lesions (the *principals* of management).

The management of skin disease in LE patients is complicated by the fact that the same type of lesion can occur in the presence or absence of systemic LE (SLE) involvement. It is therefore imperative when considering treatment options for the cutaneous manifestations of this disorder that one always be alert to the possible development or exacerbation of underlying systemic disease activity.

It is my feeling that a patient with any form of LE should receive the same type of initial evaluation, since even patients who have what is usually a relatively innocuous form of cutaneous LE, such as localized discoid LE (DLE), occasionally have evidence of clinically inapparent underlying systemic involvement at the time of presentation. My approach to the work-up and treatment of a new patient is outlined in Table 1. The dermatologist must decide whether he is in a position to carry out the entire evaluation alone or whether the help of an internist, rheumatologist, or other medical subspecialist should be enlisted. It is my hope that the following guidelines will allow the dermatologist who chooses to carry out the initial evaluation alone to do so more comfortably.

TABLE 1 Management of a New Patient with Cutaneous Lupus Erythematosus

Principles of management
    Confirmation of true diagnosis
    Determination of pattern and extent
       of current organ involvement
    Accumulation of data pertaining to
       prognosis

Principals of management
    Patient education
    Local medical therapy
    Systemic medical therapy

PRINCIPLES OF MANAGEMENT

My initial evaluation is designed to accomplish three goals: to confirm the true diagnosis, to determine the pattern and extent of organ involvement so that immediate treatment can be planned, and to accumulate data pertaining to the prognosis to facilitate the development of a long-term management plan. The approach I take to the interview, physical examination, and laboratory analysis of a new LE patient to achieve these goals is discussed sequentially.

Medical History

It is important to establish the duration of the LE related symptoms, since this fact alone can yield prognostic information. Many of the organs that eventually are affected by the LE process in a given patient often show signs of involvement within the first 2 years after the onset of the clinical illness. A drug history should be taken, since certain drugs (e.g., hydralazine, procainamide) are capable of inducing an LE-like illness. This is not a critical point in a patient who has cutaneous LE lesions as the only disease manifestation, since the skin is usually spared in the classic form of drug induced LE. The thiazides appear to be an exception to this rule, since some of these drugs appear to be capable of eliciting photosensitive forms of cutaneous LE, such as subacute cutaneous LE (SCLE). A family history should also be taken. If this is positive for LE or a related illness, one should consider the possibility of a genetic complement component deficiency (e.g., heterozygous or homozygous C2 or C4 deficiency). It has been my impression that LE skin lesions in patients who are genetically complement deficient tend to be more refractory to medical management.

A review of systems should be carried out to uncover symptoms or signs suggestive of systemic LE target organ involvement. Has the patient experienced hair loss, oral ulcers, skin lesions, joint pains, malaise, easy fatiguability, recurrent fevers, or Raynaud's phenomenon? If so, have any of these symptoms been made worse by exposure to sunlight? Has there been any evidence of involvement of the neurologic (headaches, seizures, psychosis), cardiopulmonary (pleuritic chest pain, dyspnea), or vascular (purpuric or urticarial skin lesions, unexplained abdominal pain) system?

Physical Examination

The patient's vital signs should be assessed. Evidence of hypertension could reflect underlying renal involvement. I next begin to characterize the clinical type and pattern of any skin involvement present. This information alone might yield significant insight into the relative risk of concurrent systemic disease activity or the possibility of its developing (Table 2). However, one must always be cognizant of the possibility that any rule concerning prognosis that has ever been formulated from statistical analyses of LE population data can be broken by the course of illness seen in the very next patient.

**TABLE 2 Suggested Screening Laboratory Determinations in a
New Patient with Cutaneous Lupus Erythematosus**

Hematologic tests
Complete blood count with differential and platelet count
Erythrocyte sedimentation rate
Prothrombin and partial thromboplastin times

Blood chemistry tests (SMA-12)
Serum creatinine
Total serum protein (globulin)

Urinary tests
Routine urinalysis

Serologic tests
Antinuclear antibody assay
Anti-Ro/SS-A antibody assay
Serologic test for syphilis (VDRL)

Miscellaneous tests
Total hemolytic complement (CH_{50})
C4

Is there any evidence of LE specific skin disease? Does the patient have a photosensitive symmetrical malar erythematous reaction ("butterfly" rash, i.e., acute cutaneous LE)? If so, her chance of having concurrent, potentially serious SLE activity, particularly renal disease, would be quite high (I refer to this hypothetical patient as a woman in view of the high female preponderance of LE). Does she have only classic scarring DLE lesions limited to the face and scalp (i.e., localized DLE, the most common form of chronic cutaneous LE)? If this were the case, her chance of having significant SLE activity concurrently or in the future would be considerably smaller. Her risk of having SLE or developing it would be somewhat greater if she had discoid lesions both above and below the neck (generalized DLE). In addition, the presence of periungual telangiectasia, lupus panniculitis (lupus profundus, if there is overlying DLE activity), or oral mucosal LE lesions in addition to localized DLE lesions would also significantly increase her risk of having or eventually developing systemic involvement. Does she have nonscarring, papulosquamous, or annular skin lesions in a widespread photorelated distribution that would be compatible with SCLE? If so, she would have approximately a 50 percent chance of having underlying evidence of SLE, although a life threatening form of systemic illness would be unlikely. If there is any confusion about the identity of skin lesions in such a patient, a punch skin biopsy specimen should be examined for characteristic LE specific histopathologic changes, focused at the dermal-epidermal junction. Direct immunofluorescence examination of a skin lesion biopsy specimen could also yield important diagnostic information.

Are there any LE nonspecific skin lesions (vascular lesions, sclerodactyly, calcinosis cutis, bullous lesions)? If so, the patient is also at increased risk of having or developing disease outside the skin.

The patient should next be examined for evidence of musculoskeletal, neurologic, ophthalmologic, cardiovascular, pulmonary, abdominal, or lymphatic system abnormalities that might reflect underlying SLE activity.

Radiologic Examination

A chest x-ray view should be obtained if there is historical or physical evidence to suggest cardiopulmonary disease. If she were to require systemic treatment with corticosteroids, a baseline chest x-ray view or a tuberculin skin test would be helpful in assessing the risk of reactivation of subclinical tuberculosis.

Laboratory Examination

The laboratory can be used during evaluation in a new case of cutaneous LE to confirm the presence of underlying SLE, to assess the risk of development of systemic disease activity if not initially present, and to help identify the type of systemic disease that may be present initially or that might develop.

A large number of laboratory tests can detect the presence or the risk of systemic involvement in cutaneous LE. However, a smaller number of relatively inexpensive determinations can serve as an efficient screening battery during the initial evaluation (Table 3). Pending the results of these screening assays, others can be ordered to gain a clearer picture of the overall illness and to guide future treatment.

If a low hemoglobin level is detected during the screening tests, a direct and indirect Coombs assay could confirm the presence of autoimmune hemolytic anemia. Leukopenia (particularly lymphocytopenia) or thrombocytopenia suggests SLE, as would a markedly elevated erythrocyte sedimentation rate (more than 50 mm per hour). A prolonged prothrombin time or activated partial thromboplastin time (suggestive of a circulating lupus anticoagulant) or a biologic false positive VDRL reaction could reflect the presence of anticardiolipin antibodies, which occasionally are found in the absence of abnormal levels of antinuclear antibodies (ANA). A patient with LE who has circulating anticardiolipin antibody would be at increased risk for recurrent thromboembolic phenomena and spontaneous abortions.

**TABLE 3 Relationships Between Cutaneous and Systemic
Manifestations of Lupus Erythematosus**

Type of Skin Lesion	Risk of Systemic Disease
LE specific	
Acute cutaneous LE	High
Subacute cutaneous LE	Intermediate
Chronic cutaneous LE	
Discoid LE	Low
Hypertrophic LE	Low
Lupus panniculitis (profundus)	Intermediate
Oral mucosal LE	Intermediate
Palmar-plantar LE	
LE nonspecific	
Vascular disease	Intermediate-high
Vasculitis	
Livedo reticularis	
Periungal telangiectasia	
Raynaud's phenomenon	
Alopecia	
Scarring	Low
Nonscarring	Intermediate-high
Sclerodactyly	Intermediate-high
Calcinosis cutis	Intermediate-high
Bullous lesions	Intermediate-high

Smoldering LE nephritis should be suspected if qualitative proteinuria or urinary sediment abnormalities are detected or if the serum creatinine level is elevated. Quantitation of proteinuria (24 hour urine collection) and the glomerular filtration rate (Glofil clearance) are then indicated. The creatinine clearance is not always a reliable index of glomerular filtration rates in LE patients with nephritis. If the serum globulin level is high, serum protein electrophoresis could confirm the presence of hypergammaglobulinemia, a hallmark of SLE.

A positive ANA assay would be of obvious value in screening for the possibility of systemic disease. When carried out on a substrate of human origin, this is a very sensitive test for SLE. However, to insure detection of the rather rare, truly ANA negative SLE patient, one should also screen for the presence of precipitating anti-Ro/SS-A antibody. A patient with anti-Ro/SS-A antibody is likely to have Sjögren's syndrome or widespread photosensitive forms of cutaneous LE such as SCLE. Such a patient would also be at a somewhat increased risk of delivering an infant with neonatal LE. If the ANA titer is significantly elevated, particularly with a peripheral ANA pattern, an assay for double stranded DNA antibody should be carried out. If detected, the risk of having or developing renal involvement would be considerably higher. This risk is even greater if the C4 or total hemolytic complement level (CH_{50}) is abnormally depressed (assuming of course that the patient does not have a genetic complement component deficiency). A high homogeneous ANA titer could indicate the presence of antihistone antibody, which might reflect the presence of a drug-induced LE syndrome. If a very high ANA titer (greater than 1:1280) in a speckled or particulate pattern is found, one should suspect the presence of one or a combination of the extractible nuclear antigen (ENA) antibodies (e.g., anti-

nRNP, anti-Sm). The presence of anti-Sm antibody would confirm that the patient has SLE in view of its high specificity for this disease. The patient's overall systemic illness could be relatively milder and less likely to include renal involvement if anti-nRNP antibody is present.

If after this series of laboratory examinations there remains some confusion about the presence of underlying SLE, one might consider examining a nonlesional skin biopsy specimen by direct immunofluorescence for immunoglobulin or complement components along the dermal-epidermal junction. If three or more such components were identified in relatively sun protected skin, the diagnosis of SLE would be considerably more likely. In addition this finding would place the patient at increased risk of developing LE nephritis.

At this point the decision to enlist the aid of a rheumatologist, internist, neurologist, or nephrologist to assist in the management of the patient can be made depending upon the overall pattern of illness uncovered during the initial evaluation. Follow-up laboratory determinations should be considered at 6 month intervals to detect progression to systemic disease in a patient with cutaneous LE or to gauge the extent and activity of systemic involvement in such a patient known to have SLE. The patient should be instructed to report any new symptoms as soon as possible, since the development or increase in systemic disease activity is rarely asymptomatic.

PRINCIPALS OF MANAGEMENT

Patient Education

Any specific medical regimen that might be of value

in treating cutaneous LE lesions is always more effective if the patient understands certain things about the disease. Both the patient and the physician should understand that emotional and physical stress can aggravate LE, including its cutaneous manifestations. It is always stressful to learn that one has a chronic, poorly understood, potentially life threatening, and incurable disorder such as lupus erythematosus.

I have found that the best way to begin allaying the anxiety (which itself can aggravate the disease process) that naturally follows the diagnosis of LE is to educate the patient about the particular variety of the disorder; the patient's family should be a part of this educational process. Lay literature describing the disease in simplistic terms published by patient support groups such as the Lupus Foundation of America often can facilitate this process. In addition, active participation in groups such as this seems to be of great value to many LE patients. Such groups usually can be located by contacting the local chapter of the Arthritis Foundation. Patients should be advised to avoid reading the often outdated "worst case senerio" descriptions of the disease frequently found in publications in public libraries.

The issue of prognosis also should be addressed at this point. Although a heterogeneous disorder such as LE is never bound by absolute rules, it does tend to follow several general patterns (see foregoing discussion of principles of management). Even if the predictable course is a relatively severe one, most patients find some strength and comfort in knowing about the possible direction that the disease might take. On the basis of the results of the initial evaluation it is often possible to reassure the patient with cutaneous LE that the symptoms of the disease can be controlled and that there is little chance that the disease will take a severe course. It is also comforting for the patient to hear that the mean 10-year incidence of survival in SLE is approximately 90 percent and that most patients today can expect to live a completely normal life span.

The patient should be made aware of the drugs and environmental agents capable of exacerbating LE. Some authorities believe that supplemental estrogens in any form can be detrimental. Others, while acknowledging the indisputable evidence that these drugs can worsen the disease process in experimental animal models, note that there is little basis for believing that the same is true for human LE. It would seem to me prudent to recommend that the patient avoid unnecessary exposure to exogenous estrogens. However, this is a difficult issue to be dogmatic about when considering the use of oral contraceptive therapy. In this situation one must balance the possible detrimental effect of pregnancy on LE against the risk of exacerbating LE by this effective form of birth control. The patient also should understand that any form of trauma to the skin can predispose to the development of new skin lesions (the Koebner reaction). Thus any form of self-manipulation of lesions should be avoided.

There is less disagreement regarding the deleterious effect of ultraviolet light exposure on most forms of LE. White fluorescent light bulbs of the type commonly used to light the home or office present relatively little risk in this regard, since extraordinary circumstances are required to accumulate enough UVB exposure (the portion of the electromagnetic spectrum most responsible for aggravating the cutaneous or systemic manifestations of LE) from this source to be significant. High intensity exposure to UVB or UVA light from the suntan parlor type of bulbs, however, does represent a finite risk and should be avoided. Natural sunlight also presents a clear risk, and common sense measures should be used to avoid unnecessary exposure. Patients should be advised to avoid direct sunlight exposure between 10 AM and 4 PM whenever possible, since more UVB light passes through the atmosphere during this time interval. Activities that involve exposure to sunlight reflected from water, sand, or snow should especially be curtailed during this time of day. Physical protection obtained with the use of broad brimmed hats and long sleeved shirts should be combined with the regular use of water resistant chemical sunscreens with the highest sun protective factors available. Sunscreens are most effective if applied at least 30 minutes before exposure. The regular use of make-up containing sunscreens can offer further protection. Potentially photosensitizing drugs such as tetracycline, thiazides, and piroxicam (Feldene) should be avoided.

Medical Management

The results of the initial evaluation dictate whether the patient is a candidate for local measures alone or whether more aggressive systemic therapy is indicated. Patients with only localized DLE lesions often can be managed with topical or intralesional corticosteroid therapy alone. One or a combination of the aminoquinoline antimalarial drugs is usually sufficient to control the disease in most patients with generalized DLE or SCLE. Even in SCLE, patients with mild systemic involvement often can be managed with antimalarial drugs alone, since these drugs are capable of controlling the musculoskeletal as well as cutaneous manifestations of LE. However, patients with acute cutaneous LE usually require systemic corticosteroid therapy or other forms of immunosuppressive therapy in view of the relatively strong association between this form of skin involvement and significant systemic disease activity. Even in such patients antimalarial drugs can have a steroid sparing effect on the cutaneous and musculoskeletal manifestations of the disease. Recent preliminary data suggest that diaminodiphenyl (dapsone) is effective therapy in some patients with the SCLE form of lupus erythematosus.

An overview of the specific drugs that can be of therapeutic value for the cutaneous manifestations of LE can be found in Table 4. With a few exceptions, the different varieties of LE specific skin lesions respond in a similar fashion to these various drugs. For example, many patients with DLE or SCLE in whom local therapy fails or is impractical respond to one or a combination of the aminoquinoline antimalarial drugs. However, the real challenge in managing cutaneous LE is finding something that is

**TABLE 4 Specific Medical Therapy
Useful in Treating Cutaneous
Lupus Erythematosus**

Local therapy
  Topical therapy
    Sunscreens
    Potent fluorinated corticosteroids
      Flurandrenolide (Cordran) tape
      Betamethasone dipropionate (Diprolene)
      Clobetasol propionate (Temovate)
  Intralesional therapy
    Corticosteroids
      Triamcinolone acetonide suspension
      (Kenalog)

Systemic therapy
  Aminoquinoline antimalarial drugs
    Hydroxychloroquine sulfate (Plaquenil)
    Chloroquine phosphate (Aralen)
    Quinacrine hydrochloride (Atabrine)
  Corticosteroids
    Prednisone
  Dapsone
  Retinoids
    Isotretinoin (Accutane)
    Etretinate (Tigason)
    Etretin (Ro-10-1670)
  Thalidomide
  Clofazamine
  Gold
    Auranofin (Ridaura)
    Gold sodium thiomalate (Myochrisine
    injection)
    Aurothioglucose (Solganal)
  Attenuated androgens
    Danazol (Danocrine)
  Cytotoxic immunosuppressive drugs
    Azathioprine (Imuran)
    Cyclophosphamide (Cytoxan)
    Methotrexate

relatively safe and efficacious for patients whose lesions do not respond to antimalarial therapy alone.

Local Medical Therapy

Potent fluorinated topical corticosteroid therapy (e.g., fluocinonide [Lidex], flurandrenalide [Cordran] tape) has been of some value in patients with localized forms of DLE and SCLE. However, the newer, more potent drugs such as betamethasone diproprionate (Diprolene) and clobetasol propionate (Temovate) may be of even greater value. The potency of these preparations is so great that care must be observed to avoid both local and systemic side effects. Cyclic therapy (2 weeks on, 2 weeks off) can decrease the risk of such complications. Prolonged use of these drugs on the face or in the body fold areas presents the greatest risk of cutaneous side effects (atrophy, telangiectasia). For those not responding to topical therapy, intralesional therapy with long acting corticosteroid suspensions can be of value. Injection of triamcinolone acetonide suspension (2.5 mg per milliliter) through a 27- or 30-gauge needle every 3 to 4 weeks is generally safe. Higher concentrations are more effective but can result in local subcutaneous atrophy

or hypopigmentation. However, this risk might be more acceptable in a DLE patient, considering that the disease itself is likely to produce scarring if not suppressed in some way. Special care should be taken to avoid intravascular injection when treating lesions around the eyes, since there have been reports of vision loss resulting from retinal artery crystal embolization under these circumstances. Patients who are left with scarring and postinflammatory pigmentary disturbances should be made aware of the value that especially formulated make-ups such as Dermablend or Covermark can offer for masking the permanent dystrophic residua this disorder can produce. In addition a wig can be of great psychologic benefit in a patient with irreversible scarring alopecia.

Systemic Medical Therapy

If the patient has evidence of renal, vascular, or central nervous system disease, there should be no hesitation in initiating aggressive treatment with systemic doses of corticosteroids (prednisone, 60 to 80 mg per day orally). Were such a patient to require high dose systemic corticosteroid therapy for any length of time, consideration should be given to adding a steroid sparing drug, such as azathioprine or cyclophosphamide. In addition, calcium with or without vitamin D supplements should be given during long-term steroid therapy. I would suggest that such a patient be managed in concert with the appropriate medical subspecialist.

If the disease is expressed predominantly in the skin or musculoskeletal system, less aggressive management would be indicated. Following a baseline ophthalmologic examination in preparation for antimalarial therapy, such a patient could be started on hydroxychloroquine sulfate (Plaquenil), 400 mg per day for 4 weeks followed by a dosage reduction to 200 mg per day for maintenance. If there is no improvement within 6 to 8 weeks with this regimen, the dosage could be increased again to 400 mg per day for an additional 4 weeks.

If an adequate response has not been achieved at this point, one might consider adding quinacrine hydrochloride (Atabrine), 100 mg per day, after normal glucose-6-phosphate dehydrogenase levels have been confirmed. The risk of retinal toxicity with quinacrine is minimal compared to that with other antimalarial drugs. As an alternative one could consider replacing the hydroxychloroquine with chloroquine phosphate (Aralen), 250 mg per day, since some physicians believe that chloroquine is more effective than hydroxychloroquine in certain patients with cutaneous LE. However, current data suggest that chloroquine has a greater potential for producing retinal toxicity than does hydroxychloroquine. The ophthalmologic examination should be repeated at 6 month intervals while the patient is taking chloroquine or hydroxychloroquine. Antimalarial drugs, particularly quinacrine, also can produce cutaneous (hyperpigmentation, lichenoid eruptions, annular erythematous reactions), hematologic (leukopenia, thrombocytopenia, simple anemia, and rarely aplastic anemia), and gastrointestinal (nausea, vomiting) side effects. Quinacrine also can produce a reversible yellow coloration of the skin in fair skinned patients. It has been suggested that the hematologic toxicity of dapsone and the antimalarial drugs can be additive or possibly even synergistic. I therefore avoid using these drugs concurrently.

Some authorities treat cutaneous LE with a combination of antimalarial drugs and intermediate dose systemic steroid therapy (prednisone, 20 to 40 mg per day) in an attempt to bring the disease activity under control as soon as possible. Because of the increased risk of potentially devastating bone complications in LE patients treated with corticosteroids (i.e., avascular necrosis), I prefer to reserve corticosteroids for patients whose disease does not respond to any of the other drugs listed in Table 4.

There are several other options for patients who do not respond to single drug or combination antimalarial therapy. Dapsone (100 to 200 mg per day in divided oral doses twice daily) has been reported to clear symptoms in some antimalarial refractory DLE and SCLE patients. I find this drug to be better tolerated when started at lower dosages (25 to 50 mg per day) and increased by 25 mg increments weekly.

Both isotretinoin (Accutane) and etretinate (Tigason) have been reported to be of value in refractory cutaneous LE. My experience with isotretinoin (1 mg per kilogram per day) has been that it is of only limited value in cutaneous LE. Any beneficial effect seems to disappear as soon as the drug is withdrawn. Great care must be used when treating a female of child bearing age with either of these drugs, considering their great potential for teratogenicity. There is some promise that the active metabolite of etretinate, etretin (Ro 10-1670), could be safer in this regard and might also be effective in cutaneous LE.

Thalidomide has also been reported by a number of investigators worldwide to be of value in difficult cases of cutaneous LE. However, because of an alarming frequency of cases of neurotoxicity (predominantly sensory neuropathies, sometimes permanent) in LE patients treated with this drug, it is currently impossible to obtain the drug for the treatment of LE. The antileprosy drug clofazimine has also been suggested to be of value in the management of refractory cutaneous forms of LE. The unsightly red staining of the skin that results from therapeutic doses of this drug limits its usefulness.

There have also been reports that the new oral gold preparation auranofin (Ridaura) has been of value in some refractory cases of cutaneous LE. The parenteral administration of gold, one of the classic treatments for cutaneous LE prior to the corticosteroid and antimalarial era, might also be considered in particularly difficult cases. The old concern that gold might potentiate the development of LE nephritis probably arose from a lack of understanding that gold can be nephrotoxic when used to treat any disorder. Recent studies have shown that auranofin does not precipitate or exacerbate LE renal disease. Oral gold therapy has fewer side effects than parenteral gold therapy, but unfortunately it appears to be less efficacious as well in disorders such as rheumatoid arthritis. The proper role of this drug in the management of cutaneous LE remains to be determined. Anecdotal reports have suggested that attenuated androgens such as danazol (Danocrine) might be of some value in certain female patients with therapeutically refractory forms of LE. However, it has also been suggested that this and related drugs can precipitate or aggravate SLE in male patients.

If it does become necessary to resort to the use of corticosteroids in LE patients who have predominantly cutaneous disease, several points should be kept in mind. When using these drugs, one's goal should be to limit their use to the short-term control of acute exacerbations of disease activity, relying on one or a combination of the approaches discussed for long-term management. Once symptoms begin to abate, the dosage should be tapered to 15 mg per day or less as soon as possible. Attempts should be made to convert to an alternate day regimen whenever possible, although LE patients frequently experience "miniflares" during the off days.

As a final resort, one of the cytotoxic immunosuppressive drugs might be justified occasionally in a patient with particularly severe, widespread skin disease. However, when dealing with LE patients whose disease is expressed predominantly in the skin, one should never forget to consider the possibility that the complications of treatment might be worse than the disease itself.

NEONATAL LUPUS ERYTHEMATOSUS

ROSEMARIE WATSON, M.D.

The neonatal lupus erythematosus (NLE) syndrome affects the majority of infants in utero, at birth, or within the first 2 months of life. The two major clinical manifestations of this disorder are congenital heart block and lupus dermatitis, which may be seen singularly or together in the same infant. Additional systemic manifestations that have been described less frequently include hepatomegaly, splenomegaly, pneumonitis, lymphadenopathy, and hematologic abnormalities (leukopenia, anemia, and thrombocytopenia). The Ro(SS-A) antibody, a serologic marker for this syndrome, is present in over 95 percent of the mothers and infants with this disorder. Rarely other autoantibodies are seen in this disorder in addition to Ro antibody, notably La(SS-B) and U_1RNP antibodies. The syndrome is believed to be caused by the transplacental passage of autoantibody from the mother to the fetus. Whereas many of the initial reports of NLE were of infants born to mothers with an overt connective tissue disease, i.e., SLE or Sjögren's syndrome, it is now evident that the majority of mothers (60 percent) are asymptomatic.

In the approach to the management of this disorder, several factors must be considered: the management of the lupus dermatitis, the management of cardiac disease and hematologic abnormalities in the neonate, the management of the Ro positive pregnant woman, the therapeutic approach to the mother of a neonatal lupus infant, and the risk to other siblings.

LUPUS DERMATITIS

Of the infants destined to develop lupus dermatitis, the majority present at birth or more commonly within the first 2 months of life. Photosensitivity is a component of this syndrome. The rash has a predilection for exposed sites, and there are reports of its development after a specific sun exposure. Sun avoidance in all infants born to Ro positive mothers, particularly during the first 3 months of life, is thus recommended. Should a rash develop, treatment with an emollient and 1 percent hydrocortisone three times daily may hasten resolution. The rash resolves spontaneously, often by age 6 months. Scarring is rare, but telangiectasia and pigmentary changes have persisted in some. The infant who presents with lupus dermatitis should be evaluated for the presence of bradycardia, lymphadenopathy, and organomegaly. A complete blood count is recommended to rule out anemia, leukopenia, or thrombocytopenia. Electrocardiography may detect underlying complete or incomplete heart block, which may be masked on physical examination by an adequate ventricular rate.

COMPLETE HEART BLOCK IN THE NEONATE

A recent study revealed that some 80 percent of the infants born with complete heart block manifest the neonatal lupus syndrome. Maternal serum examination for Ro antibody determines the diagnosis.

When complete heart block is isolated, the prognosis is good. Many infants do not require any specific treatment. If the bradycardia becomes symptomatic, pacemaker insertion is indicated. It is clear that there is a subset of these infants who do not do well. The mortality in infants with complete heart block is estimated at approximately 20 percent. The infants who succumb are those with cardiomyopathy or associated structural heart defects. The cardiologist directs treatment in those situations.

MANAGEMENT OF HEMATOLOGIC ABNORMALITIES

Leukopenia and thrombocytopenia generally resolve spontaneously, usually within the first 2 weeks of life. Purpura has been described, and on rare occasions platelet transfusion is required when thrombocytopenia is severe.

MANAGEMENT OF THE Ro POSITIVE PREGNANT WOMAN: COMPLETE HEART BLOCK IN UTERO

The physician should be aware that the risk of a Ro positive mother delivering an infant with NLE is probably low (less than 10 percent). Mothers who are HLA-DR_3 positive appear to be at higher risk, although the magnitude of the risk is unknown at this time. Ro antibody production appears to be controlled by genes associated with the HLA-DR_2 and DR_3 phenotypes. Mothers who are DR_3 positive tend to produce higher titers of this antibody, which may be a factor in expression of the disease.

The early detection of complete heart block in utero can be facilitated by monthly ultrasound examinations of the fetus from the eighth week of life on. If bradycardia is found, dual M mode electrocardiography is advised to monitor the fetal heart rate and possible development of cardiomyopathy. Many infants found to have complete heart block in utero have been followed to term and delivered otherwise healthy with isolated complete heart block. Therapeutic possibilities should be considered when the dual M mode electrocardiogram shows increased heart size or congestive heart failure. Experience suggests that these are the infants with a high mortality.

Because the syndrome is caused by the passage of antibody from the mother to the fetus, some therapeutic possibilities arise: steroid treatment of the mother to treat inflammation of cardiac tissue in the infant and plasmapheresis of the mother to remove the offending antibody. To my knowledge, there has been only one instance in which the mother was thus treated while the infant was still in utero (Buyon JP, et al. Arth Rheum 1987; 30:144–149). An experimental therapeutic regimen of thrice weekly plas-

129

mapheresis and high dose dexamethasone therapy was instituted in the management of a fetus who was documented to have complete heart block, myocarditis, and pericardial effusion in the 24th week of gestation. The mother was positive for La antibody; Ro antibody was not detected. The corticosteroid employed was dexamethasone, because it is not metabolized by the placenta and is thus directly available to the fetus. In this infant the authors stabilized the cardiac status and the infant tolerated delivery at week 31. Cesarean section was performed at this time because of diminishing placental function. At birth no myocarditis was found and the pericardial effusion cleared in 1 week; however, complete heart block persisted.

Plasmapheresis seems a sensible approach in the second and third trimesters because it is during these periods that the majority of antibodies cross the placenta. This mode of treatment has been used safely to treat mothers with antirhesus antibodies and anti-P blood group antibodies and also to treat flares of systemic lupus in pregnant women. The problems associated with plasmapheresis must be weighed against the possible benefits. These problems include possible induction of premature labor, reduction of nutrients supplied to the fetus, and an overall decrease in the antibodies reaching the fetal circulation. These risks did not pose any practical problems in the case just described.

The question arises, "Should a mother who has already had an infant with complete heart block undergo plasmapheresis at the onset of her second pregnancy in order to avoid the possibility of a second child with complete heart block?" Since the risk of having a second child with complete heart block appears to be on the order of 25 percent, it would appear to be more prudent to follow the fetus and to delay the decision about introduction of therapy until fetal bradycardia develops. To date, complete heart block once detected is irreversible. If a mother has a second child with complete heart block, the risk of her having a third with the same condition is sufficiently high to warrant consideration of plasmapheresis early in the next pregnancy. All infants born with complete heart block should be evaluated for pneumonitis, lymphadenopathy, organomegaly, and hematologic abnormalities (i.e., leukopenia, thrombocytopenia, anemia) because these are other features of the neonatal lupus syndrome.

MANAGEMENT OF THE MOTHER OF A NEONATAL LUPUS INFANT

Approximately 40 percent of the mothers have overt disease at the time of birth of a neonatal lupus infant. The patient should be evaluated for the presence of a connective tissue disorder by a careful history and physical examination. We note that mothers of neonatal lupus infants not only are at risk of developing lupus but also may develop Sjögren's syndrome. The potential risk of development of a connective tissue disease is probably high. In a follow-up study of 21 neonatal lupus families (15 percent of the reported cases; McCune, et al. Ann Intern Med 1987; 106:518–523), J Rheumatol, in press), 50 percent of the mothers were initially asymptomatic but in a 4½ year follow-up, 80 percent had symptoms suggestive of connective tissue disease. A long interval (reported cases up to 16 years) may intervene between delivery of an NLE infant and the development of maternal connective tissue disease. Some of these women have reported increased fetal wastage, although McCune et al found that the incidence of spontaneous abortion (6/53, 11.3 percent) did not differ significantly from that in a large control group (76/706, 10.6 percent).

RISK FOR SIBLINGS

Mothers should be advised that the chance of having a second infant with neonatal lupus is low. The risk of further sibling involvement has been estimated at 25 percent based on a prospective study in which three of 12 live births after the birth of the first child with neonatal lupus resulted in another affected child. It is not clear why this is so, because the maternal influences appear to be unchanged in each pregnancy. The mother of an infant with complete heart block may subsequently deliver a second infant with complete heart block, complete heart block with lupus dermatitis, or lupus dermatitis alone.

RISK OF CONNECTIVE TISSUE DISEASE IN THE NEONATAL LUPUS INFANT

The prognosis appears to be excellent, particularly for those with lupus dermatitis. The dermatitis resolves at 6 months and the infants remain well. Complete heart block is irreversible, but many of these infants have gone on to lead productive lives. There are, however, six case reports in the literature of neonatal lupus infants going on to develop connective tissue disease, notably, systemic lupus erythematosus, Sjögren's syndrome, and rheumatoid arthritis later in life. In one infant the onset of rheumatoid arthritis was at age 4½ years. The other reports occurred in the teenage years and early twenties. Thus, the infant's pediatrician should be alerted to this possibility for the future.

While we are still in the dawn of therapeutic intervention for infants affected with neonatal lupus erythematosus, this area remains an exciting challenge for specialists involved in the care of these mothers and their infants.

DERMATOMYOSITIS

IRA N. TARGOFF, M.D.

Dermatomyositis is characterized by proximal muscle weakness with elevated muscle enzyme levels and a typical rash. Electromyography and muscle biopsy are used to help confirm the diagnosis. A clinically similar myopathy, which occurs without the rash, is referred to as polymyositis. Polymyositis can be confused with other conditions (sporadic dystrophies, infections, and other inflammatory myopathies, such as inclusion body myositis), but the diagnosis is less of a problem with dermatomyositis when the rash is characteristic, although infections mimicking dermatomyositis (echovirus infection in agammaglobulinemic patients, or occasionally toxoplasmosis) must be recognized and treated accordingly. Juvenile dermatomyositis, dermatomyositis-polymyositis associated with malignant disease, and dermatomyositis-polymyositis occurring as part of an overlap syndrome are additional subgroups that can be distinguished. Unless indicated, the discussion in this article applies to the uncomplicated adult case of dermatomyositis. The therapy of polymyositis is similar.

Dermatomyositis and polymyositis have long been thought to have an autoimmune pathogenesis, since they produce an inflammatory pathologic picture, occur in overlap syndromes with other connective tissue diseases, and are associated with immunologic abnormalities. The general approach to therapy therefore has been to use corticosteroids as the first line of therapy and cytotoxic immunosuppressive drugs (usually methotrexate or azathioprine) if the steroids fail. These drugs appear to be very effective in many cases, with some dramatic, even lifesaving responses following their administration. Randomized, prospective, placebo controlled trials of most of these drugs in order to document their efficacy are lacking, but most authorities believe that they have activity in this disease, at least in improving strength and function. Unfortunately the disease sometimes recurs or chronic activity persists despite therapy.

In most cases of dermatomyositis in which weakness is clinically recognized, it should be treated. Therapy is usually started with 1 mg per kilogram per day of prednisone. If there is no initial response in a patient with severe disease, additional benefit might be realized by raising the dosage to 1.5 mg per kilogram per day. A further increase in the dosage is unlikely to result in significant benefit but increases the risk of side effects. Dosages of up to 2 mg per kilogram per day have been recommended in children. We use prednisone (or methylprednisolone) as the steroid preparation. Long-acting steroids such as dexamethasone should be avoided, because they are more likely to induce steroid myopathy and have a greater likelihood of causing side effects with prolonged therapy. If hydrocortisone is used, particular attention must be paid to avoiding hypokalemia. There are no absolute contraindications, but great care must be taken when administering steroids to patients with diabetes, hypertension, infection, or peptic ulcer disease.

Some retrospective studies in the literature seem to indicate that high single dose, alternate day corticosteroid therapy is effective as initial therapy for some patients with polymyositis or dermatomyositis, with a lower incidence of side effects than with daily therapy. I do not initiate therapy with this type of regimen. Effective initial therapy is important in patients with significant weakness. This regimen has not yet been studied systematically and should be considered less reliably effective; it should not be used in severe cases.

Single dose daily administration of prednisone is also considered less apt to cause side effects than divided doses and can be used initially in many cases, particularly in those with a slower onset. In more severe cases steroid therapy in the higher dosage range should be started with divided doses. These more severe cases include patients with pharyngeal (or facial) involvement and a suppressed gag reflex, leading to danger of aspiration; respiratory muscle involvement, which may pose the danger of respiratory failure; difficulty with speech; signs of cardiac involvement; systemic signs such as fever; extreme or rapidly developing weakness; and those who have indications for more intensive therapy related to associated conditions (such as severe manifestations of systemic lupus erythematosus). After the patient is out of acute danger, the steroid therapy should be consolidated to a single daily dose. Although at least one study has indicated an improved long-term outcome by beginning therapy with an immunosuppressive drug in association with prednisone, we do not do this routinely. Many patients respond and remain well after treatment with prednisone alone and thus avoid this increased risk.

Side effects are a serious problem with prolonged high dose prednisone therapy. As in other situations, it regularly leads to Cushing's syndrome and adrenal suppression and may lead to diabetes, hypertension, or severe opportunistic infections. Extended steroid therapy may lead to cataracts, ischemic necrosis of bone, and accelerated atherosclerosis. Osteoporosis can be a major problem, and patients who require long-term steroid therapy probably should take calcium supplements (500 to 1,000 mg of calcium and 400 units of vitamin D daily with a regular diet would be reasonable, checking the urinary calcium level periodically). Peptic ulcer is a possible danger and prophylactic therapy is often given concomitantly.

Of particular concern in cases of dermatomyositis are complications that could lead to muscle weakness. The mineralocorticoid effects of steroids could lead to the development of hypokalemia, which, although easily dealt with if recognized, could lead to muscle weakness. Steroids also can lead directly to a myopathy characterized by type II fiber atrophy, without inflammation or elevation of the creatine phosphokinase level. When this effect is prominent, the condition ("steroid myopathy") may be mistaken for worsening of the underlying dermatomyositis, leading the physician to raise the dose of steroids. Steroid myopathy is suggested by the recurrence of weakness without a parallel rise in the creatine phosphokinase level. Further support can be obtained, if necessary, by a repeat muscle biopsy. One can try lowering the steroid dosage and observing the patient for evidence of improvement.

In addition to medication, there are other initial therapeutic considerations. In severe cases hospitalization is indicated to allow close monitoring of initial progress and detection and management of complications. Care must be taken to avoid aspiration in patients with dysphagia or loss of the gag reflex, and measures such as the use of a feeding tube or parenteral alimentation may be necessary. Patients with severe respiratory involvement sometimes may require mechanical ventilation. Occasionally heart involvement leads to significant block that requires a pacemaker or congestive heart failure requiring treatment (this often develops later). In children, bowel perforation is another danger. During the hospital stay the patient also should begin passive range of motion exercises to maintain mobility and avoid contractures. Active exercise should be discouraged during the acute period. Some assistance also should be provided in coping with the activities of daily living during the period of severe disability.

It is crucial to monitor the progress of muscle disease on a regular basis, by both physical examination and muscle enzyme determinations. Severely affected patients should be reassessed every 2 to 4 weeks, and at first even more frequent visits may be necessary. Patients taking high doses of steroids also must be monitored for side effects (diabetes, hypertension, fluid accumulation, electrolyte abnormalities). The muscles involved initially, as well as the shoulder and pelvic girdle muscles, facial muscles, and neck muscles, should be tested directly. Muscle strength should be recorded on a graded scale so that the results can be compared over many months. Other useful measures include measuring the ability to stand from a lying position or to rise from a chair without use of the arms, and the length of time that the arms can be held horizontally or the head raised off the bed. The progress of the rash (except for vasculitis) and the heliotrope coloration should not be used to assess the therapeutic response.

The creatine phosphokinase level is elevated initially in most patients with dermatomyositis, and its level fluctuates with disease activity, making it a helpful guide to therapy. A rise sometimes can predict a flare. It should be measured as part of the diagnostic work-up and during the follow-up period, as part of each clinical evaluation. The creatine phosphokinase level may be elevated by intramuscular injections or even by vigorous muscular activity. An elevated level occurring shortly after such events cannot be interpreted. The usefulness of isoenzyme levels is unclear. Some reports claim that the creatine phosphokinase MB isoenzyme is associated with cardiac involvement. An elevated MB isoenzyme level might raise the suspicion of this complication, but it is not a reliable marker, because both false negative and false positive results are well documented.

The initial creatine phosphokinase level may be normal despite active disease (noted in 4 to 30 percent in various series, and in less than 10 percent in my experience).

In a few of these cases the level of another muscle enzyme (such as aldolase) is elevated and may be used in following the activity of the muscle disease. Another enzyme occasionally may be more helpful even if the creatine phosphokinase level is elevated. The 24-hour urine creatine excretion is a sensitive indicator of disease activity, and the level can be elevated when enzyme levels are normal. The serum myoglobin level correlates well with activity and has also been used for this purpose. Other laboratory tests are not usually used in following the progress of muscle disease, nor are electromyography or biopsy. Although some have found the erythrocyte sedimentation rate helpful, it does not correlate with activity.

The response time is variable. Some patients report subjective improvement within 2 weeks. Most patients show improvement within 4 to 6 weeks, but up to 3 months of full dose therapy may be necessary. Those with a slow onset and chronic activity often respond more slowly than those with acute disease. If no significant decrease in the creatine phosphokinase level or increase in strength has occurred by 3 months, the addition of a cytotoxic drug should be considered. It may need to be considered earlier with very severe or acute disease or a severe steroid side effect. Some patients will have lost some strength permanently and will not recover completely even after suppression of all disease activity. This must be recognized in order to avoid unnecessarily prolonged therapy. High doses should be continued, however, at least as long as progressive improvement continues and until the creatine phosphokinase level returns to normal. Most responders achieve these goals within 3 to 4 months, but it may take 6 months. Improvement in strength tends to lag behind a decrease in the creatine phosphokinase level. Normalization of the creatine phosphokinase level is not by itself enough to define a response, since it may occur with steroid therapy in the absence of recovery of strength and in the presence of continuing muscle inflammation. Persistent disease activity also should lead to consideration of cytotoxic drugs.

As the therapeutic goals are achieved, the prednisone dosage should be tapered. Tapering to a moderate dosage can be relatively rapid, but tapering below 20 mg per day should be done slowly. The initial daily steroid dosage may be tapered to about 30 to 40 mg per day by decreasing the daily dosage by 5 mg every week. After achieving this moderate dosage the daily dosage is lowered by 5 mg every 2 weeks to 20 mg per day, then by 2.5 mg every 2 to 4 weeks until the level is 10 mg per day, and then by 1 mg every 2 to 4 weeks to zero. Maintenance on low dosage therapy may be required for some time. In our experience daily low dosage regimens have been more effective than alternate day regimens in maintaining remissions in dermatomyositis, and so we generally taper by gradual reduction of the daily dosage as described.

Dosing is routinely converted to alternate day therapy by some, and this could be particularly useful if steroid side effects occur. This can be achieved by a number of regimens. As an example, after achieving a moderate daily dosage, the dosage is doubled on the first day, and then the dosage on the next and subsequent alternate days is gradually lowered (e.g., by 5 mg every 4 to 6 days until 20 mg on the alternate day is reached and then by 2.5 mg every 6 to 8 days, although the rate of tapering is tailored to the individual). Once alternate day therapy is achieved, the alternate day dosage is lowered very gradually. It should be remembered that a given dosage on alternate days is not likely to be as effective as half that dosage every day. The speed of the tapering for all regimens should be modified to fit the response of the individual patient.

Flares of activity, as determined by recurrent weakness or elevation of the creatine phosphokinase level, are frequently encountered during tapering. Should signs of a flare occur, the prednisone dosage should be raised back to a level above that which last maintained control of the disease, but usually only part of the original dosage need be restored. Tapering should not resume until the clinical and laboratory signs of recurrent disease have resolved, and it is wise to taper more slowly. Therapy may need to be extended for long periods. Although some patients may be able to stop steroids in 6 months, others may require therapy for 3 to 5 years or more. Although only one-quarter of the patients respond to the initial course of prednisone and continue to do well, the majority can be managed with steroids alone. The long-term consequences of such prolonged therapy must be considered.

Cytotoxic drugs are often used when the steroid dosage cannot be tapered without a resulting flare of disease activity, if the response to steroids is inadequate (see foregoing discussion), or if severe steroid toxicity develops. The optimal timing of the introduction of these drugs has not been established and depends to some extent on the severity of the disease. A number of cytotoxic drugs have been used in the treatment of dermatomyositis or polymyositis with reported responses, including azathioprine, methotrexate, cyclophosphamide, chlorambucil, and most recently cyclosporine A, although none are FDA approved for this condition. Azathioprine and methotrexate are used most often. They generally cause fewer side effects, and there is more reported experience than with cyclophosphamide or chlorambucil. Either azathioprine or methotrexate may be used first, for there is no established basis for favoring either as a general rule. I usually begin with methotrexate, except in patients with preexisting lung, kidney, or liver disease or alcoholism.

Methotrexate may be given intravenously or orally in dermatomyositis. Intramuscular injections are generally avoided in patients with myopathy, particularly when the creatine phosphokinase level is being monitored. Oral therapy with daily doses of methotrexate has been associated with more complications (cirrhosis and pneumonitis) than intravenous therapy. Intermittent weekly oral doses used in psoriasis (given weekly in three doses separated by 12-hour intervals), and more recently in rheumatoid arthritis, have been less toxic than daily oral dosing. The dosages conventionally used in dermatomyositis have been higher, however, and at this dosage level intravenous administration is probably best until more information is obtained.

Usually therapy is begun with a small dose (10 to 15 mg) as a test, and the dosage, administered weekly, is gradually increased to 0.4 to 0.8 mg per kilogram per week, up to 30 to 50 mg per week. (If given orally, it should also be taken weekly, usually in divided doses.) With each weekly dose, an assessment is made of the progress, measured by clinical examination and muscle enzyme determinations and watching for possible side effects, including nausea, diarrhea, stomatitis, rash, infection, pneumonitis, hepatitis, and myelosuppression. Should mild transient elevations of liver enzyme levels occur (distinct from muscle induced rises in SGOT or LDH levels), therapy may be cautiously reinstituted at a lower dosage with careful monitoring, but cessation of therapy must be considered in cases of higher or persistent elevations (the cirrhosis reported in psoriasis may occur without liver enzyme abnormalities). The patient should be warned against consuming alcohol, and the drug is best avoided when hepatic disease exists. Impairment of renal function can cause dangerous accumulation of methotrexate; if it is used at all, dosage adjustment is required. All nonsteroidal anti-inflammatory drugs, probenecid, and certain other drugs should be used with caution while methotrexate is being administered.

A response may be seen in as little as 4 to 6 weeks, but over 4 months may be necessary. Half to three-fourths of the patients requiring methotrexate improve. A response allows reduction of the steroid dosage, after which the methotrexate dosage may be tapered by extending the interval between doses—first to every 2 weeks, then every 3 weeks, then every month, and finally discontinuation. The dosage often can be tapered before a cumulative dosage of 1.5 g is reached, but more may be required. If extended use is necessary, some recommend a liver biopsy at the 1.5 g level.

Azathioprine is used orally at a level of 1.5 to 2 mg per kilogram per day, up to 150 to 200 mg per day. Complete blood counts should be monitored closely, at 1 to 2 week intervals for the first 1 to 2 months and then at 2 to 4 week intervals. The dosage should be lowered (or discontinued) if the white cell count falls below 3,000 per cubic millimeter. (If the patient is taking allopurinol, the dosage of azathioprine must be lowered to 25 percent of the usual dosage.) Beneficial effects may be expected in half the patients requiring the drug, but they may take as long as 6 to 9 months to become apparent. Following a response the prednisone dosage should be tapered first, with careful follow-up at least every month. When the patient's condition has been stable with azathioprine alone or with low dosages of prednisone for 2 to 3 months, the azathioprine dosage may be tapered slowly over a 4 to 6 month period. Side effects include nausea and vomiting, myelosuppression, and opportunistic infections. Hypersensitivity reactions may occur, including allergic hepatitis, and pulmonary fibrosis may rarely be seen. Increased risk of malignant change, which occurs in renal transplant patients taking azathioprine, is a concern.

Cyclophosphamide has been used in dermatomyositis and polymyositis, usually given orally at a level of 1.5 to 2.5 mg per kilogram per day with hydration (a single morning dose facilitates hydration). It is associated with hemorrhagic cystitis (which may be severe), an increased risk of malignant disease, infertility, and hair loss, in addition to myelosuppression and other side effects. Although the drug is apparently quite effective, these relatively frequent and severe side effects limit its use. Chlorambucil also has been used in refractory patients with, reportedly, some success, but it also carries a risk of malignant disease and other side effects. A number of case reports describe dramatic benefits from the use of cyclosporine A. Experience is limited at this time, but this drug is quite promising for the future.

If the patient is refractory to more conventional therapy, various experimental approaches may be tried. A number of reports, including large series, have described responses with the use of plasmapheresis, along with cyclophosphamide or chlorambucil and usually prednisone. Controlled trials are needed to determine whether plasmapheresis really adds anything to the regimen, but it might be considered in refractory cases with acute courses. "Pulse steroids," the administration of 0.5 to 1.0 g of methylprednisolone intravenously (over 30 to 45 minutes) on each of 3 consecutive days (or similar protocols), have been used, but long-term benefit has not been demonstrated. Various unusual side effects have been reported with this therapy, including fatal sepsis and arrhythmias. One report describes benefit from the use of "intensive immunosuppression" with antilymphocyte globulin, azathioprine, and high dose steroid therapy. As a last resort, total body irradiation has been used successfully in a few cases.

Acute untreated dermatomyositis is commonly incapacitating and may be life threatening, and systemic therapy directed at the myopathy is usually required. This therapy is usually effective for the skin disease, and thus therapy directed at the rash is not usually necessary, but local use of steroid creams is sometimes prescribed. Rarely hydroxychloroquine has been used for the skin disease, but it should not be expected to have any effect on the muscle disease. One report describes improvement in a patient with dermatomyositis and digital vasculitis after taking antiplatelet drugs. Calcinosis develops in some patients (usually children) and may remain as a long-term sequela of juvenile dermatomyositis. Satisfactory treatment of the calcinosis remains elusive, and the many reported therapies have been disappointing. The latest suggested therapy, low dose warfarin, remains to be proven. Occasionally a patient may present with the classic rash of dermatomyositis without evidence of clinical muscle disease. As long as this situation persists, the therapies described would be inappropriate, but these patients must be followed closely, since the rash sometimes precedes the myopathy.

With these therapies, improved general medical care, and possibly other factors, the prognosis in dermatomyositis is better today than in the past, the current 8-year survival being over 70 percent. In the presence of malignant disease the prognosis for the malignant disease may determine the outcome, but it should not be assumed that resection of the malignant tumor will cure the dermatomyositis or that the responsiveness of the dermatomyositis is dependent on response of the malignant disease. Other factors suggesting a less favorable outcome include older age, cardiac involvement, and impairment of the muscles of swallowing or respiratory function. The prognosis for muscle function is worse in patients with a chronic progressive course. Thus, with available therapy, most improve and many recover, but some do not respond, a number relapse, some permanently lose some function, and some develop significant side effects. An effective specific therapy is still needed.

MIXED CONNECTIVE TISSUE DISEASE

MORRIS REICHLIN, M.D.

Mixed connective tissue disease (MCTD) was described in the early 1970s by Sharp and associates as an overlap syndrome with features of systemic lupus erythematosus, polymyositis, and scleroderma. The clinical picture was quite pleomorphic, with variable numbers of features of each of the constituent diseases. No fixed clinical criteria for disease definition have been set. The consistent unifying feature of the syndrome was serologic: high titers of antibody to the nuclear RNA protein antigen, now known to be composed of U1 RNA and seven proteins composing an RNA protein particle, with antigenicity residing in several of the polypeptides. Recent research suggests that antibody to a 68-70KD nuclear matrix derived protein may be a specific marker for this syndrome. Controversy has surrounded the definition and even the existence of this syndrome, but that is not to be the focus of this discussion. Something must be said about disease definition so that one knows for which patients the described treatments are being recommended. For the purpose of this article, mixed connective tissue disease is defined primarily by the serologic criterion of antibodies to the nuclear RNP antigen accompanied by features of one or more of the following diseases: systemic lupus erythematosus (SLE), scleroderma, and polymyositis.

In that vein, my approach to these patients has been to follow the empirically developed guidelines for the treatment of the constituent diseases that compose the syndrome. The independent value of defining the disease is in the determination of the specific antibody that carries with it a somewhat more benign prognosis than that of the average patient with any of the three constituent diseases under discussion. If one is dealing with a disease with a benign prognosis, one should be more reserved in utilizing aggressive treatment, but as in all such matters some patients could present with what appears to be a serious complication. In any case, certain of the constituent complications generally require therapy for their resolution, which usually consists of systemic corticosteroid therapy. Table 1 lists the various features of the three constituent diseases that compose MCTD. They are listed for the first eight manifestations in order of increasing gravity, and therefore the applied therapies are more powerful and concomitantly more dangerous. On the right side of the table in shorthand terms are the suggested therapies.

ARTHRITIS

Arthritis is extremely common in patients with MCTD: it occurs in 80 to 90 percent of the patients. In general, the arthritis is indistinguishable from that which occurs in SLE. It is a rheumatoid-like arthritis in distribution and in character except that the arthritis is largely

TABLE 1   Features of Constituent Diseases that Compose MCTD

Arthritis	Nonsteroidal anti-inflammatory drugs, aspirin
Erosive arthritis	Remittive drugs, Plaquenil penicillamine, Imuran
Dermatitis	Local steroids, sun avoidance, sunscreens, antimalarial drugs for extensive disease
Raynaud's phenomenon	Cold avoidance Minipress, nifedipine
Pleuritis, pericarditis, peritonitis	Nonsteroidal anti-inflammatory drugs, if uncomplicated; steroids if accompanied by fever, general systemic signs and symptoms
Hemolytic anemia, thrombocytopenia	Steroids
Nephritis	Same as in lupus; depends on lesion, extent of disease
Central nervous system disease	Steroids
Polymyositis	Steroids
Scleroderma involvement	Same approach as in scleroderma; penicillamine may be useful in rapidly progressive skin disease, may prevent internal organ involvement; steroids may be useful in inflammatory lung disease

nondestructive and nonerosive and tends accordingly to be nondeforming. The frequency of distribution is similar to that in rheumatoid arthritis, and involvement of the hands and feet is most common, followed by involvement of the wrists, elbows, shoulders, knees, ankles, and hips.

The treatment is in every way similar to that of the rheumatoid patient with nonerosive nondestructive disease—physical therapy, rest, and one of the nonsteroidal anti-inflammatory drugs or aspirin. I do not use Motrin in these patients, since a number of patients with SLE have developed aseptic meningitis while receiving this drug. The response is usually similar to that seen in rheumatoid disease, one-half to two-thirds of the patients responding promptly after such therapy and requiring nothing else for this manifestation of the disease.

Perhaps as many as one-third of the patients develop a chemically manifest hepatitis with the use of aspirin. This is unfortunate in some cases, since a number of the patients who have chemical hepatitis have responded well to the aspirin. On the other hand, it is prudent to discontinue the aspirin under these circumstances. Although I know of no long-term follow-up of such patients in whom the use of aspirin has been continued, clearly this would constitute an experiment that would be difficult to justify, since there are other drugs that are generally effective even if considerably more expensive.

A small proportion of patients with antibodies to nuclear RNP develop erosive destructive arthritis, which is in my experience always rheumatoid factor positive. I approach these patients with exactly the same philosophy as in patients with erosive destructive rheumatoid arthritis. The first drug I use in such patients is Plaquenil, and I employ it in dosages of two 200 mg tablets a day with ophthalmologic monitoring every 6 months. If retinal problems occur, the drug must be discontinued. This must now be very rare. If the patient responds within the first 2 to 3 months, I reduce the dosage to one tablet a day and sustain that for an indefinite period of time. On the other hand, I do not give up on the prospect for success with Plaquenil until the patient has been taking two tablets a day for a minimum of 5 to 6 months.

If Plaquenil fails, I use penicillamine in a manner entirely analogous to that employed for rheumatoid arthritis. I prefer penicillamine rather than gold because of convenience and an impression that allergic reactions to gold are somewhat more frequent than those to penicillamine in lupus patients. I deliberately have not used gold in such patients, but have had a number of patients referred to me with severe gold reactions who turned out to have antinuclear RNP positive polyarthritis. Obviously a great deal of patient selection is involved in such observations, but they do influence one's behavior.

If penicillamine fails after an appropriate period of treatment, usually not less than 6 months and after achieving a total dosage of 750 mg per day, one is faced with the same difficult situation that is faced in rheumatoid arthritis patients who fail both conservative therapy and remittive drug therapy. At this point I favor the use of Imuran in the same dosages recommended for rheumatoid arthritis. This dosage is between 1 and 2 mg per kilogram per day to induce a remission and then a lower dosage for maintenance, determined empirically by the clinical response. Other modalities for progressive destructive arthritis in such patients are completely empiric, and there is little experience with them.

DERMATITIS

The treatment of dermatitis is, in my experience, identical to that for the various forms of dermatitis in lupus patients. Indeed the skin lesions are indistinguishable from those in lupus patients. Guidelines are similar in terms of approach and management. When photosensitivity accompanies the development and perpetuation of the lesions, the usual precautions should be taken for sun avoidance with appropriate hats, clothing, and the use of sunscreens. I encourage my patients, even when they are not demonstrably photosensitive, to take at least reasonable precautions—hats and medium levels of sun block—if they are going to be exposed to the sun. On the other hand, for patients who are very photosensitive and who must occasionally go into the sun, there are now very effective sun blocks, and any one with a rating of 15 is usually sufficient.

For acute and intermittent erythematous eruptions, local steroid therapy is usually effective. Various grades of creams can be used, but simple 1 percent hydrocortisone creams at the outset are usually effective. However, creams with triamcinolone are used in more difficult cases. Simple local measures usually are adequate in less severe cases. When skin disease is more widespread, as in the variant known as subacute cutaneous lupus (which also occurs in patients with antinuclear RNP, although not nearly as frequently as in patients with antibodies to Ro/SS-A), Plaquenil is effective and only rarely fails to control such lesions. The mode of administration is similar to that used for the erosive polyarthritis already described.

Clearly, some patients with difficult and progressive arthritis and widespread dermatitis may be well controlled with Plaquenil alone. In my experience, few patients have skin disease so difficult to control that systemic steroid therapy is either warranted or necessary. However, this occasionally occurs and steroids are then used in whatever dosages are necessary to control the skin disease. One generally treats for a relatively short period of time to bring the skin lesions under control, that is, with 1 mg per kilogram per day for 7 to 10 days, followed by a sharp reduction in dosage until the dosage is found that controls the skin disease. The exception is the rare patient who has widespread vasculitic lesions of the skin. In such patients steroids in whatever dosage is required are effective. One begins with 1 mg per kilogram per day to bring the lesions under control and then determine the minimal dosage required to control that aspect of the disease.

RAYNAUD'S PHENOMENON

The cardinal principle of management is cold avoidance and appropriate clothing at the time of year when this becomes a problem. Bothersome as they may be for people who are particularly sensitive, gloves should be worn when cold things are removed from the refrigerator or when it is necessary to handle cold objects. Many drugs have been used in the treatment of Raynaud's phenomenon and most are disappointing, although all have been said to be effective at one time or another in individual patients. These include phenoxybenzamine, guanethidine, methyldopa, and reserpine.

I no longer use any of these drugs in the management of Raynaud's phenomenon, and in difficult situations I now first use nifedipine in dosages of 10 mg three times a day, increased to 20 mg three times daily if necessary. If nifedipine is ineffective, Minipress is my next choice. Minipress in dosages of 1 mg three times daily increased to 2 or 3 mg three times daily may be used depending on the response. The first 1 mg tablet of Minipress should be taken at night by the few patients who experience syncope as a reaction to the drug. I find nifedipine particularly useful and have noted rapid healing of small skin lesions resulting from vasoconstriction in patients with Raynaud's phenomenon. I am confident that this drug—like all the others—is not uniformly effective, but it is probably one of the better drugs developed in recent years for the treatment of Raynaud's phenomenon in this and other clinical settings.

SEROSITIS

Serositis comprises mainly pleuritis and pericarditis and rarely peritonitis, in order of decreasing frequency of occurrence. I will focus on the first two. They are common in patients with this form of lupus or overlap syndrome. Pleuritis occurs in 50 to 60 percent of such patients: roughly half these patients also have pericarditis. A number of patients have isolated pericarditis.

In the usual situation involving pleuritis, the decision regarding the mode of treatment depends largely on the clinical setting. If it is an isolated phenomenon, with pleural pain and minimal effusion without other signs of systemic illness, nonsteroidal anti-inflammatory drugs can be effective. I usually use Indocin in dosages of 50 mg three times daily for the first 2 days or until symptoms are brought under control; the dosage is then reduced to 25 mg three times a day.

If the pleuritis is accompanied by other signs of systemic disease and the patient is ill with fever, gastrointestinal symptoms, and so on, I consider this an indication for systemic steroid therapy. Steroids should be used for as short a period of time as is necessary to bring these symptoms under control. One may start with 1 mg per kilogram per day until the signs and symptoms of pleuritis are controlled, the appetite improves, and the patient is afebrile. Thereafter, the steroids are rapidly tapered to whatever dosage is required to maintain the patient in an asymptomatic state. When pleuritis is accompanied by significant fluid accumulation, steroids are almost always necessary for resolution.

An approach similar to that for pleuritis is possible with pericarditis. However, I have seen two patients with antinuclear RNP alone who presented with cardiac tamponade related to pericarditis and required pericardiocentesis for improvement of the cardiovascular status. Patients are then treated with steroids in a manner and dosage similar to what has been described for the treatment of pleuritis accompanied by fluid in the pleural cavity or systemic signs and symptoms.

HEMATOLOGIC INVOLVEMENT

Hematologic complications are common in MCTD. A patient may have hemolytic anemia, thrombocytopenia, or leukopenia. It is an error to consider leukopenia an indication for therapy of any type. It is extremely common, and although the granulocyte and lymphocyte count—both of which are usually depressed—do rise with steroid treatment. I have followed patients with low white counts for many years who do not seem to have unusual problems with infection and are best left alone. On the other hand, Coombs positive hemolytic anemia with a hemoglobin count of less than 10 g per deciliter in females or less than 12 g per deciliter in males is to me an indication for steroid treatment.

The approach to this, as well as to platelet counts less than 100,000 mm³, is in all respects similar to the recommendations made for autoimmune hemolytic anemia or idiopathic thrombocytopenic purpura. In both instances, steroids are the mainstay of treatment and are used—as they are for the other manifestations—at a level of 1 mg per kilogram per day until there is normalization of either the hematocrit or the platelet count; in some instances normalization may occur within a few days, especially the platelet count. However, in both instances I have sustained the dosage of medication at the milligram per kilogram level for a minimum of 3 to 4 weeks before beginning a reduction to the lowest dosage that will sustain the hemoglobin or platelet count in the normal range. Blockade of the reticuloendothelial system and loss of rapid destruction of red cells or platelets, which are characteristic of both these syndromes, probably occur in a few days. On the other hand, it has been shown in autoimmune hemolytic anemia that several weeks are required to reduce effectively the production of autoantibody, which is ultimately responsible for the shortened life span of red cells, and presumably similar considerations would apply in idiopathic thrombocytopenic purpura.

RENAL AND CENTRAL NERVOUS SYSTEM INVOLVEMENT

I come now to two manifestations that are only rarely found in patients with the overlap under discussion with antibodies to nuclear RNP, and so I will discuss them only briefly. One is glomerulonephritis, and the other is various forms of central nervous system (CNS) disease, such as generalized seizures, psychosis, and other CNS manifestations, such as stroke, transverse myelitis, or an encephalitis-like picture with coma. Serious renal and CNS diseases are rare in my experience in patients who truly only have antibodies to nuclear RNP. I hold the view that this syndrome is a variant of lupus with a certain coincident expression of the other two diseases in question (scleroderma and myositis). The precise serologic definition of these patients is an essential part of the initial evaluation. Lupus patients who have only antibodies to nuclear RNP rarely, if ever, develop nephritis or CNS disease. However, patients with antibodies to nuclear RNP accompanied by antibodies either to single-stranded DNA or to the Ro/SS-A antigen that are not detected in routine laboratory examinations frequently develop nephritis. In my opinion, much of the literature about glomerulopathies and CNS disease in MCTD is probably confounded by incomplete serologic studies, which have ignored antibodies to single-stranded DNA and the Ro/SS-A antigen. Other antibodies that occur with a lesser but definable frequency and are often missed in routine laboratory examination are low levels of antibodies to Sm and native DNA, and patients with such serologic profiles have, in my experience, the same morbidity from nephritis and CNS disease as any other lupus patient.

Thus precise serologic definition is, I believe, the key to the frequency of appreciation of these complications in MCTD. If MCTD is defined by antibodies to nuclear RNA protein alone, then serious nephritis and CNS disease are rare. One manifestation in the nervous system that has been described frequently in patients of this type is trigeminal neuropathy, or tic douloureux, which does indeed occur with an as yet undetermined frequency. The management of this problem is not defined, but steroids may not be an effective approach.

The next manifestation of the disease to consider is polymyositis. I refer the reader to the chapter on *der-*

matomyositis for details, because the treatments for dermatomyositis and polymyositis are indistinguishable. The mainstay of treatment of polymyositis when significant weakness is present is corticosteroids. Steroids are used at an initial dosage of 1 mg per kilogram per day. Higher dosages are rarely required for a good clinical effect, although divided doses (20 mg three times daily) may be used for the first week or two in acutely ill or profoundly weak patients.

Two guidelines are followed to assess the efficacy of treatment: the myogenic enzymes that appear in serum and the clinical assessment of strength, including creatinine phosphokinase, or CPK, which is by far the most important, and under certain circumstances, aldolase, LDH, and SGOT, all of which appear in the serum in polymyositis. A rare patient in whom the clinical picture is clear-cut and serum enzyme levels are normal shows an elevation of the urinary creatine level. In the most favorable clinical situations, a reduction in serum myogenic enzyme levels and increased strength occur simultaneously at similar rates. If maximal strength is regained and the serum enzyme levels return to normal, the dosage of corticosteroids may be reduced over 6 to 8 weeks until 20 mg per day is reached; thereafter the dosage may be reduced 10 percent per week until the steroids are no longer given, if there is no flare of the disease.

The preferred drug for treatment is prednisone. Triamcinolone preparations should be avoided, since there seems to be an increased incidence of steroid myopathy with the use of that steroid preparation. As with all steroid usage, an ulcer regimen should be instituted when the dosage of prednisone exceeds 20 mg per day. It is my clinical impression that patients with polymyositis and antibodies to nuclear RNP are more responsive to steroids and are more frequently capable of sustaining a remission in the absence of steroids than patients with polymyositis with other serologic markers. Most patients with polymyositis and antinuclear RNP also have features of lupus and are only rarely encountered with polymyositis alone. Should steroid therapy fail, other drugs used are methotrexate or Imuran.

SKIN DISEASE

The management of the scleroderma manifestations of the disease is perhaps the most difficult part of the treatment of this overlap syndrome. Because no effective proven treatment of the scleroderma process is available, there are no specific therapies to describe. I do not use steroids for the treatment of hand swelling or skin thickening in such patients. There is no evidence that steroids alter the ultimate outcome, but they do expose the patients to risks.

There are several other manifestations of the scleroderma aspect of the disease in these patients that merit comment. One is the rapid development of skin disease, the second is pulmonary fibrosis, and the third is the late development of pulmonary vascular lesions with pulmonary hypertension and right sided heart failure. The latter complication is rare, occurs 10 to 30 years after onset of the skin disease, and is extremely serious, since there is no known effective treatment. Rapid progression of skin disease in general is associated with a poor prognosis in scleroderma because of concomitant internal organ involvement, and demonstrably failing pulmonary function with x-ray findings of infiltration is also of concern to the physician.

For the sclerotic features of skin disease the empiric treatment given by most physicians is penicillamine, based on the retrospective studies of the Pittsburgh group that showed a decrease in the expected frequency of internal organ complications in patients whose scleroderma was treated with penicillamine. The penicillamine is used in similar fashion to that described for rheumatoid arthritis. One begins with one 250-mg tablet per day and maintains that for 2 months. Barring any adverse effects, the dosage is raised to 500 mg a day for 2 months and ultimately to a maximum of 750 mg per day. I have not yet encountered a patient with antibodies to nuclear RNP whose skin disease was so widespread and rapidly progressive as to warrant the use of penicillamine.

PULMONARY DISEASE

A number of patients develop pulmonary infiltrative disease, and here again we are in a gray zone. My procedure is as follows: Two examinations that are made if one is concerned about the activity of the pulmonary disease are pulmonary lavage to look for neutrophils and gallium scanning to look for increased uptake in the lung as a manifestation of inflammation. If the pulmonary lavage contains more than 10 percent neutrophils and the patient is not a smoker and is found to have a positive gallium scan, I use prednisone in a dosage of 1 mg per kilogram per day for 1 month and then repeat the lavage and the gallium scan. If there has been a favorable effect as reflected by these tests, the prednisone dosage can be reduced and the examinations can be repeated at a less frequent interval. The other manifestations of the disease, such as calcinosis, telangiectasias, the skin hardening per se, and gastrointestinal involvement, are not to my knowledge responsive to any specific treatment.

Certain maneuvers are useful in the management of specific complications, such as esophageal reflux and the malabsorption of the sclerodermatous bowel, which is frequently due to bacterial overgrowth. The latter may respond to antibiotic treatment, but for these specific situations there are no general systemic treatments of proven value. In my experience almost all patients with scleroderma features with antinuclear RNP have a limited form of the disease known as the CREST syndrome. These patients have calcinosis, Raynaud's phenomenon, esophageal motility disturbances, and telangiectasias but in general do not have widespread skin involvement or internal extensive organ involvement. The usual form of the disease is therefore a limited, extremely chronic one in which late complications may include proliferative endarteritic lesions of the pulmonary vasculature and biliary cirrhosis for which no treatments are known to be effective.

There is no overall treatment for mixed connective tissue disease. The treatment is tailored to the manifestations of the individual constituent diseases. The overall prognosis in these patients tends to be good, and a conservative stance is warranted except in clinical circumstances in which more aggressive treatments are indicated.

REITER'S SYNDROME

FRANK C. ARNETT, M.D.

Reiter's syndrome (disease) is classically defined as the triad of nongonococcal urethritis, nonbacterial conjunctivitis, and arthritis. Several distinctive mucocutaneous lesions also occur frequently, including keratodermia blennorrhagica, circinate balanitis, painless oral ulcers, and onychodystrophy.

Many patients, however, do not manifest the classic triad but present with a lower extremity oligoarthritis often accompanied by "sausaging" of digits, heel pain, or one or more mucocutaneous features (incomplete Reiter's syndrome). The histocompatibility antigen HLA-B27 is present in 75 percent of the cases. The disease is often preceded by acute gastroenteritis or sexually acquired urethritis.

THERAPY

Musculoskeletal Manifestations

The articular manifestations of Reiter's syndrome usually constitute the major clinical problems requiring therapeutic intervention. An intense sterile synovitis most commonly affects the knees, ankles, and small joints of the feet, usually in an asymmetrical oligoarticular pattern. Upper extremity and sacroiliac joints may also be involved. In addition, inflammation at bone sites where tendons or fascia inserts (enthesopathy) may give rise to often disabling pain, especially in the heels or along the pelvis, spine, or ribs. Although cartilage and bone destruction may ensue, there appears to be a greater tendency toward new bone formation and fusion across joints, with severe contractures a potential complication. Thus, therapy should be aimed at pharmacologic suppression of inflammation and, once maximized, an active program of physical therapy to preserve joint mobility and function.

The potential course and prognosis of the disease must also be recognized in guiding both physician and patient through the principles of management. The majority of patients have a self-limited illness lasting several months to a year, with full recovery the general rule. Relapses occur in less than one-third but often after many disease-free years. Less than 20 percent of the patients have a relentlessly destructive arthropathy resulting in significant disability, most often from severe foot deformities.

Nonsteroidal anti-inflammatory drugs (NSAID), potent inhibitors of prostaglandin-mediated inflammatory pathways, constitute the foundation of pharmacologic therapy. Suppression of synovial inflammation is the ultimate goal. This is clinically reflected by decreased joint swelling, heat, and pain as well as improved overall function.

Indomethacin is an excellent first choice. Four divided doses totaling 100 to 200 mg per 24 hours are usually necessary. A more convenient schedule of sustained-release indomethacin, 75 mg every 12 hours, is also available. Tolmetin, 400 mg three times daily, may be equally useful, as may naproxen, 375 to 500 mg twice daily, sulindac, 200 mg twice or three times daily, or piroxicam, 20 mg per day. Salicylates and the proprionic acid-derived drugs, such as ibuprofen and fenoprofen, are generally less effective in Reiter's syndrome than in other arthritides such as rheumatoid arthritis. It must be emphasized, however, that there is a wide range of patient variability with respect to clinical improvement and tolerance with these drugs. Thus, a patient may require sequential trials of several drugs before the optimal one is found. Narcotic analgesics should be assiduously avoided because of their addictive potential.

Once pain and objective signs of inflammation are significantly reduced according to both the patient's and the physician's observations, an active program of physical therapy should be initiated to maintain joint mobility and function and muscle strength. In the meantime NSAID therapy is continued until the disease runs its course. The most frquent toxic effect of all these drugs relates to their potential for causing upper gastrointestinal intolerance. Nausea, dyspepsia, gastritis, or frank peptic ulcer disease may ensue. It is often wise to instruct the patient to take the medication at mealtimes and, in some cases, to follow each dose with an antacid 1 hour later. H2 blockers to reduce gastric secretion are occasionally necessary.

Allergic reactions to NSAID therapy, usually skin rashes, are uncommon but dictate discontinuation of the offending drug and cautious substitution of another. Individuals who are sensitive to aspirin, however, especially those with nasal polyps and asthmatic reactions, usually demonstrate cross sensitivities to all these prostaglandin inhibitors. Such patients should not be challenged with any of these drugs. Those with mild joint disease may respond to nonacetylated salicylates (sodium or choline salicylate) or acetaminophen; however, a more potent alternative (to be described) may be necessary. Moreover, all NSAID therapy must be used with caution in patients with renal insufficiency, since further deterioration may be induced. Sulindac may be less nephrotoxic than the others.

Phenylbutazone is probably the most potent and most effective medication for the arthritis and enthesiopathic manifestations of Reiter's syndrome. Its use is tempered, however, by its potential for causing serious or even fatal idiosyncratic bone marrow suppression. Its use is justified in the seriously ill patient with function-threatening disease who has not responded to other NSAID therapy. Moreover, it appears to be tolerated by patients with aspirin-NSAID hypersensitivity, although it should be instituted under observation in case a similar asthmatic diathesis is precipitated. A dosage of 200 mg three times daily for 2 to 3 days is often desirable to suppress highly active disease, but the dosage then should be lowered to 200 mg twice daily for several weeks. Thereafter an attempt is made to taper to a 200 to 300 mg per day maintenance schedule. Diligent hematologic monitoring with complete blood counts, including platelet counts, is mandatory—weekly at first for several months, then at 2 week intervals, and finally monthly if long-term therapy is required. Other less serious reversible adverse reactions include painful oral ulcers, salt and water retention (a potential with all forms of NSAID therapy), parotitis, allergic reactions, upper gastrointestinal symptoms, and hepatotoxicity.

Systemic corticosteroid therapy is rarely used for the arthritis of Reiter's syndrome and appears to be less effective than in other arthritides. Occasionally prednisone may prove useful in low dosages of 5 to 10 mg per day in patients with continuing disease already taking maximal NSAID dosages or in the rare patient who is intolerant to NSAID therapy. On the other hand, intra-articular corticosteroid injection of a refractory joint such as the knee may prove effective in quieting the inflammation. More than three injections in the same joint in 1 year is not recommended.

Immunosuppressive drugs such as the folic acid antagonist methotrexate should be reserved for the most severe and refractory cases of joint or cutaneous disease. A starting dosage of 2.5 mg orally every 12 hours for three doses (7.5 mg total) at weekly intervals is recommended. If there is no response after 2 to 3 weeks, the amount of drug can be doubled to 5 mg every 12 hours for three doses (15 mg total weekly). Higher dosages of 20 to 35 mg per week have been used but usually require intravenous administration and are often accompanied by significant toxicity. Even at low doses, chemical evidence of hepatic dysfunction should be sought frequently by liver function tests. Liver biopsy to detect occult cirrhosis should be performed every 2 years if continuous therapy is needed. In addition, hematologic parameters of bone marrow function must be monitored frequently. Other adverse reactions include oral ulcers, gastrointestinal intolerance, allergic reactions, pruritus, and hypersensitivity pneumonitis.

Another immunosuppressive drug, the purine antimetabolite azathioprine, has been used recently for severe cases. The recommended daily dosage is 1.5 to 2.0 mg per kilogram given orally. Again serious hematologic and hepatic toxic effects are potential risks, although liver damage does not occur in the absence of blood chemistry abnormalities as with methotrexate. The rare but real potential for oncogenic sequelae (lymphoma or leukemia) in response to azathioprine therapy, as documented in renal transplant recipients, justifies caution in regard to its frequent use.

Another precautionary note must be added in regard to all the immunosuppressive drugs, including corticosteroids. There are increasing reports of an association of Reiter's syndrome with the acquired immunodeficiency syndrome (AIDS). Fatal opportunistic infections and Kaposi's sarcoma have emerged during immunosuppressive treatment of Reiter's disease in some patients with asymptomatic or unrecognized HIV infection. Clinical and/or serologic exclusion of this possible coexisting infection is now necessary prior to instituting therapy with any of these drugs.

Nonpharmacologic therapy includes a major role for physical therapy. During an acute attack or phase the inflamed joint may require complete rest with splinting for optimal comfort and to prevent contracture. As inflam-

mation subsides or is suppressed, passive range of joint motion should be initiated, followed by active exercises to preserve function and maintain or restore muscle strength. If the spine is involved, the potential for fusion identical to that in ankylosing spondylitis must be recognized. Thus, extension exercises for lumbar, thoracic, and cervical spinal segments should be instituted.

Heel or forefoot involvement may present significant mechanical impediments to walking and standing. Corticosteroid injections into the Achilles tendon or plantar aponeurosis insertions are rarely effective. Instead proper footwear, including shoes or orthotics that direct maximal weight to noninvolved areas, often can provide some relief.

Ocular Features

The conjunctivitis is usually mild and transient, requiring no therapy. When eye involvement is severe, ophthalmologic consultation is advisable. Acute anterior uveitis, heralded clinically by severe ocular pain, photophobia, and erythema, occurs in approximately 20 percent of the patients and is an ophthalmologic emergency. The lesion usually responds to topical corticosteroid therapy, but systemic administration may be necessary. Although uveitis is most often a self-limited complication responsive to appropriate therapy, prolonged or repeated episodes or a chronic course may threaten vision.

Genitourinary Features

The urethritis is often subtle, manifested by mild dysuria and a scant mucopurulent discharge. Nonetheless Gram staining and culture for concomitant gonorrhea are mandatory. Symptoms of prostatitis are not infrequent, but vigorous prostatic massage should not be performed because of evidence suggesting that it might exacerbate the arthritis. It is unclear whether antibiotics are effective in clearing the genitourinary tract, since this manifestation is usually self-limited and transient. Nonetheless a 10 to 14 day course of tetracycline, doxycycline, or erythromycin is worthy of trial, since *Chlamydia trachomatis* can be cultured from the urethra in over 30 percent of the cases.

Mucocutaneous Features

Keratodermia blennorrhagica, the distinctive skin lesion of Reiter's syndrome, frequently appears first on, and remains limited to, the soles or palms. Although short lived and in need of no treatment in the majority of cases, skin lesions occasionally become widespread. Keratodermia is clinically and histologically indistinguishable from pustular psoriasis, and when treatment becomes necessary, the same guidelines as those given in the article on psoriasis can be applied.

Circinate balanitis also clears spontaneously in the majority of patients. Occasionally, when it is persistent or recurrent, topical corticosteroid therapy may be used judiciously. Overuse may produce undesirable thinning of the glans penis. Circumcision may be necessary if phimosis becomes a complication of this lesion.

The oral ulcers are usually painless and transient. Treatment is rarely necessary, but topical therapy with corticosteroid in an oral paste vehicle (Orabase HCA) may be used effectively.

Cardiac Features

Variable degrees of heart block and aortic valvular regurgitation occur rarely in Reiter's disease, usually after a prolonged and severe course. Referral for cardiologic management is required when electrocardiographic evidence of heart block is found or an aortic murmur is heard. Such patients may require pacemaker implantation or aortic valve replacement.

SJÖGREN'S SYNDROME

NORMAN TALAL, M.D.

Patients with Sjögren's syndrome require a team approach to management and thus need to be seen regularly by a rheumatologist, an ophthalmologist, and a dentist. Close follow-up is required to detect significant functional deterioration, superimposed signs of disease complications, or significant changes in the course of the disease. Regular outpatient visits with serial observations of pertinent laboratory parameters may allow for the early diagnosis of extraglandular complications or malignant change.

It is a misconception that Sjögren's syndrome is a rare disease. Rather it is a neglected disease, adding greatly to the distress of the patient. There is nothing minor about the symptoms of dry eyes and dry mouth, which can cause great morbidity and suffering for the patient.

TREATMENT OF THE GLANDULAR DISEASE

Ophthalmologic Manifestations (Keratoconjunctivitis Sicca)

There may be an accumulation of thick ropy secretions along the inner canthus owing to a decreased tear film and an abnormal mucus component. Related complaints include erythema, photosensitivity, eye fatigue, decreased visual acuity, and the sensation of a "film" across the field of vision. Desiccation can cause small superficial erosions of the corneal epithelium. Slit lamp examination may reveal filamentary keratitis (filaments of corneal epithelium and debris) in severe cases. Conjunctivitis caused by *Staphylococcus aureus* is a complication.

The low level of humidity in air conditioned environments may make these symptoms worse. Similar problems arise in windy or dry climates. Cigarette smoking and drugs with anticholinergic side effects may also increase symptoms. The drugs most frequently implicated are phenothiazines, tricyclic antidepressants, antispasmodics, and antiparkinson and decongestant medications. Many of these are available over the counter.

The mainstay of treatment for dry eyes is lubrication through the use of artificial tear drops, which can be used as often as necessary (generally every 1 to 3 hours). A variety of such drops are readily available without prescription, differing primarily in viscosity and preservative. The thicker, more viscous drops require less frequent application, although they can cause blurring and leave a residue on the lashes. Many patients prefer the thinner drops, which require more frequent application. A patient generally tests several different preparations to determine the one that is best for him. An apparent failure to respond to artificial tears may actually reflect eye irritation resulting from the topical application of preservatives such as benzalkonium chloride, chlorbutanol, or thimerosal. Also available are lubricating ointments, which may produce significant blurring and are best used at night to provide protection over a longer period.

A slow release tear is on the market under the trade name Lacrisert. It is a polymer of hydroxypropyl cellulose and comes as a cylinder, which is inserted every 6 to 12 hours below the inferior tarsal margin. It absorbs the tears, slowly dissolves, and releases polymer. It is particularly useful in patients who otherwise would use tear substitutes as frequently as every 15 minutes.

Other steps can be taken to preserve tears if tear substitutes are insufficient to control symptoms. Water-tight swimmer's goggles can be helpful in creating a moist chamber effect by preventing evaporation. They also protect against wind and dust particles. The same effect can be achieved with ordinary food plastic wrap taped over the eyes. Commercial "bubble" bandages are also available.

Soft contact lenses may also help to protect the cornea, especially when filaments are a problem. However, the lenses themselves require wetting, and patients must be followed carefully because there is an increased risk of infection. Such lenses are invaluable in the management of corneal ulcers, which can arise as a complication of keratoconjunctivitis sicca.

Punctal occlusion is another method of conserving the few tears produced. This procedure should be considered only in severe cases when there seems little likelihood of a spontaneous increase in tear flow. Stents have been devised as a nonsurgical means of occlusion; this is a good way to predict the success of surgical occlusion.

Autonomic stimulation of tear flow has been relatively neglected as a form of therapy because the eyedrops have generally worked well. Sympathomimetic and parasympathomimetic drugs, especially the muscarinic drugs, serve to stimulate tear flow. Pilocarpine taken orally has been reported as being successful, as have bromhexine and psysalaemin.

In patients with a relative excess of mucin production and formation of filaments, a mucolytic drug such as acetylcysteine has been found to be useful. However, other investigators have failed to confirm this.

Topical steroid use for the corneal ulcers of Sjögren's syndrome has been associated with a worsening of the clinical course and is not recommended.

Two new approaches to topical therapy have recently been suggested. One is the use of dilute sodium hyaluronate. This compound has recently been approved for intraocular surgery, and investigators have advocated a 10 percent diluted solution for topical use. Another group of investigators has developed a procedure for taking the patient's own serum and using this as an artificial tear (Fox et al, 1984). Both these possibilities are somewhat tedious and need further study before final recommendations can be made.

Salivary Disease

Xerostomia is often the initial symptom of Sjögren's

syndrome. However, it is a common and subjective clinical complaint with a wide variety of etiologies, including emotional factors, sialodochitis, chronic sialadenitis, various drugs already listed, irradiation, and dehydration. It is best considered a relatively nonspecific finding requiring further evaluation by careful history, physical examination, and often labial salivary gland biopsy to confirm the presence of significant lymphocytic infiltrates attaining a focus score compatible with autoimmune exocrinopathy (i.e., Sjögren's syndrome).

Complaints resulting from dryness of the mouth are varied. The "cracker sign" describes the difficulties encountered in trying to eat dry foods without sufficient lubrication. A positive "cracker sign" is almost diagnostic of true Sjögren's syndrome. Many subjects require frequent ingestion of liquids. They may resort to carrying water bottles or candy in the purse or pocket. Additional features include oral soreness, adherence of food to buccal surfaces, fissuring of the tongue, and dysphagia. Angular cheilitis associated with superimposed candidiasis may occur. The patient may lose the ability to discriminate foods on the basis of taste and smell. Dental caries is accelerated. The parotid gland enlarges in many patients secondary to cellular infiltration and ductal obstruction. Usually asymptomatic and self-limited, the enlargement can be recurrent and associated with pain or erythema. Local heat and analgesics are often helpful. Because of the potential risk of malignant disease, ionizing irradiation of the parotid glands is not recommended.

The treatment of xerostomia associated with Sjögren's syndrome is difficult. No single highly effective method is currently available, and most efforts are aimed only at palliation. Before any treatment program is started, it is important to identify contributing factors, such as mouth breathing, heavy smoking, and drugs with anticholinergic side effects that further decrease salivary flow. Stimulation of salivary flow by sucrose free, highly flavored lozenges or chewing gums, the use of lemon flavored drinks, and dietary counseling to avoid particularly dry foods also may be of assistance. Most patients discover that it is helpful to carry water, sugarless lemon drops, or chewing gum. These must be sugar free because of the risk of rampant dental caries. Fluids ad libitum should be utilized for all meals and snacks, which should also begin and finish with highly flavored substances, which tend to stimulate salivary flow. The consumption of large amounts of water during the day, although symptomatically helpful, may produce nocturia that interrupts sleep patterns and leads to fatigue.

Artificial saliva substitutes offer additional palliation. Mucin containing saliva substitutes seem to be more effective than substitutes based on carboxymethyl cellulose or polyethylenoxide. Mucins tend to protect against desiccation, provide for lubrication and cleaning, and appear to have some antimicrobial effect. Saliva substitutes, however, should be utilized sparingly with only the minimal volume necessary for oral lubrication. This usually consists of no more than 2 ml before and after meals, at bedtime, and following oral hygiene. The materi-al also can be applied to any removable intraoral appliance to facilitate more sustained release.

Topical or oral treatment with stannous fluoride enhances dental mineralization and retards damage to tooth surfaces. In cases of rapidly progressive dental disease the fluoride can be applied directly to the teeth from plastic trays that are used at night. The latter method may be inconvenient but provides better exposure of gingival margins to the fluoride.

Increased salivary flow may be induced by potassium iodide or parasympathomimetic drugs such as pilocarpine or neostigmine, systemically or as a mouthwash; varying degrees of success have been noted. A battery powered electronic device for stimulating salivary flow has been developed recently and is currently under study. Bromhexine, a synthetic alkaloid originally used as a mucolytic agent in cough syrups, has been tried with limited success (Frost-Larsen et al, 1978; Nahir et al, 1981).

Increased moisture applied to the upper airways by the use of normal saline sprays and humidifiers at night may reduce respiratory symptoms and alleviate mouth breathing. In some cases nasal irrigation with normal saline proves helpful.

Vaginal dryness is treated with lubricants such as K-Y jelly, and dry skin is treated with moisturizing lotions.

TREATMENT OF EXTRAGLANDULAR DISEASE

The systemic administration of corticosteroids and immunosuppressive drugs is used only to treat potentially life threatening disease, often involving the lung or kidney. They are not recommended for the treatment of dry eyes and dry mouth. No controlled studies have been performed because relatively few patients require systemic treatment.

A diffuse interstitial pneumonitis resulting from lymphocytic infiltration and fibrosis may cause severe exertional dyspnea. Obstructive disease (in the absence of smoking) may result from lymphocytic infiltration surrounding small airways. Pulmonary function tests should be performed and monitored twice per year to determine the extent of functional impairment. Lung biopsy should be performed before treatment is started. There is a better chance for therapeutic success if a highly cellular infiltrate is found. Conversely, one may decide against treatment if only scar tissue is present on lung biopsy.

Treatment is usually initiated with corticosteroids in dosages of 0.5 to 1 mg per kilogram daily. As the patient improves, the dosage can be tapered to a maintenance level at 50 percent of the starting dosage. If there is no apparent response within 3 to 6 months, steroids should be discontinued and a trial of cyclophosphamide considered; a level of 100 mg per day is a good starting dosage. Cyclophosphamide has succeeded when other immunosuppressive drugs have been tried first and failed. Although the risk of lymphoma is an important theoretical consideration, in our experience it has not appeared in patients with Sjögren's syndrome treated with cyclophosphamide.

The most common renal abnormalities in Sjögren's

syndrome involve the tubules, particularly overt or latent renal tubular acidosis. Potassium and bicarbonate are generally sufficient to control the hyperchloremic acidosis. Steroids were successful in one patient (El-Mallakh et al, 1985), but we prefer cyclophosphamide (100 mg per day) on the basis of personal experience. Peripheral and cranial neuropathy has been associated with vasculitis involving the vasa nervorum. Although there is little information concerning the treatment of this complication, bolus cyclophosphamide in a dose of 0.5 to 0.75 g per square meter may be of benefit.

The incidence of lymphoma is increased 44-fold in Sjögren's syndrome. Pseudomalignant or malignant lymphoproliferation may be present initially or may develop later in the illness. Most lymphomas belong to the B cell lineage, although the histologic appearance is variable. A diminution in previously elevated immunoglobulin levels and a loss of autoantibodies may precede malignant transformation. Pseudolymphoma is an intermediate stage in this transition from benign to malignant lymphoproliferation.

The distinction between lymphoma and pseudolymphoma may be difficult even for highly experienced pathologists. Some patients with pseudolymphoma may not require treatment if there is no functional compromise. If there is, treatment of pseudolymphoma with corticosteroids or cyclophosphamide is often successful. Treatment of lymphoma and decisions regarding chemotherapy or radiation therapy should be guided by experienced oncologists. In general, these lesions are highly refractory to treatment.

USE OF NONSTEROIDAL DRUGS AND OTHER MEDICATIONS IN SJÖGREN'S SYNDROME

Treatment of secondary Sjögren's syndrome is usually directed at the associated disease. The treatment of rheumatoid arthritis or systemic lupus erythematosus is not altered because of the concomitant presence of Sjögren's syndrome. The sicca complex is generally milder and managed as already discussed. Arthralgias or myalgias are managed with salicylates or nonsteroidal anti-inflammatory drugs.

SCLERODERMA

THOMAS A. MEDSGER Jr., M.D.

The term scleroderma describes a spectrum of diseases, including systemic sclerosis, a multisystem disorder, and localized scleroderma of the morphea or linear scleroderma type. All these conditions are characterized by a proliferation of fibroblasts and excessive production of connective tissue proteins (collagen and glycosaminoglycans) in the affected tissues, often associated with a mononuclear cell inflammatory infiltrate.

In systemic sclerosis it is important to distinguish three major subtypes in order to consider therapy (Table 1). Patients with diffuse scleroderma are at risk of developing serious articular and life threatening renal and myocardial involvement early in the disease course. In contrast, individuals with limited scleroderma (often called the CREST syndrome variant) most often have a prolonged indolent course before developing one or more visceral complication. Finally, in some patients the primary or prominent manifestations are those typically ascribed to another disease (e.g., systemic lupus erythematosus or polymyositis-dermatomyositis). Along with certain key clinical features, serum autoantibody determinations are of considerable assistance in determining the patient's classification.

THE ROLE OF THE PHYSICIAN

The physician should discuss the nature of systemic sclerosis with the patient and his family, who are often unreasonably pessimistic. The chronicity of the disease and the tendency for some features to worsen with time can be explained without using the devastating term "progressive." An explanation using diagrams of the blood vessels, skin, and esophagus and other illustrations helps to establish a good relationship between physician and patient, which is crucial in this chronic demanding disease. It is important to state unequivocally that scleroderma is not considered hereditary, infectious, or contagious.

Alteration of facial and hand appearance can lead to an unattractive body image, fear of increased dependence on others, and depression. The support system needed to cope in this circumstance is strengthened by the reassurance of the physician, acceptance and encouragement by family members and loved ones, and the assistance of patient support groups in the community. Realistic work goals must be set for patients who are employed, and disability and job stress alterations should be recommended to employers.

The natural history of the scleroderma variants, and the recommended follow-up vary (Fig. 1). The patient with long-standing, uncomplicated, limited scleroderma should be reassured and infrequent evaluations planned (every 1 to 3 years). Attention should be directed to the potential complications of pulmonary arterial hypertension, intestinal malabsorption, and biliary cirrhosis. In contrast, the patient with rapidly progressive diffuse scleroderma should be carefully examined every 2 to 3 months, with special emphasis given to symptoms and signs signalling the development of finger and other joint contractures or cardiac or renal disease. The latter patients, with their tendency to develop early visceral involvement, are candidates for the aggressive use of potential "remittive" agents.

EVALUATING THE LITERATURE

There is an impressively long list of vitamins, hormones, pharmaceutical products, and surgical procedures that have been employed in systemic sclerosis, nearly all of which have been abandoned after initial periods of enthusiasm but later, more critical examination. It is important to make clear to the patient that no drug or combination of drugs has been proved to be of value in adequately controlled prospective trials, nor are any

---

TABLE 1 Classification of Scleroderma

Systemic sclerosis (progressive systemic sclerosis; systemic scleroderma)

    Diffuse scleroderma. Symmetrical widespread (diffuse) skin involvement affecting distal extremities and face as well as proximal extremities and trunk; tendency for rapid progression and early appearance of visceral involvement

    Limited scleroderma (CREST) syndrome. Relatively limited (restricted) skin involvement, often confined to fingers and face; prolonged delay in appearance of internal manifestations, certain of which are distinctive (e.g., pulmonary arterial hypertension and biliary cirrhosis); prominent calcinosis and telangiectasis

    Overlap syndrome. Either diffuse or limited scleroderma and typical features of one or more other connective tissue diseases

Localized scleroderma

    Morphea. Single or multiple (generalized) plaques

    Linear scleroderma. Linear bands of skin involvement; includes scleroderma *en coup de sabre* (with or without facial hemiatrophy)

Eosinophilic fasciitis

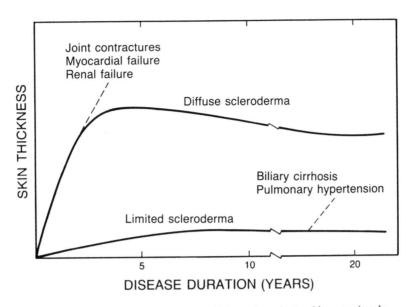

Figure 1 The natural history of skin thickness in patients with systemic sclerosis with diffuse and limited scleroderma and the timing of associated complications.

generally accepted as being useful in systemic sclerosis.

The physician should understand that many methodologic errors have flawed reports of therapeutic interventions in systemic sclerosis. These include the tendency of authors to indiscriminantly lump together patients with diffuse and limited disease; the absence of control or comparison groups; the use of subjective (e.g., the frequency and severity of Raynaud's phenomenon or dysphagia) rather than objective criteria for the determination of improvement or deterioration; and studies of inadequate duration (a minimum of 2 years is recommended).

THERAPEUTIC ALTERNATIVES

Understanding current concepts of the pathophysiology of systemic sclerosis is important in assessing the potential therapeutic approaches. The likely sequence of events and the proposed loci of drug action are depicted in Figure 2. Activated mononuclear cells accumulate in the skin and other sites and elaborate cytokines, which stimulate fibroblasts to produce excessive amounts of procollagen and mucopolysaccharides. The end result is overproduction of collagen, which leads to organ dysfunction. Similar deposits occur in the subintimal areas of blood vessels, narrowing lumina and contributing to ischemia. Platelet aggregation also occurs, and a serum factor cytotoxic to endothelial cells has been demonstrated.

Beneficial results of therapy might therefore be gained from suppressing the appearance or function of mononuclear cells in affected tissues; blocking synthesis or transport mechanisms in overactive fibroblasts; enhancing solubilization or breakdown of extracellular collagen; or protecting vascular endothelium, dilating vessels, and enhancing blood flow.

A summary of the currently accepted therapeutic choices for systemic sclerosis is presented in Table 2. The uses of these modalities are described in more detail in the following sections.

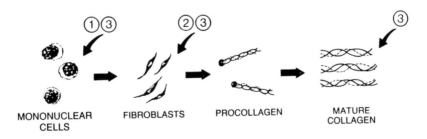

Figure 2 Immune mechanisms in the pathogenesis of systemic sclerosis. The proposed location of action of certain drugs is indicated. 1, Immunosuppressive drugs. 2, Colchicine. 3, D-Penicillamine.

Anti-inflammatory Drugs

Anti-inflammatory drugs and corticosteroids have proved to be disappointing in the treatment of this disorder. Corticosteroids are helpful in inflammatory myopathy and symptomatic serositis and may result in short-lived improvement in the early "edematous" phase of cutaneous disease. An occasional patient with inflammatory alveolitis improves following such therapy, but other visceral involvement is unaltered. In high dosages (equivalent to dosages of prednisone of 20 mg per day or more) corticosteroids may precipitate "scleroderma renal crisis."

D-Penicillamine

D-Penicillamine is my choice as the most beneficial drug available today. It has several effects on collagen metabolism, including acceleration of collagen turnover by cleaving intermolecular disulfide bonds and inhibition of collagen biosynthesis, and is an immunosuppressive drug (Fig. 2). A number of uncontrolled trials of D-penicillamine in systemic sclerosis have been reported, including those claiming significant improvement in England, Denmark, and the Soviet Union. We have been prescribing D-penicillamine with increasing frequency over the past 15 years, limiting its use primarily to patients with diffuse scleroderma and early disease (less than 5 years after the onset).

Our method is to administer D-penicillamine orally, 250 mg per day (on an empty stomach to achieve adequate absorption), raising the dosage every 2 to 3 months to a maximal daily dosage of 1,000 mg. If there is improvement, which is usually apparent only after 12 to 24 months, we recommend continuing the maximal dosage until no further amelioration is evident. At that time a slow reduction is begun to a maintenance dosage of 250 mg daily. Because we have seen several severe relapses after discontinuation of D-penicillamine, we recommend continuing this low dosage for a minimum of 10 years (Fig. 3).

By retrospective analysis we have studied 159 patients receiving D-penicillamine for a minimum of 6 consecutive months and a comparison group of 115 individuals not receiving the drug. During a mean follow-up interval of 38 months, the degree and extent of skin thickness determined by physical examination decreased considerably more in the D-penicillamine patients than in the comparison group (p=0.07). The rate of new visceral organ involvement was also reduced, especially in regard to the kidney (p=0.001). Primarily for this reason, the 5 year cumulative survival rate was 88 percent in the D-penicillamine group and 66 percent in the comparison group (p < 0.01). Established pulmonary involvement may also be ameliorated.

Many disturbing side effects of D-penicillamine have been reported, including fever, loss of taste (may remit spontaneously), nausea and anorexia, rash, leukopenia, thrombocytopenia, aplastic anemia, the nephrotic syndrome, myasthenia gravis, and pemphigus. Up to one-fifth of the patients may be forced to discontinue the drug. Fewer toxic reactions occur when the drug is administered in the "go low, go slow" fashion already outlined. Careful monitoring of the white blood cell and platelet counts and the urine protein level is recommended.

Colchicine

Colchicine has been found to interfere with microtubular transport and extrusion of procollagen from fibroblasts and to stimulate collagenase production. It is given orally in doses of 0.5 mg once or twice daily and is safe and well tolerated, save for diarrhea, but should be used with caution in individuals with hepatic or renal failure. Both short-term (3 months) and uncontrolled long-term (over 3 years) benefits have been reported, but in our experience and that of most other investigators, results have been disappointing.

Immunosuppressive Drugs

Because of mounting evidence that immune processes, both humoral and cell mediated, play an important role in the pathogenesis of systemic sclerosis, various forms of immunosuppression have been proposed. Our policy

TABLE 2 Therapeutic Choices in Subsets of Patients with Systemic Sclerosis

	Diffuse Scleroderma	Limited Scleroderma
Corticosteroids	+ (polyarthritis, pericarditis, or myositis)	0
Immunosuppressive drugs	±	0
Colchicine	±	0
D-Penicillamine	+	0 (except severe pulmonary fibrosis)
Vasoactive drugs	+	+
Apheresis (plasma, lymphocytes)	?	0

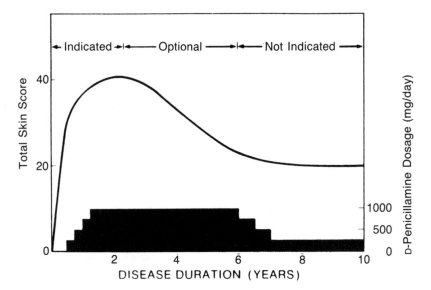

Figure 3 The use of D-penicillamine in systemic sclerosis with diffuse scleroderma. The drug should be begun early in the disease course but generally is not recommended in late stage disease. The dosage is incrementally increased to a maximum of 750 to 1,250 mg per day, maintained until no further cutaneous improvement is detected, and finally tapered slowly to a maintenance dosage of 250 mg per day. A minimum of 10 years of therapy is recommended.

is to use cytotoxic therapy only in severe, life threatening, or disability threatening disease in which D-penicillamine has failed, provided informed consent has been obtained and close surveillance is undertaken for adverse effects. Typical regimens consist of azathioprine, 100 to 150 mg per day, cyclophosphamide, 100 to 150 mg per day, or chlorambucil, 4 to 8 mg per day, with appropriate monitoring of toxicity.

Manipulation of the immune system is not without hazard. Bleomycin-induced scleroderma, graft versus host disease in immunosuppressed bone marrow transplant recipients, and systemic sclerosis in patients receiving chemotherapy for carcinoma of the breast have been described. These phenomena suggest that immunologic alteration in fact may produce a systemic sclerosis-like illness. Furthermore, the risk of late developing malignant disease in patients treated with immunosuppressive drugs is as yet unknown. We have seen three such examples 6 and 8 years after courses of cyclophosphamide (both histiocytic lymphoma) and 9 years after chlorambucil (acute myelocytic leukemia). The role of apheresis has not yet been clarified.

Vasoactive Drugs

We consider vasodilators to be adjunctive rather than primary therapeutic drugs. Less than half the patients with systemic sclerosis benefit in any sustained way from these drugs. We prescribe them for patients with recurrent digital tip ulcerations or those in whom Raynaud's phenomenon interferes with work or life style. Often their use can be limited to the winter months.

The new calcium-channel blocker nifedipine signifi-

cantly reduces the number and severity of attacks of Raynaud's phenomenon and results in a faster digital skin temperature recovery time after a cold challenge. The proper dosage is 10 to 20 mg three times daily. If this fails, we choose prazosin, 1 to 5 mg twice daily. In cases of impending gangrene, we perform a cervical sympathetic block on the affected side and, with the vessels maximally dilated (when fingertip temperatures reach a peak), inject phentolamine, 1.0 mg, slowly into the brachial artery.

SUPPORTIVE MEASURES

The local complications of systemic sclerosis can be managed in a variety of ways to minimize pain, inconvenience, and disability (Table 3). We advise patients to avoid undue exposure to cold and digital tip trauma. Using a hat and clothes that provide central warmth in cold weather serves to induce peripheral vasodilation. The room temperature may need to be maintained at 78° F. Tobacco smoking should be discouraged. Special lotions and bath oils, lanolin or petrolatum lubricants, and humidification of room air may be used to relieve excessive skin dryness. Frequent bathing and household detergents may aggravate this condition.

Digital tip ulcers should be considered ischemic in origin and treated primarily with vasodilators. Ulcerations over the proximal interphalangeal joints and elbows are attributable to stretching and atrophy of the skin and repeated trauma. Both types of ulcerations may be less painful when covered with ointment and immobilized and protected by a plaster finger cast. If these lesions become infected (typically with staphylococci), half-strength hydrogen peroxide soaks and gentle local manual or enzymatic

TABLE 3 Management of Local Complications of Systemic Sclerosis

Raynaud's phenomenon	Common sense Vasodilators
Digital tip ulcers	Vasodilators Cervical sympathetic blockade Finger casts Analgesics
Calcinosis	Surgical excision
Arthritis, tenosynovitis	Physical therapy Nonsteroidal anti-inflammatory drugs Surgical reconstruction
Myositis	Corticosteroids Physical therapy
Gastrointestinal tract Dysphagia, heartburn	Physical maneuvers Antacids, H2 blockers Metoclopramide
Esophageal stricture	Esophageal dilatation Gastroplastic surgery
Malabsorption	Broad spectrum antibiotics Dietary supplements
Lung Interstitial inflammation, fibrosis	Corticosteroids D-Penicillamine Immunosuppressive drugs
Pulmonary hypertension	Vasodilators Supportive measures

Heart
  Pericarditis
  Arrhythmias
  Congestive failure
	Corticosteroids
	Standard drugs
	Diuretics, digitalis

Kidney	Antihypertensive drugs Dialysis Transplantation

debridement are employed; oral doses of antibiotics are sometimes recommended. Deeper infections, such as septic arthritis or osteomyelitis, must be treated more radically with intravenous antibiotic therapy, excision of infected and devitalized tissue, joint fusion, and rarely amputation. In circumstances in which ischemia is present alone without infection, autoamputation is preferable for maximal preservation of viable tissue. However, if pain is intolerable, careful surgical amputation may minimize the period of disability.

The combined effects of skin, joint, and tendon changes in scleroderma lead to immobility, atrophy, and contracture. Movement is necessary to retain normal skin pliability and nutritional circulation. Daily massage of the skin, facial exercises, and joint range-of-motion exercises should be taught by a physical therapist and performed by the patient with the physician's strong encouragement. This is especially true in the early stages of diffuse scleroderma when contractures may develop and progress with alarming rapidity. Articular symptoms may be decreased by heat (paraffin), exercises, salicylates, and other nonsteroidal anti-inflammatory drugs. Surgical reconstruction in the hand, including arthrodesis, capsulotomy, and arthroplasty, has been reported but is not com-

monly performed because of concerns regarding healing. We have successfully treated severe contractures of the proximal interphalangeal joints with traumatic ulcerations by bone removal (shortening) and arthrodesis in a more functional position, with excellent wound healing.

The typical indolent noninflammatory fibrotic myopathy does not progress rapidly and fails to respond to corticosteroids; it is thus better left untreated, except by physical therapy to prevent contractures. Inflammatory myositis requires standard doses of corticosteroids. When this therapy is either ineffective or not tolerated owing to toxicity, we generally add an immunosuppressive drug in doses similar to those already outlined. There is no proven effective medical therapy for calcinosis in patients with scleroderma, although surgical excision of large calcareous masses and the removal of smaller deposits that interfere with hand function may be helpful in selected instances.

Persons who have difficulty in swallowing should learn to chew slowly and thoroughly and to avoid foods likely to cause substernal dysphagia (e.g., meat, bread). Metoclopramide, 10 to 20 mg taken 30 minutes before each meal and at bedtime, may improve esophageal motility in some patients. Nifedipine, a smooth muscle relaxant, theoretically may aggravate esophageal symptoms. Alcohol has a similar effect. Reflux esophagitis can be minimized by multiple small feedings during the day rather than fewer larger meals, sitting upright for 1 hour after each meal, elevation of the head of the bed on 4 to 6 inch blocks, antacids given 45 to 60 minutes after each meal and at bedtime, and histamine (H2) receptor blockade with either cimetidine, 300 mg three times daily before meals and at bedtime, or ranitidine, 150 mg twice daily. If esophageal reflux is demonstrated, even asymptomatic patients should be treated prophylactically as already discussed. For esophageal stricture, dilatation is now safely performed in outpatients and is gratifying because of the prompt, often complete and prolonged improvement. Rarely excision of a stricture and correction of gastroesophageal reflux by gastroplasty combined with fundoplication must be considered.

In patients with small intestinal malabsorption, diagnostic oral barium studies may result in severe obstipation and impaction of the contrast material. Diarrhea due to bacterial overgrowth in the proximal small bowel can be documented by culturing the duodenal or upper jejunal contents for aerobic and anaerobic microorganisms. Improvement may follow the administration of tetracycline, 250 mg four times daily for 10 to 14 days, but the underlying hypomotility is unaffected. Other helpful drugs include ampicillin, 250 mg four times daily, metronidazole, 250 mg three times daily, and Bactrim D-S, twice daily. Two week antibiotic rotations interspersed with periods of time with no antibacterial therapy are helpful in preventing the development of bacterial resistance and overgrowth of *Candida albicans*. Metoclopramide most often is ineffective. Dietary supplements should include an increase in calories without bulk and the administration of calcium, medium chain triglycerides, iron, and vitamin B. Episodes of intestinal pseudo-obstruction or pneumatosis intestinalis with (benign) pneumoperitoneum are best managed by nonsurgical decompression, bowel rest, and hydration. Antibiotics may minimize the excessive formation of gas by gut bacteria. If malnutrition ensues, hyperalimentation is required and has been used successfully in the home for 2 years or more in many instances.

A high-roughage diet, Metamucil for added bulk, and stool softeners may decrease the obstipation that occasionally complicates colonic dysmotility, since increased intraluminal pressure facilitates emptying. Rarely is insertion of a rectal pessary for recurrent rectal prolapse necessary.

Bronchoalveolar lavage studies suggest that inflammatory alveolitis is a precursor or occurs concomitantly with pulmonary interstitial fibrosis. In some instances pulmonary function has substantially improved with the use of corticosteroids alone or combined with immunosuppressive therapy, but the long-term effects of such interventions are unknown. In our experience D-penicillamine, after prolonged administration, stabilizes or decreases established pulmonary disease, and we have prescribed it in symptomatic patients with deteriorating lung function. Individuals with pulmonary interstitial fibrosis who have bacterial bronchitis or pneumonitis require prompt and vigorous antibiotic treatment, and prophylactic influenza and pneumococcal pneumonia vaccines are recommended.

No effective therapy is available for pulmonary arterial hypertension and subsequent right sided cardiac failure. Nasal oxygen administration, anticoagulation, digitalis, and diuretics may retard the progress of this complication, but death is almost inevitable.

Symptomatic pericarditis should be treated with nonsteroidal drugs or short term corticosteroid therapy. Pericardiocentesis or creation of a pericardial window rarely may be indicated in order to abort or treat tamponade. Patients who develop primary myocardial failure often respond poorly to digitalis and easily become intoxicated with this drug; thus greater reliance is placed on the use of diuretics. There is no evidence that corticosteroids alter this process unless active myocarditis (arrhythmia, elevated serum MB creatine kinase fraction, abnormal endomyocardial biopsy results) can be demonstrated. The role of coronary vasodilators is uncertain, but their use is reasonable. We use D-penicillamine as a last resort. Left ventricular heart failure secondary to the severe hypertension of renal involvement responds only to blood pressure reduction.

The availability of new, very potent antihypertensive drugs and improved dialysis methods and care have dramatically reduced the mortality due to renal involvement. Early recognition of this complication and aggressive therapy with such drugs as hydralazine, methyldopa, propranolol, minoxidil, and the angiotensin converting enzyme inhibitor captopril often, but not always, reverse this process. We favor the immediate administration of captopril as the therapy of first choice. When medical management fails, intervention with peritoneal dialysis or hemodialysis is indicated, but this is not always successful. Technical problems include reduced peritoneal clearance, limitation of vascular access, and limited shunt flow due to a combination of structural and vasospastic disease of large and small vessels. Many instances of successful renal transplantation have been reported, but histologic changes typical of "scleroderma kidney" have been found in a transplanted organ and an allograft.

LOCALIZED SCLERODERMA

In the majority of instances localized scleroderma is active for less than 2 years and does not recur. Therapy is generally indicated for the following reasons: persistence or recurrence of the disease 2 or more years after the onset; facial involvement, especially in a child; and extension of a lesion across a joint line that threatens to cause contracture or impairment of the circulation. Antimalarial drugs (hydroxychloroquine, 200 to 400 mg per day, with ophthalmologic toxicity monitoring every 3 to 6 months) or para-aminobenzoic acid (6 to 12 g daily orally) may be helpful. Our routine is to use combined therapy with oral corticosteroid therapy (prednisone, 10 to 30 mg per day, tapering and discontinuing after 6 months) and D-penicillamine (250 mg daily on an empty stomach, increasing every 3 months to a maximum of 750 mg per day) until there have been no new lesions or activity in old lesions for at least 1 year. Intralesional steroid therapy may be helpful.

EOSINOPHILIC FASCIITIS

Fasciitis is self-limited in most patients, with spontaneous improvement over a 2 to 5 year period. Corticosteroids in modest dosages (prednisone, 5 to 20 mg per day) often provide prompt and substantial symptomatic relief and may be discontinued after 6 to 18 months. In some cases of persistent uncontrolled disease, proved by repeat biopsy to have an inflammatory component, we have added D-penicillamine or an immunosuppressive drug, but we cannot comment about their usefulness because of the few individuals so treated. The physician should be aware that in a rare patient with fasciitis, thrombocytopenia or aplastic anemia of immunologic origin may develop during the course; periodic hematologic monitoring is thus recommended.

RAYNAUD'S PHENOMENON

FREDRICK M. WIGLEY, M.D.

Raynaud's phenomenon is characterized by episodes of vasospasm of the vessels of the digits of the hands and feet in response to both cold and emotion. The precapillary vasoconstriction is manifest by cutaneous pallor followed by cyanosis and then, on recovery, rubor secondary to hyperemia. The initial phase of pallor may be transient and often is not observed by the patient. Cyanosis persists until rewarming, following which a period of approximately 15 minutes passes before gradual return to normal color. Attacks may begin in one or more fingers but typically spread to the other digits symmetrically and bilaterally. During the phase of pallor and cyanosis, patients may experience a pins and needles sensation, blunting of normal sensation, and cold damp skin. Occasionally episodes are painful, particularly if the attack is prolonged or there is continuous exposure to cold. Other peripheral parts of the body may be involved, including the tips of the ears, nose, areas of the face, or the nipples. Patients with migraine headaches, primary pulmonary hypertension, and atypical angina (Prinzmetal's angina) have an increased prevalence of Raynaud's phenomenon. These associations suggest that Raynaud's phenomenon is the cutaneous manifestation of a generalized vasospastic disorder.

CLASSIFICATION

Raynaud's phenomenon may occur as the sole clinical problem (Raynaud's disease, idiopathic Raynaud's disease, primary Raynaud's disease) or in association with another process (Table 1). In approximately 40 percent of the patients presenting to an internist there is a defined secondary cause, the most common being a connective tissue disease. Disturbances of neurovascular supply, proximal vascular lesions, hematologic disorders, exposure to vibratory tools, certain vasoactive drugs, and a variety of miscellaneous disorders need to be carefully considered in the differential diagnosis. Obviously management of a treatable secondary process may improve or eliminate the Raynaud episodes.

Primary Raynaud's phenomenon is seen most commonly in young women who are otherwise healthy. Symptoms are limited to bilateral symmetrical Raynaud's phenomenon, which is rarely severe. Digital pitting or superficial ulceration of the fingertips with sclerodactyly may complicate the course in 10 to 15 percent of these patients. The presence of abnormal nailfold capillaries or positive antinuclear antibodies (particularly anticentromere antibodies) may herald the development of active connective tissue disease. Approximately 4 to 20 percent of the patients who initially are thought to have primary Raynaud's phenomenon develop signs or symptoms of connective tissue disease. This transition usually occurs within 2 to 3

TABLE 1 Classification of Raynaud's Phenomenon

Primary
  Idiopathic (Raynaud's disease)

Secondary
  Connective tissue disease
    Systemic sclerosis (90%)
    Systemic lupus erythematosus (20%)
    "Mixed connective tissue disease" (75%)
    Dermatomyositis (20%)
    Rheumatoid arthritis (10%)
  Extrinsic neurovascular compression
    Carpal tunnel syndrome
    Thoracic outlet syndrome
  Intrinsic arterial disease
    Arteritis
    Occlusive vascular disorders
  Hematologic disorders
    Cryoglobulins
    Polycythemia
    Paraproteins
  Occupational injury (vibration white finger syndrome)
    Vibratory tools
  Drugs and toxins
    Ergotamine
    Beta-adrenergic blockade
    Polyvinyl chloride exposure
    Sympathomimetic drugs
  Other associations
    Primary pulmonary hypertension
    Migraine headaches
    Atypical angina
    Reflex sympathetic dystrophy

years but may take many years from the onset of Raynaud's phenomenon. Frank ulceration, distal digital amputation, and scleroderma with loss of hand function occur primarily in patients with an underlying connective tissue disease such as systemic sclerosis.

MANAGEMENT

The treatment of Raynaud's phenomenon generally has been disappointing (Table 2). This lack of response probably reflects the fact that the pathogenesis is incompletely understood, and cases usually represent a heterogeneous group of disorders. Patients with primary Raynaud's phenomenon usually have mild episodes, which are more frightening than problematic. Drug treatment is not necessary; the attacks are rarely associated with sequelae and frequently they decrease over time. By contrast, patients with systemic sclerosis have structural abnormalities of the digital vessels and noncompliant skin, making their response to treatment less successful and local tissue complications common.

Although no ideal therapy has been defined, aggravating factors need to be avoided. Cold and emotional stress are major provocators of attacks in every diagnostic category (see later discussion). Smoking should be stopped because of the reflex vasoconstriction induced by nicotine. Ergotamine and sympathomimetic drugs can induce peripheral vasospasm. Approximately 50 percent of the

**TABLE 2 Nondrug Management of
Raynaud's Phenomenon**

Educate and reassure
  Delineate psychosocial status
  Define precipitating factors
  Establish behavioral modification
Avoid cold
  Avoid rapidly changing temperatures
  Wear loose fitting, warm clothing
  Keep entire body warm
  Adjust life style
Eliminate aggravating factors
  Stop smoking
  Avoid drugs (ergotamine, beta-blockers, sympathomimetics,
    bleomycin, birth control pills)
Rapidly reverse vasospasm
  Rewarm quickly

patients taking nonselective beta-blocking drugs develop Raynaud-like episodes, probably because of interference with the beta-receptor induced vasodilation. Studies have suggested that the selective beta-blockers labetalol and pindolol can be substituted when beta-blockage is essential. Oral contraceptive administration should be avoided on the theoretical basis of hormonal influences on vasospasm and the potential increase in fibrinogen levels while these drugs are being taken.

Education

Education and reassurance reduce inappropriate anxiety and eliminate misconceptions regarding this condition. Informing the patient of the nature, significance, and precipitating factors in the disorder often reduces the number and intensity of attacks without the use of other treatment modalities. Following an initial evaluation the patient can be instructed to maintain a diary recording the circumstances that precipitate an attack, the length of attack, and the factors that seem to end the episodes. A review of the diary with the patient serves as a means of defining the intensity and character of the affliction.

Allied health professionals also can help by gathering information pertaining to the patient's current psychosocial situation as well as providing support and education. Patients who clearly identify emotional upset as a causative factor benefit a great deal from nondrug support, which involves the physician and the family. Stressful situations should be reduced in the home and at work. Psychotherapy in the form of biofeedback or behavioral adaptation has been advocated by some and may be helpful in anxious patients with mild to moderate uncomplicated Raynaud's phenomenon. Sedative medications are usually not necessary and have no direct effect on the peripheral vasculature.

Cold

Cold is the most common and most intense factor that triggers attacks of Raynaud's phenomenon. Patients note that attacks are precipitated by rapidly changing tempera-

tures, as in walking into an air conditioned room, placing a hand into the refrigerator, or walking by open freezers in the markets. Patients should be instructed to avoid cold exposure and to dress warmly when it is necessary to go into the cold. Loose fitting clothing is most effective. It is important to keep the whole body warm, not just the hands and feet. Episodes can be precipitated by a general body chill, such as one induced by an ice pack placed on the neck, even if the hands are warm. Mittens are better than fingered gloves. Daily activities can be adjusted to avoid the cold. For example, another family member may do the frozen food shopping. A phone call to an employer may be helpful to adjust working temperatures or to move the patient from an outdoor to an indoor job during the winter months. Moving to a warm climate is usually not necessary, nor is it totally effective because of the many sources of cold exposure in our daily lives.

There is increasing evidence that cold adaptation occurs both in normal individuals and in patients with Raynaud's phenomenon. Graded exposure to cold has been suggested as a form of treatment, but its efficacy has not been proved and the methodology is unclear. Gentle and rapid warming of the extremities is an effective means of reversing the cold induced vasospasm. Patients discover that running warm (not hot) water over the digits, using a hair dryer, or placing the hands close to the body ends an attack. Rapidly swinging the arm in a wide circle has been reported to stop an attack in some cases. Prolonged vasospasm should be avoided because abnormal nutritional blood flow may result in ischemic changes. Patients therefore should be encouraged to end attacks by rewarming whenever possible.

Drug Treatment

Patients with mild noncomplicated Raynaud's phenomenon are most likely to respond to vasodilators but should be treated only with nondrug modalities. Repeated painful attacks (more than once daily), digital ulceration, or cutaneous changes such as early sclerodactyly warrant consideration for drug intervention. Patients who have repeated episodes that alter hand function or who must work in cold environments also may be considered for drug treatment. Patients with systemic sclerosis are thought to have cold induced vasospasm in renal, pulmonary, and cardiac vessels. However, there is no direct evidence that early treatment of Raynaud's phenomenon prevents the systemic sequelae of this disorder. Similar consideration has also been given to patients with migraine headaches, pulmonary hypertension, and atypical angina.

A large number of drugs have been used to treat Raynaud's phenomenon by either directly or indirectly causing peripheral vascular dilation (Table 3). Unfortunately only a few have been critically studied in appropriately blinded, placebo controlled trials. In addition, drug toxicity frequently limits the use of a potent vasodilator. It is important to carefully review reports about an effective drug in the treatment of Raynaud's phenomenon because episodes are seasonal and highly variable. Studies need to be placebo controlled and done in the winter months

TABLE 3 Drugs Reported to be Effective in Raynaud's Phenomenon

Alpha-adrenergic receptor blocking drugs
    Phenoxybenzamine
    Tolazoline
    Prazosin

Beta-adrenergic receptor stimulus
    Terbutaline

Adrenergic neuronal blocking drugs
    Reserpine
    Guanethidine
    Methyldopa

Direct smooth muscle relaxants
    Isoxsuprine
    Papaverine
    Nitrates
    Nylidrin
    Naftidrofuryl oxalate
    Calcium-channel blockers

with measurement of both subjective and objective responses.

Potent vascular alpha-receptor blockers nave been used alone and in combination with adrenergic neuronal blocking drugs. Phenoxybenzamine and guanethidine have been reported to produce symptomatic relief, but no controlled studies have been done. Significant side effects, including postural hypotension, reflex tachycardia, nasal congestion, impotence, lassitude, and incontinence, have made these unproven drugs impractical.

Prazosin, a specific adrenergic alpha-receptor antagonist, has been reported to reduce the number of attacks in several controlled studies. However, at a dosage of 1 mg twice daily the clinical improvement has tended to vanish in 1 to 2 months. In addition, intolerance to higher dosages of the drug has made many patients discontinue therapy. The general experience is that prazosin is rarely effective for long-term therapy.

The oral and intra-arterial administration of reserpine has been suggested as being effective in the treatment of Raynaud's phenomenon owing to its capacity to deplete norepinephrine from sympathetic nerve terminals. Oral reserpine therapy is not effective and often leads to significant side effects. Recent controlled studies have shown that the intra-arterial administration of reserpine is no more effective than a saline placebo in both short and long-term follow-up. Reserpine and other adrenergic neuronal blocking drugs should not be used in the treatment of this condition.

Although most direct smooth muscle relaxants and beta-receptor stimulants have not been effective, the development of drugs that interfere with the entry of calcium into vascular smooth muscle has led to a new and exciting approach to the treatment of Raynaud's phenomenon. These calcium-channel blockers have been shown to relax vascular smooth muscle, thus reducing peripheral vascular resistance and increasing peripheral blood flow. In addition, the calcium-channel blockers may have other secondary effects in that they have been shown to reduce platelet activation, which occurs in some patients with Raynaud's phenomenon.

Several controlled studies have been done with calcium channel blocks in the treatment of Raynaud's phenomenon. Nifedipine has been the most extensively studied, but diltiazem, verapamil, nicardipine, and nisoldipine also have been investigated. Verapamil was found ineffective in dosages of 40 to 80 mg four times daily in a group of patients with severe Raynaud's phenomenon. Nicardipine was not effective in one study and only minimally different from placebo in another. Nisoldipine (not available) was effective at a dosage of 20 mg daily in a 3 week trial.

Nifedipine is used at a dosage of 10 to 20 mg three or four times daily. Approximately 60 percent of the patients experience a decrease in the symptoms of Raynaud's phenomenon—both fewer and less intense attacks. A great deal of variability in response has been seen in all studies, partially explained by the fact that patients with primary Raynaud's phenomenon respond, whereas those with secondary Raynaud's phenomenon (particularly systemic sclerosis) do not. The ideal dosage and the duration of effect are unknown; one study found nifedipine to be less effective after 5 weeks of therapy.

Diltiazem has also been shown effective at dosages of 30 to 120 mg three times daily. When starting therapy with a calcium-channel blocker a test dose (nifedipine, 10 mg; diltiazem, 30 mg) should be given while the patient is in the office and vital signs and symptoms should be monitored. Following documentation of tolerance, graded increases can be made at 1 to 2 week intervals until clinical effectiveness or intolerance occurs. If no response is documented at maximal dosages, the drug should be discontinued.

It has been difficult to measure objective improvement in digital flow following treatment with the calcium-channel blockers. One study found a decrease in skin temperature recovery time following cold provocation by nifedipine. However, another demonstrated a paradoxical fall in digital pressure and flow acutely following a dosage of nifedipine. The clinician is best served by careful clinical assessment and a patient diary documenting the number of attacks and symptoms in order to measure the effectiveness of therapy.

Nifedipine is the most potent peripheral vasodilator of the calcium-channel blockers and is associated with a high prevalence of minor vasodilatory side effects (rarely causing drug stoppage). These side effects are even more frequent in patients with Raynaud's phenomenon. Similar side effects also can occur with other calcium-channel blockers and include orthostatic dizziness, lightheadedness, cutaneous flushing, headaches, disorientation, and mild peripheral edema. Lowering of the lower esophageal sphincter pressure can occur and can aggravate or cause esophageal reflux. This is particularly a problem in patients with systemic sclerosis who commonly have severe reflux.

Diltiazem has been reported to decrease the lower esophageal sphincter pressure less than nifedipine. Calcium-channel blockers should also be avoided if the patient is pregnant or is planning on becoming pregnant, a common situation in young women with Raynaud's phenomenon. The medication may not be necessary in the summer months when cold provocation is less likely. Occasionally a patient finds that periodic use 1 to 2 hours before an intense cold exposure is better tolerated than continuous use. Unfortunately patients with severe Raynaud's phenomenon are less likely to improve than those with primary mild Raynaud's phenomenon.

A number of new drugs have been studied in the treatment of Raynaud's phenomenon (Table 4). Vasodilatory prostaglandins (PgE and PgI) given by central intravenous infusion have been effective for up to 6 weeks following 72 hour infusion. The topical administration of prostaglandin analogues may provide a more practical mode of delivery. The topical use of nitrates (1 percent glyceryltrinitrate ointment, Nitroderm patch) has been tried, but few controlled studies have been carried out. Ketanserin, a serotonin receptor inhibitor, has been used with limited success. Dazoxiben, a thromboxane synthetase inhibitor, was not effective in one large controlled study. Fibrinolytic therapy

TABLE 4 New Modes of Treatment

Vasodilatory prostaglandins
    PgE and prostacyclin infusion
    Topical use of PgE analogues

Serotonin receptor inhibition
    Ketanserin

Antagonist of renin-angiotensin
    Captopril

Thromboxane synthetase inhibitors
    Dazoxiben

Fibrinolytic drugs
    Stanozolol

Plasmapheresis

Evening primrose oil

with stanozolol, an anabolic steroid, has been reported effective but is not recommended. Plasmapheresis, captopril, dextran infusion, and evening primrose oil have all been reported as successful modalities of treatment, but controlled trials are needed to confirm their effectiveness. Pentoxifylline (Trental) has been studied because of its potential for improving the rheologic properties of blood, but it was not effective. Few studies have been done using combinations of vasodilatory drugs, and therefore there is no evidence that they should be used.

Surgical Treatment

Surgical sympathectomy was once popular for the treatment of Raynaud's phenomenon but was disappointing because improvement was only transient and the condition returned with the same intensity in a relatively short period. Neither ganglionectomy nor preganglionic surgery has improved the results. Surgical morbidity and significant postural hypotension have been reported.

Digital sympathectomy recently has been reported as a successful mode of treatment, but no control studies have been done. Sympathectomy has been largely abandoned and should be considered only for the short-term relief of an intractable course complicated by digital ulceration that has failed to respond to medical treatment. Local digital block has been used for transient acute effects in patients with digital tissue compromise. Occasionally surgical intervention is necessary for some forms of Raynaud's phenomenon (carpal tunnel syndrome, thoracic outlet syndrome, or occlusive vascular disease). Local debridement and antibiotic treatment may be necessary if ischemic ulceration becomes secondarily infected. Whirlpool treatments have proven the most effective method of ulcer care.

TEMPORAL ARTERITIS

MARC C. HOCHBERG, M.D., M.P.H.

Temporal arteritis, also known as giant cell arteritis, and the closely related clinical syndrome, polymyalgia rheumatica, are common rheumatic diseases in the elderly population affecting about 1 of every 2,000 persons aged 50 and above. These two conditions may occur individually or together, and appropriate management depends on the nature of this relationship. Therefore, I will briefly review their distinctive clinical features before discussing their management as separate entities.

CLINICAL FEATURES

Polymyalgia Rheumatica

Polymyalgia rheumatica (PMR) presents with pain and stiffness in the neck, shoulder and hip girdles, upper arms, and thighs in persons aged 50 and above (Table 1). Usually the symptoms have developed over several days to weeks, often following a flulike syndrome. Most patients note malaise or fatigue, and low-grade fever, weight loss, or mild depression may be present. These signs and symptoms of systemic illness, as well as the laboratory findings of an elevated erythrocyte sedimentation rate often accompanied by a mild normochromic normocytic anemia, help differentiate PMR from simple hypertrophic spondylosis affecting the cervical and lumbar spine.

Giant Cell Arteritis

Giant cell arteritis (GCA) may occur in 15 to 40 percent of the patients with PMR or as an isolated syndrome. The hallmark of GCA that brings the patient to medical attention is headache, often unilateral and accompanied by scalp tenderness and tenderness or erythematous swelling (at times, plaques) over the ipsilateral temporal artery. Jaw claudication and visual symptoms, including diplopia, blurring, transient field cuts, and blind spots, are also common. Blindness is fortunately rare. Systemic symptoms, including weight loss, fever, and PMR, may also occur. The diagnosis of GCA is confirmed by temporal artery biopsy.

MANAGEMENT

Polymyalgia Rheumatica

The most effective drugs for treating PMR are corticosteroids. Although some authors have reported that nonsteroidal anti-inflammatory drugs (NSAID) are effective in PMR, I am reluctant to use NSAID therapy for two reasons: the intimate relationship between PMR and GCA, and the fact that almost all PMR patients I have treated have already failed to benefit from several different forms of NSAID therapy before they were referred to me.

The key decision in treating patients with PMR is the choice of a starting dose of prednisone. This depends on whether one is dealing with PMR alone or in combination with GCA. I believe that this decision can be made on a clinical basis; the physician must take a complete history and perform a physical examination, searching for signs and symptoms of GCA. If these are present, confirmation of the diagnosis of GCA with temporal artery biopsy should follow. The patient should be managed, even with negative biopsy findings, as if he had GCA (see later discussion). If signs and symptoms of superimposed GCA are absent, the patient can be managed as an uncomplicated case of PMR.

In this instance I usually start with prednisone, 20 mg per day, in a single daily dose and continue until symptoms resolve and the sedimentation rate falls into the normal range. Generally symptoms abate first; however, if the steroid dosage is reduced too early, the disease will flare, necessitating an increase in dosage. In most patients the sedimentation rate returns to normal; in some it may stabilize in the range of 20 to 40 mm per hour. In this instance it is useful to exclude other causes for such an elevation, including occult infections (especially urinary tract or periodontal infections) and dysproteinemic states, such as benign monoclonal gammopathies and multiple myeloma.

When the patient has responded, after about 4 weeks of therapy with 20 mg per day, I begin to slowly taper the prednisone dosage at a rate of 2.5 mg per day every 4 weeks; 20 mg per day for 1 month, then 17.5 mg per day for 1 month, then 15 mg per day for 1 month, carefully following symptoms and the laboratory parameters of disease activity. When the dosage reaches 10 mg per day, I begin reducing by increments of 1 mg per day every 4 weeks as tolerated. Most patients require a maintenance dosage, arbitrarily defined as that below which symptoms recur—between 5 and 10 mg per day for several months to years to control musculoskeletal symptoms.

Another aspect of the treatment of patients with PMR that bears note is the role of physical therapy. Patients with neck and proximal limb girdle pain and stiffness may develop weakness and limitation of motion of affected joints. Thus, they are likely to benefit from a prescribed regimen of local moist heat, ultrasound, range of motion exercises, and muscle strengthening exercises. The joint

TABLE 1 Frequency of Clinical Features in Patients with Polymyalgia Rheumatica and Giant Cell Arteritis*

Polymyalgia Rheumatica		Giant Cell Arteritis	
Pain and stiffness		Headache	++++
Neck	++++	Temporal artery	
Shoulder girdle	++++	swelling or tenderness	+++
Hip girdle	+++	Polymyalgia rheumatica	+++
Malaise, fatigue	++	Jaw claudication	++
Weight loss	+	Weight loss	++
Fever	+	Visual symptoms	++
Arthritis	+	Fever	+
Depression	+		

* +,<25%; ++, 25 to 49%; +++, 50 to 74%; ++++,≥75% of the patients.

involvement in patients with PMR rarely leads to difficulties with activities of daily living, and supports and other devices are rarely needed.

I will comment on corticosteroid side effects, their prevention, and management later.

Giant Cell Arteritis

The approach to the treatment of patients with GCA is straightforward: Give prednisone early, initially in high dosages—1 mg per kilogram per day or 60 mg per day—and divide the dosage for the first couple of weeks of therapy until the symptoms resolve and the sedimentation rate begins to fall. Then the prednisone dosage can be converted to a single daily dose and maintained at the same level until the sedimentation rate returns to normal or stabilizes. If the sedimentation rate stabilizes in the mildly elevated range, evaluation for other comorbid conditions should be performed (see previous discussion).

Again, once the patient is asymptomatic and the laboratory abnormalities have been corrected, the dosage of prednisone can begin to be tapered at a rate of about 5 mg per day every 4 weeks. Once again careful follow-up is necessary in order to recognize early flares of disease activity so that the prednisone dosage can be increased as needed. After such a flare has been treated and symptoms and signs again have responded, prednisone tapering may be pursued at the same rate. Once the prednisone dosage reaches 20 mg per day, tapering should be carried out at increments of 2.5 mg, and when the dosage reaches 10 mg per day, at increments of 1 mg. As in patients with PMR, most patients require a maintenance dosage of prednisone for several months to years.

COMPLICATIONS OF THERAPY

The potential complications of corticosteroid therapy in patients with PMR and GCA are myriad (Table 2). However, some are of particular concern given the elderly age of this patient population with its frequent comorbidity.

Myopathy

Proximal muscle weakness, similar to that which occurs in patients with polymyositis and dermatomyositis, can develop with high dose prednisone therapy. Steroid myopathy is differentiated from myositis by the presence of normal skeletal muscle enzyme levels in serum and the presence of specific type II fiber degeneration without inflammation on muscle biopsy. Steroid myopathy is best treated with an aggressive physical therapy program concurrent with prednisone tapering.

Osteoporosis

Osteoporosis is the bane of the elderly white female and is associated with increased risk of hip, wrist, and vertebral fracture and increased mortality. Since most patients with PMR and GCA are white (more than 90 percent) and female (about 70 percent), osteoporosis is usually

TABLE 2 Potential Adverse Effects of Corticosteroids in Polymyalgia Rheumatica and Giant Cell Arteritis

Organ System	Adverse Effect
Cutaneous	Acne, hirsutism, purpura, striae
Musculoskeletal	Myopathy, osteoporosis, ischemic necrosis
Gastrointestinal	Peptic ulcer disease, pancreatitis
Cardiovascular	Hypertension, accelerated atherosclerosis
Ophthalmic	Cataracts, glaucoma
Central nervous system	Psychosis
Endocrine-metabolic	Iatrogenic Cushing's syndrome, glucose intolerance, hyperlipemia, obesity, sodium retention, hypokalemia, hypercalciuria
Immunosuppressive	Increased risk of infection

found as a comorbid condition. Furthermore corticosteroid therapy can lead to or accelerate osteoporosis in part by decreasing calcium absorption and increasing calcium excretion. Therefore I treat all my female patients with supplemental calcium (1,000 to 1,500 mg per day) and vitamin D (50,000 units, 2 or 3 days a week). I refer women with fractures related to osteoporosis to their gynecologists for consideration for supplemental estrogens as well. Obviously all patients are encouraged to eat a well balanced, healthy diet and maintain a moderate level of physical activity.

Peptic Ulcer Disease

Moderate to high dose corticosteroid therapy (20 mg per day or more) has been associated with an increased risk of peptic ulcer disease. In patients without history of ulcer disease or upper gastrointestinal bleeding, I do not prescribe any specific prophylactic regimen. In patients with such a history, however, I prescribe a cytoprotective drug, such as sucralfate, 1 g four times a day, or cimetidine, 400 mg twice a day, in an attempt to prevent recurrence of ulcer disease. In patients who develop an ulcer while taking prednisone for the treatment of PMR and GCA, the ulcer requires aggressive management with a combination of sucralfate (already discussed) and cimetidine, 800 mg once daily at bedtime. These drugs are then continued indefinitely, even after ulcer healing, as long as the patient takes prednisone therapy.

PROGNOSIS

Polymyalgia rheumatica and giant cell arteritis are disorders wherein symptoms respond promptly to therapy, and almost all patients, except those who have developed irreversible visual loss, note a complete return to normal with appropriate treatment. Most patients with PMR and GCA require continued therapy for several years with a maintenance dosage of prednisone, usually 5 to 10 mg per day; some patients go into remission and can discontinue prednisone after prolonged tapering. Neither of these disorders is associated with decreased survival compared to that expected for an age and sex matched population.

HYPEREOSINOPHILIA

JOHN B. HARLEY, M.D., Ph.D.
BARBARA H. BJORNSON, M.D.

An exhaustive diagnostic evaluation may fail to find the cause in a case of eosinophilia. If in addition there have been more than 1,500 eosinophils per microliter in the peripheral blood for more than 6 months in a patient with definite organ injury, the criteria are satisfied for the diagnosis of idiopathic hypereosinophilic syndrome. This designation encompasses patients with different manifestations. End organ involvement commonly includes many organs—the central or peripheral nervous system, heart, vasculature, hematologic system, lungs, skin, gastrointestinal tract, and more rarely muscles and kidneys. With such a wide range of possibilities, it is not surprising that a flexible and responsive approach is needed in treating patients with this disorder.

These cases are unified by the inability to discover a cause for the eosinophilia. Careful evaluation, however, has revealed two separate groups of patients. One group has a collection of findings consistent with a myeloproliferative disease, which in its most severe form has been termed eosinophilic leukemia. These patients are likely to have immature forms in the peripheral blood, thrombocytopenia, fibrosis in the bone marrow, splenomegaly, high serum vitamin B_{12} levels, and morphologically abnormal eosinophils, which are more vacuolated and hypogranular than those in normal individuals. These abnormal eosinophils are usually seen only in the peripheral blood, while normal eosinophils and eosinophil precursors are found in the bone marrow. These patients are also likely to have endomyocardial fibrosis (Löffler's syndrome).

The second form of idiopathic eosinophilia appears to be a reactive eosinophilia that has the characteristics of an immunologic disease. These patients have a tendency to have high IgE levels, lymphadenopathy, and idiopathic angioedema. The peripheral blood eosinophils are normal in appearance with few or no vacuoles and are normally granulated. These patients with apparent reactive disease are more likely to respond to corticosteroid therapy than are those with myeloproliferative eosinophilia.

The medical literature before the mid-1960s recorded a nearly uniformly fatal outcome for patients with the idiopathic hypereosinophilic syndrome, with an average survival of 9 months. Attempts to treat these patients with aggressive chemotherapy had not increased survival; consequently, with the recognition that the eosinophil was responsible for the clinical manifestations, therapeutic regimens were established in which reduction of eosinophilia became the goal. With this strategy, average survivals of 9 years or more are now common in these patients.

Even after excluding all known causes of eosinophilia (Table 1), it is important for prognostic reasons to determine whether eosinophilia is more likely to be the reactive or the myeloproliferative type. To do this, patients are followed closely after the initial presentation with physi-

TABLE 1 Disorders Associated with Eosinophilia

Secondary eosinophilia
  Parasitic diseases
    Strongyloidiasis
    Trichinosis
    Schistosomiasis
    Filariasis
    Toxocara
    Other tissue invasive helminths

  Allergic diseases
    Asthma
    Atopic dermatitis
    Seasonal rhinitis
    Allergic eosinophilic gastroenteritis
    Allergic bronchopulmonary aspergillosis
    Allergic drug reactions

  Connective tissue diseases
    Systemic necrotizing vasculitis
      Polyarteritis nodosa
      Allergic angiitis and granulomatosis
    Fasciitis with eosinophilia
    Rheumatoid arthritis
    Systemic lupus erythematosus
    Scleroderma
    Wegener's granulomatosis

  Neoplastic diseases
    Hodgkin's disease
    T cell lymphomas
    Acute or chronic myelogenous leukemia
    Adenocarcinoma

  Immunodeficiency diseases
    Wiskott-Aldrich syndrome
    Hyper-IgE with recurrent infection
    Selective IgA deficiency

  Other diseases and iatrogenic causes
    Angioimmunoblastic lymphadenopathy
    Dermatitis herpetiformis
    Irradiation disease
    Graft versus host disease
    Administration of Il-2

Primary eosinophilias
  Idiopathic hypereosinophilic syndrome
  Idiopathic reactive hypereosinophilia
  Idiopathic myeloproliferative hypereosinophilia

cal examination, chest x-ray examination, urinalysis, complete blood count with differential and platelet counts, chemistry profile, serum protein electrophoresis, quantitative immunoglobulin levels, including immunoglobulin E and serum vitamin B_{12} levels, bone marrow aspirate and biopsy examinations, and two dimensional cardiography as needed. With idiopathic reactive eosinophilia, the patient generally has an easier clinical course; the disease is usually easily controlled with corticosteroids. Meanwhile those with the more myeloproliferative disease are more likely to have cardiovascular complications and to be more refractory to therapy.

The clinical manifestations observed in patients with the idiopathic hypereosinophilic syndrome are due to either direct tissue invasion by eosinophils or end organ damage mediated by the granular contents of the eosinophil. In support of the contention that the eosinophil is, in fact, responsible for the organ damage in these patients is the

159

observation that patients with long-standing eosinophilia secondary to a well defined cause, e.g., parasitic disease, may have similar patterns of organ involvement. Hence, the goal of treatment is to decrease the total number of circulating eosinophils.

THERAPY

Many patients require no therapy at all. Indeed instances of persistent eosinophilia have been documented for more than 20 years without evidence of clinical consequences. Usually the eosinophilia in these patients is accidentally discovered, and they generally have had absolute eosinophil levels of less than 5,000 per microliter. Although an occasional patient may develop organ involvement after prolonged eosinophilia (an example of mitral valve stenosis after 24 years of eosinophilia is known), the risks of therapy are greater than is the disease for these patients.

Patients who have organ involvement (Table 2) and in whom the disease severity justifies the risk of initiating corticosteroid therapy are initially treated with 1 mg per kilogram of prednisone per day (usually a total dosage of 60 mg is used). This is frequently done as a 3-month trial both to reinforce the diagnostic impression and to determine the effectiveness of therapy. Patients with reactive eosinophilia often respond with a decrease in the peripheral eosinophilia to at least half by the end of the first week. Those with the mild myeloproliferative form may be resistant, or they may initially respond and later become refractory. After about 4 weeks the daily prednisone therapy is tapered to alternative day therapy. If there is no evidence of clinical deterioration, the trial is usually continued for 3 months before it is abandoned. Prednisone is terminated in those who have no response, whereas in those who show evidence of maintaining a response to prednisone, an effort is made to lower the dosage to obtain maximal benefit with the least risk.

When prednisone fails, hydroxyurea is usually added to the regimen (see Table 2), and patients are treated with 500 mg per day for the first 1 to 2 weeks. Then the dosage of hydroxyurea is gradually increased to achieve desired suppression of the eosinophilia. In most patients 1 g per day is sufficient, although a few require more. However, in most of these patients the toxicity of hydroxyurea (especially thrombocytopenia, neutropenia, and anemia) intervenes and prevents the use of higher dosages. Some patients do well with 2 g every other day or 3 g every third day when 1 g per day is necessary to suppress the hypereosinophilia but is not tolerated in a daily dosage schedule because of toxicity. Since hydroxyurea affects eosinophil production, a period of adjustment is required before changes in the therapy can be evaluated. A week or more must elapse before determining whether a change in the hydroxyurea dosage has had the desired effect.

Some patients with idiopathic eosinophila have a concurrent vasculitic syndrome. Many of these have responded to prednisone alone, but a few have required cytotoxic therapy. Cyclophosphamide at a level of 1 to 3 mg per kilogram per day has been an effective drug. The dosage of this drug is titered to maintain the peripheral white blood cell count between 3,000 to 4,000 cells per microliter or in order to maintain an absolute neutrophil count of 1,500 to 2,000 cells per microliter. Any use of cyclophosphamide must be accompanied by an effort to keep the patient well hydrated so that the complication of hemorrhagic cystitis can be avoided. Like hydroxyurea, cyclophosphamide may cause thrombocytopenia, neutropenia, and anemia, which may require decreasing or discontinuing this therapy altogether.

A few patients may develop eosinophil counts that are extremely high (up to or exceeding 100,000 eosinophils per microliter). These patients often develop neurologic findings and are in great danger of cerebrovascular injury from presumed stasis. Usually these patients are treated with vincristine, hydroxyurea, and prednisone to gain control of the disease as rapidly as possible. Leukophoresis also may be used to cause a precipitous fall in the number of peripheral eosinophils. Vincristine is usually given in doses of 1.4 mg per square meter (not exceeding 2 mg) that are repeated in weekly intervals for up to six doses. Patients with the idiopathic hypereosinophilic syndrome seem to be more sensitive to vincristine induced neurotoxicity. This is especially true in elderly patients; thus the dose should be reduced to 1 mg to reduce the likelihood of neurotoxicity. A clinical crisis with very high eosinophil counts is often controlled with only one dose of vincristine, although occasionally repeated doses are necessary. Any decision to continue therapy must be considered carefully, since the risk of neurotoxicity increases with each dose. These patients are treated concurrently with hydroxyurea so that the reduced eosinophilia can be maintained. This strategy has been almost uniformly successful in sufficiently controlling the eosinophilia to allow recovery from transient neurologic symptoms.

In some cases increasingly immature myeloid forms begin to appear in the peripheral blood, and the disease appears indistinguishable from acute nonlymphocytic leukemia. Such patients are currently treated with standard acute nonlymphocytic leukemia chemotherapy regimens, but the incidence of complete response and the duration of remission tend to be poor in patients with eosinophilic leukemia. In a few instances bone marrow transplant has been attempted.

The cardiac disease is characterized by endocardiomyofibrosis with superimposed organizing thrombosis and accounts for many of the difficulties found in these patients. They may present with an unexplained deterioration in cardiac pump function or have advancing atrioventricular valve incompetence or peripheral emboli. Congestive heart failure is usually responsive to standard therapy, which traditionally has included digoxin and diuretics. Unloading agents have not been particularly helpful, although trials in individual patients are warranted. There has been very little experience with the calcium-channel blocking drugs in this disease. The valvular disease usually involves the atrioventricular valves, because the organizing thrombosis leading to the fibrosis restricts the movement of the chordae tendineae and leads to valvular incompetence. The progress of atrioventricular valve disease is unpredictable. In some patients cardiac func-

TABLE 2 Therapeutic Strategy in the Idiopathic Hypereosinophilic Sydrome

I. In the absence of clinical crisis
  A. Observation with no therapy
  B. Prednisone if warranted by organ involvement
    1. With improvement maintain lowest does of prednisone
    2. In the absence of improvement use
      a. Hydroxyurea, if no evidence of vasculitis is present
      b. Cyclophosphamide, if vasculitis is proven

II. Clinical crisis may require a combination of
  Prednisone
  Hydroxyurea
  Leukophoresis
  Vincristine
  Anticoagulation
  Embolectomy
  Valve replacement or thrombectomy
  Treatment of congestive heart failure

tion is stable indefinitely; in others it is slowly progressive; but for a few unfortunates, it deteriorates rapidly and leads to severe congestive heart failure in a period of weeks. Though a desperate therapy, valve replacement with porcine heterografts along with ventricular thrombus excision and dissection of areas of fibrosis has been successfully employed in a few patients.

Multiple emboli may also be a manifestation of the cardiac disease. It is easy to imagine that endocardial clot formation and necrotic organizing thrombi might dislodge and embolize to any organ. One-fifth of the patients have cerebrovascular accidents. There are no data to justify treating these patients with anticoagulants, and there are examples of patients who continue to embolize after being treated with anticoagulants. Nevertheless clinicians experienced with this disorder usually choose to give anticoagulants to patients using the standard therapy with heparin in the acute situation and subsequently long-term warfarin sodium therapy. Once a patient is anticoagulated, it is important to re-evaluate the patient at least every 6 months to determine whether continued anticoagulation is necessary. Sometimes two dimensional echocardiographic changes are present, which may be used to follow these patients.

Patients may also develop serious noncardiac problems. Central nervous system disease may be manifest by the deterioration of intellectual function or personality change, which is usually most severe at presentation. Peripheral neuropathy with peripheral sensory polyneuropathy is especially common. These patients have decreased sensation in a stocking glove distribution. Patients with these manifestations are found in both the reactive and myeloproliferative forms of the disease, and they may have central nervous system dysfunction with relatively low numbers of eosinophils (less than 5000 eosinophils per cubic micrometer). In many patients the neurologic manifestations may respond to prednisone therapy alone; it is usual for a patient to show long-term improvement, unless the patient has had a cerebrovascular accident.

Pulmonary disease may pose other difficulties. When pulmonary disease is a presenting feature in a patient with idiopathic eosinophilia, additional diagnostic possibilities must be reinvestigated, including allergic pulmonary aspergillosis, allergic angiitis and granulomatosis, lymphoma, sarcoidosis, and parasitic disease. In some patients fibrotic pulmonary changes are found along with endomyocardial fibrosis. When a prednisone trial is attempted, it is important to follow pulmonary function closely.

Eosinophilia may eventually resolve and require no therapy in some patients. This has occurred even in patients with what initially appears to be the more aggressive myeloproliferative disorder. Therapy is designed mainly to control disease manifestations by reducing eosinophil levels. Although this strategy is more palliative than curative and does not appear to specifically interfere with the underlying cause of the disease, it does have the potential for ultimate success.

ERYTHEMA NODOSUM

MARK E. UNIS, M.D.

Erythema nodosum is a distinctive clinical entity believed to represent a hypersensitivity reaction to a variety of stimuli and associated diseases. A typical patient presents with the sudden onset of crops of tender, painful, erythematous to purplish subcutaneous, usually pretibial, nodules, biopsy specimens of which show a predominantly septal panniculitis.

Although many cases are idiopathic, several associated diseases listed in Table 1 have been reported frequently. A history, physical examination, and appropriate laboratory evaluation are performed to exclude these associated diseases. If the history and physical findings are unremarkable except for cutaneous findings, a minimal initial evaluation would include a complete blood count, erythrocyte sedimentation rate, and chest x-ray examination. If there is an associated underlying disease, treatment or control of the underlying disease usually improves the erythema nodosum.

PREFERRED APPROACH

Evaluation of any particular pharmacologic therapy in patients with erythema nodosum is difficult because of the tendency for spontaneous remission to occur in this disease. Nonetheless there are several modes of therapy that I have found effective. Nearly all patients with erythema nodosum find relief of symptoms with rest and leg elevation. The preferred approach includes attempts at treatment or control of an underlying disease, if present, bed rest, leg elevation, and pharmacologic therapy, usually potassium iodide or nonsteroidal anti-inflammatory drugs (NSAID).

TABLE 1   Erythema Nodosum Associated Diseases

Sarcoidosis
Inflammatory bowel disease
    Crohn's disease
    Ulcerative colitis
Collagen vascular diseases
Drugs
    Birth control pills
    Sulfonamides
    Antibiotics
    Bromides
Behçet's syndrome
Infections
    Streptococcal infection
    Atypical mycobacterial infection
    Fungal infections
    Viral infections
    Chlamydial infections
Pregnancy
Lymphoma and leukemia

Potassium Iodide

Although there are no established guidelines for the use of potassium iodide in treating erythema nodosum, the medication seems to inhibit mononuclear phagocytes, and this may be the reason for the response of erythema nodosum to therapy with iodides. The reason for their effectiveness is unclear, especially in light of the fact that iodides and bromides have been reported to induce erythema nodosum. I usually prescribe potassium iodide as the 300 mg enteric coated tablet taken three times daily with meals. Symptomatic improvement usually begins within a few days after starting therapy. If tablets are unavailable, a saturated solution of potassium iodide, 5 to 8 drops orally three times daily in juice or water, may be substituted.

Potassium iodide has a bitter taste. Dyspepsia and heartburn may result from its administration, and small bowel ulcerations have been associated with administration of the enteric coated potassium iodide preparations.

Potassium iodide is contraindicated during pregnancy because it can induce fetal goiter. Occasional patients display hypersensitivity reactions to iodides, including angioedema, fever, arthralgia, lymphadenopathy and eosinophilia.

Other effects of iodides are chronic and may include thyroid adenoma, goiter, and myxedema because the drug suppresses thyroid function. Chronic iodism may occur after prolonged treatment, and symptoms may include salivary gland enlargement, increased salivation, coryza, pain in the teeth and gingiva, swelling of the eyelids, headache, and pulmonary edema. Acne may develop or iododerma may occur.

In general, I do not use potassium iodide in chronic or refractory cases of erythema nodosum.

Nonsteroidal Anti-inflammatory Drugs

I have found several nonsteroidal anti-inflammatory drugs useful in the therapy of erythema nodosum. Their mode of action is not known, but it is believed that inhibition of prostaglandin synthesis by metabolites of NSAIDs may be involved in the anti-inflammatory action of these drugs.

The NSAID I most frequently prescribe is indomethacin in doses ranging from 25 to 75 mg orally three times daily with meals, depending on the age and size of the patient and the severity of the disease. Indomethacin is the most likely of the NSAIDs to cause gastrointestinal disturbance, including dyspepsia, ulceration, perforation, and hemorrhage. Patients should be monitored carefully for development of these problems. Indomethacin can precipitate renal insufficiency, particularly in those with pre-existing renal or hepatic dysfunction. Using the drug for only 2 or 3 weeks of continuous therapy in erythema nodosum usually helps avoid these problems.

Ibuprofen, 400 to 800 mg orally three or four times daily, also may be effective, but I have found it less useful than indomethacin. In general, gastrointestinal side effects are much less frequent with ibuprofen than with other nonsteroidal anti-inflammatory drugs. Its relative safety and efficacy in inflammatory diseases have been well established, as it has been a commonly prescribed medication.

Clinoril 200 mg orally daily or twice daily, might be considered for chronic or recurrent erythema nodosum. Many rheumatologists consider Clinoril to be the most efficacious NSAID with a good safety profile.

All nonsteroidal anti-inflammatory drugs are capable of causing adverse gastrointestinal reactions and platelet dysfunction and are contraindicated in aspirin sensitive patients.

MISCELLANEOUS THERAPIES

Aspirin can be effective in treating erythema nodosum, usually in doses of 10 to 15 grains taken orally every 4 hours. Use of enteric coated preparations again decreases the frequency of side effects, but the efficacy of nonsteroidal anti-inflammatory drugs seems to be greater.

I have had success in one patient with chronic and refractory erythema nodosum by treating with intermittent courses of phenylbutazone. It is usually prescribed in doses of 100 mg three or four times daily with meals. If there is no improvement in the condition within 1 week,

the drug should be discontinued. When improvement is obtained, the dosage should be promptly decreased to the minimal effective level necessary to maintain relief, not exceeding 400 mg daily because of the possibility of cummulative toxicity, particularly in terms of bone marrow depression. Aplastic anemia and agranulocytosis have occurred in patients taking phenylbutazone. Like the nonsteroidal anti-inflammatory drugs, phenylbutazone causes gastrointestinal distress and may cause fluid retention. The patient should fail to respond to nonsteroidal anti-inflammatory drugs before one tries phenylbutazone.

I have treated four patients with colchicine, 0.6 mg orally twice daily, and I have had clinical responses in two patients. The most common side effects are nausea, diarrhea, and headache. Long-term use and high doses may be associated with bone marrow depression, among other complications.

I have not found systemic steroid therapy necessary in the treatment of patients with erythema nodosum, but I would not have any reservations about using steroids in patients who are unresponsive to any of the modalities listed, provided the erythema nodosum was not associated with infection. A burst of prednisone, 40 to 60 mg daily tapered over 2 to 3 weeks to avoid chronic side effects would be appropriate.

LIGHT RELATED DISORDERS

SUNBURN

JENNY L. STONE, M.D.
DAVID J. ELPERN, M.D.

Sunburn is a trauma to the skin that triggers a classic wound healing response. The exact pathophysiology of sunburn remains to be determined. However, prostaglandins, histamine, and kinins appear to be involved in promoting the inflammatory response to the burn. In addition, photons are believed to impart direct damage to endothelial cells of dermal vessels. The treatment of sunburn attempts to decrease pain and inflammation and promote normal wound healing.

FIRST DEGREE SUNBURN

A first degree sunburn produces a painful erythema, which appears 2 to 6 hours after sun exposure, peaks at 24 to 36 hours, and fades in 72 to 120 hours (assuming predominant UVB damage). Damage to the epidermis promotes dehydration of the affected skin. Treatment then consists of the following:

1. Emolliants (nonirritating) such as Aquaphor or Eucerin help decrease dehydration.

2. Aspirin may be used for its analgesic and antiprostaglandin activity.

3. Aloe gel (the clear gel from the center of the leaf) is often suggested by local emergency rooms. Aloe is applied topically within several hours after the sunburn. This substance does appear to contain a bradykinin inhibitor and an antiprostaglandin. Aloe moisturizes but may also sensitize.

4. Systemic cortiosteroid therapy should be considered for an extensive burn. Although no studies have proven steroids to be therapeutic for sunburn, many Hawaiian dermatologists have found steroids to be effective if therapy is started 36 hours or less after the burn. Use prednisone, 20 mg orally three times for 2 to 3 days, or Celestone, 1.5 to 2 cc (9 to 12 mg) intramuscularly for one dose in an adult. Occasionally a petite individual develops some degree of mania with this dose of prednisone.

5. Analgesics such as Tylenol 3, Percodan, or Percocet may be needed for extensive painful burns.

6. Antihistamines may be considered for an exceptionally pruritic burn, although they have not proven to be efficacious.

7. Topical anesthetic application is not recommended because these drugs are not particularly effective and have a potential for causing sensitization.

SECOND DEGREE SUNBURN

A second degree sunburn produces vesicles and bullae, which may present either intact and fluid filled or broken. This type of burn is treated similarly to a second degree thermal burn with the following modalities in addition to those already listed:

1. Wet dressings are applied to the burn with milk and water (50:50) or saline (1 teaspoon of salt per pint of water) solution twice or three times daily for 15 to 20 minutes at a time. Therapy is continued until the vesicles or bullae have dried.

2. Leave most intact bullae and vesicles alone. Consider rupturing and debriding extremely large bullae that are likely to break imminently.

3. Debride broken bullae and apply Silvadene. (Note: Silvadene is contraindicated in term pregnancy and in newborns less than 1 month old because of the danger of kernicterus. Substitute another antibacterial cream or ointment.) Use wet dressings with sterile saline twice daily and reapply Silvadene twice daily covering (optional) with a nonadherent dressing. Continue the treatment until the lesions have re-epithelialized. Encourage the oral intake of fluids because fluid loss may be significant, depending upon the surface area involved.

4. Consider hospitalization for an extensive second degree sunburn in an elderly or debilitated patient.

The best treatment for sunburn is prevention. Counseling the patient about proper sunscreen use may help prevent future burns. Generally a sunscreen with a sun protection factor (SPF) of 15 or higher is recommended for skin types 1 and 2 (patients who always burn or who burn initially and gradually tan). SPF 15 sunscreen is also recommended for the face of patients with type 3 skin (burn occasionlly, tan easily). People with type 3 skin should use at least an SFP 10 sunscreen on other areas. Sunscreens must be applied after swimming or excessive perspiration.

POLYMORPHOUS LIGHT ERUPTION

JOHN H. EPSTEIN, M.D.

Polymorphous light eruptions (PMLE) are idiopathic photodermatoses. However, there is disagreement about the acceptable morphologic presentations for inclusion under this heading. For our purposes here we include patterns ranging from small papular, papulovesicular, and eczematous eruptions to large papules, plaques, and prurigo types of lesions. It is likely that the clinical problems designated as PMLE represent more than one disease entity. Unfortunately definitive mechanisms for distinguishing such entities are lacking.

Action spectrum studies have led to more complications. In our experience and that of a number of observers the primary offending rays fall in the UVB range (290 to 320 nm). However, we have been able to reproduce the eruptions at test sites with UVC (less than 290 nm) and with alpha particles (ionizing radiation).

With the advent of high energy UVA irradiators some investigators have noted adverse responses to UVA as well as UVB radiation. In addition there appears to be a certain PMLE population sensitive only to UVA energy. From a therapeutic point of view this wavelength dependency leads to variations in sunscreen efficacy.

One other issue concerning therapeutic responses relates to the activity of the disease and the degree of photosensitivity of the patient. In our experience patients with the small papular and eczematous eruptions are significantly more photosensitive than those with the large papular and plaque variety. Also the more active the disease process, the more photosensitive the patient. This again relates to how well the patient responds to therapy and what therapy will be effective.

THERAPEUTIC ALTERNATIVES

The treatment varies with the type of eruption, the extent and severity of the process, and the specific responsiveness of the individual. As noted in Table 1, the alternatives include photoprotection, anti-inflammatory medications, and antimitotic therapy.

Protective measures consist of the use of protective clothing, avoiding exposure at specific times, the topical use of sunblocks and sunscreens, and the systemic use of photoprotective medications.

Hats, gloves, and other protective clothing with a close knit weave are most useful, especially in people who cannot avoid sun exposure because of their occupations and those who are very photosensitive.

Avoiding sun exposure in the mid-day between 10 AM and 3 PM eliminates almost all the UVB radiation in most parts of the world. This would be of value in a UVB reactor but not in a person sensitive to UVA, which does not decrease in intensity so greatly early and late in the day.

Topically applied sunblocks reflect the sun's rays and if used in thick enough layers can protect against most radiation. Zinc oxide and titanium dioxide are used most commonly. Unfortunately if applied thickly, they present as white pastes and are not cosmetically acceptable. The introduction of other colors (red, green, blue) have made them more acceptable to children at least. Makeup, used cosmetically by women as a rule, does afford some blocking protection, can be worn over sunscreens, and helps keep them in place.

Topically applied sunscreens are transparent, cosmetically acceptable, sun protective agents that absorb the offending rays. Only the most potent ones with sun protective factors (SPF) of 15 or over should be used. They usually contain combinations of PABA or PABA esters and benzophenones and overt their primary protective effects in filtering out UBV rays. Thus they are most effective in UVB reactors, especially those who are not exquisitely photosensitive. In patients who are allergic or photoallergic to PABA, the combination of benzophenones and other chemicals, such as cinnamates, provides an effective sunscreen. Although sunscreens containing benzophenones have some effect in absorbing UVA radiation, they do not provide much help for patients who are significantly sensitive to UVA. The methoxy-dibenzoylmethanes, which have gained more extensive use in Europe, do absorb better in the UVB range and may add to our choices for protection.

TABLE 1 Therapy in Polymorphous Light Eruption

Photoprotection
  Protective clothes
  Avoid mid-day sun
  Sunblocks and sunscreens
  Betacarotene
  PUVA?

Anti-inflammation
  Dermatologic principles
  Topical corticosteroid therapy
  Systemic corticosteroid therapy
  Antimalarial drugs
  Thalidomide
  PUVA?
  Azathioprine (antimitotic)

Sunscreens applied in the morning 1 hour before venturing into the sun can prevent reactions in less sensitive patients, who then can enjoy their vacations or weekends with little more precaution.

Systemic protection with oral doses of betacarotene (30 to 90 mg in childhood, 90 to 180 mg in adults), possibly in combination with canthaxanthin, has been reported to be of value in PMLE. However, I have not had success with betacarotene as yet. The mechanism of its action may well relate to quenching of free radicals and singlet oxygen activity rather than its action as a direct physical screen.

Topical corticosteroid therapy is of use in PMLE as in most inflammatory eruptions. In addition, general dermatologic care including cool wet dressing and soothing baths is useful for these reactions.

Systemic corticosteroid therapy is needed at times to control severe extensive eczematous eruptions. This may be combined with hospitalization. Unfortunately these patients are usually extemely photosensitive and frequently do not avoid the sun when they are discharged from the hospital. Thus flares occur shortly thereafter, and relatively high doses are needed to control the chronic disease. Intralesional corticosteroid therapy (5 mg per cubic centimeter) can be used for resistant plaque or lichenified lesions. Potent topically applied corticosteroids also can be tried in such lesions.

The antimalarial drugs chloroquine and hydroxychloroquine (Plaquenil) are most effective in the least photosensitive eruptions. Thus they are most effective in large papule and plaque reactions. However, they also are valuable in small papular lesions that require a great deal of exposure to induce. I have a number of patients who just take the medications on vacation or weekends when they are going to be exposed a great deal. We always have the patient obtain an ophthalmologic examination before and at regular intervals during such therapy. Generally 250 to 500 mg of chloroquine or 200 to 400 mg of Plaquenil for 1 to 2 weeks of vacation or over weekends controls the eruption in these individuals. Some patients require 1 tablet every second or third day for control in the summer months. In my experience the antimalarial drugs are of little value in the more photosensitive, small papular and eczematous reactions.

Thalidomide has proved to be most effective in the treatment of the Latin American Indian patient with PMLE. Unfortunately legal restrictions have prevented its evaluation in other forms of the problem. Also we have not had experience with its use in the United States.

Psoralens and UVA (PUVA) have been shown to be effective in active disease, even in very photosensitive patients. This treatment must be done very carefully, starting with 1 joule or less even in deeply pigmented patients. It is frequently necessary to use systemic corticosteroid therapy to control severe flares at the beginning of such therapy. This beneficial effect does not appear to be due to increased melanin and stratum corneum protection but may well be due to effects on the cellular infiltrate. By contrast, PUVA, when used before the usual spring flares, has been useful in producing "hardening" and thus reducing or preventing such reactions. This has proven to be most effective in patients who experience flares in the spring and improve as the summer progresses.

The exquisitely photosensitive patient with chronic eczema, who is usually but not exclusively a male over the age of 50, presents a severe therapeutic problem. In my opinion at least some of these patients represent the result of having chronic PMLE. Some respond to PUVA, as noted. However, many do not. Sunscreens are of little value, and systemic corticosteroid therapy usually requires high maintenance doses. Recently azathioprine has proven to be a most effective therapy for this problem. A dosage of 50 mg twice a day is used for several months. A complete blood count, platelet counts, and liver function tests should be done. Improvement frequently requires 2 to 4 months to be obvious. At least some patients can discontinue the medication after 6 to 8 months of therapy.

PREFERRED APPROACH

It should be noted that PMLE appears to be a most common idiopathic photodermatosis. However, many of the patients have mild flares on one or two occasions in the spring and are then no longer bothered with the problem until the next year. These people rarely seek medical help for their problems. The following approach concerns the treatment of the more severe cases in patients who wish therapy.

The initial history and examination are most important in determining the character, degree of sensitivity, and (if possible) the relationship to UVA exposure. Phototesting, when possible, also aids in these determinations. If the patient is a primary UVB reactor and is not very photosensitive, the disorder might be controlled with the faithful use of a potent sunscreen. More extensive disease in a sensitive patient may require protection with clothing such as gloves, hats, closely woven shirts, avoidance of the mid-day sun, and the like. Betacarotene can be tried, but I have had little success with it to date.

Potent topical corticosteroid therapy should be used on exposed areas except for the face. If the eruption is severe and or extensive, especially if it is eczematous, systemic corticosteroid therapy (30 to 60 mg of prednisone) may be needed. Also small amounts of intralesional (5 mg per cubic centimeter) triamcinolone therapy can be used for chronic lichenified and plaque lesions.

Systemic antimalarial therapy is most effective in the large papule and plaque lesions or the less photosensitive, small papular reactions. Usually 200 mg of Plaquenil twice daily for 1 to 2 weeks with tapering to one dose every second to fourth day controls the process for the summer months. A number of patients need only take the medication, 200 mg per day, for 1 to 2 weeks when they are on vacation or over weekends during the summer and in ski season when they are exposed to a great deal of sun. Ophthalmologic examinations are obtained, as noted previously.

Thalidomide is not available in the United States for general use; thus it will not be discussed further.

If the foregoing measures are not effective, PUVA therapy may be attempted. Starting at low doses with corticosteroids is necessary in most of these patients, since they are the most photosensitive individuals. This can be used effectively with gradually increasing doses in a number of patients.

Finally azathioprine, 50 mg twice a day, has proven to be of great value in the chronic, severe, very sensitive eczematous photoreactors. Monitoring of hematologic and liver parameters should be done. Usually improvement begins in 2 months or so. Thus one must be patient in using this therapy.

PHOTOALLERGIC CONTACT DERMATITIS

RICHARD D. GRANSTEIN, M.D.
ERNESTO GONZALEZ, M.D.

Photoallergic contact dermatitis (PCD) is an immune response to an offending exogenous chemical, in which participation of the immune system is necessary for the response to occur and in which photons are required with the chemical for immunologic activation. An epidemic of PCD occurred in the 1960s as a result of the use of the potent photoallergen tetrachlorsalicylanilide as an antimicrobial agent in soaps. Other halogenated salicylanilides and related compounds are still used in some toiletries, although their photosensitizing potential seems to be low. More recently musk ambrette and 6-methylcoumarin, contained in perfumes and other fragrance containing toiletries, have been implicated as a cause of PCD; this has required the U.S. Food and Drug Administration to remove 6-methylcoumarin from the market.

PCD is to be distinguished from phototoxic chemical photosensitivity states in which photosensitized damage occurs directly and does not involve the immune system. There is considerable controversy over this distinction in the clinical literature. Numerous drugs and chemicals have been reported in the past to be photoallergens, despite little or no evidence for immunologic involvement in the induced photosensitivity. Phototoxic reactions are characterized by occurrence on the first exposure to the offending agent, with a high incidence among those exposed (theoretically 100 percent if the dose of the chemical and radiation is sufficient) and with subsequent exposures at untreated sites mimicking the time course and intensity of the first exposure. By contrast, photoallergic reactions require previous exposure for sensitization to oc-

cur, with subsequent exposures resulting in more severe reactions than the initial exposure. The incidence of photoallergic reactions among those exposed is low, and the dose of chemical required to elicit the reaction in sensitive individuals is usually quite low. Table 1 summarizes these differences. In addition, many, if not most photoallergic agents are also phototoxic, yielding some confusion. Table 2 lists the major agents commonly implicated in PCD.

TABLE 1 Characteristics of Photocontact Dermatitis

Characteristic	Photoallergic	Phototoxic
Occurs on first exposure	No	Yes
Requires previous sensitization	Yes	No
Incidence	Low	High
Dose of agent needed to elicit	Low	High
Flare at nonexposed, previously involved site	Possible	No
Skin changes	Eczematous	Similar to sunburn

In recent years several animal models have been developed to study mechanisms involved in PCD. These models, utilizing guinea pigs or mice, have shown that PCD is a cell mediated immune response that can be induced in a naive animal by the adoptive transfer to T-lymphocytes from sensitive animals. Indeed PCD appears to be immunologically identical to ordinary allergic contact dermatitis except for the requirement for photons for initiation or elicitation of the response. In animal models it has been demonstrated that irradiation of chlorpromazine or sulfanilamide in vitro results in the production of a photoproduct that is capable of inducing or eliciting ordinary allergic contact dermatitis and that is cross reactive with induced PCD to these agents. Thus, in PCD the mechanism of antigen formation to these agents appears to be the generation of a hapten photoproduct.

Two other mechanisms have been proposed to account for the generation of the antigen in PCD. A photon could

TABLE 2 Agents Reported to Induce Photoallergic Contact Dermatitis *

Halogenated phenols
    Tetrachlorsalicylanilide
    Tribromosalicylanilide
    Dibromosalicylanilide
    Multifungin
    Trichlorocarbanilide
    Bithionol
    Fenticlor
    Hexachlorophene
    Buclosamide (Jadit)
    Chloro-2-phenylphenol
Drugs
    Promethazine hydrochloride
    Chlorpromazine hydrochloride
    Sulphonamides
    Diphenhydramine
    Quinine
    Benzocaine

Sunscreens
    Para-aminobenzoic acid (PABA)
    Glyceryl PABA
    Digalloyl trioleate
    Mexenone
    Cinnamate

Various chemicals
    Moquizone
    Quindoxine
    Thiourea
    Musk ambrette
    6-Methylcoumarin
    Stilbenes
    Sandalwood oil

* Inclusion of some of these agents is based on a single or very few reports.

be necessary for the binding of a hapten to a carrier protein, or the photon with the chemical may alter a host protein, which becomes antigenic. There are no current experimental data to support these mechanisms.

CLINICAL DESCRIPTION

The majority of photoallergic reactions are eczematous. Early changes are acute eczema with vesiculation, which may progress to bullae, with scaling, crusting, and excoriations as variable features. In the chronic stage thick lichenified plaques are present. Urticarial papular and lichenoid eruptions have also been reported as photoallergic reactions, but these are unusual responses described in isolated case reports. The histology of the eruption is that of a spongiotic dermatitis with intercellular edema in the epidermis with or without vesicle formation, depending on the clinical pattern. A dense perivascular dermal lymphohistiocytic infiltrate is present, identical to that found in allergic contact dermatitis. Some authors believe that a biopsy in some cases may make it possible to distinguish a photoallergic reaction from a phototoxic one. The differences observed are those that distinguish allergic contact dermatitis from a primary irritant contact dermatitis.

PCD can occur at any age and in either sex. Males are more commonly affected than females, although it has been postulated that this may reflect differences in exposure to photoallergens. As in other diseases, the history and physical examination should begin the evaluation of the patient. The patient usually presents with a rash, restricted to exposed sites, which he attributes to sunlight exposure. The initial eruption frequently occurs a few days after long exposure to sunlight, but subsequent eruptions may occur within hours after exposure. The face, V of the neck, and dorsum of the hands and arms are usually involved. The areas behind the ears (Wilkinson's triangle), under the chin, between the fingers, and in the skin folds are usually spared. Facial involvement is sometimes surprisingly patchy. The actual distribution of the eruption and the time course are determined, of course, by the dose and site of exposure to the chemical and radiation. When a localized area is exposed to the offending agent as well as the relevant wavelengths of radiation and PCD ensues, a distant, previously involved area may demonstrate a flare of activity.

The differential diagnosis includes phototoxic reactions, contact dermatitis (especially airborne contact dermatitis), photosensitive eczema, and the eczematous form of polymorphous light eruption. Photoallergic reactions also may be a consequence of drugs administered systemically.

In addition to the physical findings and history, photopatch testing can be useful in making a diagnosis. There is no standard procedure, but the approach to testing is uniform. A battery of known photosensitizers is applied in duplicate to small areas of the back, and all sites are covered by an opaque material. Table 3 lists standard photoallergy testing materials. Substances to be tested are prepared in petrolatum at the concentrations listed in Table 3.

TABLE 3 Photopatch Testing Agents

Benzocaine	5% in petrolatum
Chlorpromazine	0.1% in petrolatum
Diphenhydramine	2% in petrolatum
Hydrochlorothiazide	1% in petrolatum
Musk ambrette	5% in petrolatum and 5% in alcohol
6-Methylcoumarin	10% in alcohol
Sandalwood oil	1% in petrolatum
Sulfanilamide	5% in petrolatum
Tribromosalicylanilide	1% in petrolatum
Bithionol	1% in petrolatum
Buclosamide (Jadit)	10% in water
Fenticlor	1% in petrolatum
Hexachlorophene	1% in petrolatum
Tetrachlorsalicylanilide	1% in petrolatum
Trichlorocarbanilide	1% in petrolatum
Quinine	1% in petrolatum
Para-aminobenzoic acid	1% in petrolatum
Cinnamate	1% in petrolatum
Benzophenone (Piz Buin sunscreen)	Commercial preparation as is

After 24 hours one set of the applied substances is exposed to UVA (320 to 400 nm) radiation, because the action spectrum for most photoallergens is thought to be in this range. We use a bank of PUVA fluorescent bulbs filtered through mylar (to remove wavelengths below 320 nm) as the source of radiation in our clinic. The exposure dose is usually 10 J per square centimeter, a dose empirically selected because it is below the minimal erythema dose for most individuals and is presumed to be sufficient to elicit a photoallergic response. However, if the patient's minimal erythema dose for UVA is at or below this level, a lower exposure dose is used. We believe that it is mandatory to do phototesting prior to photopatch testing to ensure that a proper dose of UVA radiation is selected (see later discussion). The sites are then re-covered. Twenty-four and 48 hours later the sites are examined for a reaction. Erythema, edema, and vesiculation are considered positive responses that are graded on a 1+ to 4+ scale of severity. Positive responses of equal intensity at both the nonirradiated and the irradiated sites are interpreted as ordinary allergic contact dermatitis. A positive response at an irradiated site, or in the presence of allergic contact dermatitis, an enhanced response at the irradiated site are interpreted as being consistent with photocontact allergy.

Phototesting in which the minimal erythema dose to UVA and UVB radiation is determined may be helpful in differentiating idiopathic photosensitivity states from PCD (Table 4) and is necessary for determining the dose of radiation to use in photopatch testing, as already mentioned. All patients referred for photopatch testing undergo phototesting prior to photopatch testing. This is performed by exposing small areas of nonsun-exposed (buttock) skin to graded doses of radiation, shielding these sites from light exposure, and examining these areas 24 hours later. In our experience the skin type of the patient is not a reliable indicator of the "normal" minimal erythema dose. Generally a minimal erythema dose below 20 mJ per square centimeter for UVB or 20 J per square centimeter for UVA radiation is considered abnormal, depending on the cir-

TABLE 4 Interpretation of Phototesting

Condition	MED to UVA	MED to UVB	Photopatch Test
PCD	Normal	Normal	Positive
Photosensitive eczema	Normal or decreased	Usually decreased	Negative
Persistent light reaction	Normal or decreased	Decreased	Positive
Actinic reticuloid	Usually decreased	Normal or decreased	Positive or negative

cumstances and characteristics of the patient. We also examine sensitivity to visible radiation by exposing nonsunexposed skin to graded doses of radiation from a tungsten lamp, shielding these areas from light exposure, and examining them 24 hours later. Any reaction is considered abnormal.

There are limitations to the use and interpretation of the photopatch test. Radiation sources used vary, but most investigators use a source with a main emission spectrum in the UVA range because, as already mentioned, the action spectra of photoallergic reactions to most chemicals are included in this waveband. However, the action spectra of some reactions probably involve UVB (280 to 320 nm) radiation. Therefore, a solar simulator that emits both UVA and UVB radiation is sometimes used. However, because UVB radiation is much more erythemogenic than UVA radiation, problems of dosimetry occur when using a solar simulator source for photopatch testing.

A suberythemal dose of radiation, chosen by testing the patient, is administered when the solar simulator is employed. To increase the probability of detecting a response, a dose of radiation just below the minimal erythema dose could be employed at each of several suspected wavelengths. This could clearly result in very large and impractical amounts of testing.

Other problems of phototesting include determining the amount of photosensitizer to apply and differentiating allergic contact dermatitis from photoallergic contact dermatitis when both occur. In addition, allergic contact dermatitis to some agents could be increased by exposure to ultraviolet radiation. Another problem relates to the possibility that photoallergic contact dermatitis to some chemicals might result from exposure to visible radiation. Finally, the differentiation of phototoxic responses from photoallergic responses can be difficult, although biopsy of test sites can sometimes distinguish these reactions, as already mentioned. Risks and complications of photopatch testing include inadvertent photosensitization to test agents, discomfort at positive test sites, occasional flares of disease activity at sites of previous involvement, and false-positive or false negative results due to incorrect amounts of chemical or radiation. Despite these caveats, in many circumstances photopatch testing can be very helpful in identifying the offending agent in a patient with PCD.

THERAPY

Avoidance of the offending agent is, of course, the single most important therapeutic maneuver. Thus, it is im-

portant to identify the offending agent if at all possible. This often can be done by means of the history, but when the history is ambiguous, photopatch testing can be useful. If more than one chemical is implicated by the history, photopatch testing can determine which among them is responsible for the eruption. It also can be used as a confirmatory test when the history suggests only one offending chemical, and occasionally it is useful in diagnosing photosensitivity states when the history does not clearly implicate any substance. Once an offending agent is identified, it is crucial to tell the patient what substances in his environment may contain that chemical or a cross reactive substance. In our clinic we provide the patient with a written list of common materials containing the agent to which he is sensitive.

The avoidance of sunlight can be important in the treatment of acute photoallergic contact dermatitis. This often must be extended beyond the period of acute dermatitis because the offending chemical may persist in the skin for some time. In severe cases confinement to a darkened room for several days may speed recovery. Since most offending agents are activated by exposure to wavelengths above 320 nm, sunlight penetrating window glass can aggravate the dermatitis. When the offending chemical cannot be identified, avoidance of sunlight may become a mainstay of treatment.

The utility of sunscreens is limited by the fact that most transparent sunscreens do not protect against photons of wavelengths in the UVA range. Although some of these agents, especially those that contain benzophenones, afford some protection above 320 nm, the most useful sunscreens are those that form an opaque barrier to all photons of solar radiation. These agents contain opaque powders, such as titanium oxide, kaolin, zinc oxide, or talc. Unfortunately these are usually not as cosmetically acceptable as sunscreens that are invisible. It should also be pointed out that some sunscreens, notably those that contain paraminobenzoic acid and its esters, can produce allergic contact dermatitis and sometimes, although rarely, photoallergic contact dermatitis. In addition, various inactive components of these preparations, such as preservatives and fragrances, may produce ACD or PCD.

Symptomatic Therapy

The acute treatment of photoallergic contact dermatitis is similar to that of ordinary allergic contact dermatitis. For vesicular and weeping areas, astringent soaks are appropriate as is topical steroid therapy. It is crucial to keep open areas clean to prevent superinfection. We often prescribe astringent soaks, such as Domeboro's solution, three or four times a day. If large areas are weeping, we also may advise the patient to clean these areas with an antimicrobial cleansing agent, such as Hibiclens antimicrobial cleanser, twice a day. Antihistamines may be helpful for pruritus. In severe cases a short course of systemic steroid therapy can be given. As already implied, removal of the offending photosensitizer and related compounds eliminates the problem once the acute eruption has resolved.

Persistent Light Reaction

A small number of patients with PCD display photosensitivity without apparent continuing exposure to a chemical or a cross-reacting agent to which they are demonstrably sensitive. This condition, termed persistent light reaction, was first recognized as a consequence of tetrachlorsalicylanilide exposure. Since that time it has been observed as a consequence of other photosensitizers. The eruption is a chronic eczematous dermatitis initially restricted to light exposed sites. Patients display marked photosensitivity with a lowered minimal erythema dose to UVB radiation, often to UVA radiation, and sometimes to visible light. Photopatch testing reveals a strongly positive response to a photoallergen. This disorder can be disabling, and severe depression and suicide have been reported among patients with photosensitivity states.

Various hypotheses have been presented to account for this condition. One is that patients continue to encounter the photoallergen or a cross-reacting substance. Another is that an induced photoantigen persists in the skin, and a third is that a normal skin constituent has undergone an alteration and has become antigenic, with subsequent exposure to ultraviolet radiation producing the same or a similar photoproduct without further exposure to an offending chemical. This last possible mechanism is perhaps, supported by the observation that tetrachlorsalicylanilide can photo-oxidize proteins. None of these hypotheses completely explains the broad spectrum of photosensitivity observed in some patients or the abnormal sensitivity of uninvolved skin on phototesting.

The treatment consists of using sunscreens, avoiding sun exposure and, when necessary, fluorescent light exposure. Topical and systemic steroid therapy is useful, especially for acute eruptions. Suppression of persistent light reaction (PLR) by 8-methoxypsoralen and sunlight has been reported. We find this interesting, because a patient with actinic reticuloid was treated in our clinic with PUVA and did very well for a prolonged period.

Patients with actinic reticuloid, photosensitive eczema, and PLR generally share a number of characteristics. They are usually male, middle-aged or older, and the eruption is usually eczematous. The relationship among these three disorders is not clear. For this reason it has been proposed by some authors that the present nomenclature be abandoned and that the term "chronic actinic dermatitis" with appropriate subdivisions be used to classify these diseases.

PHOTOTOXIC DERMATITIS

EDWARD A. EMMETT, M.B., B.S., M.S.

Phototoxicity designates an increased reactivity of the skin to ultraviolet or visible radiation produced by a chemical on a nonimmunologic basis. Each response is governed by a dose-response relationship between the intensity of the reaction and both the concentration of the inciting chemical in the target area of the skin and the amount of radiation of the appropriate wavelengths to which the skin is exposed. Phototoxic reactions can be elicited in all people exposed to a phototoxic agent provided the dose of the substance and the light exposure are sufficient. In this respect they differ from photoallergic reactions, which occur only in previously sensitized individuals.

Phototoxic reactions may be caused by systemic or topical administration of a variety of medications, as listed in Table 1, or other chemicals that contact the skin such as cosmetics, plants and fruits, and industrial products, as listed in Table 2. These lists are far from complete and the number of possible phototoxic photosensitizers is large. All, however, appear to act by absorbing ultraviolet or visible radiation, which initiates photochemical reactions culminating in dermatitis. Most phototoxic reactions result from UVA (longer UV) radiation.

Phototoxicity caused by orally administered medications is usually characterized by erythema and papules or edema followed by scaling, sharply confined to light-exposed areas such as the face and the V of the neck. Shaded areas such as behind the ears, the submental region, and fold areas of the face are spared. Vesiculation and bullae

TABLE 1 Medications Leading to Phototoxic Reactions

Sulfonamides
  Sulfanilamide, sulfacetamine, sulfadiazine, sulfaguanidine, sulfapyridine

Sulfonylureas
  Tolbutamine, chlorpropamide

Antibiotics
  Nalidixic acid, meclocycline (dimethylchlortetracycline), doxycycline, oxytetracycline

Thiazides and related sulfonamide diuretics
  chlorothiazide, hydrochlorothiazide, furosemide

Phenothiazines
  Chlorpromazine, thioridazine, trimeprazine

Nonsteroidal anti-inflammatory drugs
  Benoxaprofen, diroxicam

Oral contraceptive therapy

Psoralens

Coal tar and fractions

TABLE 2 Sources of Contact Phototoxic Reactions

Cosmetics
  Perfumes and perfumed cosmetics, aftershaves

Plants
  Celery, lime, meadow grass, St. John's wort

Industrial chemicals
  Coal tars and pitches, UV curing agents

may occur with more severe reactions. However, the clinical picture may vary depending both on the inciting agent and on the method and site of skin contact. Phototoxic reactions from fruits or plants (phytophotodermatitis) are frequently bullous with a streaked pattern reflecting the type of contact. In milder cases of phytophotodermatitis only hyperpigmentation may be seen. Psoralens in cosmetics or perfumes (berloque dermatitis) and oral contraceptive therapy may produce mottled or reticulate hyperpigmentaton on the facial area. Other types of lesions seen in phototoxic reactions include papular reactions mimicking lichen planus, cutaneous changes similar to those of porphyria cutanea tarda, onycholysis, and ocular keratoconjunctivitis. Ocular cataracts are a theoretical risk, particularly from UVA and oral psoralen therapy.

The most important feature of management of phototoxic dermatitis is the avoidance of clinical episodes by avoidance of the chemical, the inciting radiation, or both. In the case of patients taking photosensitizing medications, avoidance of the inciting radiation is a key measure.

Since most phototoxic reactions are elicited by UVA light, protection should be afforded against these wavelengths. Direct or strong reflected sunlight should be avoided. Whereas solar UVB radiation is much stronger in the middle of the day (10 AM to 2 PM before accounting for daylight saving), UVA radiation is relatively intense throughout more of the day; moreover UVA radiation passes through ordinary window glass. Hats, gloves, and clothing provide protection; the degree of protection is related to the tightness of the weave and to a lesser extent the color of the fabric.

Commercial sunscreens are often effective only against UVB radiation and are thus ineffective in most phototoxic reactions. Benzophenone-containing sunscreens are efficacious against UVA, although the degree of protection is less than we are accustomed to in dealing with UVB exposure. Sun protectives containing opaque shields such as titanium dioxide protect against all wavelengths but are less pleasing cosmetically. Of products in the latter category I find Doak Solar Cream useful. Only opaque sunscreens protect against visible light elicited reactions; such reactions include oral-contraceptive induced melasma. Patients being treated with oral doses of psoralens should wear UVA protective sunglasses. In extreme cases other steps can be taken to reduce UVA exposure. These can include the use of UV free bug lights for illumination and shielding the subject from the sun and from artificial light sources using UV absorbing plastic screens. The necessary duration of these precautions depends on the pharmacokinetics of the drug or chemical. In the case of oral psoralen therapy, for example, increased UVA susceptibility is generally negligible 1 day after administration.

UVA tanning sources pose a new danger for those exposed to phototoxic agents. Both patients and all clients at tanning salons need warnings about the dangers of phototoxic reactions.

Avoidance of the causal chemical is critical with cosmetics, industrial products, plant photosensitizers, and the like. Toxicologic testing is now available to identify chemical photosensitizers before use so that there can be adequate precautionary labeling of commercial products. Frequently repeated phototoxic reactions are undesirable and in some instances (e.g., coal tar pitch or psoralens and UVA) may be a risk factor for skin cancer.

The treatment of phototoxic reactions after they have occurred is nonspecific and depends on the severity and extent of injury. Bullous and weeping reactions require wet dressings with water or aluminum acetate (Burow's) solution. Aspirin may reduce discomfort, but in very painful reactions stronger analgesics may be required. As the eruption heals, moisturizing preparations should be applied. Topical corticosteroid therapy may reduce the immediate discomfort and erythema, but this relief is temporary and symptomatic and the subsequent damage is not reduced. Rarely, in very severe reactions, additional supportive therapy including hospitalization, replacement of fluid loss, and extensive nursing care may be necessary. Systemic steroid therapy may be given but is not usually dramatically effective.

XERODERMA PIGMENTOSUM

JOHN J. DiGIOVANNA, M.D.

Xeroderma pigmentosum (XP) is a rare autosomal recessive disorder characterized by progressive degeneration of the skin, eyes, and nervous system. At an early age these patients sustain severe actinic damage to the sun exposed areas of the skin and eyes. Some also develop neurologic abnormalities. The parents of affected individuals, obligate heterozygotes, are clinically normal but may have an increased risk of developing skin cancer.

The progressive skin and eye damage seen in patients with this disorder appears to be the result of progressive DNA damage that is not properly repaired. This damage is largely due to environmental mutagens such as ultraviolet (UV) light and certain chemical agents. Just as patients with XP are sensitive to certain agents that damage DNA, so are their cultured cells. In vitro, cells cultured from patients with XP have defects in the capacity to repair DNA damage resulting from exposure to UV radiation, certain mutagenic chemicals (e.g., benzo [a] pyrene derivatives found in cigarette smoke), and drugs (e.g., psoralens, cancer chemotherapeutic drugs).

From cell fusion studies it has been determined that all patients with XP do not have genetically identical DNA repair defects. Fusion of two fibroblast lines derived from patients with different defects allows some degree of correction (i.e., complementation) of the abnormality. The capacity of different abnormalities to correct or complement each other has made it possible to classify patients with XP into complementation groups. Currently nine complementation groups have been described.

The progressive neurologic degeneration has also been thought to be due to unrepaired DNA damage that has resulted in neuronal cell death. Since neurons do not divide, and are therefore not replaced, this damage would lead to progressive neuronal loss and would be manifested as progressive neurologic degeneration.

We do not know how to correct or improve the DNA repair defects that have been associated with this disease. Therapy therefore is directed at three levels:

Protection: prevention of DNA damage by minimizing exposure to relevant known and suspected mutagens.

Surveillance: careful monitoring aimed at early detection of the disease resulting from chronic degenerative changes in the skin, eyes, and nervous system.

Management: therapy for the premalignant, malignant, and nonmalignant degenerative changes that are identifed.

The large number of neoplasms that develop in this disease makes therapy difficult and often disfiguring. In addition, metastasis from cutaneous malignant tumors is often a cause of early death in these patients. Adopting strict measures of UV light protection from infancy on has been shown to prevent the most severe skin and eye abnormalities in a few patients. Therefore, prevention of degenerative changes by protection from UV radiation is the cornerstone of XP therapy and probably can prolong the life expectancy of these patients. Patients with XP are also thought to be at increased risk for the development of internal malignant disease, and thus environmental carcinogens (e.g., cigarette smoke) also should be avoided.

It is important to establish the diagnosis of XP as early as possible, after which the patient should be protected from UV radiation by all possible means. Once an individual is diagnosed with XP, the patient's close relatives should be examined. Any mildly affected individuals who could thereby be identified could institute protective measures very early.

CLINICAL MANIFESTATIONS AND MANAGEMENT

Dermatologic Manifestations

Clinical Dermatology

The hallmark of XP is a marked sensitivity to sun and other UV light exposure, resulting in the early development of cutaneous damage. Some, but not all, patients have acute photosensitivity, which can be severe, with the development of vesicles and blisters. During infancy patients may present with an exaggerated acute sunburn reaction after exposure to small amounts of UV light. Later they develop extensive solar damage on sun exposed areas. At an early age these patients develop the actinic changes usually associated with chronic exposure. Freckle-like, hyperpigmented macules and dryness of the skin usually begin to develop before the age of 2 years. Actinic keratoses and cutaneous neoplasms often develop before the age of 10. The disease is often fatal within the first 2 decades because of metastases from cutaneous squamous cell carcinoma or malignant melanoma.

The term xeroderma pigmentosum, or parchment skin, typifies the xerotic and atrophic qualities of the actinically damaged skin in these individuals. By the time these patients reach young adulthood, their skin usually is covered with freckle-like hyperpigmented macules. These occur in many shades, varying from brown to black, and vary in size up to more than 1 centimeter in diameter. These are interspersed with hypopigmented atrophic areas. Telangiectasias are common, as are angiomas. These changes result in a poikilodermatous skin, with damage being most severe in sun exposed areas and relative sparing of the axilla, buttocks, and groin. Actinic keratoses, keratoacanthomas, basal cell carcinomas, and squamous cell carcinomas may be numerous, but malignant melanomas also occur. Neoplasms of the oral cavity (especially the tip of the tongue, because of relative UV light exposure), sarcomas, and other malignant tumors are also found

Prevention

Sources of Exposure. Patients with XP and their families must be educated to recognize the acute and long-term hazards of UV exposure. Optimally they should accept the necessity for constant protection, recognize the known sources of exposure, and utilize the measures known to decrease exposure. The most significant risk occurs with exposure to radiation in the UVC (200 to 290 nm) and UVB (290 to 320 nm) ranges. In terms of DNA repair defects, cells from patients with XP are most sensitive to UVC radiation. Since short wavelength UVC does not penetrate intact skin very effectively, it is not known how much actually reaches the basal cell layer to damage the dividing cells. UVB and UVA radiation penetrates more deeply into the skin. UVB radiation is the most significant risk, and sunlight exposure is the major hazard.

In addition to sunlight, germicidal lamps, artificial sunlamps, and to a small extent the common cool white fluorescent bulbs can be noxious sources. Common fluorescent bulbs emit small amounts of UVC radiation, which is effectively filtered by covering with light diffusers made of solid plastic, but not those made of metal that have hatched openings. These sources may also emit some UVA, which is not filtered by the thin glass bulb. The newer, high intensity visible light sources such as mercury arc and halide lamps are usually encased in a double envelope. These sources generate UVB and UVC radiation which is usually filtered but can leak out if the envelope is broken.

Long wave UV or UVA light is found in sources such as sunlight that has passed through window glass and incandescent lamps. Compared with UVC radiation, UVA causes less DNA damage to cells, but it penetrates skin much more deeply. UVA is also thought to potentiate the carcinogenic capacity of UVB. Therefore, UVA radiation cannot be assumed to be innocuous to these patients.

All patients with XP should adopt prudent measures for UV radiation protection (Table 1). The amount of time spent outdoors during the day should be minimized, especially on sunny days and during mid-day (10 AM to 2 PM) when UV radiation is most intense. Whenever possible, outdoor activities should be planned to occur in the morning, late afternoon, or evening, and in the shade. Significant UV exposure can occur on overcast days. Clouds can preferentially filter visible and infrared light more than UV. With less brightness and warmth, there is the appearance of being shaded from the sun while deceptively allowing UV to penetrate. The environment influences the amount of light reaching the skin. Sand and snow, which reflect light, increase the amount of light reaching the skin. When one is outdoors, protective clothing should be worn, such as shirts with long sleeves, long pants, and broad brimmed hats. Significant amounts of UV can penetrate loosely woven, light colored cloth, and thus two layers of

TABLE 1 Measures for UV Protection

Adopt a sun sheltered life style to minimize exposure.
  Limit daytime outdoor activities.
  Reschedule daytime outdoor activities to avoid mid-day
    sun (10 AM to 2 PM).
  Close vehicle windows during daytime travel.
Wear protective clothing: glasses, hairstyles, wide brimmed
  hats, long sleeved shirts, long pants, two layers of cloth-
  ing when possible.
Institute daily application of a high SPF sunscreen.

clothing should be worn whenever possible. Long hair styles can be used to protect the skin of the forehead, ears, and neck. When one is traveling during daylight, vehicle windows should be kept closed; this serves to decrease the amount of UV light reaching the interior of the vehicle.

Sunscreens. Coincident with the greater public interest in protection from sun exposure to prevent wrinkling and skin cancer, there has been a great increase in the diversity and quality of commercially available sunscreen preparations. Sunscreens are now rated on a numerical scale according to their protective factor (SPF). When wearing a sunscreen with an SPF of 15 compared to no protection, an individual can be exposed to 15 times the amount of UV and develop the same redness. Sunscreens with high SPFs (e.g., 15 to more than 30) have recently become available. The active agent is usually para-aminobenzoic acid (PABA) or its derivatives, sometimes in combination with other agents. Several PABA-free sunscreens are also available, usually containing benzophenones or cinnamates. The great variety of commercially available sunscreens in a wide range of vehicles (alcohol based, lotions, creams, and sticks) insures that a cosmetically acceptable preparation can be found for virtually every patient.

All patients with XP should routinely apply a high SPF sunscreen daily to protect against unrecognized sources of exposure. This is easily done as part of a morning ritual upon awakening. The sunscreen should be reapplied after washing or excessive sweating. Other make-up or cosmetics can be applied over the sunscreen. Opaque corrective cosmetics, such as Covermark or Dermablend, can be used to cover unsightly pigmentary abnormalities and surgical scars and also act as an additional blocking agent. When applicable, opaque blocking agents such as thick make-up or titanium dioxide or zinc oxide containing preparations can be used. Sunscreens also should be applied to the lips, and many commercially available lipsticks, balms, and lubricants for chapped lips contain effective sunscreens.

The administration of psoralens followed by exposure to UVA radiation (PUVA) has been used in other diseases to induce pigmentation, thereby hardening the skin and providing protection from UVB damage. This therapy should not be used in patients with XP. PUVA causes the type of DNA damage that XP cells do not repair normally and might cause an increase in skin cancer in these patients.

Chemoprevention. Since preventing skin tumors avoids significant morbidity and mortality, there has developed a great interest in cancer chemoprevention. Currently there are studies under way at many institutions that have been designed to assess the capacity of a variety of agents (retinoids, β-carotene, trace elements) to prevent the development of cancer. To date no drug has been proven safe and effective in the prevention of skin cancer. Two retinoids, isotretinoin and etretinate, have been studied in a small number of patients with XP and other disorders at high risk of skin cancer and have shown some effect in both therapy and prevention.

To assess the efficacy and safety in this disorder, a

long-term chemoprevention study of high dose isotretinoin is currently under way at the National Cancer Institute. Although there are significant mucocutaneous and bone toxicities associated with this therapy, early results suggest that the drug can decrease the incidence of skin cancer in some patients. It is not yet know whether long-term therapy is needed, and the optimal dose has not been determined. Therefore this treatment cannot yet be recommended. However, this approach offers these patients hope for the future.

Surveillance

Physicians and patients should take an aggressive role in regularly conducting frequent thorough examinations to strive for the earliest detection of premalignant and malignant skin lesions. Optimally a family member who can be taught to recognize suspicious lesions should examine the patient weekly. All skin surfaces, including the scalp, oral cavity, and covered areas, should be examined. Any suspicious lesions should be reported to the dermatologist. In addition, the patient should be examined by a dermatologist at regular frequent intervals (e.g., every 3 months).

Keratotic lesions that are indurated or thicker than usual should be subjected to histologic examination to rule out the presence of keratoacanthoma or squamous cell carcinoma. Small pearly papules are often basal cell carcinomas. Hyperpigmented lesions that are large (larger than 6 mm), indurated, irregular in shape or color, notched, or changing in size or sensation should undergo biopsy to rule out melanoma. A 4 to 6 mm punch biopsy specimen can be effective in establishing the diagnosis of a pigmented lesion without subjecting the patient to an unnecessarily extensive procedure. These patients develop so many unusual pigmented lesions that it is not practical to attempt excisional biopsy of every suspicious pigmented lesion.

An extensive set of baseline color photographs can greatly facilitate the identification of changing lesions. A photograph album can be made using standard 3 by 5 inch prints. Multiple close-up views should be taken of the cancer prone, sun exposed areas. Several overviews of larger areas are necessary in order to locate the lesions seen in the close-ups. All lesions suspected of being malignant should undergo histologic examination. Areas that are not suspicious enough to require biopsy but that may be questionable can be circled with a felt tipped marker, photographed, and followed. If lesions are to be followed, it is often helpful to number them to facilitate later identification and to include a metric ruler in the photograph to establish the size so that changes can be identified.

Management

Premalignant lesions such as actinic keratoses are usually treated with standard therapies such as cryotherapy with liquid nitrogen or curettage and electrodesiccation. Extensive areas of keratosis can be treated with a course of topical 5-fluorouracil therapy. Care should be taken to insure that all potentially malignant areas are re-moved before application of 5-fluorouracil. A short course of topical 5-fluorourcil therapy can be partially effective in treating a tumor. If the superficial part undergoes necrosis and is re-epithelialized, deeper residual tumor can remain to grow more extensively downward and laterally along tissue planes.

In some patients with large areas of severely sun-damaged skin, dermabrasion or dermatome shaving has been used to remove the superficial, more damaged epidermal layers. The rationale for this procedure is to allow epidermal replacement with cells arising from the deeper adnexal structures, which have suffered less UV damage. A few patients have undergone replacement of the most damaged areas of skin (face) with grafts taken from covered, less actinically damaged areas.

Skin cancers should be treated without delay using standard techniques such a curettage and desiccation, surgical excision, or cryosurgical ablation, but care should be taken to conserve tissue for future therapy, particularly on the face and eyelids. The early and adequate removal of all tumors is extremely important. Owing to the extensive poikilodermatous changes and scarring in these patients, it is often difficult to identify recurrences, which if persistent can result in extensive tissue destruction. Plastic surgical excision of tumors in some patients has resulted in minimal deformity even after many dozens of procedures. For extensive procedures that require grafting, donor sites should be chosen from sun protected areas, such as the buttocks, which are less likely to develop new skin cancers. Because patients with XP, as their cultured cells, do not react abnormally to X irradiation, standard radiation therapy techniques can be used safely.

For large or recurrent lesions and lesions in locations where there may be a high risk of recurrence (such as the nasolabial fold), Mohs chemosurgery is an effective method for combining tumor removal with tissue sparing. After removal of a layer of tissue, it is divided into sections, each of which is examined by frozen section. Additional tissue can be selectively removed from only those areas with residual tumor. In patients with severe actinic damage, many areas of the epidermis appear abnormal, and on frozen section care must be taken to differentiate this from residual tumor.

Ophthalmologic Manifestations

Clinical Ophthalmology

As in the skin, the UV exposed parts of the eye are also susceptible to actinic damage, degeneration, and subsequent malignant change. The eyelids, periorbital areas, cornea, and conjunctiva are at risk. Most patients with XP have photophobia and some degree of conjunctivitis. With UV exposure these patients develop dryness of the conjunctiva and are susceptible to keratitis. Atrophy of the eyelids can lead to progressive deformity such as ectropion or entropion. In addition, structural deformity and tissue loss resulting from periocular malignant disease may lead to complete loss of the eyelids. Eyelid deformity can exacerbate the conjunctival inflammation and corneal dryness, which can progress from keratitis to corneal ulceration, scarring, and eventual opacification.

The eyelids, conjunctiva, cornea, and sclerae develop benign hyperplastic keratotic, pigmentary, inflammatory, and vascular lesions similar to those that develop in the skin (keratoses, papillomas, hyperpigmented macules and patches, telangectases, and angiomas). These lesions can undergo malignant degeneration.

Prevention

Shielding the UV exposed portions of the eye and periocular skin can reduce acute and chronic ophthalmologic morbidity. Whenever patients with XP are out of doors during daylight hours, they should wear sunglasses or prescription glasses designed to block UV radiation. Such UV blocking sunglasses are currently in vogue and available in most large department stores. Sunglasses should be chosen that are labeled to state that they totally block UV. Glasses with side shields to add further protection are preferable, and these are commercially available in several styles and are cosmetically acceptable.

Several measures can decrease the progression of conjunctivitis and keratitis. Methylcellulose eyedrops, preferably without added chemical vasoconstrictors, should be used frequently. As lid deformity progresses, ophthalmic ointments may be necessary to keep the cornea moist. This is especially important at night in patients with poor occlusion of the lids in whom exposure can easily lead to dryness and keratitis. In patients with severe lid deformity soft contact lenses may be indicated.

Surveillance

Frequent ophthalmologic examination at regular intervals is important to preserve vision in these patients. In addition, any observed new growths or symptoms should be promptly assessed by a physician. Burning or vision abnormalities should alert the patient to the possibility of keratitis or corneal abrasion and protective measures should be taken. Frequent careful examination of the eyelids and periorbital skin in addition to all surfaces of the conjunctiva and cornea is necessary to identify neoplasms promptly.

Management

The importance of lubrication in the therapy of dry eyes has been already discussed in the section on prevention. Conjunctivitis should be evaluated by an ophthalmologist and treated with appropriate antibiotics. For severe keratitis, temporary patching of the affected eye may be necessary. In severe cases in which corneal scarring and opacification have led to blindness, corneal transplantation may restore vision.

Patients with XP tend to develop numerous neoplasms on the eyelids and periorbital skin, which may lead to loss of structural integrity of the lids and eventually may threaten vision. It is therefore important that lesions in this area suspected of being neoplasms be subjected to biopsy and histologic examination as early as possible, when small, in an effort to remove them with minimal tissue loss.

Neurologic Manifestations

Clinical Neurology

About 20 percent of the patients with XP develop progressive neurologic degeneration. This may begin in infancy or may not start to develop until the second decade. In some patients involvement may be limited to diminished or absent deep tendon reflexes, but can include motor abnormalities, sensorineural deafness, or mental retardation. Only a few patients have the most severe neurologic involvement constituting the De Sanctis-Cacchione syndrome, which includes microcephaly, mental deterioration, motor abnormalities, sensorineural deafness, and retardation of growth and sexual development.

Prevention

At the present time it is not known how to prevent the development of neurologic degeneration in XP.

Surveillance

Patients with XP should be examined by a neurologist at an early age, with the frequency of follow-up examination dependent on the presence and degree of neurologic abnormality. Decreased or absent deep tendon reflexes may be an early manifestation. Audiologic assessment, including audiography, is indicated to detect early hearing loss and monitor progression. Early detection of hearing loss and intervention may prevent poor school performance, behavioral problems, or social withdrawal, which can occur with undetected slow hearing loss.

Management

Hearing loss may be improved with a hearing aid. Other neurologic impairments such as motor abnormalities (e.g., spasticity) or seizures are treated as indicated.

XERODERMA PIGMENTOSUM REGISTRY

XP is a very rare disease with severe multisystem involvement, which is also of academic interest in understanding the mechanisms involved in carcinogenesis. Advances in the understanding and treatment of this disease depend on the accumulation of clinical data from many patients. To assist in this goal, a registry of patients has been created. This registry collects clinical information about patients with XP and provides educational materials to physicians. All patients with this disease should be reported by writing to the Xeroderma Pigmentosum Registry, c/o Department of Pathology, Room C520, Medical Science Building, UMDNJ—New Jersey Medical School, 100 Bergen Street, Newark, NJ 07103.

ERYTHROPOIETIC PROTOPORPHYRIA AND PORPHYRIA CUTANEA TARDA

FREDERICK D. MALKINSON, M.D., D.M.D.

ERYTHROPOIETIC PROTOPORPHYRIA

Erythropoietic protoporphyria (EPP) is the most common porphyria of bone marrow origin. It is inherited as an autosomal dominant trait and results from a deficiency of the enzyme heme synthase (ferrochelatase), which converts protoporphyrin to heme by incorporation of the ferrous ion. Red blood cell, plasma, and fecal protoporphyrin levels are substantially increased, providing disease markers for diagnosis. Urine porphyrin and porphyrin precursor levels are normal, and EPP activity is unaffected by environmental factors or medications.

EPP usually appears in childhood but may first develop, or be recognized, in young or older adults. Accumulation of protoporphyrin in plasma and skin causes photosensitization in the light energy range of 380 to 560 nm, inducing the various skin changes that characterize the disease. Photosensitization-induced lesions have been linked principally to the generation of proinflammatory oxygen species by photoexcitation of protoporphyrin molecules. Skin changes occur principally on the nose, cheeks, and dorsa of the hands. The patient's most common complaint is painful burning, often noted within minutes after sunlight exposure. Pruritus, erythema, and edema are frequently associated; petechiae are occasionally seen. Vesicle formation may occur, resulting in shallow, depressed scars. Longer term, chronic sunlight exposure produces characteristic thickening and wrinkling of the skin over the dorsa of the interphalangeal joints and the knuckles. About 10 percent of the patients are found to have protoporphyrin containing gallstones at a relatively young age. Five to 10 percent of the patients develop rapidly progressive, fatal hepatic failure associated with cirrhosis and jaundice. This complication appears to be related to protoporphyrin deposits, which produce persistent cell-damaging toxic and inflammatory changes in the liver parenchyma and bile ducts.

The treatment of choice for the cutaneous photosensitivity manifestations in EPP is the oral administration of beta-carotene (Solatene). Outside the United States a synthetic carotenoid, canthaxanthin, has been admixed with beta-carotene to reduce the resultant skin discoloration. The treatment effects of beta-carotene are probably related to the compound's capacity to quench singlet oxygen, produced by photoexcited protoporphyrin, and to trap free radicals. Beta-carotene has no effect on the basic metabolic disorder in EPP. The compound does not function primarily as a sunscreen and, interestingly, has little effect in most patients with other photosensitive porphyrias. This observation may relate to the fact that, in EPP, protoporphyrin is largely deposited in and around blood vessels and that both beta-carotene and protoporphyrin are hydrophobic compounds. In other forms of porphyria, especially those characterized by uroporphyrin and coproporphyrin deposits in skin, these porphyrins are hydrophilic and are much more diffusely distributed in tissue.

Beta-carotene is usually administered to adults in oral dosages of 60 to 200 mg daily to obtain serum concentrations of 600 to 800 μg per 100 milliliters. In a few individuals daily dosages up to 300 mg may be needed. For children a dosage range of 25 to 150 mg daily is employed, depending on the patient's weight. A treatment period of 1 to 3 months is required to obtain the maximal sunlight tolerance effects produced by beta-carotene. Such tolerance usually increases by a factor of at least 3, but for some patients it may range as hgih as 30-fold. Beta-carotene reduces or eliminates the skin symptoms and lesions of EPP in up to 90 percent of cases. Ancillary measures such as increased use of sun-protective clothing should also be encouraged. Substantially reduced sunlight exposure is not usually feasible, however, and sunscreens provide little protection.

Therapy with beta-carotene may be continued for periods of up to several years. Systemic side effects are nil, and the mild hypertriglyceridemia occasionally seen in patients with EPP has been shown to be unrelated to the medication. However, essentially all patients develop a yellow-orange skin color within 1 month or so after starting treatment. This color change is most pronounced where the stratum corneum is thickest. Although the efficacy of the drug can be demonstrated by altered thresholds for skin reactivity induced by artificial light tests, such test results are variable. Correlative effects are often absent even in individuals responding well to treatment. Finally, in patients given beta-carotene dosages of 300 mg daily to obtain blood levels of 800 μg per 100 milliliters for up to 3 to 4 months and in whom no increased sun tolerance is seen, the treatment should be discontinued.

All patients with EPP should be followed for long periods. Intake of alcoholic beverages should be sharply restricted when indicated. Liver function tests should be monitored at 6- to 12-month intervals because of the potential complication of fatal hepatic failure. The development of abnormal liver function test results usually warrants liver biopsy in these patients, particularly as a baseline finding for the management of possible hepatic disease and failure. Since greatly increased protoporphyrin levels (over 2,000 μg per deciliter for erythrocytes and more than 50 μg per milliliter for plasma) may be seen in accompanying liver disease and particularly in hepatic failure, this determination should also be made.

The uses of other forms of treatment for EPP have met with infrequent or only partial success. A small number of patients have improved following treatment with washed packed red blood cell transfusions or with plasmapheresis and red blood cell exchanges. Increased sunlight tolerance in these cases was correlated with reduced erythrocyte and serum protoporphyrin levels. However, the substantial risks involved in the repeated transfusions of blood products are too great to make this treatment feasible.

The development of abnormal liver function test results or the precipitous onset and rapid progression of hepatic failure to fatality, reported in over 20 cases of EPP, have elicited a variety of treatment approaches. Cholestyramine, a nonabsorbable anionic resin, can be given in doses of 4 g up to several times daily to interrupt the enterohepatic circulation of protoporphyrin, thereby reducing its levels in plasma and in the liver. Its use has yielded some encouraging results in the treatment of early hepatic dysfunction. A similar, newer, perhaps more effective therapy is the administration of activated charcoal, 60 g as a slurry with cold water three times daily, over a period of weeks to months. In patients with hepatic failure, hypertransfusion, or the intravenous administration of hematin, has been aimed at inhibition of the heme synthetic pathway with resultant sharp reductions in protoporphyrin production and, perhaps, mobilization and reduction of protoporphyrin deposits in the liver. Although these different treatment approaches are not well established because of their variable effects and the few cases treated to date, they deserve further trials and evaluation.

Recently effective treatment for one EPP patient with hepatic failure was demonstrated with the use of alternating courses of carbonyl (purified elemental) iron and ferrous sulfate. Carbonyl iron is relatively nontoxic and can be used in far higher doses than standard ferrous sulfate therapy. It was postulated that increased intracellular iron in this patient might have either enhanced her reduced ferrochelatase activity or increased nonenzymatic heme formation, with consequent reductions in protoporphyrin blood and tissue concentrations. A 3-month course of treatment produced marked decreases in free erythrocyte and stool protoporphyrin levels, with the return of liver function to normal. This therapeutic result may well hold promise for other patients with this grave, potentially fatal complication of EPP and should be evaluated in additional cases. Finally, for patients with hepatic failure who are unresponsive to the various treatment approaches described, liver transplantation should be considered.

PORPHYRIA CUTANEA TARDA

Porphyria cutanea tarda (PCT) is the most common form of porphyria in the United States and in Europe. Most cases are of sporadic origin, but some are familial and are inherited as a dominant autosomal trait. PCT is a hepatic form of porphyria and is characterized by a deficiency of the enzyme uroporphyrinogen decarboxylase (UDC), which progressively decarboxylates uroporphyrinogen to coproporphyrinogen. In these patients there is reduced enzyme-substrate affinity, increased enzyme inhibition by ferrous ion, and, perhaps, enhanced enzyme instability. UDC deficiency results in marked elevations of uroporphyrinogen, its successively decarboxylated products (7, 6, 5-carboxylated intermediates), and the 4-carboxyl compound, coproporphyrinogen. Nonenzymatic oxidation of porphyrinogens results in porphyrin com-

pounds that are water soluble and highly photosensitizing, especially at wavelengths of about 400 nm and, less so, in the range of 500 to 650 nm. The UDC enzyme defect is present in the liver in all forms of the disease, but is also found in red blood cells, fibroblasts, and other cell lines in familial PCT (50 percent enzyme activity) and in the rare, severe homozygous variant, hepatoerythropoietic porphyria (HEP; 10 percent enzyme activity). Increased plasma porphyrin levels induce a diagnostic and marked elevation of urine uroporphyrin excretion, with a smaller increase in coproporphyrin, regularly reversing the ratios of these compounds found in normal urine.

PCT usually appears in adults; the onset is rare in children, but it occurs in infancy in HEP. The common skin findings are increased fragility in light-exposed areas in all patients, vesicles and bullae, hypertrichosis, especially on the upper cheeks and temples, hyperpigmentation, periorbital violaceous erythema and conjunctival injection, and, least commonly, localized morphea-like lesions, which may also occur in light protected areas. Milia and atrophic scars are prominent secondary lesions. The diagnosis of PCT is made on the basis of characteristic cutaneous findings and typical porphyrin excretion abnormalities in the urine.

Abnormal liver function test results are found in over half the patients with PCT, and porphyrin deposits may be present in the hepatocytes. Siderosis (hepatic iron overload) and chronic hepatitis or cirrhosis may accompany the disorder. The incidence of diabetes mellitus or an abnormal glucose tolerance test result is significantly increased in PCT. Concomitant lupus erythematosus is a rare finding. Over a dozen patients have been found to have hepatocellular carcinoma at the time of onset of PCT. Also in several series 15 to 40 percent or more of the patients developed hepatocellular carcinoma up to 20 years or more after the onset of PCT symptoms. Male sex, age over 50, and the presence of cirrhosis are all frequently associated factors in patients developing tumors.

The treatment of PCT first involves the elimination of possible environmental and other agents that induce or exacerbate the disease. These may be primary factors in sporadic cases or critical ancillary factors, increasing disease susceptibility in patients with familial UDC deficiency. Ethanol and estrogens are the most common agents that induce or exacerbate PCT. The oral intake of iron supplements has been found in rare patients. Polychlorinated aromatic hydrocarbons (hexachlorobenzene, di- and trichlorophenols) are hepatotoxic and may induce PCT, although the etiologic role of 2, 3, 7, 8-tetrachlorodibenzo-p-dioxin (TCDD) has recently been questioned. Each of these incitants appears to reduce UDC activity. Elimination of these agents alone, together with the avoidance of sunlight, usually results in gradual but substantial clinical and biochemical improvement. Without the addition of active therapy, however, complete remission seldom occurs. Notable exceptions are patients with PCT induced by short-term (less than 1 year) estrogen therapy or, sometimes, by chlorinated hydrocarbon exposure. Nonetheless careful avoidance of inciting factors almost certainly accelerates the response to the major therapeutic alternatives for PCT.

The most widely used treatment technique is phlebotomy. The mechanism of action of this therapy has not been precisely defined. The usual explanation for it is the mobilization and depletion of hepatic iron stores, which depress UDC activity. Removal of a circulatory factor inducing porphyrinogenesis has been suggested but not demonstrated. Phlebotomy is most conveniently carried out in a local blood bank, but can be performed in the office with plastic blood-drawing bags. The procedure employs repeated removals of 500 ml of whole blood every 7 to 14 days until the hemoglobin level is 10 to 11 g per 100 milliliters or the serum iron level is 50 to 60 μg per 100 milliliters. The total blood volume removed usually ranges from 2 to 16 liters. Clinical remission times vary widely, but on the average remission occurs within 6 months after the initiation of treatment. This is generally seen when urine uroporphyrin excretion rates fall below 1,000 μg per 24 hours. The urine porphyrin levels then continue to fall progressively long after the phlebotomies have been stopped. Nearly normal 24-hour urine uroporphyrin levels (100 μg per 24 hours or less) or normal urine total porphyrin levels (about 400 μg per 24 hours) are found in several months to 1 year. By this time, aberrant liver function test results are also often normal.

The first skin changes to disappear are blister formation, followed by skin fragility. Hypertrichosis and hyperpigmentation resolve over a period of several months to 1 year or more. The localized sclerodermatous lesions are the slowest to disappear and may persist for 1 to 2 years or longer.

Side effects of phlebotomy therapy in otherwise healthy patients are almost nil. Weakness or fatigue occurs occasionally. Clinical remission times are variable, lasting many months to years, but averaging 2½ to 3 years. Exacerbations are preceded by progressive rises in urine porphyrin excretion and may be hastened by re-exposure to ethanol, estrogens, or other inciting factors. Retreatment when the 24-hour urine uroporphyrin level rises to 500 to 600 μg per 24 hours prevents the reappearance of clinical lesions. The response to a second course (or repeated courses) of treatment is usually as complete as that to the initial therapeutic experience.

For some patients phlebotomy is contraindicated because of anemia, cardiac disorders, pulmonary disease, or rarely, poor venous access. In these patients and in those averse to the idea of phlebotomy therapy, the use of chloroquine or hydroxychloroquine therapy should be undertaken. Hydroxychloroquine is the drug of choice, since side effects, especially retinopathy, are almost certainly less frequent with this drug. The mechanism of action of these 4-aminoquinolines is apparently related to the drugs' high avidity for water soluble complex formation with porphyrin molecules. This complex mobilizes large amounts of porphyrins from the liver, which are excreted in the urine. There is also evidence that chloroquine and hydroxyloroquine increase urinary excretion of iron, but whether hepatic iron stores are significantly depleted by long-term administration of these drugs has not been demonstrated. The mechanism for the prolonged disease remission that

may follow treatment with one of these antimalarial compounds is unknown.

For other disorders the recommended dosages of hydroxychloroquine are 200 to 400 mg daily and for chloroquine, 250 mg daily. However, in PCT these customary dosage levels are often hepatotoxic and may induce central lobular necrosis. Toxicity is associated with abdominal pain, fever, nausea, and vomiting. These symptoms apparently result from high hepatocyte levels of the antimalarial compound or of the antimalarial-porphyrin complex. However, initial low dose drug therapy, followed by gradually increasing doses to speed treatment results, is effective, and the larger dose induced side effects are almost invariably absent.

For hydroxychloroquine this author suggests the following treatment course. Hydroxychloroquine, 100 mg every other day or three times weekly, is given for the first month. The dosage is increased to 200 mg every other day, or three times weekly, for the second month, following which 200 mg can be given daily. If clinical or biochemical responses are slow, the hydroxychloroquine dosage can be raised to 300 to 400 mg daily, 5 to 6 months after initiating treatment. Complete clinical and biochemical remission times are comparable to those seen with phlebotomy, ranging from 5 to 13 months (average, 9 to 12 months). Relapse incidences are also similar to those seen following phlebotomy, with up to 50 percent or more of the patients requiring retreatment in about 3 years. Some patients may be disease free for 6 to 7 years or longer, however. In about 15 patients treated once or repeatedly with hydroxychloroquine, we have seen excellent treatment results with no instance of hepatotoxic symptoms or retinopathy. Others have used lower dosages, giving hydroxychloroquine at a dosage of 200 mg two to three times weekly throughout the course of therapy.

If chloroquine is administered, an initial dosage schedule of 125 to 250 mg two to three times weekly can be used. This dosage is usually maintained throughout the treatment course, but can be carefully raised after 2 to 3 months, not to exceed dosages of 250 mg daily or every other day. Remission times and durations are comparable to those seen with hydroxychloroquine. Although combined therapy with phlebotomy and chloroquine has been used to accelerate treatment results, there appears to be no great advantage to increasing the complexity of therapy.

When 4-aminoquinoline treatment is used, a baseline complete blood count, urinalysis, serum hepatic transaminase level, and ophthalmologic examination should be done. Patients can be clinically reassessed every 2 to 2½ months; total 24-hour urine porphyrin levels should be obtained along with repeat blood tests. Ophthalmologic examination should be carried out every 6 months. Treatment is continued until the urine uroporphyrin level falls to 100 μg per 24 hours. Thereafter the 24 hour urine porphyrin level should be reexamined at 6 to 12 month intervals. Elevations of uroporphyrin levels above 600 μg per 24 hours presage clinical relapse and treatment should be reinstituted.

Side effects of antimalarial treatment are rare at the

dosages recommended. The incidence of retinopathy should be essentially nil, especially with hydroxychloroquine, if the foregoing dosage ranges are carefully observed. In children, antimalarial therapy should be avoided or undertaken very cautiously at extremely low dosage levels.

THERMAL INJURY

ANDREW M. MUNSTER, M.D., F.R.C.S.
(Eng., Edin), F.A.C.S.

Thermal injury occurs as a result of an energy transfer from a heat source to the body. The peripheral circulation, surface pigmentation, the presence or absence of other insulating material, such as hairs, natural skin oil, or cornified layers of surface epithelium, and the total water content of the tissues are other factors of major influence in thermal injuries. Partial thickness (second degree) burns are characteristically caused by a flash, scalding and brief exposure to flame. Full thickness (third degree) burns are the result of exposure to flame for more than very brief periods of time, immersion scalds, chemicals, direct contact, or electricity; they can be caused by less significant thermal transfers in the very elderly or the very young in whom the thickness of tissue is less than that of persons in the prime of life.

CLASSIFICATION

Major burns include second degree burns of over 20 percent of the total body surface (15 percent in children); burns of the face, hands, perineum, or feet; electrical and chemical burns; burns complicated by respiratory tract damage, fractures, or extensive soft tissue injuries; and burns in patients with pre-existing disease such as diabetes, congestive heart failure, or chronic renal dysfunction who have decreased ability to resist infection, and in whom management of fluid shifts may be a major problem despite relatively smaller burns. Patients with major burns should be referred to burn centers.

Moderate burns include second degree burns of 15 to 20 percent of the total body surface in adults and third degree burns of less than 10 percent of the total body surface. Such patients may be treated at community hospitals.

Minor burns include second degree burns of less than 15 percent of the total body surface and third degree burns of less than 2 percent of the total body surface. Such patients may be treated as outpatients if social circumstances allow.

INITIAL TREATMENT

First, a good airway must be secured and associated injuries checked for. The burn wound is carefully inspected and palpated, and areas of second and third degree burns are charted. Pain often accompanied by anxiety and fear, should be treated with analgesics, preferably by the intravenous route. Sterile gloves, a gown, a mask, and a cap should be worn. After the wound has been washed, loose necrotic epithelium is cut away. Large blisters are broken and thoroughly debrided; if intact and small, they may be protected with a sterile dressing that is bulky enough to absorb the fluid contents should the blister break prior to the next change of dressing. Tetanus prophylaxis should be administered as appropriate.

RESUSCITATION

The key alteration leading to the need for fluid resuscitation is increased capillary permeability resulting in loss of colloid, water, and electrolytes, not only into the burn wound but elsewhere into the tissues as well. This leads to the "third spacing" of a large amount of volume, which cannot be reversed by any method of resuscitation until the capillary wall has healed well enough to retain colloid once again, enabling the plasma osmotic pressure to begin returning toward normal, a process usually complete by 2 to 4 days after the burn. The objective of fluid resuscitation is to maintain normal cardiovascular parameters while the healing process takes place, without fluid overloading.

Formulas are only a guideline. The final rate and method of administration must be individualized for each patient.

Patients with burns of less than 15 percent of the total body surface in adults, and 10 percent in children, usually can be resuscitated by the oral administration of fluids. Patients with burns larger than that usually require intravenous resuscitation and the placement of a Foley catheter to measure hourly urine output. We recommend the Parkland formula, which uses Ringer's lactate solution:

First 24 hours = 4 ml × weight of patient in kg × percentage of burn:

Example: a 70 kg man with a 55 percent burn: 4 ml × 70 kg × 55 percent = 15,400 ml in the first 24 hours, or ½ of 15,400 = 7,700 cc given in the first 8 hours; ½ of 15,400 = 7,700 cc in the next 16 hours.

Requirement for second 24 hours: colloid 0.5 ml per kg per percent + D5W 2,000 + ½ of first day's Ringer's lactate.

Successful resuscitation is signaled by:

1. Maintenance of normal sensorium.
2. Adequate urine output: 30 to 50 ml per hour in adults, 1 ml per kg per hour in children younger than 3 years of age, and 15 to 25 ml per hour in children older than 3 years.
3. Normal blood pressure.
4. Good skin turgor.
5. Normal central venous pressure.

Fluid orders should be revised hourly for the first 8 hours after admission and no less frequently than every 4 hours for the remainder of the first 24 hours.

MANAGEMENT OF THE WOUND

The object of topical antibacterial therapy is to reduce the possibility of colonization and invasion of the burn wound by pathogenic bacteria. The most popular topical therapy is currently silver sulfadiazine, 1 percent aqueous cream, applied to the wound twice daily and protected with light dressings. The characteristics of the other topically applied drugs are summarized in Table 1.

DRESSING CHANGES

Most topical therapy requires changing dressings and reapplication twice daily. As much of the previous application as possible should be gently cleaned off prior to application of the fresh cream. The following is a list of standard dressing techniques:

1. Regular dressings over topical creams. Light wrap with one layer of gauze bandage (Kling, Kerlix), leaving maximal mobility while protecting the burned limb.
2. Wetted down dressings. These are suitable for the application of silver nitrate, especially if the patient is allergic to sulfonamides. The dressing is changed daily —an inner layer (Adaptic, Veriflo) followed by a burn dressing (16 ply, coarse mesh gauze) held in place by Kerlix, wetted down every 4 hours.
3. Wet to wet dressings. These dressings are suitable for areas requiring moderate nonsurgical debridement and cause least pain to the patient. The inner layer is fine mesh gauze. The next layer of burn dressing is held in place by Kerlix bandages. The entire dressing is wetted down with a solution containing bacitracin and polymyxin; the dressing is changed every 8 to 12 hours.
4. Wet to dry dressing. The inner layer is coarse mesh gauze (4 by 4's) held in place by Kerlix. The bandage is wetted down initially with a solution of bacitracin and polymyxin, allowed to dry, and removed every 8 hours. This technique is painful and may cause some bleeding, but it is extremely effective in debriding

residual dermal debris because the eschar adheres to the dressing. These patients should be medicated prior to dressing changes.

SURGICAL APPROACH TO THE WOUND

Early surgical excision of the burn wound is gaining in popularity. According to proponents, the eschar should not be allowed to go on to natural separation, a process taking 3 to 4 weeks and then followed by dressing, biologic dressings, and finally autografting. Rather, early excision and wound closure should be performed. The patient is taken to the operating room within the first 5 to 7 days after admission, the eschar is excised by surgical means, and immediate closure of the wound with cutaneous autografts is carried out. If donor sites are inadequate, allograft coverage may be used. The advantages of this technique include early wound closure, early mobilization, reduced time of hospitalization, and in very large burns a chance of forestalling inevitable colonization, invasion, and septic death.

The disadvantages include the exposure of an ill and unstable patient to a major surgical procedure with its accompanying hazards of major blood loss and anesthesia, the risk of technical failure, and the creation of new donor areas, which are a potential source of sepsis, should the operation fail.

It is our present practice to immediately excise deep second degree burns in areas of important function such as the back of the hand, small (less than 10 percent) third degree burns, moderate size (less than 20 percent) third degree burns in elderly people who do not do well when

TABLE 1 Commonly Used Topical Drugs

Name	Advantage	Side Effects	Dressing Orders
Silver sulfadiazine (Silvadene)	Broad antibacterial action, painless, washable	Only fair penetration of eschar; chance of sulfonamide sensitivity (rash); absorption into fetal circulation unknown and thus is contraindicated in pregnancy; occasional leukopenia (reversible upon discontinuation)	Apply twice daily; cover with light layer of Kling or Kerlix bandage on extremities; leave face and chest open
Mafenide (Sulfamylon)	Excellent antibacterial action, particularly against gram-positive organisms and clostridia, and also gram-negative organisms; rapid eschar penetration	Painful; sulfonamide sensitivity (rash); carbonic anhydrase inhibition leading to an acid load, which has to be compensated for by lungs and kidneys	Leave face, chest, and abdomen open; one light layer of gauze, dressings elsewhere; apply twice daily
Aqueous silver nitrate solution	Universal antibacterial action	Poor penetration of eschar; leeching of chloride into dressings with potential hypochloremic alkalosis; marked staining of tissues, equipment, linens, and floor	All areas to be dressed with thick layer of burn dressings and gauze bandage; wet down with silver nitrate solution every 4 hours; change dressings daily
Iodophors (e.g., Efodyne)	Universal antibacterial action	Poor penetration of eschar; marked staining of tissues; iodine absorption	Apply twice daily and dress with light layer of gauze dressing
Topical bacitracin cream	Transparent, cosmetically acceptable, easy to apply	Limited antibacterial action; poor eschar penetration; rapid development of resistance; conjunctivitis develops if in touch with conjunctiva	Should be applied only to small areas of cosmetic importance, e.g., second degree burns of face; leave open; apply twice daily

placed in bed for a period of several weeks, and very large burns when nonoperative therapy would lead to certain septic death.

Without question, the results of excisional therapy in small and moderate size burns are excellent. There is also accumulating evidence that the mortality in very large burns can be reduced by this technique.

Care of the Donor Site

Care of the donor site is directed at the prevention of infection, and the best way to achieve this is to prevent maceration and moisture. Donor sites are usually covered with fine mesh gauze or a biologic dressing and kept dry.

Most commonly the donor site is covered with fine or coarse mesh gauze, either unimpregnated or impregnated with a topically applied antiseptic such as scarlet red, after which it must be kept exposed and dry with the help of heat lamps. After 7 to 10 days the fine mesh gauze peels off and the donor area will be healed.

SPECIAL CARE FOR SPECIAL AREAS

Face

Superficial burns of the face are often best left exposed without topical therapy. The lips should be treated with bacitracin to prevent cracking. For deeper burns topical chemotherapy with silver sulfadiazine is advised.

Ears

Deep second degree burns of the ears must be protected from excessive pressure, which potentially leads to chondritis. This is accomplished by using topical chemotherapy and a fluffy type of occlusive dressing while avoiding the use of a pillow for sleep until the burn is healed.

Eyes

Fluorescein staining should be performed for a suspected corneal burn and the eye treated with Neosporin (ophthalmic). All patients with suspected eye injuries are referred to an ophthalmologist within 24 hours.

Hands

Burned hands should be elevated for the first 48 to 72 hours to minimize swelling. A bulky dressing or a splint may be necessary to maintain the hands in the position of function. Exercises to preserve mobility should begin as soon as they can be tolerated.

Lower Extremities

The feet and lower extremities should be elevated for the initial 48 to 72 hours or until the major swelling sub-

sides. An early balance must be obtained between rest and elevation of the part and exercise and weight bearing. Elastic support should be continued for up to 2 to 3 months after wound closure.

Subsequent Care

The resulting healed dry wound may benefit from a mild cream, such as lanolin or Eucerin, applied twice daily.

AFTER-CARE OF HEALED BURNS

Pruritus is a common complaint and, when severe, is difficult to treat. Benadryl, 25 mg three times daily, may be of some help. Hypertrophic scarring occurs rarely in small burns, but may follow spontaneous healing of deep partial thickness injuries; this is a continuing process as long as the scar is biologically active. These scars can be minimized during their development by using a pressure stocking or sleeve (Jobst garments).

NUTRITIONAL SUPPORT

Aggressive management of the nutritional needs of patients with major burns is an essential cornerstone of clinical care. Without adequate nutritional support, the burn wound will not heal and host defenses against invasive sepsis are compromised.

On admission the caloric requirement is calculated. (Curreri formula: calories per day = 25 × kg body weight + 40 × percent burn.) In a patient with burns not exceeding 20 percent if healing is expected soon, the oral intake may approach the required calories. Daily weight measurement is imperative in monitoring the patient's progress. In a patient with large burns, nutritional support must be initiated as soon as the period of paralytic ileus is over and the gastrointestinal tract is capable of resuming normal function.

If the combination of oral and enteral feedings does not meet the caloric requirements for prolonged periods of time or because of gastrointestinal complications, or if the patient is unable to tolerate enteral feedings, intravenous hyperalimentation may be necessary.

Vitamins and minerals are usually included in the commercially available enteral formulas. If the patient is unable to tolerate enteral feeding, he should receive these supplements intravenously.

INHALATION INJURIES

Inhalation injuries include the inhalation of superheated air with injury to the respiratory tract usually sustained in a closed spaced fire, and the inhalation of noxious products of incomplete combustion, particularly of nylon and polyvinyl products. Also included is the inhalation of carbon monoxide and accompanying cyanides and cyanates. Hot steam inhalation also can lead to thermal damage of the lower respiratory tract.

Carbon monoxide inhalation occurs most frequently in house fires and should be suspected in any individual who has been involved in a fire and is unconscious, with no other demonstrable cause. Blood carboxyhemoglobin levels should be determined immediately and endotracheal intubation instituted with the administration of 100 percent oxygen.

Upper airway injury is the most immediately dangerous and insidious respiratory complication in patients with smoke inhalation, and laryngeal edema is its most feared component. Progressive hoarseness is a danger signal of the imminent onset of upper airway obstruction. Admission blood gas levels and chest x-ray findings are usually normal. In the patient with an appropriate history and facial burns, increasing hoarseness is an indication for immediate endotracheal intubation and the administration of humidified oxygen via the endotracheal tube.

CURLING'S ULCER

The incidence of Curling's ulcer, once a common and feared complication of major burns, has diminished markedly over recent years owing to the routine institution of antacid therapy and enteral feedings.

Major complications such as hemorrhage have been described as early as 12 hours following a major burn. Because of the diminished inflammatory response in the burn patient, perforation of a Curling's ulcer is commonly accompanied by a paucity of clinical signs compared with those of a perforation in an otherwise healthy individual. It is our practice to administer Maalox, 30 cc every 2 hours, through the nasogastric tube even during the initial period of paralytic ileus. If the patient is unable to tolerate enteral feedings, we administer ranitidine in doses of 50 mg given intravenously every 6 hours. With an appropriate combination of antacid therapy, the incidence of Curling's ulcer should be less than 1 percent in the burn patient population.

SEPTIC THROMBOPHLEBITIS

Septic thrombophlebitis is a life-threatening complication in the burn patient. Although it is usually seen in a vein that has been cannulated with a plastic cannula for several days, we have seen it in a vein cannulated with a steel butterfly needle for only 2 hours. The onset may be delayed as long as 10 to 12 days after removal of the intravenous cannula.

If there is pus exuding from an intravenous puncture site or there is fever of unknown origin, the diagnosis should be confirmed by biopsy of the suspicious vein under local anesthesia. A portion of the vein should be sent for pathologic examination and a portion for microbiologic culture. Once the diagnosis is confirmed, extensive excision of the vein and its tributaries under general anesthesia in the operating room is mandatory. Appropriate antibiotic therapy must be instituted preoperatively.

REHABILITATION

Psychosocial support, early attention to mobilization by trained physical and occupational therapists, and long-term follow-up by experienced members of the burn team are mandatory to accomplish the return of the patient with a major burn to a useful productive existence.

FUNGAL INFECTIONS

DERMATOPHYTE INFECTIONS

EVAN R. FARMER, M.D.

ESTABLISHING THE DIAGNOSIS

Dermatophytes are superficial fungi that infect the stratum corneum of the skin, hair shaft, or nail. They normally do not invade the viable tissue of the epidermis but still can elicit an inflammatory response, depending upon the immune competence of the host and prior exposure to the organism. The presence of a dermatophyte infection should always be suspected when scaling is a component of the lesion or when there is hair loss or nail dystrophy. The diagnosis of a dermatophyte infection should always be established prior to initiation of therapy by either direct visualization of the fungus on a potassium hydroxide wet mount or culture.

Since the fungus lives in keratin, scales, hair, or nail clippings can be placed on a glass slide with a drop of 20 percent potassium hydroxide in water, a coverslip applied, and the slide gently warmed with a flame and then examined for hyphae or spores. The addition of dimethyl sulfoxide or dyes to the potassium hydroxide solution may facilitate identification of the organism, but I do not find these additives a significant help. Similarly scale, hair, or nail may be placed on Sabouraud's medium or Dermatophyte Test Medium and incubated at room temperature. The culture should be examined weekly for growth of the fungus; identification is made on the basis of the morphology of the colony. If no growth has occurred by 6 weeks, the culture can be considered negative. Currently the most common dermatophyte cultured is *Trichophyton rubrum*, accounting for approximately 75 percent of the isolates.

The presence of a dermatophyte infection should always be considered in patients who present with erysipelas or lymphangitis of the lower extremities, especially those who have recurrent episodes. Since the bacterial infection can mask the dermatophyte infection, the patient should be reevaluated once the bacterial infection has resolved if the dermatophyte infection could not be documented on the initial presentation.

SITES OF INVOLVEMENT

Dermatophyte infections are named according to the anatomic site involved, generally irrespective of the specific fungus with only a few exceptions. For example, tinea capitis is an infection of scalp hair that may be due to either *Trichophyton tonsurans* or *Microsporum canis*. Tinea pedis, an infection of the feet, may be due to *Trichophyton rubrum*, *Trichophyton mentagrophytes* or *Epidermophyton floccosum*. Conversely, tinea imbricata is an unusual dermatophyte infection in the United States caused by *Trichophyton concentricum* and generally is seen in patients who have traveled for a prolonged period in the Far East or South America or who are immigrants to this country. This disorder is named for the imbricate or concentric pattern on the skin. (See Table 1 for designation of the sites and common dermatophytes.)

Tinea versicolor is a common disorder, of worldwide distribution, usually affecting large areas of the trunk and extremities and occasionally the hair follicles. The disease is caused by *Malassezia furfur* and is characterized by distinctive hypopigmented (rarely hyperpigmented) scaling macules that become confluent over large areas. The organism is somewhat difficult to culture but is easily demonstrated by a potassium hydroxide wet mount.

EVALUATING THE PATIENT

Once the diagnosis is established, the patient should be evaluated for predisposing factors such as atopy (asthma, hay fever, atopic dermatitis), diabetes mellitus, or immune deficiency. Patients with atopy tend to have chronic dermatophyte infections and tend to be infected with *Trichophyton rubrum*. The infection is difficult to eradicate, and it is difficult to prevent recurrences. Presumably these patients have an immune defect that permits dermatophyte infections to persist, although they are able to handle most other infections. Patients with diabetes mellitus, particularly when the blood sugar level is not under control, tend to have dermatophyte infections, especially in the groin region. Infection in this area may coexist with *Candida* and *Corynebacterium* infections of the skin. Immune deficiency may be primary, or as a result of an underlying disease, such as cancer, connective tissue disease, or genetic disease, or it may result from the

TABLE 1 Dermatophyte Infections

Site	Designation	Dermatophyte
Scalp	Tinea capitis	*Trichophyton tonsurans* *Microsporum canis**
Body	Tinea corporis	*Trichophyton rubrum* *Trichophyton verrucosum**
Body	Tinea versicolor	*Malassezia furfur*
Groin	Tinea cruris	*Trichophyton mentagrophytes* *Trichophyton rubrum* *Epidermophyton floccosum*
Feet	Tinea pedis	*Trichophyton mentagrophytes* *Trichophyton rubrum* *Epidermophyton floccosum*
Face	Tinea facei	*Trichophyton rubrum*
Beard	Tinea barbae	*Trichophyton rubrum* *Trichophyton mentagrophytes* *Trichophyton verrucosum** *Microsporum canis**
Nails	Tinea unguium	*Trichophyton rubrum* *Trichophyton mentagrophytes*
Follicles	Majocchi's granuloma	*Trichophyton rubrum*
Follicles	*Malassezia* folliculitis	*Malassezia furfur*

* Transmitted from animals.

administration of immunosuppressive drugs. Detection and treatment of an underlying immune deficiency disease and minimizing iatrogenic immunosuppression help in the management of the dermatophyte infection.

COINFECTION

As mentioned, dermatophyte infections may coexist with other fungal infections, especially in the diabetic or immunocompromised patient. Bacterial infections also may compound dermatophyte infections, particularly in the toe webs or skin folds. These infections may be due to either gram-positive or gram-negative micro-organisms and should be suspected whenever there is maceration or lesions are malodorous. Gram staining of the debris and culturing may be helpful in identifying these bacteria.

Corynebacterium infection may coexist in the groin and occasionally on the feet and can be detected by the presence of a coral-red fluoresence on examination with Wood's light. The patients tend to respond much more quickly to therapy for dermatophyte infection if these secondary infections are also treated.

THERAPY

The goals of therapy are to eradicate the fungus with a specific antifungal drug, to minimize the inflammatory response to the fungus when appropriate, to prevent recurrent disease, and to prevent transmission of the fungus.

Topical Therapy

Antifungal drugs in current use can be divided into those that are applied topically for localized disease and those that are given systemically for widespread, resistant, or adnexal (hair, nail) disease. The drugs that are

most effective topically belong to the imidazole group and include 1 percent clotrimazole (Lotrimin, Mycelex), 2 percent miconazole (Monistat), and 1 percent econazole (Spectazole). These drugs are available in cream, solution, and lotion forms. One percent ciclopirox (Loprox) and 1 percent haloprogin (Halotex) are other effective drugs. Tolnaftate (Tinactin) and Desenex are over the counter drugs that are useful for mild disease but are much less effective than the prescription drugs in my experience. I generally use the cream preparation for most patients with localized disease and the solution preparation on hair-bearing skin, especially on the pubic region or genitalia. I have not found the powder formulations to be particularly helpful.

I recommend that the patient apply the cream twice daily to the affected area, rubbing it in well because these are vanishing creams. The skin does not have to be hydrated as when using a corticosteroid topically because the depth of penetration of the drug is not so critical. If there is maceration, I recommend comfortable temperature, tap water soaks using a small basin, linen, or terry cloth for 5 to 15 minutes before application of the cream. If there is maceration, I evaluate for *Candida* or bacterial infection and treat it at the same time. *Candida* infection of the skin usually responds to one of the imidazole drugs, but if the infection is in the groin or perineal region, I also prescribe a 7 to 10 day course of nystatin, 500,000 units orally four times daily. Nystatin vaginal suppositories (one twice daily) are also useful in women with dual *Candida* infections. For bacterial infection I usually take a culture and initiate therapy with enteric coated erythromycin, 500 mg twice daily for 10 days, and alter the drug, depending on the response, using cultures as a guide.

Dermatophyte infections usually respond quickly to

this therapy, with clinical cures in 2 to 3 weeks and negative cultures in 4 to 6 weeks. Therefore, I usually expect to treat the patient for about 6 weeks with reevaluation at 3 weeks and again about 6 weeks if there is clinical activity at 3 weeks. If there is little or no response to this topical approach, I reevaluate for the presence of the fungus by potassium hydroxide examination and culture, evaluate for the presence of an associated bacterial infection, reevaluate for immune deficiency, consider alternative diagnoses, and review the patient's understanding and actual application of the drug.

For very inflammatory infections with significant pruritus, I add triamcinolone cream, 0.1 percent twice daily, for the first 7 days to be used concomitantly with topical application of the antifungal drug. Alternatively I may begin with Lotrisone cream (betamethasone dipropionate plus clotrimazole) for the first week and then switch to clotrimazole alone.

Systemic Therapy

Currently there are two systemically administered drugs—griseofulvin and ketoconazole—for use in the United States for dermatophyte infections, but other drugs are under investigation and show promise. Systemic therapy is indicated for the following situations: failure of topical therapy, widespread disease when topical therapy is impractical, infection of hair and hair follicles on either the scalp or the body as a folliculitis, and infection of the nails. (See the chapter on *nail disorders* for the therapy of onychomycosis, tinea unguium.)

Griseofulvin is available in several different preparations, but I usually use the microsize tablets, 500 mg twice daily, for an average sized adult and adjust the dose downward for a smaller individual or child. Griseofulvin suspension is also available for children. In my experience the most common side effects of griseofulvin are headaches and gastrointestinal upset. These usually resolve in spite of continued therapy if the patient can tolerate the discomfort. Less frequent but potentially serious side effects include allergic reactions, photosensitivity, exacerbation of lupus erythematosus, and alteration of warfarin metabolism. The safety of griseofulvin in pregnancy has not been demonstrated.

Griseofulvin resistant dermatophytes are a problem and should be suspected if there is no clinical response within 1 month. An alternative explanation for the lack of response may be poor absorption of the drug or noncompliance. If resistance is most likely, I consider using ketoconazole at this point. Griseofulvin should be taken with food, and I usually recommend it with milk. Complete eradication of dermatophyte infections may take much longer than 1 month, especially if there is adnexal involvement; treatment should continue until there is a clinical cure, usually for several months. Confirmation of eradication of the infection can be made by a negative potassium hydroxide examination or culture.

Ketoconazole is the other currently available drug and in contradistinction to griseofulvin is effective against a wide variety of fungi in addition to dermatophytes. It is usually given in a single daily dose of 200 to 400 mg and generally is well tolerated. It is useful in mixed fungal infections with dermatophytes and *Candida*. It is also effective in tinea versicolor.

At present, when systemic therapy is indicated, I begin with griseofulvin, except for widespread tinea versicolor, and reserve ketoconazole for griseofulvin treatment failures. Ketoconazole, although generally well tolerated, may induce nondose-related hepatitis in 1 in 10,000 to 15,000 patients; transient elevation of liver function test results occurs more frequently, requiring careful laboratory monitoring. If these abnormalities are more than minor or are persistent, the drug should be discontinued immediately and the patient carefully monitored until the test results return to normal. If the test results do not normalize quickly or levels continue to rise after discontinuing the drug, consultation with a liver specialist may be indicated. Females and patients over 50 years of age seem to be most at risk for the complication of hepatitis. Liver function tests should be carried out prior to therapy and frequently for the duration of therapy. I usually carry out liver function tests every 2 weeks for the first 3 months and then monthly. The median time for the development of hepatitis is day 28 after the initiation of therapy. Ketoconazole also alters testosterone metabolism and may cause gynecomastia. The absorption of ketoconazole may be decreased when it is given in conjunction with cimetidine. Allergic reactions to ketoconazole have been reported, including a lichenoid eruption of the oral mucosa. Its safety in pregnancy has not been established. On the positive side, there seems to be minimal dermatophyte resistance to ketoconazole to date, and it may be more effective than griseofulvin in the treatment of tinea unguium and peristent *Trichophyton rubrum* infections.

TINEA VERSICOLOR

Tinea versicolor differs from tinea corporis in that in spite of widespread involvement, it usually responds well to topical therapy. My first choice is selenium sulfide lotion, 2.5 percent (Selsun), applied daily for 10 minutes and thoroughly washed off. Selenium sulfide can cause an irritant dermatitis if not completely removed. Applications should continue for 1 week with a second course in 1 month. Alternative regimens include clotrimazole cream, 1 percent twice daily for 7 days or 50 percent propylene glycol in water twice daily for 14 days. For patients who have extensive or recurrent tinea versicolor I now use a short course of ketoconazole, 200 mg daily for 7 to 14 days. Ketoconazole is also more effective than the topical approach for *Malassezia furfur* folliculitis.

IMMUNE REACTIONS

Two types of immune reactions are associated with dermatophyte infections—kerion and id reactions. A kerion is an acute pustular reaction forming an abscess-like lesion on the scalp in tinea capitis or in the beard in tinea barbae. The lesion is believed to be an immune reaction to dermatophyte antigen and not simply a rupture of the fungus into the dermis with a subsequent foreign-body response. A kerion responds best to a three-fold approach.

First, the fungus should be treated with either griseofulvin or ketoconazole because it usually does not respond to topical therapy. Second, these lesions tend to become secondarily infected with bacteria, and systemic antibiotic therapy, as with enteric coated erythromycin, 500 mg twice daily, or dicloxacillin, 500 mg twice daily, for 7 to 10 days is helpful. Third, I use a short course of prednisone, 0.5 to 1.0 mg per kg per day tapering to zero over 2 to 3 weeks. I continue the griseofulvin or ketoconazole for 2 to 3 months or until resolution of the dermatophyte infection occurs.

Most id reactions are manifested by a pruritic papulovesicular eruption, predominantly on the hands and feet, but it may become widespread. Id reactions occur most frequently in patients with inflammatory tinea pedis. Many patients have only toe web infections, and the id reaction involves the palms and soles. It is the id reaction that brings most of these patients to the physician. The id reaction by definition is an immune response and is potassium hydroxide and culture negative for dermatophytes. Once the dermatophyte infection has cleared, the id reaction spontaneously resolves. However, since eradication of the dermatophyte may take several weeks, I treat the id reaction with topical corticosteroid therapy, such as triamcinolone cream, 0.1 percent, or fluocinonide cream, 0.05 percent (Lidex), four times a day. The corticosteroid is applied following hydration of the affected area by soaking or compressing with cool tap water. An antihistamine at bedtime, such as hydroxyzine, 25 to 50 mg, or diphenhydramine, 25 to 50 mg, is helpful for the first 2 to 3 days. For severe id reactions a short course of prednisone, 0.5 to 1.0 mg per kg per day tapering to zero over 2 to 3 weeks, is indicated.

PREVENTION

Once a dermatophyte infection has been cleared, especially in patients with chronic widespread infection, prevention of a relapse or reinfection is desirable. In my experience the topical use of an antifungal drug, although probably effective, is not practical, and patients discontinue its use after a short time.

Recently I have been using 400 mg of ketoconazole in a single dose every 2 weeks, and it has been effective without side effects so far. I monitor liver function test results every 6 months. I have had no experience with griseofulvin used in a similar manner.

Since most dermatophyte infections occur in the groin region or feet, I recommend cotton underclothing and socks as well as a drying powder, such as Johnson's Baby Powder or Zeosorb, to decrease the moisture needed to promote fungal growth. Bathing and thorough drying after swimming or other sports activities are also helpful.

Spread of a dermatophyte infection to another family member normally is not a problem except in the case of tinea capitis. An individual's susceptibility to the organism seems to be the predominant factor. However, with tinea capitis the spores may be spread to other children, and thorough daily shampooing of the hair minimizes the number of loose spores. I also recommend restricting the use of combs, brushes, and towels to the patient alone. Notification of the local public health agency and the school nurse is also helpful in controlling spread.

Because some fungi are acquired from animals, especially dogs and cats (e.g., *Microsporum canis*), pets should be inspected and treated by a veterinarian.

CANDIDIASIS

JAMES G. MARKS Jr., M.D.

Candidiasis is a fungal infection of the skin, the mucous membranes, or the viscera caused by *Candida albicans* or another *Candida* species. This yeast microorganism is a normal inhabitant of moist skin, mucous membranes of the mouth and vagina, and the gastrointestinal tract. It becomes pathogenic when environmental conditions allow transformation from the yeast form to the filamentous form, resulting in an inflammatory response. Factors that predispose to the development of candidiasis include moisture, occlusion, pregnancy, diabetes mellitus, immunosuppression, and medications such as birth control pills and systemic antibiotic therapy. The diagnosis can be confirmed with a potassium hydroxide preparation that demonstrates yeast and filamentous hyphae.

Therapy for candidiasis should be focused on reducing nonspecific predisposing factors such as moisture and occlusion as well as prescribing specific antifungal drugs. The polyene (nystatin, amphotericin B) and imidozole (clotrimazole, econazole, miconazole, ketoconazole) antifungal drugs work by interfering with the functioning of the candidal cell membrane. The polyene antibiotics bind to ergosterol in the membrane, causing leakage of essential cellular constituents. The imidazoles work similarly, but in this case by inhibiting ergosterol synthesis. The imidazoles also disrupt liposomes and block cytochrome C peroxidase activity, which is toxic to fungal organisms.

INTERTRIGINOUS AND DIAPER CANDIDIASIS

The physical appearance of candidiasis is similar in both adults and infants when it involves the intertriginous areas of the perineum, axilla, breast, or under a diaper. The infected skin has a central beefy red, scaling patch that is characteristically surrounded by satellite pustules and papules.

The treatment is first aimed at reducing local conditions, particularly moisture, that enhance the growth of *Candida albicans*. Topical therapy is undertaken with a polyene or an imidazole antifungal drug twice a day.

I prefer using an imidazole (clotrimazole, miconazole, ketoconazole, econazole), since it is occasionally difficult to differentiate between candidiasis and a dermatophyte infection. In this case an imidazole covers both organisms, whereas nystatin or amphotericin B is effective only against *Candida*. I prescribe a cream, applied sparingly twice a day until there is no more redness or scaling; this generally requires a week or two. Treatment is rarely interrupted by side effects such as irritation, itching, or burning. Allergic contact dermatitis in response to these drugs is rare. Imidazoles are available in creams, solutions, or lotions. Nystatin is available in an ointment, cream, lotion, or powder. Amphotericin B is available in a cream, lotion, or ointment for topical application. The ointments are best avoided for intertriginous infections, since they may contribute to maceration.

PARONYCHIA

Chronic paronychia is characterized by loss of the cuticle, tenderness, swelling, erythema of the proximal nail fold, and separation of the nail fold from the plate with deformity of the nail plate. Trauma and exposure to water must be stopped to cure chronic paronychia. Nystatin, amphotericin B, or imidazoles are required for weeks to months. I prefer an imidazole lotion or solution to deliver the medication under the nail fold and nail plate. Alternatively a solution of 2 percent thymol in alcohol applied twice daily has been successful in some recalcitrant cases. Chronic oral ketoconazole therapy, 200 mg daily, may be necessary if topical treatment fails, heeding the precautions to be mentioned.

THRUSH

Candidiasis of the oral cavity—thrush—presents as adherent white patches on the oral epithelium, which when scraped off leave an erythematous base. Thrush usually affects newborns and immunosuppressed adults. The angles of the mouth (angular chelitis) may also be involved, particularly in patients who drool or have a malocclusion. The usual therapy for thrush is nystatin oral suspension, 200,000 units (2 ml) for infants and 500,000 units (5 ml) for adults, swished and swallowed four times daily. Nystatin is virtually unabsorbed after oral administration and thus is nontoxic. In patients in whom nystatin fails, a clotrimazole troche dissolved in the mouth two to four times a day is generally successful.

If topical treatment fails, oral ketaconozole therapy 200 mg daily, is prescribed for 1 to 2 weeks. Gastric acidity is necessary for dissolution and absorption of ketoconazole. Antacids, anticholinergics, and H2 blockers such as cimetidine therefore should not be administered concomitantly. The most frequently reported adverse reaction to ketoconazole is nausea or vomiting, which occurs in 3 percent of the patients taking the drug. An uncommon (1 in 15,000 patients) but serious side effect is idiopathic hepatitis, which is unrelated to the daily dosage, the cumulative total dosage, or the duration of therapy. Periodic liver function tests are warranted in patients treated for long periods with ketoconazole. With large dosages of ketoconazole (greater than 400 mg daily), adrenal and gonadal synthesis of steroid hormones is inhibited, resulting in decreased production of cortisol and depressed serum testosterone levels in men, manifested as gynecomastia and decreased libido. Recurrence or resistance to treatment suggests an underlying disease, which should be investigated.

VULVOVAGINITIS AND BALANITIS

Vaginal candidiasis causes itching and irritation accompanied by a whitish curdlike discharge and inflammation and satellite lesions on the vulvae. Involvement of the glans penis (balanitis) is evidenced by moist red papules and pustules, which when ruptured leave a peeling edge. Vaginal candidiasis is treated with nystatin or imidazole vaginal cream or tablets once daily for 1 to 2 weeks.

Ketoconazole, 200 mg daily for 1 week, is also effective. Candidal balanitis responds to the topical application of nystatin or imidazole cream twice daily. Besides the predisposing factors mentioned previously it is important that the sexual partner be evaluated and treated for candidiasis if there is recurrent infection.

DISSEMINATED CANDIDIASIS

This life threatening infection characteristically occurs in the immunosuppressed patient who is febrile and fails to respond to multiple antibiotics. The cutaneous manifestations are single or multiple erythematous to purpuric papules and nodules, which occur on the trunk and extremities. The diagnosis can be confirmed by obtaining a skin biopsy specimen for fungal stains and cultures. Because of the severe systemic nature of this infection, the drug of choice is amphotericin B administered intravenously. A test dose of 1 mg in 20 ml of 5 percent dextrose is given intravenously followed with 0.3 mg per kilogram on the first day and increased to 0.6 mg per kilogram on the second and subsequent days. The recommended concentration of the intravenous infusion is 1 mg per 10 milliliters given over approximately 6 hours. The addition of 100 units of heparin to the intravenous solution may reduce the incidence of thrombophlebitis.

Nephrotoxicity is a common predictable adverse reaction. Renal function therefore must be followed closely with at least weekly blood urea nitrogen and serum creatinine determinations. Anaphylactoid reactions, hypotension, arrhythmias, and convulsions have occurred after rapid infusions. Weekly hemograms and serum potassium determinations are recommended. It is important that no other medications be added to the infusion of amphotericin B, with the exception of heparin.

Flucytosine (5-fluorocytosine) with amphotericin B is occasionally used for disseminated candidiasis. Flucytosine is never given by itself because resistance readily develops. Treatment should be continued for 1 to 2 weeks unless toxicity dictates a shorter course. The usual dosage of flucytosine is 37.5 mg per kilogram orally every 6 hours. The principle toxic effects are nausea, vomiting, thrombocytopenia, leukopenia, enterocolitis, and hepatic dysfunction.

Oral therapy with ketoconazole, 400 mg daily, has also been recommended, but because of possible sanctuary organs (central nervous system and kidney), this is not a first therapeutic choice.

CHRONIC MUCOCUTANEOUS CANDIDIASIS

HOWARD M. LEDERMAN, M.D., Ph.D.
JERRY A. WINKELSTEIN, M.D.

The term chronic mucocutaneous candidiasis (CMCC) describes a clinical syndrome of persistent severe candidal infections involving the skin, mucous membranes, hair, and nails that persist despite what would generally be considered adequate treatment. A key to the management of patients with CMCC is the realization that the syndrome may be the presenting symptom of a variety of underlying diseases that have in common deficiencies of cell mediated immunity. Thus, some patients with CMCC may have an underlying primary immunodeficiency disease that affects T-lymphocytes (e.g., severe combined immunodeficiency or DiGeorge's syndrome). In a second group of patients, CMCC may occur because cell mediated immunity has been depressed as the result of other infections (e.g., acquired immunodeficiency syndrome caused by HIV infection), lymphoreticular neoplasms (e.g., lymphoma or thymoma), or immunosuppressive drugs (e.g., cyclophosphamide or prednisone). Recognition of these underlying disorders is critical in the patient with CMCC because each of these disorders carries different therapeutic and prognostic implications.

In still a third group of patients, CMCC results from what appears to be a more limited primary defect in immunity—the inability to mount a cell mediated immune response to *Candida*. Such patients demonstrate diminished or an absence of in vitro T cell proliferative responses to *Candida* antigen and have cutaneous anergy to *Candida*, although proliferative responses to mitogens and other antigens are generally normal. Candidal infections in these patients occur most frequently on the oral mucosa as well as on fingernails and toenails. Although oropharyngeal infections may progress to involve the esophagus, deep visceral involvement or disseminated candidiasis is rare, if it occurs at all. In this particular clinical setting, CMCC is often accompanied by endocrinopathy (diabetes mellitus, hypoparathyroidism, adrenocortical insufficiency, thyroiditis, and gonadal failure) or autoimmune diseases (autoimmune hemolytic anemia, idiopathic thrombocytopenic purpura, and autoimmune neutropenia). Endocrinopathy and autoimmune disease may precede the candidiasis or vice versa, and the full spectrum of disease in a given patient may not be expressed for months to years.

THERAPY

As previously discussed, the first goal of therapy in any patient with severe or persistent candidiasis should be to identify a possible underlying or associated condition. Mucocutaneous candidal infections that are severe or persistent, even if they are localized, should alert the physician to the possibility of underlying immunodeficiency and an evaluation of the patient's immune status should be undertaken. Similarly, a search for associated endocrinopathy and autoimmune disorders should be performed.

Nystatin

Although nystatin has been the primary drug used for mucous membrane candidal infections, its role in chronic mucocutaneous candidiasis is limited. This antibiotic is produced by *Streptomyces noursei* and exerts its antifungal effect by binding to sterols in the fungal cell membrane and thereby interfering with membrane function. Nystatin can be used topically two to three times per day for the treatment of monilial infections involving the skin and mucous membranes. It also can be given by mouth for infections of the oral mucosa. The usual oral dosage is 400,000 to 800,000 units per day in newborn infants, 1 to 2×10^6 units per day in older infants and children, and 2 to 3×10^6 units per day in adults, given in four divided doses. One-half of each dose should be directed toward each side of the mouth, and the preparation should be retained in the mouth as long as possible before swallowing. Nystatin is not effective in the treatment of candidal onychomycosis, and it generally has been ineffective in patients with chronic mucocutaneous candidiasis. Indeed many patients with CMCC are first identified because of a lack of response to oral or topical therapy with nystatin.

Clotrimazole

Clotrimazole is a topical antifungal drug that does have a role in the treatment of chronic mucocutaneous candidiasis. Clotrimazole is a synthetic imidazole derivative, which alters the cell membrane permeability of fungi by binding to phospholipids in the membrane. There have been no clinical reports of acquired resistance developing in initially susceptible fungi. A major disadvantage of this drug is that it is a potent inducer of hepatic microsomal enzymes, such as cytochrome P_{450}, which results in accelerated metabolism of the drug. Systemic administration of clotrimazole for several days induces hepatic enzyme formation to the extent that serum drug levels and chemotherapeutic effects are rapidly diminished. The role of clotrimazole is therefore limited to topical therapy of the skin or mucous membranes. In addition, as is the case with nystatin, clotrimazole is not effective for the therapy of onychomycoses.

Clotrimazole is used orally in the form of a lozenge for the topical treatment of oropharyngeal candidiasis. The usual adult dosage is one 10-mg lozenge five times per day for 14 days. Longer or even prolonged therapy may be necessary in severe infections or in a patient with multiple recurrences of candidiasis in whom no treatable underlying disease can be identified. To achieve the maximal therapeutic benefit, lozenges should be slowly dissolved in the mouth. Therefore this form of therapy should be limited to patients who are able to comprehend and follow instructions.

Clotrimazole is not currently recommended for use in children under the age of 3 years. However, there has been some experience with this drug in small infants. In such patients a clotrimazole lozenge or suppository can be inserted tightly into the slit tip of a pacifier and given to the infant to suck four times a day. Clotrimazole is also available as a 1 percent cream and a 1 percent lotion for topical use two to three times per day.

Skin irritation or sensitization occurs occasionally, leading to erythema, edema, pruritus, or a burning sensation. Mildly elevated liver enzyme levels have been reported in approximately 15 percent of the patients receiving clotrimazole. Liver function tests should therefore be performed in patients undergoing prolonged therapy or those with preexisting hepatic impairment.

Ketoconazole

Topical therapy of skin and mucous membrane infections, using either nystatin or clotrimazole, is generally not fully effective in CMCC. Furthermore, such patients frequently have candidal infections of the nails that are resistant to any topical treatment. The introduction of ketoconazole has been, therefore, a major therapeutic advance.

Ketoconazole is an imidazole derivative, which has broad spectrum antifungal activity. It appears to exert its antifungal activity by blocking the demethylation of lanosterol and thereby interfering with the synthesis of ergosterol. As a result, membrane permeability of the fungus is altered and purine transport is inhibited.

Ketoconazole is useful in patients with chronic candidal infections of the skin and mucous membranes that have been resistant to therapy with nystatin or clotrimazole. However, ketoconazole should not be used for the treatment of acute visceral or systemic candidiasis, because improvement occurs very slowly, generally over a period of weeks to months. For example, improvement in oral candidiasis is usually not apparent until after 10 days of therapy, and a minimum of 3 months of treatment is usually required before any improvement is noted in onychomycoses.

The usual adult dosage of ketoconazole is 200 mg per day given as a single daily oral dose. If improvement is not achieved after an appropriate period of time, the dosage may be increased up to 400 mg but should continue to be given as a single daily dose. There are insufficient data at present to indicate whether dosages higher than 400 mg per day result in an improved clinical response. The usual dosage for children over the age of 2 years is a single daily dose of 3.3 to 6.6 mg per kilogram. Studies have not been performed to establish the appropriate dosage for children under the age of 2 years. Treatment should be continued until all clinical and laboratory evidence of fungal infection has disappeared. Patients with CMCC usually require long-term maintenance therapy.

Hepatic toxicity has been reported in patients taking ketoconazole. Approximately 10 percent of the patients treated with this drug have mild, and clinically unapparent, elevations in serum transaminase or alkaline phosphatase levels. These elevations are usually transient and resolve even with continued administration of ketoconazole. Clinical symptoms of hepatitis (jaundice, nausea, malaise, or anorexia) develop in approximately 1 in 10,000 patients treated with ketoconazole, usually as the result of hepatocellular toxicity. Rare patients have evidence of cholestatic injury or mixed hepatocellular and cholestatic injury. Predisposing factors appear to be female gender and age over 40 years. This injury appears to be limited and reversible as long as ketoconazole therapy is immediately discontinued. In a few patients who have continued to receive the drug, there has been massive and fatal hepatocellular necrosis.

It is therefore recommended that patients receiving ketoconazole have liver function tests (measurement of serum AST, ALT, bilirubin, and alkaline phosphatase levels) performed biweekly for the first 2 months and then monthly or bimonthly for the duration of therapy. Patients with minor asymptomatic elevations in liver enzyme levels should be followed closely. Ketoconazole therapy should be discontinued immediately if liver enzyme levels progressively rise or if any clinical symptoms of hepatitis occur.

Several other potential side effects should be considered. The concomitant administration of ketoconazole and phenytoin may alter the metabolism of both drugs, and the administration of ketoconazole with cyclosporine causes decreased metabolism of the latter. Finally, ketoconazole, particularly when used at dosages exceeding 800 mg per day in adults, inhibits testosterone and adrenal steroid synthesis. Gynecomastia, oligospermia, decreased libido, and impotence have been reported.

Despite these limitations, ketoconazole is probably the most effective antifungal drug currently available for use in CMCC. It should be remembered, however, that control of candidiasis in these patients requires continuous therapy. There are insufficient data at present to predict the efficacy or side effects occurring after multiple years of ketoconazole therapy, nor can the incidence of drug resistance be predicted.

Amphotericin B

Since the introduction of ketoconazole, amphotericin B generally has not had a role in the therapy of patients with CMCC. It is an antifungal drug that is effective in the therapy of candidal infections of the mucous membranes, skin, and nails in patients with CMCC. Unfortunately relapses are the rule in these patients, and long-term therapy with amphotericin B is generally impractical because of the requirement for intravenous infusions and the significant risk of renal impairment.

There are, however, several specific indications for the use of amphotericin B in patients with CMCC. It is an alternative therapy in patients who have developed hypersensitivity or hepatic damage as a result of ketoconazole therapy. Furthermore, the response to amphotericin B is generally more rapid than the response to ketoconazole. Amphotericin B, with or without flucytosine, should therefore be considered for the rare patient with CMCC who has developed deep visceral infection, such as perforation of the esophagus with extension into the chest cavity.

Intravenous therapy with amphotericin B is usually initiated with a dose of 0.25 mg per kilogram administered over a 6 hour period. The daily dosage should then be increased gradually over 3 to 5 days to 0.5 to 0.6 mg per kilogram daily. It may also be administered as a double dose (not to exceed 1.5 mg per kilogram) given every other day. In critically ill patients, the initial escalating dosages may be given over a 1- to 2-day period. The duration of therapy depends on the clinical response but usually ranges from 4 to 8 weeks.

The most significant side effect of amphotericin B is renal damage, which is related to both the daily dosage and the total dosage of the drug. Hypokalemia may be an early manifestation.

SYSTEMIC MYCOSES

JOHN P. UTZ, M.D.

The systemic mycoses exclude fungal infections of the skin (dermatophytoses) or of the mucous membranes alone (such as thrush due to *Candida* species), although these two tissues may occasionally be the site of entry of the causative fungus. The systemic mycoses do include those with a primary focus in the lung (principally blastomycosis, coccidioidomycosis, cryptococcosis, histoplasmosis, paracoccidioidomycosis) and those (for example, aspergillosis, candidosis, cryptococcosis, and phycomycosis) occurring as opportunistic infections in patients immunocompromised congenitally (as with hypogammaglobulinemia), by disease (Hodgkin's, lymphoma, leukemia, diabetes mellitus, or AIDS) or by treatment (such as with corticosteroids, azathioprine, cyclosporine, or antineoplastics).The systemic mycoses include, lastly, those of subcutaneous origin (from injury or inapparent puncture) and character (chromomycosis, mycetoma, and sporotrichosis). No matter what the site of entry, the responsible fungi commonly spread to other organs, by either the hematogenous or, less frequently, the lymphatic route.

EPIDEMIOLOGY

The epidemiologic aspects of the 11 fungal diseases just cited are highly different and complex. For diagnostic purposes it is important to know where the patient has lived or visited. For practical purposes coccidioidomycosis occurs only in residents in or visitors from the southwestern United States (Arizona, California, Nevada, New Mexico, Texas, Utah), and paracoccidioidomycosis occurs only in those in or visiting from South or Central America. The sex of the patient is less helpful, even though such diseases as blastomycosis, chronic cavitary histoplasmosis, and cryptococcal meningitis are five to ten times more frequent in men. In Filipinos and blacks coccidioidomycosis is far more likely to disseminate than in whites.

DIFFERENTIAL DIAGNOSIS

With a few exceptions the systemic mycoses are chronic infections, the prototype of which is tuberculosis. They may mimic sarcoidosis as well, and, curiously, there is a repeatedly observed association of that disease with a concurrent mycosis. A second setting is in a less chronic infection (for example, a persisting pneumonia), especially one that does not seem to be responding to treatment for a presumptive bacterial origin. The opportunistic mycoses occur in the compromised patient, and in such, the picture can be more acute, can be characterized by fever, or occasionally can suggest a gram negative bacterial sepsis. In mycetomas (Madura foot) the diagnosis rests on careful microbiologic study, since that disease may be due to one bacterium alone or to a farrago of microorganisms. Other abnormal conditions include unexplained lymphadenopathy, hepatosplenomegaly, altered mental status, chronic lymphangitis, and chronic cellulitis.

DIAGNOSIS

The diagnosis is established unequivocally by culture of the fungus (and its identification) from a "deep" patient specimen: blood, urine, cerebrospinal fluid, bone marrow, or surgical biopsy of a lesion. With few exceptions (such as candidosis and aspergillosis), when the fungus is a commensal of man or a common saprophyte of nature (but especially the patient's hospital room or the microbiology laboratory), the diagnosis is made by culture and identification from sputum, bronchoscopy material, or draining pus. Microscopic examination of fresh, unstained, or specially stained material is less certain but more immediately helpful.

Owing to the variety and distinctive microscopic forms of the fungi, the resourcefulness in staining, and the experience and expertise of the pathologist, the diagnosis is almost as sure when the typical forms are seen microscopically with special stains (such as Brown-Brenn, periodic acid–Schiff, methenamine silver, alcian blue, mucicamine, or Grocott's) of histopathologic material. The unfortunate aspect of this method is that such biopsy material frequently is not cultured as well.

An important aspect of this method is that although the etiologic agent is established, the activity of the disease is not. In the classic case of a pulmonary nodule (coin lesion) the forms seen may represent old dead fungi rather than viable ones. To resolve this question, a consideration *before* therapy is undertaken, requires a careful study of the patient. Such study usually takes three forms. The first is obtaining the proper patient specimens and culturing them or, in selected instances, inoculating them into laboratory animals. Culture from such specimens establishes activity. Secondly, there are a great many tests that indicate inflammatory activity: leukocyte count, differential, erythrocyte sedimentation rate, serum globulin, serum enzymes, and hemoglobin (or hematocrit or erythrocyte count). In coccidioidomycosis the pattern of the absence of delayed cutaneous hypersensitivity (to coccidioidin or spherulin) and the presence of an important titer of antibodies (measured by a variety of techniques) indicate progressive disease. Also among the tests are serial roentgenograms or perfusion or computerized scans of abnormalities previously present, undertaken to search for signs of activity, either healing or worsening. Thirdly, other underlying disease must be diagnosed. Impaired cellular or serologically mediated immune mechanisms, diabetes mellitus, sarcoidosis, or malignant disease (with attendant antineoplastic therapy) may tip the balance in favor of antifungal therapy, even when the evidence for activity is inconclusive or, occasionally, even absent.

THERAPY

Palliative or symptomatic care has its place. Cough that disturbs rest (histoplasmosis), headache from chronic meningitis (cryptococcosis), and painful orchitis (blastomycosis) can be greatly relieved by such kindly and attentive measures as antitussives, analgesics, and a suspensory. Complaints and appropriate assistive measures are legion.

Surgery can be invaluable, first in obtaining proper specimens, aseptically and from deeper tissues, for diagnosis. In addition, such care can be a great help to the patient, again symptomatically, for example, casting in painful synovitis or osteomyelitis (sporotrichosis or blastomycosis). Surgery can also be critical; no amount of any antifungal agent may be curative in the presence of a well encapsulated abscess or an avascular necrotic lesion (coccidioidomycosis). Lastly, and most importantly, such therapy can be lifesaving; many lives of patients with meningitis have been saved, 2 or even 4 weeks before the diagnosis was made, by placing a ventriculovascular, ventriculoperitoneal, or ventriculopleural shunt.

CHEMOTHERAPY

Despite the value of surgery, the quintessential therapeutic regimen for fungal, as well as other microbiologic infections is chemotherapy, based on successful studies in vitro and in vivo and investigational controlled testing in diseased patients. (The latter needs saying, since so many of the earliest reports were based on an unproved or questionable diagnosis, a self-limited prognosis, an irrationally selected drug without known measurable activity, and an anecdotal setting.)

Despite the dismal start of chemotherapy and late appearance of some of the drugs, there are eight antimycotic drugs in use today. Selection from among them is based on the diagnosis, past successful or unsuccessful therapy, and a few contraindications, either partial or absolute. Table 1 depicts the first and second choices of therapy.

Some modes of therapy are as follows:

1. Potassium iodide, given as a saturated solution, 1 g per milliliter, and diluted in water or other substance to disguise the taste. Begin with 1 ml four times daily and increase to 3 to 4 ml four times daily. When iodism (coryza, skin rash, nausea) occurs, stop treatment for a few days and cut dose slightly. Continue therapy for

TABLE 1   Chemotherapy of the Systemic Mycoses

Infection	Primary Therapy	Secondary Therapy
Actinomycosis*	Penicillin	Tetracycline, erythromycin
Aspergillosis		
Allergic bronchopulmonary	Corticosteroids	
Aspergilloma, pulmonary	Observation	Surgery, amphotericin B transtracheally or percutaneously
Systemic	Amphotericin B IV	Ketoconazole or flucytosine†
Blastomycosis		
Acute pulmonary (especially in localized outbreaks)	Observation	Amphotericin B IV
Invasive, progressive, or systemic	Amphotericin B IV	Hydroxystilbamidine isethionate or ketoconazole†
Candidosis		
Chronic mucocutaneous	Ketoconazole	Amphotericin B IV
Septicemia	Amphotericin B IV	Flucytosine†
Meningitis	Flucytosine†	Amphotericin B IV
Endocarditis	Amphotericin B IV	Surgery
Bladder infection	Amphotericin B IV with or without intravesicular use	Flucytosine† or ketoconazole
Chromomycosis	Flucytosine	Amphotericin B intralesionally
Coccidioidomycosis		
Progressive	Amphotericin B IV	Ketoconazole
Meningitis	Amphotericin B intrathecally	Amphotericin B IV or miconazole or ketoconazole or transfer factor
Cryptococcosis		
Pulmonary	Observation	Flucytosine†, amphotericin B IV
Meningitis	Amphotericin B IV combined with flucytosine	Amphotericin B IV or intrathecally, or flucytosine separately, or miconazole
Other	Flucytosine†	Combined therapy
Histoplasmosis		
Progressive disseminated Chronic cavitary	Ketoconazole	Amphotericin B IV
Mycetoma	Amphotericin B† or flucytosine† or ketoconazole†	Surgery
Nocardiosis*	Sulfonamide	Cotrimoxazole or amikacin
Paracoccidioidomycosis	Ketoconazole	Amphotericin B IV or sulfonamide
Phycomycosis	Amphotericin B†	Surgery and correction of diabetic ketoacidosis
Sporotrichosis	Potassium iodide	Amphotericin B IV

* Not a mycosis, but historically dealt with by mycologists.
† Based on in vitro sensitivity.

4 to 6 weeks after lesion(s) heal or are stable.

2. Sulfonamides. A number are effective. My choice is generic sulfadiazine. Sulfamethoxazole-trimethoprim (cotrimoxazole) is currently modish, but why use two drugs if one suffices? The dosage (for sulfadiazine, 4 to 6 g daily) should be adjusted to achieve a serum level of 10 mg per deciliter.

3. Penicillin. For actinomycosis give penicillin in the usual dosage for anaerobic infections, that is 10 to 12 million units of penicillin G intravenously. As the patient improves and discharge is contemplated, reduce the dosage to 2 g per day; then switch to the oral route with 2 g per day of phenoxymethyl-penicillin. Continue treatment for at least 3 months after lesions have healed or become stable. In one patient whose infection relapsed twice after such a program, I have continued treatment through the twelfth year and until death from other cause. Usually treatment is given for 6 to 12 months to achieve the 3 months of stability recommended.

In patients allergic to penicillin, 2 g per day of erythromycin or tetracycline can be substituted. Amikacin has recently been reported useful, though the intramuscular route of administration is less convenient.

4. Hydroxystilbamidine isethionate. For nonprogressive cutaneous blastomycosis this drug is an acceptable alternative to amphotericin B. Begin with an initial dose of 25 mg in 250 milliliters of 5 percent glucose in water intravenously over a 2 to 3 hour period and increase by daily increments of 25 mg until an optimal dosage of 225 mg is reached. The arbitrary total dosage—based on a VA cooperative study—is 8 g. The drug is deposited in skin and liver, and abnormal liver function test results are a relative contraindication. Side effects are hypotension, when the drug is infused too rapidly, anorexia, nausea, headache, and rash.

5. Amphotericin B. My initial dose is 1 mg. Under the rare circumstances when disease appears to be life threatening, give 1 mg in 50 milliliters of 5 percent glucose solution in water slowly over 2 hours, and follow that with the residual 9 mg in 450 milliliters of fluid. Follow directions carefully in suspending vial contents and adding to 5 percent glucose solution. Final concentration should not exceed 10 mg per deciliter. Protection from light is not necessary, however. Although an infusion time of only 45 minutes is employed by some, lingering anxiety and awareness of cardiotoxicity in man and dogs with such rapidity lead me to use an infusion time of 2 to 6 hours, depending on patient tolerance. Increase the daily dosage by 5-mg increments.

Opinion varies about the optimal daily dosage of the drug, and the duration of therapy. One school recommends a daily dosage (20 to 30 mg) meant to give serum levels two to three times the expected minimal inhibitory concentration, and a 10-week course. Another school recommends an optimal daily dosage of 1 mg per kilogram (not to exceed 50 mg), a total dosage of 1.5 to 3 g, usually administrable over a 4- to 6-week course. The lesser period of hospitaliza-

tion, and lesser expense, are purchased at the price of greater toxicity. For some infections, for example, *Candida* spp., septicemia, mucocutaneous esophageal, or urinary tract infection, smaller total dosages (10 to 355 mg) over 4 to 18 days have been successful.

If reactions (fever, chills, sweats, malaise, anorexia, nausea, and vomiting) are severe and repeated, give 25 mg of hydrocortisone intravenously at the beginning of the infusion. Aspirin and antihistaminics are less effective but occasionally useful. Measure renal function twice weekly. The creatinine clearance is the most sensitive measurement, but serum creatinine or blood urea nitrogen (BUN) determinations are usually preferable for reasons of ease and completeness of collection. Interrupt therapy for a few days if creatinine goes over 3 or BUN over 50 mg per deciliter. Mannitol does not reduce nephrotoxicity in humans. Use scalp vein needles to minimize the risk of phlebitis, and if the latter is a problem, use heparin (1,000 units per infusion). Determine potassium levels twice weekly and correct hypokalemia by oral supplementation. I advise documenting the predictable fall in hemoglobin or hematocrit, but anemia is rarely severe, oral iron therapy is ineffective, and transfusion is unnecessary. The significance of pulmonary infiltrates when amphotericin is given with granulocyte transfusions has not been settled. Caution is indicated.

For intrathecal use at lumbar, cisternal, or ventricular reservoir (Ommaya) sites, give 0.1 to 1.0 mg diluted in at least 5 milliliters of sterile water, and in the cerebrospinal fluid in the syringe. Inject slowly and no more frequently than two to three times weekly. For intra-articular use inject 5 to 15 mg once. For nebulization or percutaneous injection into a pulmonary cavity use 50 mg in 50 milliliters of glucose solution. For intravesicular use dilute 50 mg in 1,000 milliliters of irrigating fluid.

6. Flucytosine. Give 150 mg per kilogram per day orally in four equally divided doses. In cases of renal failure adjust the interval between doses according to creatinine clearance: every 6 hours when 40 or greater, every 12 hours when between 40 and 20, and every 24 hours when between 20 and 10 ml per minute. When less than 10, adjust by serum level (optimal: 50 to 75 μg per milliliter).

The commonest side effects are gastrointestinal and usually mild: nausea, vomiting, and diarrhea. However, enterocolitis and bowel perforation have been reported. Thrombocytopenia, leukopenia, and anemia occur in about 5 percent of the patients, but more frequently—and occasionally with fatal outcome—with serum concentrations in excess of 100 μg per milliliter. The latter is more apt to occur when renal excretion (equivalent to that of creatinine) is reduced by concurrent intravenous use of amphotericin B. Less frequently encountered side effects are headaches, hallucinations, somnolence, and vertigo. Elevated serum transaminase and alkaline phosphatase values are the basis for claims of hepatotoxicity.

7. Miconazole. The current limited recommended range

of dosage (25 to 30 mg per kilogram per day) hardly reflects the past practices of giving 200 to 1,200 mg intravenously, in either saline or glucose solution, every 8 hours over a 30- to 60-minute period of infusion. The duration of therapy has been of almost equal variability, and stabilization of laboratory and clinical findings has been the customary criterion for stopping treatment.

The most common side effects have been nausea, vomiting, and pruritus. However, more serious side effects, such as anaphylaxis and cardiac and respiratory arrest, have been reported. Hyperlipidemia, lipoproteinemia, interference in granulocyte function, anemia, and ''other hematologic abnormalities'' have been attributed to the castor oil vehicle.

8. Ketoconazole. The dosages initially employed were only 200 or 400 mg (one or two tablets) daily (or, in the second instance, sometimes twice daily). As treatment failures began to occur, the dosage was increased progressively to 1,200 mg daily. As new side effects appeared, there has been diminishing enthusiasm for higher dosages. In sum, the optimal dosage is still unsettled.

The oral route of administration has permitted, for the first time, the concept of long-term (6 months, 1 year, 18 months) therapy similar to that for tuberculosis. Ironically, this concept of prolonged therapy is appearing in an era of intensive study of short course therapy (9 months or less) with isoniazid, rifampin, and other drugs for tuberculosis.

Increasing use of the drug has, as in many classic cases, revealed abnormalities not encountered in the earliest trials. For example, elevated transaminase (aspartate aminotransferase) values had been seen in about one-third of the patients, but values had exceeded 100 in less than 5 percent and had been considered unimportant. More recently, however, biopsies have revealed enlarged portal tracts, mononuclear cell infiltrations, and piecemeal necrosis, all suggestive of chronic active hepatitis (type II reaction, National Institutes of Health classification). Gynecomastia, loss of libido, and impotence were then observed. Inhibition of adrenal steroid and testosterone synthesis was then described in a patient with a 1,200 mg daily dosage. Oligospermia and azoospermia persisted for 3 weeks after discontinuation of the drug. Lastly, ketoconazole has been shown to impair the hepatic metabolism of cyclosporine (in a renal transplant recipient), with an increase in serum trough levels from about 100 to about 3,000 mg per milliliter and attendant impairment of renal function. Again, evaluation of toxicity (and efficacy) is evolving, and the role of this newest drug awaits definition.

PREVENTION AND PROPHYLAXIS

A vaccine for the prevention of coccidioidomycosis is currently being evaluated, but otherwise no progress has been made in immunization.

With the increasing problem of opportunistic infections in immunocompromised patients, it should be expected that antifungal prophylaxis would be attempted, notably in patients with pancytopenia, bone marrow depression, and immunoparalysis, deliberately or unintentionally evoked. Among the drugs discussed, oral doses of amphotericin B in a nonabsorbable form, in combination with cotrimoxazole, resulted in fewer overall infections and fewer local *Candida* spp. infections. No systemic infections occurred in either the treatment or the control group. In combination with cephalothin-gentamicin-carbenicillin, amphotericin B seemed to prevent superinfections and ''control undetected fungal invasion.'' However, in another study, ketoconazole was superior to nystatin-amphotericin B in protecting against fungal infection, again in an immunocompromised group of patients.

PARASITIC INFECTIONS AND INFESTATIONS

LEISHMANIASIS

SAMUEL L. MOSCHELLA, M.D.

Leishmaniasis, a group of clinically distinguishable diseases, results from the infection of man with different species of parasitic protozoa of the genus *Leishmania*. Many species of the parasite have been found in the tropics and subtropics. Each has different sandfly vectors and animal reservoirs and exhibits different types of behavior in humans.

Leishmaniasis is essentially a zoonosis and is found in an environment that varies from the humid rain forests of South and Central America to the dry savannas of Africa south of the Sahara and the deserts of the Middle East. It is transmitted by sandflies of the genera *Phlebotomus, Lutzomyia,* and *Psychodopygus* within which the organisms develop flagellate promastigote forms. The human and various mammalian hosts are infected by the bite of an infected sandfly. The parasites, because of the different biochemical milieu, develop into the nonflagellated amastigote stage (Leishman-Donovan body) and proliferate by binary fission within cells of the mononuclear phagocytic system.

It is almost impossible to differentiate the species of *Leishmania* that cause disease in humans from one another on the basis of morphology, even ultrastructurally, in either the amastigote or promastigote stage. The taxonomy of *Leishmania*, which was originally based on traditional approaches, such as the behavior of the parasites in humans, geographic distribution, involvement with different animal reservoirs, and transmission by different species of sandflies, is now considered inadequate. The current taxonomy utilizes biochemical techniques, such as a species identification by isoenzymes and kinetoplast DNA analysis, the position of the isolate in the gut of experimentally infected sandflies, and developing immunologic techniques, such as the use of monoclonal antibodies.

The clinical manifestations of leishmaniasis depend on a complex and intriguing interaction of the virulence factors and tropism inherent in the parasite and the genetically determined host defense mechanism. The clinical expressions of human disease are self-healing localized ulcers, persistent or recurrent cutaneous lesions, widely disseminated progressive skin lesions, destructive mucous membrane lesions, or, in the case of visceral leishmaniasis,

hepatosplenomegaly and anemia resulting from involvement of the entire reticuloendothelial system.

The diagnostic studies include demonstration of the amastigote (2 to 4 mm) by Giema stained smears made from prints of skin biopsy or needling of an ulcer base, culture utilizing the Novy-MacNeal-Nicholle (NNN) medium or Difco agar with 10 percent defibrinated rabbit blood kept at 23° C, hamster inoculation of nose and hind foot, and the leishmanin skin test.

At least 10 species of human *Leishmania* are currently accepted (Table 1). The clinical expressions of cutaneous leishmaniasis can be divided into those due to Old World species and the others due to New World species.

OLD WORLD SPECIES

In the urban form, *L. tropica* causes the oriental sore after an incubation period longer than 2 months and usually over 1 year. Clinically it is characterized by few nodules or plaques, which ulcerate; secondary satellite nodules may be seen. Usually many organisms are found in the lesions. Man and dogs are the host reservoirs. *L. tropica* infection protects against reinfection. The lesions heal spontaneously. However, two chronic expressions exist: the chronic cutaneous lupoid type persists for many years, and the recidivans type recurs for years with clinically complete or incomplete healing. Both harbor few organisms, are characterized by a tuberculoid histopathology and delayed hypersensitivity skin response to vaccines, and are resistant to therapy. If the lesions are in cosmetically unimportant sites, specific (antimonial) treatment usually can be avoided.

L. tropica major causes furunculoid lesions, which ulcerate, can number more than 30 lesions, and may be associated with satellite lymphatic nodules as well as lymphadenitis. The host reservoir is rodents. Infection protects against reinfection and infection with *L. tropica*.

L. aethiopica usually causes a single lesion on an exposed area and rarely diffuse cutaneous leishmaniasis, which can resemble clinically nodular lepromatous leprosy and unlike the localized lesion is chronic, disseminated, and resistant to therapy.

NEW WORLD SPECIES

The *L. mexicana* complex infection behaves much like Old World cutaneous leishmaniasis by causing self-healing lesions. However, when the pinna is affected by *L. mexicana mexicana,* the resultant lesion has been described as the chiclero ulcer, which is destructive and persistent. Both *L. mexicana amazonensis* and rarely *L. mexicana mexicana* can cause diffuse disseminated leishmaniasis.

The four parasites of the *L. brasiliensis* complex cause more chronic and long-lasting, small, self-healing to large intractable ulcers. However, the mucocutaneous type, which is characterized clinically by chronic and progressive "metastatic" mucosal lesions that are refractory to treatment, results mainly from infection with *L. brasiliensis brasiliensis* and infrequently by *L. brasiliensis panamensis.*

The *L. donovani* complex consists of *L. donovani, L. infantum,* and *L. chagasi* and causes a potentially fatal systemic disease. A primary cutaneous ulcerative lesion has been described in African patients. A cutaneous relapsing form of kala-azar called postkala-azar dermal leishmaniasis appears shortly after treatment of the disease in patients in Africa, but may be delayed for up to 2 years in patients in India. The condition clinically resembles lepromatous leprosy and is characterized by nodules and pigmented macules.

THERAPY

Since the current biochemical and immunologic techniques necessary to identify the species and subspecies of the genus *Leishmania* are not readily available but are necessary to direct more effective attitudes and approaches to therapy, an unsatisfactory but the only practical solution is an educated guess based on where the patient was infected, the course of the disease, the numbers of organisms present in the lesions, and the histopathology of the lesions.

The indications for "specific" systemic therapy with antimonial drugs when one is confronted with the simple "ulcerative" type are (1) ulcers in cosmetically or vital sites, such as the periorbital area; (2) an ulcer that shows no evidence of healing after several months and even local extension or dissemination; (3) evidence of lymphatic spread such as satellite lesions, a sporotrichoid pattern or lymphadenitis, or both; (4) evidence suggesting infection with members of the *L. brasiliensis* complex because of their refractoriness and persistence and potential for metastatic mucosal lesions; (5) the chiclero ulcer; (6) the *L. tropica* infection because of the potential development of the chronic cutaneous type (the so-called lupoid or recurring so-called recidive type); and (7) the ulcers of *L. aethiopica* and *L. mexicana amazonensis* infections because of their potential for the development of diffuse disseminated cutaneous leishmaniasis.

The chronic (lupoid) type of leishmaniasis and the recurring (recidive) type, both of the Old World type of disease, require not only several more intensive and prolonged courses of antimonial therapy but also an adjunctive trial course of intralesional or systemic corticosteroid therapy if the response to antimonial drugs alone is poor.

If no reponse is apparent to intensive and recurrent courses of antimony therapy, the mucosal disease may require a trial of amphotericin. For cutaneous lesions that are self-limited without the potential for chronicity, simple excision, cryosurgery, local heat, or the topical application of an ointment containing 15 percent paromomycin sulfate and 12 percent methylbenzethonium chloride in white paraffin (available from Teva Pharmaceutical Industries Ltd., Jerusalem) applied twice daily for 80 days may reduce the scarring and morbidity. If cryosurgical therapy is to be used, an ice ball measuring up to 2 mm outside the margin of the lesion should be produced with a freeze time of 60 to 90 seconds. Surgical modalities of treatment may also be tried with localized lesions that fail to respond to antimonial drugs.

The pentavalent antimonial drugs, sodium stibogluconate (Pentostam) and meglumine antimoniate (Glucantime), are the primary drugs of choice for systemic

TABLE 1 Species of Leishmaniasis: Clinical Presentation and Geographic Distribution

Species	Clinical Expression	Principal Geographic Foci
L. tropica	Simple cutaneous leishmaniasis; leishmaniasis recidivans; visceral leishmaniasis	Mediterranean, Europe, Africa, Middle East, West Asia, India
L. tropica major	Simple cutaneous leishmaniasis	Israel, USSR, Iran, Sahara Africa, West Asia, India
L. aethiopica	Simple cutaneous leishmaniasis; diffuse cutaneous leishmaniasis	Ethiopia, Kenya, Tanzania, Namibia
L. mexicana mexicana	Simple cutaneous leishmaniasis	Mexico and Central America
L. mexicana amazonensis	Simple cutaneous leishmaniasis; diffuse cutaneous leishmaniasis	Brazil, Venezuela, Colombia
L. brasiliensis brasiliensis	Simple cutaneous leishmaniasis; mucocutaneous leishmaniasis	Brazil (south of Amazon), Bolivia, Peru (east of Andes)
L. brasiliensis panamensis	Simple cutaneous leishmaniasis	Panama and Costa Rica
L. brasiliensis guyanensis	Simple cutaneous leishmaniasis	Goyanas and Brazil (north of Amazon River)
L. brasiliensis peruviana	Simple cutaneous leishmaniasis	Peru (west slopes of Andes)
L. donovani	Visceral; postkala-azar disseminated leishmaniasis	India, China, Kenya, Sudan, Mediterranean basin, Brazil, Venezuela, Paraguay

therapy. Pentostam may be obtained from the Center for Disease Control, Atlanta, Georgia, and Glucantime is available in most Latin American countries. Pentostam is supplied in 100 ml vials containing 100 mg of antimony base. In the past, for skin ulcers that were considered to be best treated systemically, the drug was given in dosages of 10 mg (0.1 ml) per kilogram of body weight not to exceed a 6.0 ml total dosage for 10 days followed by a rest period of 10 to 14 days before this regimen was repeated if the response was not effective. For such patients the currently advocated dosage is 15 to 20 mg per kilogram given for 20 days.

Patients with the chronic and resistant types of leishmaniasis, such as the chronic lupoid or recidivans type, the mucocutaneous types, and the chiclero ulcer, should be treated with an antimonial drug, 25 to 30 mg per kilogram daily, for 20 days or more. For the diffuse disseminated type of disease, 30 to 60 days of such therapy is prescribed.

Amphotericin B is the second line drug to be used in disease resistant to antimony, especially the mucocutaneous and diffuse disseminated types. The drug is administered as recommended for the therapy of the deep mycoses, by intravenous administration slowly in 5 percent dextrose in water over 4 to 6 hours, starting with 0.1 mg per kilogram daily and slowly increasing to 1.0 mg per kilogram until 1 to 3 g is given. The amount prescribed depends on the clinical response and toxicity. Rifampin may be used orally in dosages of 600 to 1,200 mg daily in conjunction with antimonial drugs at the lower or higher dosages in an attempt to improve therapeutic effectiveness.

The adverse reactions to antimonial drugs are pain at the injection site, local thrombosis, anorexia, nausea, vomiting, headache, myalgia, arthralgia, urticaria, or an anaphylactoid reaction or both, electrocardiographic changes, bradycardia and serious arrhythmias, syncope, renal and hepatic injury, and hemolytic anemia. The side effects of amphotericin are anorexia, nausea, vomiting, fever, chills, anemia, elevation of the blood urea nitrogen level, renal damage, hypokalemia, and local thrombosis.

CERCARIAL DERMATITIS

EVAN R. FARMER, M.D.

Cercarial dermatitis, swimmer's itch, is caused by the penetration of the skin by schistosome cercariae. These cercariae are widely distributed throughout the world in both salt and fresh water, and the disease has many local names identified with place or occupation, such as swamp itch or clam digger's itch. Sea bather's eruption is a term used to describe a similar eruption, but it differs from cercarial dermatitis in that no causal organism has been identified, it is limited to salt water, and the area of involvement is primarily the clothing covered parts.

Schistosomes have a complex life cycle in which the adult schistosome is a blood parasite of birds or mammals. The droppings of these animals contain schistome eggs, which develop into a miracidium stage that infests specific species of snails. In the snails the miracidia evolve into cercariae, which are released into water and normally infest birds and small mammals to complete the cycle, unless man happens to be available to act as a host.

The clinical features begin with penetration of the skin by the cercariae. This penetration may take place while the person is still in the water but may also occur as water evaporates from the skin. The initial symptom is a prickling or itching sensation that is followed by small urticarial wheals. After approximately 30 minutes these wheals develop into papules. The eruption spontaneously resolves over 1 to 2 weeks but may be complicated by excoriations and a secondary bacterial infection. These clinical manifestations are probably at least partly, if not entirely, due to an allergic response to the organism, for repeated infestations seem to cause a more severe dermatitis. In North America there is no evidence, so far, that these particular schistosomes can cause systemic disease in man.

The diagnosis is based entirely on the history and clinical findings because the cercariae cannot be identified.

THERAPY

The mainstay of therapy is recognition of the disease and reassurance of the patient that it is a self-limited disorder; otherwise treatment is symptomatic. Calamine lotion, an over-the-counter drug, provides some relief of the itching. Menthol, 0.25 percent, or phenol, 0.5 percent, added to a lotion such as Lubriderm is soothing and antipruritic for mild cases. The topical use of corticosteroids, such as triamcinolone cream, 0.1 percent, applied several times a day helps to diminish the inflammation. Antihistamines such as hydroxyzine, 25 to 50 mg, or diphenhydramine, 25 to 50 mg, every 4 hours or at bedtime are helpful in providing relief of the pruritus. In severe cases a short course of prednisone, 0.5 to 1.0 mg per kilogram per day with tapering to zero over 2 to 3 weeks, is justified.

If there is a secondary bacterial infection, I recommend a 7 to 10 day systemic course of antibiotics, either dicloxacillin or enteric coated erythromycin, both in doses of 500 mg twice daily.

Prevention is the best measure. Places that are infested should be avoided, and as a general measure after swimming in fresh or salt water other than a pool, it is best to dry off immediately with a towel. This is particularly true for patients who have had prior episodes of cercarial dermatitis.

As mentioned, sea bather's eruption is similar to cercarial dermatitis except for lack of a known causal agent, limitation to salt water, and a predilection for areas covered by clothing. The disease otherwise has similar clinical features, and again there is probably an element of sensitization. The treatment is the same as for cercarial dermatitis.

SEA NETTLE DERMATITIS

EVAN R. FARMER, M.D.

Sea nettles are coelenterates, that are found in both salt and fresh water, and they possess nematocysts capable of inflicting stings on man and other animals. Approximately 100 species of the 9,000 in the phylum Coelenterata have these nematocysts, including the Portuguese man-of-war, sea nettles (jellyfish), sea anemones, and sea wasps.

The nematocysts are located on the long trailing tentacles and contain the toxic substance responsible for the stings. Each nematocyst has a spiral coil or barb that is injected into the victim along with the toxin upon contact with the sea nettle. The morphology of the nematocyst and the composition of the toxin vary from species to species. Friction and contact with fresh water are at least two of the known and common factors that cause the nematocyst to discharge its contents. Thus, the nematocyst can produce its effects both in the water or after the patient has gotten out of the water.

The toxin is a heat labile, nondialyzable protein that may work by altering ionic permeability. It seems to affect both nerves and the cardiovascular system. The local effects in the skin are probably mediated by the release of serotonin, histamine, and other mediators of inflammation. The clinical features are the result of the concentration of the toxin, the specific toxicity of the species, and the host's immune response. Most lesions are a result of toxicity, but an allergic component may play a role in a few patients.

The clinical symptoms begin with localized stinging at the site of contact, followed by a burning sensation and then itching. The first sign is an urticarial lesion that is usually in a linear pattern, which evolves into a more diffuse area of redness. Occasional cases may rapidly evolve into anaphylaxis. Other signs or symptoms include hyperhidrosis, cramps, dizziness, nausea, and vomiting. Ulceration and secondary bacterial infection occur only rarely. As the lesion resolves, postinflammatory hyperpigmentation may develop, which eventually fades. Scarring is rare unless there has been ulceration. Conjunctivitis occasionally develops, especially in children who transfer nematocysts to the eyes during crying. Death from these toxins is rare and is associated with extensive stings, anaphylaxis, or cardiac arrest.

TREATMENT

The aims of treatment are to neutralize and remove the nematocysts to prevent additional envenomation, to alleviate the symptoms induced by the toxin, and to provide life support in patients with severe reactions. Since fresh water and friction both trigger the nematocysts, it is best initially to avoid these activities until the nematocysts have been neutralized or removed. Rinsing the area of involvement with sea water as the patient emerges from the water is usually a reflex action and is helpful as long as rubbing is minimized.

The application of alcohol (any type available but generally isopropyl) provides rapid and soothing relief to the inflamed skin while neutralizing the nematocysts. An alternative is meat tenderizer, which may degrade the toxin and render it inactive. In my experience the action of meat tenderizer is not as quick or as effective as alcohol, and it also is not as readily available at the time of need. A slurry of 50 percent baking soda or talcum in water may be applied to the area to help in removing any tentacles. After applying the slurry the tentacles may be gently scraped off using the dull edge of a knife or other blunt instrument. Remember not to touch the area of involvement with an ungloved hand until the tentacles have been removed or neutralized, because the helper may quickly become a victim as well. A slurry of sand in sea water is an alternative to the baking soda.

Once the nematocysts have been neutralized, the patient should rest or at least limit the mobility of the affected part for 30 minutes in order to slow the blood flow from the area. In severe envenomation it may be necessary to apply tourniquets to the limbs to retard the venous return and dissemination of the toxin.

The local symptoms usually resolve without treatment in mild cases, but applications of a cooling lotion such as Lubriderm with 0.25 percent menthol are comforting. The topical application of lidocaine may provide some relief in more severe stings. Occasionally systemically administered medications, including aspirin, codeine, nonsteroidal anti-inflammatory drugs, and antihistamines, may be helpful, depending upon the symptoms. Anaphylaxis, shock, or cardiac arrest should be managed in the usual manner. Secondary infection, although rare, may develop several days later and should be treated with either topical antibiotic therapy, such as bacitracin ointment, or systemic doses of antibiotics, such as enteric coated erythromycin or dicloxacillin, 500 mg twice daily (in an adult) for 7 to 10 days.

Avoiding swimming in heavily infested areas is the most effective measure. This is particularly true for individuals who seem to have an allergic reaction to the toxin.

CUTANEOUS LARVA MIGRANS

BRUCE H. THIERS, M.D.

The term cutaneous larva migrans refers to the migration of larval parasites through the skin of humans (creeping eruption). The disorder is usually caused by the larvae of nematode parasites of animals other than humans (Table 1). *Ancylostoma braziliense*, the dog and cat hookworm, is most often implicated. The condition is most common in warm humid climates, and in the United States it is endemic in the Southeastern states, especially Florida, Georgia, and South Carolina.

Eggs pass from the feces of infected animals onto the soil, where they mature, molt, and eventually become infectious filariform larvae, which, upon contact, can penetrate human skin, especially through fissures and hair follicles. Pruritus develops at the site of penetration within a few hours, and an erythematous papule can be noted within 2 or 3 days. Migration of larvae usually begins shortly thereafter, although it rarely may be delayed for weeks or months. As the larvae tunnel through the lower epidermis, a serpiginous, slightly elevated, 2 to 3 mm wide erythematous tract extends out from the papule. The usual rate of migration is 1 to 2 cm per day, although with some species (e.g., *Strongyloides stercoralis*) it may exceed 10 cm per day (larva currens).

Unlike in their natural hosts, the larvae are unable to penetrate human dermis (apparently because of a lack of the appropriate collagenase enzymes). Thus, depending on the parasite involved, the disorder is self-limited, lasting a few weeks, months, or, rarely, years before migration ceases.

THERAPY

Older methods of treating the skin with physical modalities (ethyl chloride spray, carbon dioxide snow, liquid nitrogen, electrocautery, or phenol application) required sloughing of the epidermis (and with it the migrating larvae) and were only partially successful. Since then, thiabendazole, given either orally or topically, has become the treatment of choice.

Thiabendazole is usually administered orally at a dosage of 50 mg per kilogram per day (maximal daily dosage, 3 g) in 2 divided doses (25 mg per kilogram twice daily) for 2 days. The drug should be given after meals. Pruritus decreases markedly within 1 to 2 days, and tracts resolve within 5 to 7 days. The treatment may be repeated in 2 days if lesions remain active.

Oral doses of thiabendazole are poorly tolerated, with frequent side effects including anorexia, nausea, vomiting, and dizziness. A lowered dosage, 25 mg per kilogram per day (12.5 mg per kilogram twice daily), may cause fewer problems and be equally effective. Furthermore, thiabendazole competes with theophylline for sites of metabolism in the liver; thus blood levels of the latter must be monitored in asthmatic patients taking both drugs to guard against the possibility of theophylline toxicity.

TABLE 1 Cutaneous Larva Migrans

Species	Common Name	Incidence	Clinical Distinction
A. braziliense	Cat, dog hookworm	Most common	Threadlike pruritic migratory burrow; may persist for months, moving 1 or 2 cm/day
A. caninum	Dog hookworm	Common	Papular, rarely linear lesions; disappear in 2 weeks
G. spinigerum	Pig, cat stomach worm	Rare	Deep burrows; bandlike infiltrates, at times furunculoid; may be active for years
U. stenocephala	European dog hookworm	Rare	Threadlike pruritic migratory burrow; may persist for months, moving 1 or 2 cm/day
B. phlebotomum	Cattle hookworm	Rare	Papules, migration for few millimeters; clear in 2 weeks
A. ceylanicum	Cat, dog, human hookworm of Southeast Asia	Common	Usually papular initially, followed by migratory burrow
A. duodenale	Human hookworm	Common	Papulovesicular, pruritic, minimal migration in skin; disappears within 2 weeks
N. americanus	Human hookworm	Common	Papulovesicular, pruritic, minimal migration in skin; disappears within 2 weeks
S. stercoralis	Human threadworm	Rare	Urticarial band extending up to 10 cm/day; originates in perianal area; persists for weeks; recurrent for years owing to autoinoculation from intestinal infection
Strongloides species of wild animals			
S. myopotami	Rodent threadworm	Rare	
S. procyonis	Raccoon threadworm	Rare	
S. fülleborni	Old World primate threadworm	Rare	Usually papular initially, followed by migratory burrow
S. papillosus	Sheep, goat threadworm	Rare	
S. westeri	Horse threadworm	Rare	
S. ratti	Rat threadworm	Rare	
S. venezuelensis	Rat threadworm	Rare	

Modified from Little M, Farah F. Larva migrans. Unit 18-16. In: Demis DJ, ed. Clinical Dermatology. Philadelphia: Harper & Row, 1987; 2.

Because of these difficulties, the preferred approach to the treatment of cutaneous larva migrans is the topical application of a 10 percent thiabendazole suspension four times per day for 1 week. Because the larvae often can be found as far as 2 cm beyond the advancing edge of the burrow, the area of application must extend beyond the clinical limits of involved skin. Treatment may be continued an additional week if active larvae persist. Topical thiabendazole therapy appears to be as effective as systemic administration without the attendant side effects.

Antibiotics, given either topically or systemically, are prescribed as indicated. Antihistamines may be useful in relieving pruritus. Systemic corticosteroid therapy is rarely necessary.

PREVENTION

An important aspect of the treatment of cutaneous larva migrans is prevention. An attempt should be made to control cats, dogs, and other animals responsible for contaminating the soil. Anthelmintic treatment should be administered to pets to prevent or eliminate hookworm infection, and animals should be kept from excreting in areas frequented by humans. Protective clothing should be worn whenever contact with potentially infected soil is anticipated.

INFESTATIONS AND INSECT BITES

RONALD R. LITEPLO, M.D.

SCABIES

Scabies is paradoxically one of the easiest and one of the most difficult diseases to treat. Although there are several effective scabicides that can be used, the difficulty comes not only in being able to correctly recognize the disease at first but also in effecting management control procedures that will eradicate the disease in the family, nursing home, or elsewhere.

Treatment

Lindane

One percent lindane (Kwell) is still the treatment of choice for nearly all types of scabies and in nearly all age groups. It is highly effective (95 to 98 percent), easy to use, and readily available in cream, lotion, and shampoo forms. I am convinced of its safety, although there is some controversy about its safety, especially for children and pregnant women.

In order to be effective, lindane must be applied to the entire body surface area from the neck to the toes, with particular attention to the creases of the body. In children, in whom the disease may also involve the face and scalp, it should be applied from the neck up as well, care being taken to avoid the corners of the eyes and mouth. A pretreatment bath is no longer required because it probably increases percutaneous absorption. However, if an adequate drying-off period is allowed (e.g., one-half hour) prior to treatment, a bath or shower will have no adverse effects. It does inspire a sense of cleanliness and resolve, and is psychologically beneficial to the patient, who is often already feeling shamed and dirty.

Lindane is best applied at bedtime, and the patient can wear old pajamas to bed after it dries on the skin. It is imperative that handwashing be avoided before the prescribed period of time has elapsed, as this is the second most common cause of treatment failure. A touch-up application should be used if this rule is not adhered to. Inadequate application to the entire integument is the leading cause of treatment failure. Spouses or other family members can be helpful in applying the medicine to hard to reach places, and since high risk household members should also be treated simultaneously to prevent "ping-ponging," this practice is mutually beneficial. In crowded households all members should be treated.

At the end of treatment a cleansing bath is taken. Sometimes a patient may need a bland emollient or a steroid cream following treatment, depending on the severity of the symptoms. I find oral antihistamine therapy of little benefit in relieving itching in this disease. All bed linen, pajamas, underclothing, and towels should be washed in a hot cycle. Nonwashables may be dry cleaned or just not worn for up to 1 week. The mite cannot survive off the human host longer than 3 to 4 days, even under optimal conditions of temperature and humidity. Fomite control plays little role in the management of sporadic cases of scabies. This is not true, however, when it comes to institutional epidemics (vide infra).

How long lindane should be left on the skin remains controversial. The manufacturer at one time recommended 6 hours, although I have found this to be ineffective. Most authorities now recommend 8 to 12 hours, although the scientific rationale for this duration is unclear. Peak blood levels after a single application are reached in 6 hours, and there is a gradual diminution in the blood level (one-half of the peak concentration at 24 hours, one-fourth at 48 hours), even after a cleansing bath at 24 hours. Therefore there seems to be little if any reduction in blood levels from shortening the application time of lindane to less than 24 hours, and the incidence of cure falls sharply at application times less than 6 hours. There is no evidence of observable side effects at these blood levels.

Indeed, considering the paucity of reports of toxic effects (usually convulsions) following proper topical application, the safety record of lindane over the past 38 years is quite impressive. Serious central nervous system toxicity, seizures, and even death, however, have been associated with accidental ingestion or abuse or overuse of topical lindane therapy, a risk even greater in infants and young children. I tell patients or parents of young children to pay strict attention to the guidelines for treatment.

In my experience a single 24 hour application of lindane (along with the proper patient education) is more desirable than two 8 to 12 hour applications, although I cannot say that it is more effective. I see many patients who have already been given lindane unsuccessfully and improperly for their rash; and when the diagnosis is scabies (frequently it is not!), I stress the need for one total-body 24 hour application of lindane, rarely if ever requiring a follow-up application in 1 week. Since I have found this treatment to be 100 percent effective, I am much more comfortable in prescribing a mild corticosteroid cream for any residual itching that may last for 7 to 10 days even after successful treatment, without masking any new signs of partially treated scabies. In my experience this treatment is without toxicity, and side effects (which are more frequently seen in the lindane abuser) are limited to irritation of the skin.

Children are more likely to be secondarily infected, and occasionally an antibiotic against gram positive cocci is indicated. Parents need not worry if their child is a "thumb sucker," because they can fully clothe and glove the child during the night to prevent inadvertent licking. Nodular lesions of scabies may subsequently develop in the axillas or groin and are best treated with steroid creams.

Alternatives to Lindane

The safety record of lindane notwithstanding, there

are physicians who prefer a more conservative approach. When dealing with infants or young children, or pregnant or nursing mothers, the drug of second choice would be 10 percent crotamiton cream (Eurax). I recommend that it be applied to the entire skin surface daily on 2 consecutive days and that a final cleansing bath be taken 24 to 48 hours after the last application. The patient is instructed about the individual control measures already noted. Crotamiton cream may be slightly irritating, especially to denuded skin. The drug is reputed to have independent antipruritic properties, but I am not impressed. The efficacy in adults is satisfactory but less than with lindane. In children studies have shown much less efficacy, with cure rates of 70 percent following five consecutive daily applications. Human toxicity data are not well established, and along with other scabicides, its safety in pregnancy has not been substantiated.

Because of the incomplete efficacy of crotamiton in young children, some experts prefer 6 percent precipitated sulfur in petrolatum, which is applied nightly for 3 nights accompanied by a bath prior to each new application. The treatment is messy, causes staining, and has an unpleasant odor. I have had no personal experience with this form of treatment, whose safety and efficacy profile are not known.

Benzyl benzoate (20 to 35 percent) is no longer used in this country and is not commercially available. Because it is inexpensive and relatively nontoxic when topically applied, it is often widely used to eradicate scabies in endemic areas of underdeveloped countries.

On the Horizon. As of this writing, there appears to be a new scabicide on the horizon as effective as lindane, with none of its neurotoxicity. The drug is a synthetic pyrethroid called permethrin and will be available as a 5 percent cream. It is cosmetically elegant and easy to use, has no objectionable odor, and does not stain clothing. Despite a 2 percent incidence of percutaneous absorption, the drug is rapidly broken down by esterases in the skin and excreted in the urine. Its major advantages will be very low mammalian toxicity and an efficacy of over 90 percent. Since not all synthetic pyrethroids exhibit the same degree of safety and stability as permethrin, and since the drug has been used in limited situations in this country, sweeping generalizations about its safety and efficacy in broad clinical use await further study. A 1 percent permethrin cream rinse (Nix) for the treatment of head lice was approved by the FDA in 1986.

Scabies in Institutions

I have had considerable experience in handling several nursing home epidemics of scabies in the last few years, and some principles of management have become clear to me. In the first place, the presence of an epidemic is not often apparent. Many of the usually elderly, debilitated, and bedridden patients who had been diagnosed by the dermatologist-consultant as having psoriasis, eczema, exfoliative dermatitis, or drug eruptions have proved to have crusted ("Norwegian") scabies. Alternatively the nursing home personnel most likely to contract scabies

(any "hands-on" employee) develop modified or atypical disease despite adequate time for development of a full blown picture and thus are not readily recognized as scabies victims. Be assured that by the time it becomes clear that there is a problem in the home, it is far more extensive than meets the eye.

Crusted scabies is associated with myriad mites and is highly contagious. Fomite control therefore becomes a major focus of the therapeutic regimen and calls for swift and aggressive action to eradicate every last mite. The cooperation of administration, professional staff, nursing personnel, housekeeping personnel, volunteers, and visitors is essential for success. In general, efforts should be directed along several avenues: treatment of actual skin disease in both staff and patients, containment of the epidemic by physical and administrative measures, and employee-patient education through inservice discussions, handouts, and memos.

If there is a clustering of cases on one ward or floor, all the employees and all the patients on that floor are to be treated. Be sure to identify "floaters" who have spent some time on the affected ward in the preceding 2 months, especially if they have had any direct physical patient contact. Also note any recent transfers of patients from that floor to other areas within the institution. The treatments of staff and patients should be synchronized so as to prevent cross infestation. Each staff member should receive treatment as outlined in the foregoing discussion, with lindane supplied by the institution. The treatment of the ward patients is not as easily accomplished and must be organized to ensure thoroughness and prevent reinfestation. Be prepared for treatment failures.

The ward must be quarantined, and mobility for patients, staff, volunteers, and visitors must be restricted. Standard infection control procedures using "gown and glove" techniques must be instituted, and meals should be served on disposable trays. Treatment teams are mobilized and educated about the proper application of a scabicide. The patients are bathed and treated over the entire body, including the scalp and especially under the fingernails with a toothbrush. All patients should then be restricted to bed for 24 hours while the rooms and wheelchairs are cleaned and wheelchair cushions changed. One day later—24 hour application is logistically rational in a nursing home—the patients should be given cleansing tub baths, and while they are being bathed, linens and pajamas should be changed and the beds cleaned. Articles of personal clothing should be bagged and given to family members for cleaning, while soiled linen and bedclothes are bagged before being removed from the floor. Restriction on "floating" onto or off the ward for at least 3 weeks must be strictly maintained, as should the continuation of "gown and glove" techniques. Frequent handwashing should be encouraged. Visitors and volunteers should be screened before returning to the floor several days later.

In my experience it is crucial that the entire treatment protocol for the ward patients be repeated in 1 week. Others have suggested that lindane is not as effective in nursing home epidemics. In my opinion this is because thoroughness of treatment is not stressed and not because it is inherently ineffective. Since most elderly debilitated patients already lack an effective immune response, aggressive measures to combat even one undetected mite seem warranted.

Three weeks after the onset of treatment, and in 3-week cycles thereafter if needed, a critical re-evaluation of the patients must be made, paying careful attention to fresh lesions, especially at the sites of predilection. If the treatment has been successful, older lesions will already have crusted and healed by then, and thus any new suspicious clinical lesions should be considered to be recurrent scabies. All patients thus identified as treatment failures must be rerouted through the entire 3-week treatment cycle again, i.e., lindane on days 21 and 28, and restricted to their rooms. It may be useful to cluster the treatment failures in one subsection of the ward and quarantine that area only. All personnel should continue to maintain a high index of suspicion when any patient presents with a pruritic papulovesicular and scaly eruption.

PEDICULOSIS

Head Lice (Pediculosis Capitis)

Each year nearly three million Americans, most of them children, are infested with head lice. The majority of these cases are probably never seen by the dermatologist, being diagnosed and managed by the school nurse and the family doctor, respectively. It is a major problem in urban and suburban school districts among young school age children and is transmitted by direct person to person contact as well as through fomites on combs and brushes, towels, bed linens, and hats. Communal use of these types of products should be discouraged. It is no longer necessary to shave the hair unless it is densely matted.

There are a number of specific drugs for the treatment of head lice that are safe and effective. In general there is no toxicity associated with any of the drugs used, probably because they are applied to a limited area (the scalp) and left on for a short period of time. Mild side effects would include minor irritant dermatitis. After treatment the remaining nits (those not washed off by the shampoo) may be removed with forceps or a fine toothed comb ("nit comb"); often this is included in the lice treatment package kit. As a rule the child may return to school the day after this treatment, since it is not necessary to remove the dead nits. However, some school officials have been hesitant and require that the nits be at least one-quarter inch away from the scalp, indicative of no recrudescence of the disease. It is prudent to treat the other children in the household regardless of whether they are infested. Antibiotics may be required if secondary infection is present. All adults should at least be examined and treated accordingly.

Heat (wet or dry) applied to fomites is a very effective louse and nit killer. Personal articles of clothing and bed linens should be laundered in hot water and dried in a hot cycle. Nonwashables may be drycleaned (coats, hats, scarves, and sweaters); combs and brushes can be washed in hot water (130° F for 20 minutes). There are a number of synergized pyrethrin sprays available to kill lice and nits on contact on furniture, mattresses, carpets, and other non-launderable objects in the home. Although lice can survive off the host for approximately 2 days, nits die immediately. The potential for reinfestation from these sources is therefore more theoretical than real, and sprays are not indicated for pediculosis capitis.

Lindane

The 1 percent lindane shampoo is used extensively in this disease. One or 2 tablespoonfuls of the undiluted shampoo is thoroughly massaged into the scalp, left on for 5 to 10 minutes, lathered with warm water, and rinsed. Because there is some debate as to the ovicidal properties of lindane, repeat shampooing may be recommended in 5 to 7 days, but never sooner.

Malathion

Malathion, 0.5 percent lotion (Prioderm), is reported to be safe and effective in the treatment of head lice and is ovicidal as well. It is applied to the scalp, allowed to dry for 8 to 12 hours, and then shampooed out. It has not been used much since its introduction into this country in 1982. Like lindane, it requires a prescription.

Pyrethrins

Synergized pyrethrins are the main ingredient in the over the counter pediculocides (RID, A-200, Cuprex, Pronto) used in this country. They are mixed with piperonyl butoxide to potentiate the insecticidal effects. They should be applied undiluted until the scalp is entirely wet and allowed to remain on the area for 10 minutes. Then the scalp is thoroughly washed with warm water and soap, shampooed, rinsed, and dried. As with lindane, the treatment may need to be repeated in 5 to 7 days.

Permethrin, 1 percent cream rinse (Nix), is a new synthetic pyrethrin treatment for head lice, as alluded to earlier. According to the manufacturer it kills both lice and nits for up to 14 days with a single application because it is retained on the hair even with normal shampooing.

Pubic Lice (Pediculosis Pubis)

In general, pediculosis pubis ("crabs") is treated in much the same way as pediculosis capitis. The preparation is applied to the infested and adjacent hairy areas, with particular attention to the pubic mons and perianal area. In hairy individuals application should include the thighs, trunk, and axillary areas because of frequent involvement of these sites. Failure to do so will result in treatment failure in hairy individuals. All sexual contacts must be treated simultaneously, but other household members need not be treated. Clothing and linens should be hot washed and dried.

Lindane lotion is more widely used than lindane shampoo. The lotion is left on for 12 to 24 hours, followed by a thorough washing and removal of the remaining nits.

Treatment may need to be repeated in 1 week. When compared with lindane, the synergized pyrethrins produce comparable results in patients with pubic lice. Other than irritation, side effects are nonexistent.

Nits on the eyelashes are caused by pubic lice and not head lice. The usual specific drugs for lice are too irritating to be used on the eyelashes. A safe, simple, effective, and virtually nontoxic regimen consists of using petrolatum applied thickly to the eyelashes with a cotton swab or with the tips of the fingers several times a day for several days. Any nits that do not slip off spontaneously may then be removed mechanically with forceps.

Body Lice (Pediculosis Corporis)

Body lice are rarely found on the individual and then only in heavily infested persons. The louse feeds on the human host while clinging to the seams of clothing, particularly in the axilla, collar, and waistband areas. Lesions seen include linear crusted papules, numerous excoriations, and frequent secondary hyperpigmentation and bacterial infection. Lindane lotion may be used when nits on body hairs are present, but this is usually not necessary. Treatment should be directed toward "vagabondiosis" and should include proper hygiene, bathing, clean clothing and bedding, and proper nutrition. Outer garments must be dry cleaned or pressed, especially along the seams, with a hot iron. Specific therapy should include oral antibiotic therapy, antihistamines, and topical antipruritic therapy, e.g., calamine or pramoxine, or topical corticosteroid therapy.

INSECT BITES

Insect bites generally produce relatively minor skin changes, although the local response to some insect stings, as from bees, wasps, and fire ants, includes fierce burning, swelling, redness, and itching and often may be quite intense. Most of the time it is not possible to identify the culprit from the cutaneous reaction pattern. Mosquitoes produce small erythematous urticarial papules scattered diffusely on exposed sites, whereas chiggers produce similar findings although mostly on the ankles and legs.

Minor Reactions

In general these minor reactions need no treatment. The patient should be told to wash the sting site with soap and water. Ice packs bring some relief. I have tried applying a paste hurriedly made with Adolf's meat tenderizer, as others have suggested (presumably the papain enzymatically digests the venom), but the relief is not earth shattering. Since the reaction lasts for a few days, treatment should be directed against preventing patients from scratching and secondarily infecting the bites. This is especially important, but not easily done, in children. Cooling shake lotions, e.g., calamine, along with oral antihistamine therapy may be helpful. The use of preparations containing topically applied antihistamines (e.g., Caladryl) or "-caines" (e.g., Lanacaine) should be strongly discouraged

because of the high sensitization potential of these products.

Major Reactions

More significant reactions include the extensive dermal necrosis seen with brown recluse spider bites, systemic neuromuscular paralysis seen with black widow spider bites, and generalized allergic anaphylaxis from bee, wasp, and hornet stings. Treatment of the brown recluse spider bite with local or systemic steroid therapy, heparin, or early surgical excision often produces unsatisfactory results. Like the bite of the black widow, it is most effectively treated with specific antivenom when available. Neuromuscular paralysis and circulatory collapse require prompt and aggressive medical attention.

Anaphylaxis or anaphylactoid reactions usually require intravenous epinephrine therapy, parenteral doses of antihistamines, and the systemic use of steroids. Ice packs, compresses, cooling metholated lotions, systemic analgesic therapy, and oral doses of corticosteroids are used for local stings, depending on the severity of the clinical picture. Desensitization is useful for generalized reactions but not for localized ones. The desensitization procedure should be followed by periodic radioallergosorbent (RAST) or skin testing to help determine the duration of desensitization therapy.

Fleas

Flea collars for pets control light infestations, but a heavy infestation requires treatment of the home, pets, and the yard. The various indoor flea control "bombs" (or aerosol spray cans) contain varying combinations of pyrethrin, rotenone, malathion, carbaryl, or methoprene. Professional exterminators and the local veterinarian can provide invaluable advice for a lingering problem.

Prophylaxis

By far the best therapy is prevention. Susceptible individuals or those who must work outdoors should use potent insect repellents. The most effective action ingredient is diethyltoluamide (DEET), which is present in varying concentrations in different products.

In addition, avoid perfume and scented soaps. When picnicking, keep food covered and pack leftovers promptly. Dispose of trash in closed receptacles. To avoid stings, wear shoes and socks outdoors. Cover as much of the exposed parts of the body as possible. Do not wear bright colors, prints, or loose clothing that might brush against insects.

Stay away from spider webs around trees, bushes, outhouses, outdoor lighting fixtures, waste cans, and junk piles. Cleaning out attics and garages, old clothes, boxes, and woodpiles and plugging up cracks and crevices greatly help in discouraging infestation by the brown recluse spider.

BACTERIAL INFECTIONS

ROBERT M. TAYLOR, M.D.

Cutaneous bacterial infections occur when there is loss of the natural barrier function of the skin. Primary infections arise within minor cuts or hair follicles in otherwise normal skin. Secondary infection occurs within the context of pre-existing dermatitis such as atopic dermatitis in which the cutaneous barrier is severely compromised. The majority of cases of cutaneous bacterial infection are caused by gram positive cocci—*Staphylococcus aureus* and group A beta hemolytic *Streptococcus pyogenes*. Most of the therapeutic discussion in this article centers on these two organisms and the superficial pyodermas and cellulitides that they cause. Brief consideration is given to the gram positive *Corynebacterium* species and the gram negative bacteria, including *Pseudomonas aeruginosa*. A brief description of the disease entities is followed by a detailed discussion of therapeutics.

STREPTOCOCCUS PYOGENES

Impetigo

The classic lesion of nonbullous impetigo consists of a small erythematous vesicle, which rapidly breaks down and becomes covered by an abundant golden crust. Autoinoculation from one site to another is the major cause of spread of the organism. When cultured, about 40 percent of the lesions grow *S. pyogenes*, an additional 50 percent being a mixture of *S. pyogenes* and *Staphylococcus aureus*. Approximately 10 percent are caused by *S. aureus* alone. In the mixed infections *S. aureus* appears to play a minor role, apparently representing simple colonization without true infection.

The approach to therapy is twofold: topical and systemic. Topical treatment includes lukewarm normal saline compresses (1 teaspoon of table salt in 2 cups of water) to remove crusts followed by the topical application of bacitracin ointment. Compresses as well as routine cleansing of the skin should be done with disposable paper towels to avoid autoinoculation and spread to other family members. Crusts should not be forcibly removed because avulsion of underlying dermal tissue may result in scarring. Oral antibiotic treatment of impetigo is controversial, but I believe its use to be justified because of the established risk of acute glomerulonephritis following skin infection with a nephritogenic serotype of group A *Streptococcus*.

Penicillin is the drug of choice. It can be given by mouth over a 10 day period at a dosage of 25,000 to 90,000 units per kilogram per day for infants and small children in 6 hour divided increments, and 250 mg every 6 hours for adults and children over 12 years of age. If one's preference is injectable penicillin, long acting benzathine penicillin is given in one injection—300,000 to 600,000 units for infants and children weighing less than 60 pounds, 900,000 units for older children, and 1,200,000

units for adults. Defining "older children" (PDR's designation) is somewhat difficult, and my preference is to use an arbitrary weight designation: 61 to 88 pounds means an older child and 88 pounds and up means an adult. For penicillin sensitive patients erythromycin may be given orally over a 10 day period in the following manner: 30 to 50 mg per kilogram per day in 6 hour divided increments for children and 250 mg every 6 hours for adults.

Cellulitis

Streptococcal cellulitis is a poorly defined, rapidly spreading, hot, painful, erythematous, indurated lesion, which may be accompanied by systemic symptoms of chills, fever, and malaise. It may arise via a puncture wound or within an area of dermatitis; e.g., tinea pedis, stasis ulcer. Erysipelas is a clinically specific type of cellulitis whose lesion is bright red and indurated and (unlike the usual acute cellulitis) has a sharply defined, elevated border. Systemic symptoms are the rule and the patient is quite ill with a high fever.

Most cases of streptococcal cellulitis that I have encountered can be treated with the usual dosages of penicillin or erythromycin as outlined in the impetigo section. For expansive forms of either cellulitis or erysipelas, hospitalization is indicated, and aqueous penicillin G should be given parenterally at a dosage of 600,000 to 2,000,000 units every 6 hours. Local therapy consists of applying soothing normal saline compresses over the involved areas. If blister formation occurs concomitantly with the cellulitis, normal saline compresses for drying and dressings consisting of bacitracin ointment, Telfa pads, and Kerlix wrap are optimal. Bed rest is recommended to prevent trauma to the infection site and to help the patient through the acute phases of infection.

Ecthyma

Streptococcal ecthyma begins as a superficial pyoderma similar to impetigo, but subsequently involves deeper dermal tissues, producing necrosis and a superficial ulcer. Causative factors include minor trauma and poor hygiene.

Topical therapy for ecthyma consists of the application of normal saline compresses and topical dressings consisting of bacitracin, Telfa pads, and Kerlix. Gentle debridement of the ulcer base is carried out only as needed. Systemic therapy (oral or parenteral) is the same as that outlined for impetigo except that the duration of therapy is 2 weeks.

One final comment about topical antibiotic therapy. Bacitracin is an occasional sensitizer, most probably because of its "coreacting" with neomycin in preparations containing both compounds. Erythromycin ointment is a rare sensitizer but is no longer commercially manufactured except as an ophthalmic preparation. In a recently published article on contact dermatitis,[*] a topical erythromycin formulation was recommended for those not wishing

---

* Adams R&M, Fisher AA. Contact allergen alternatives: 1980. J Am Acad Dermatol 1986; 14:951–969.

to use bacitracin. The formula is as follows:

> Erythromycin powder, 0.6 g (incorporated into mineral oil)
>
> Petrolatum q.s. ad 60.0 g
>
> Shelf life: indefinite

The powder can be purchased from the following companies: Pharma-Tek (Huntington, NY) and Paddock (Minneapolis, MN).

STAPHYLOCOCCUS AUREUS

Impetigo

About 10 percent of the cases of nonbullous impetigo are caused by coagulase positive *S. aureus*. The lesion is identical to that produced by *S. pyogenes*, the possible exception being that the lesions caused by *S. aureus* may last for a shorter time, requiring less than 2 weeks to resolve. Bullous impetigo, on the other hand, is caused by phage group II staphylococci and is characterized by yellow, turbid bullae arising on normal appearing skin.

Unlike *S. pyogenes*, which is highly susceptible to penicillin, *S. aureus* is not. In fact a high percentage of *S. aureus* organisms are penicillinase producing, and if one considers *S. aureus* as the pathogen, penicillinase resistant semisynthetic penicillins should be used (e.g., cloxacillin, dicloxacillin). Erythromycin is somewhat more difficult to evaluate. In a hospital based patient population I prefer the semisynthetic penicillins rather than erythromycin; the pathogenic staphylococci acquired in hospitals are frequently penicillinase producing and resistant to a variety of antibiotics.

Cultures with antibiotic sensitivity determinations should be carried out in cases of both nonbullous and bullous impetigo in hospital based patients. For non-hospitalized patients in an office setting when *S. aureus* is suspected as the cause of nonbullous impetigo, I obtain a culture and sensitivity determination and begin systemic treatment with erythromycin as outlined for streptococcal impetigo. When there is a greater suspicion of *S. aureus* as the cause of nonbullous impetigo (i.e., a history of chronic recurrent pustular folliculitis, furunculosis, or carbunculosis), I treat in the same manner as for bullous impetigo: culture and sensitivity tests and a 10 day course of semisynthetic penicillin (dicloxacillin or cloxacillin). Systemic treatment is given as follows: dicloxacillin, 12.5 mg per kilogram per day, is given in divided doses at 6 hour increments for patients weighing less than 40 kg (88 pounds), and 125 mg is given every 6 hours for adults. Cloxacillin, 50 mg per kilogram per day, is given in divided doses at 6 hour increments for patients weighing less than 20 kg (44 pounds) and 250 mg every 6 hours for adults. For penicillin allergic patients, erythromycin is given as outlined in the *S. pyogenes* section on impetigo. For erythromycin resistant *S. aureus*, clindamycin or cephalothin is a possibility. With the latter there is a 10 percent risk of cross reactivity with penicillin. Topical therapy is the same as that outlined for impetigo.

Folliculitis

Bacterial infection of hair follicles can be superficial (Bockhart's impetigo) or deep (furuncle or carbuncle). Unlike the spreading character of streptococcal infections, follicular infections secondary to *S. aureus* remain relatively localized and are pustular rather than vesiculobullous. Recurrence may be a frequent problem in some patients, and search for the bacterial reservoir is important (nose, axillae, perineum).

After culture of the lesions, topical therapy for all forms of folliculitis consists of the application of warm normal saline compresses (1 teaspoon of table salt in 2 cups of tap water) followed by the topical application of bacitracin or erythromycin ointment and sterile absorbent gauze dressings. Incision and drainage are particularly helpful to relieve the pressure and pain often experienced with furunculosis and carbunculosis. Use of a number 11 blade with its sharp tapered end is best, and a small (2 to 4 mm) rather than lengthy incision is preferable in an attempt to prevent unsightly scarring. Moreover, the timing of incision and drainage is important, optimal drainage occurring as the lesion "points" (the papule or nodule becomes more conical than spherical). It is important to contain the purulence within the dressings, since auto-infectivity is possible in peripheral skin, especially as it becomes macerated from the suppurative fluid. Careful attention also should be given to cleansing of the hands after handling lesions or dressings and to the washing of all garments in contact with the skin in order to prevent further spread of the bacteria. This is especially true for patients with dermatoses such as atopic dermatitis and contact dermatitis. Patients with pre-existing dermatoses should receive appropriate care, including topical steroid therapy in order to prevent further colonization and subsequent infection by *S. aureus*. Fingernail trimming may be necessary in chronic scratchers to prevent the accumulation of bacteria laden debris under the nails, which may result in autoinoculation and infection.

Since clindamycin is often effective against *S. aureus*, I generally use Cleocin T topically twice or three times daily for very early lesions, such as superficial pustular folliculitis. The alcohol vehicle dries the skin and the antibiotic and alcohol are bactericidal. With nodular furunculosis or carbunculosis, systemic treatment is preferable after initial culture. I generally begin with a semisynthetic penicillinase resistant penicillin (dicloxacillin, 12.5 mg per kilogram per day in 6 hour, equally divided doses for children weighing less than 40 kg (88 pounds) and 125 to 250 mg every 6 hours for adults; cloxacillin, 50 mg per kilogram per day, is given in 6 hour, equally divided doses for children weighing less than 20 kg (44 pounds) and 250 mg every 4 to 6 hours for adults. For penicillin sensitive patients, I begin with erythromycin, 30 to 50 mg per kilogram per day, every 6 hours in equally divided doses in children up to 23 kg (50 pounds) and 250 to 500 mg every 6 hours for adults. If the organism is resistant to erythromycin, I consider oral therapy with cephalothin or clindamycin.

One comment should be made about patients who are carriers of *S. aureus*. Reservoirs for the pathogenic staphylococci may be found in the nose, axillae, or perineum. In patients who have chronic recurrent *S. aureus* folliculitis, culture of these potential reservoir areas should be done to determine whether the patient is carrying a nidus for recurrent staphylococcal infection. If so, suppression of colonization may be achieved with the topical application of bacitracin or erythromycin ointment. If successful, this method results in a decreased incidence of autoinoculation and infection by substantively reducing the number of bacteria.

PSEUDOMONAS AERUGINOSA

Gram Negative Folliculitis

Hot tub folliculitis is found as both superficial and deep necrotizing folliculitis, which frequently has been associated with *Pseudomonas aeruginosa*. Infrequently *Pseudomonas* otitis externa is associated with the folliculitis. Biopsy of a lesion for culture reveals the causative organism.

Treatment is twofold: correction of the cause of overgrowth of *Pseudomonas* and topical supportive therapy. In general, pools or hot tubs are conducive to *Pseudomonas aeruginosa* growth because of incorrect chlorine concentrations and pH levels. Ideally the pH should be 7.5, with a range of 7.2 to 7.8. The free chlorine content should be 1.0 to 1.5 parts per million with a range of 1.0 to 3.0 parts per million. Topical therapy for this self-limited disease consists of cool to lukewarm 0.25 percent acetic acid (vinegar) compresses (1 ounce of vinegar in 2 cups of water) applied every 20 minutes to affected areas followed by the topical application of Garamycin cream. In point of fact if nothing were done, most cases would clear within 7 to 14 days.

Other Causes of Gram Negative Folliculitis

A brief comment should be made about gram negative folliculitis secondary to other organisms (*Klebsiella, Escherichia, Serratia, Proteus*). Patients with acne treated with systemic antibiotic therapy (most commonly tetracycline) may develop a sudden onset of superficial folliculitis or nodulocystic lesions. The aforementioned organisms are frequently cultured from the superficial pustular component of the folliculitis. Treatment has been twofold: discontinuation of the long-term systemic antibiotic treatment and substitution of ampicillin (250 mg four times daily) or trimethoprim-sulfamethoxazole (2 tablets every 12 hours or, if using the DS form, 1 tablet every 12 hours). Therapy should be continued for 10 to 14 days after the cysts and pustules have disappeared.

CORYNEBACTERIUM INFECTIONS

Erythrasma and Trichomycosis Axillaris

Both erythrasma and trichomycosis axillaris are caused by *Corynebacterium* species, which are gram positive bacilli. In erythrasma a red, scaly, slightly wrinkled, configurate eruption occurs between toe webs and in the groin or axillae. In trichomycosis axillaris yellow, red, or black encrustations of the hairs occur in the axillae. This infection of the axillary hairs is often accompanied by an offensive body odor.

Shaving or clipping of the axillary hairs in trichomycosis axillaris is essential because the infection does not extend beneath the skin surface. In both trichomycosis axillaris and erythrasma I prescribe an erythromycin lotion topically twice daily (ATS, Staticin, Erymax) and erythromycin, 250 mg orally four times daily or 500 mg twice daily for 7 days.

LEPROSY

THOMAS H. REA, M.D.

Leprosy (Hansen's Disease) is a chronic granulomatous infection caused by *Mycobacterium leprae*. A definitive diagnosis is not possible without demonstration of acid fast bacilli or a neurologic deficit. Two kinds of phenomena in leprosy indicate the need for medical management: the infection itself requires antibacillary therapy, and the reactional states, if present, may warrant anti-inflammatory measures.

For the purpose of this discussion the granulomatous spectrum of leprosy is grouped into two broad segments, "paucibacillary" (the tuberculoid and borderline tuberculoid classes whose bacilli are difficult to demonstrate) and "multibacillary" (the borderline, borderline lepromatous, and lepromatous classes whose bacilli are easily found). Because most patients with paucibacillary leprosy are borderline tuberculoid in classification and self-healing is not reliable (as it is in true polar tuberculoid disease), antibacterial therapy is necessary. Dapsone (diaminodiphenylsulfone), 100 mg daily, is recommended for a period of 5 years. Multiple drug regimens are advocated by some physicians to reduce the time span or cost of therapy. This approach has not been proven to be either better than or equal in efficacy to that of dapsone alone.

Multibacillary disease requires therapy for life (triple drug therapy is being tried as a curative; the results of this experiment will not be known for years). At present combination chemotherapy is widely recommended, although there is no direct evidence that combination therapy is superior to dapsone monotherapy. The rationale for combination therapy comes by analogy to the treatment of tuberculosis (emergence of leprosy bacilli resistant to dapsone). As a practical matter, the unproven benefits of combination chemotherapy must be weighed against the uncertain risks of possibly more toxic multiple drug regimens. In addition, in the United States today the clinician who decides that he will treat all multibacillary disease with combination chemotherapy is conducting an experiment, because such an approach, however widely recommended, is not FDA approved. To pursue such a course the physician, according to the rules, must secure permission from an institutional review board and have the patient sign an informed consent form before proceeding.

In our clinic we select dapsone monotherapy or combination chemotherapy following complete evaluation of each patient. In particular, we consider the exact classification, bacillary load, age, and occupation. If dapsone monotherapy is chosen, 100 mg daily is recommended. If combination chemotherapy is elected, 600 mg rifampin in a single daily dose for 3 years and 100 mg of dapsone daily for life are recommended.

The erythrocyte glucose-6-phosphate dehydrogenase level is routinely evaluated and determined to be normal before beginning dapsone therapy. Because the dapsone syndrome (an infectious mononucleosis-like drug reaction) although rare, is potentially fatal, dapsone therapy is begun at a dosage of 25 mg daily and is increased in increments of 25 mg each week in conjunction with weekly clinic visits until a dosage of 100 mg daily is reached. With this schedule we have seen a few morbilliform eruptions associated with fever and malaise of moderate severity but, to date, no fatal cases.

After 4 to 6 weeks of dapsone therapy, when the danger of the dapsone syndrome has become remote, a moderate fall in the hematocrit level is to be anticipated. By virtue of a direct membrane effect, dapsone produces a hemolytic anemia, usually well compensated. Modest falls in the hematocrit level to 30 mm are not rare. Among lepromatous patients, in whom anemia of chronic disease is common, interpretation may be difficult. Falls in the hematocrit to levels below 30 mm do occur from time to time and warrant reduction in the dosage of dapsone to 50 mg per day. True idiosyncratic hemolysis from dapsone is rare.

Having avoided glucose-6-phosphate dehydrogenase deficiency, the dapsone syndrome, and hemolytic anemia, the patient may experience peripheral neuropathy months to years after the beginning of dapsone therapy. In diagnosis the differentiation of dapsone associated neuropathy from neuritis due to leprosy may be difficult. Furthermore, improvement following the cessation of dapsone therapy may take many months.

The most common serious side effect of rifampin therapy is hepatotoxicity. If liver function test results are abnormal before its use, rifampin should be administered only with great caution. We routinely monitor liver function tests after 1, 3, and 7 weeks of therapy and every 3 months thereafter. Severe idiosyncratic hepatic reactions occurring after few doses are extremely rare but must be considered as a risk of rifampin therapy. Red urine is an alarming but banal consequence of rifampin therapy.

Clofazimine (B663, Lamprene) is an acceptable drug for monotherapy or for use in conjunction with dapsone or rifampin in combination chemotherapy. Because the drug darkens the skin, patient acceptance is poor, particularly in patients with borderline lepromatous and lepromatous leprosy in whom the drug accumulates in the widespread macrophages. At its usual dosage, 100 mg daily, gastrointestinal intolerance, dry skin, and acquired ichthyosis are, in decreasing order of frequency, encountered. In larger, anti-inflammatory doses, clofazimine crystals accumulate in mesenteric lymph nodes and in the mucosa and submucosa of the gut, producing a unique enteropathy.

The clinical response is the fundamental guide to the adequacy of therapy. The timetable for a response is highly variable. In addition, when determining the adequacy of the patient response to antibacterial therapy, the clinician should be aware of the changes that could be produced by a reactional state, requiring anti-inflammatory measures not a change in antibacillary medication.

Serial biopsies are also used to determine the response

to treatment. Favorable signs include fewer solid staining and more beaded organisms, a decrease in the number of bacilli, and involution of the granulomatous architecture.

The reactional states of leprosy do not have analogous or parallel syndromes in common diseases and therefore may be conceptually difficult to grasp. The difficulty in managing reactional states and their destructiveness to tissue justify leprology as a clinical specialty and, if available, warrant the referral of patients to physicians skilled in leprosy diagnosis and management.

Erythema nodosum leprosum, a syndrome of unproven pathogenesis, occurs in over one-half the lepromatous patients under treatment, most often within 1 year after the institution of chemotherapy. A minority of lepromatous patients may present with erythema nodosum leprosum as the initial manifestation of their disease. Erythema nodosum leprosum is also not rare in borderline lepromatous individuals. Clinically this syndrome is characterized by painful tender subcutaneous and dermal nodules, fever, chills, and malaise. Arthritis, neuritis, iritis, and orchitis also may occur. Neutrophilic leukocytosis and a high sedimentation rate are the rule. Histologically a lepromatous infiltrate with the addition of neutrophils and abundant lymphocytes is characteristic.

Thalidomide is an excellent therapeutic drug, but because of its teratogenicity is contraindicated in fertile women. Most patients respond well to oral doses of 100 to 200 mg at bedtime, although an increased dosage is occasionally required. Few patients require the use of a second anti-inflammatory drug, such as glucocorticoids. In women of child bearing potential who should not receive the thalidomide, we usually begin treatment with 40 mg of prednisone administered orally daily in the morning or 40 mg of triamcinolone intramuscularly given weekly. Alternate day administration of prednisone has been disappointing. Clofazimine in the long term has anti-inflammatory properties, but large dosages (200 to 300 mg daily) are required. Clofazimine may be administered for several months before a clinical response is evident. Generally the absence of systemic symptoms is the best guide to adequate therapy, a few active local lesions being well tolerated.

Peripheral neuropathy, so commonly reported when thalidomide is used for conditions other than erythema nodosum leprosum, is unusual in the latter disorder; perhaps one peripheral neuropathy protects against another, or perhaps one is difficult to detect on the background of another. Rarely patients are prohibitively sedated by thalidomide.

Lucio's reaction, characterized by hemorrhagic infarcts evolving into ulcers, occurs in patients from Mexico and Central America with diffuse non-nodular lepromatous leprosy, the pure and primative diffuse lepromatosis of Latapi. Histologically the lesions are ischemic infarcts secondary to profound endothelial proliferation, with or without thrombosis, in the deep dermal vessels.

In our experience, which has been restricted to mild cases, the Lucio reaction may worsen with dapsone monotherapy, but to date new lesions have promptly ceased in association with rifampin therapy.

Reversal reactions putatively a delayed type of hypersensitivity response, have no uniformly accepted nomenclature. The term reversal implies that the patient moves or has the potential of moving from a posture of less resistance to one of more resistance, but the actuality of such a move is not a prerequisite to the diagnosis. In reversal reactions, formerly torpid lesions become tumid and new lesions appear rapidly; there may be an abrupt onset of neuritis and nerve trunk palsies. Iritis may occur. In our clinic approximately two thirds of the patients with reversal reactions present because of the reaction. The rest develop the reaction after the beginning of chemotherapy. The histologic changes associated with reversal reactions are not consistent and include edema within granulomas, the presence of foreign body giant cells, and desmoplasia of connective tissue.

Reversal reactions are usually amenable to 40 mg of prednisone given daily. If skin alone is involved, reversal reactions in most patients after several weeks can be managed with alternate day doses of 20 to 30 mg, with the need for anti-inflammatory therapy tapering off gradually over a 3- to 12-month period. Neuritic reactions are more difficult to manage, because they are less responsive to an alternate day regimen and often require therapy for more than 1 year. Decreased symptoms and the absence of nerve tenderness are the best guides to adequate therapy.

Ocular involvement may occur in the reactional states or as part of uncomplicated granulomatous infection. In either event management by an ophthamologist is essential.

After the first few years of drug therapy, the most common difficult problem is the management of changes secondary to neurologic deficits, in particular, contractures and trophic changes in the hands and feet. Loss of pain perception (insensitivity) leads to tissue injury, secondary infection, and further tissue destruction. Few such cycles are required to significantly impair hand and foot function, a distressingly common event but one that under optimal circumstances should be preventable. Thus, the cadre of health care professionals required to give good care for patients with Hansen's disease is large and includes orthopaedic surgeons, hand surgeons, and podiatrists, in addition to ophthalmologists, neurologists, and physical medicine and rehabilitation professionals.

A network of regional Hansen's Disease centers has been established under the sponsorship of the National Program for Hansen's Disease in Carville, Louisiana. These centers offer complete care for Hansen's Disease and its complications without charge to the patient. Assistance in evaluation for suspected Hansen's disease and examination of contacts are also performed without charge. Because of the complexities of management, whenever practical, referral of patients diagnosed with Hansen's disease to a regional center is strongly recommended. Because the patients are often poor, their receipt of care and medication without cost helps to ameliorate at least one of the burdens imposed by this potentially devastating illness. This program is no farther away than the telephone; the toll free number (1-800-642-2477) connects one to the central office.

ATYPICAL MYCOBACTERIAL INFECTIONS

REGINA ANDERSON, M.D.

Nontuberculous (atypical) mycobacterial infections in man are unusual, yet many of the offending organisms are ubiquitous. The Runyon classification divides the organisms into four groups, based on their rate of growth and pigment formation in culture (Table 1). The pathogenic organisms responsible for cutaneous infections are included in the table, but it should be noted that the supposed nonpathogens may also cause infections, particularly in immune compromised hosts.

The spectrum of cutaneous lesions is diverse. The primary lesion may be an erythematous nodule, an ulcerated plaque, or an abscess that is sterile on routine bacteriologic culture. Trauma is often a causative factor, and therefore the lesions commonly occur over the bony prominences of the hands, elbows, and knees. The patient is typically afebrile, and there are no associated systemic signs or symptoms. The presentation in the immune compromised host can be decidedly different; these individuals develop rapid local progression or dissemination of the disease process.

The diagnosis of these infections is based on a strong clinical suspicion of an infectious process, coupled with a negative bacteriologic culture and a histologic picture of noncaseating granuloma. A skin specimen for mycobacterial culture should be obtained and sent to a laboratory service (such as a state board of health) that can culture and specify atypical mycobacterial organisms. The Lowenstein-Jensen culture medium is used preferably. Light and temperature conditions must be closely controlled, as indicated in Table 1, and biochemical testing as well as microscopic morphology and phage typing also yields useful information in organism identification. Since the atypical mycobacteria have varying degrees of resistance to the antituberculous drugs, susceptibilities are routinely determined when a pathogen is identified.

THERAPY: GENERAL COMMENTS

Mycobacterium marinum not only is the most common infecting agent of the group I organisms, but it also is the most common cause of nontuberculous mycobacterial infections in nontropical countries. Infections from this organism are commonly associated with water related activities, such as exposure to fish tanks and swimming pools. A favorable response to treatment with antibacterial drugs is the rule. *Mycobacterium scrofulaceum*, from group II, causes cutaneous disease rarely and is much more often associated with lymphadenitis. Although resolution of the skin lesions may occur with antibacterial treatment, relapses occur and eradication often depends on antituberculous therapy. Skin infections produced by group III and group IV organisms also occur rarely, although they are being seen with increasing frequency in the immune deficiency states. Unfortunately these organisms are usually completely resistant to the antituberculous drugs and do not respond well to antibacterial drugs. Surgical debridement and excision therefore assume an important part of the therapeutic approach.

Because of its prevalence in tropical countries, the most common atypical mycobacterial infection in the world is due to *Mycobacterium ulcerans*. This organism produces a painless palpable subcutaneous swelling, which invades fascia and causes the development of a chronic necrotizing skin ulceration, known as the Buruli or Barksdale ulcer. Multiple modalities are recommended for the treatment of this condition. Local heat applied to the involved area (since the organism is very temperature sensitive and grows only between 30 and 33° C) and surgery with possible skin grafting are effective if done early in the course. These infections also respond poorly to both antituberculous and antibacterial therapy.

It should be emphasized that the mainstay of drug therapy for the atypical mycobacterial infections has been the antituberculous drugs. Because of their many complications and side effects, however, and the fact that weeks to months are required to identify and test the susceptibility of the specific organism, alternate therapies using antibacterial drugs have been developed. These drugs are recommended for use pending the results of microbial

TABLE 1 Runyon Classification

Group	Name	Pigment	Growth Rate	Temperature Requirements	Species Causing Cutaneous Disease
I	Photochromogens	Yellow with exposure to light	2–3 weeks	30° C 37° C	M. marinum M. kansasii
II	Scotochromogens	Yellow-orange in light and dark	2–3 weeks	37° C	M. scrofulaceum
III	Nonchromogens	No color	2–3 weeks	37° C 37° C	M. avium M. intracellulare
IV	Rapid growers	Variable	3–5 days	37° C 37° C	M. fortuitum M. cheloni
	Unclassified			30° C	M. ulcerans

sensitivity tests and are discussed here with respect to doses and adverse effects.

ANTIBACTERIAL THERAPY

When an atypical mycobacterial infection in nontropical countries is suspected, initial treatment (pending culture results) with minocycline (100 mg orally twice a day for 2 months) is recommended. It effectively eradicates *M. marinum* with minimal side effects. Dizziness and lightheadedness, which occasionally occur at the initiation of therapy, usually resolve with time. Later complications from extended minocycline usage include occasional permanent dentition staining, epidermal hyperpigmentation, and discoloration of various other tissues.

Other antibacterial drugs used for group I and group II organisms are tetracycline (500 mg orally four times daily for 2 months) and trimethoprim-sulfamethoxazole (160 mg-800 mg orally twice a day for 2 months). The adverse effects of these drugs include gastrointestinal intolerance and photosensitivity with tetracycline and the possibility of severe *E. multiforme* with trimethoprim-sulfamethoxazole.

Antibacterial therapy with erythromycin has been used in the treatment of infections in the *Mycobacterium avium-intracellular-scrofulaceum* (MAIS) complex, and doxycycline and amikacin have been used for infections due to *M. fortuitum* and *M. cheloni* with varying success.

The Buruli ulcer responds poorly to medical therapy, as noted previously. Clofazimine can be used and has been found to be effective when given in combination with antituberculous therapy. Undesirable side effects of clofazimine include a reddish discoloration of the skin and possible eosinophilic enteritis.

ANTITUBERCULOUS THERAPY

As noted previously, antituberculous drugs must be used for certain atypical mycobacterial infections that have not responded to the foregoing regimens. These drugs are classified into the bactericidal and bacteriostatic groups. The principles governing chemotherapy include the following:

1. Begin with multiple drug therapy. Select bactericidal drugs when possible. For group I and group II organisms, two drugs are adequate, whereas for group III and group IV organisms, four to six drugs are often necessary.
2. Give all drugs in full doses and administer treatment for an adequate period of time, i.e., 6 to 9 months for groups I and II and 12 to 18 months for groups III and IV.
3. Never add a single drug to a failing regimen. Select a new combination of drugs and give in full doses.

Unfortunately hypersensitivity reactions typified by fever, cutaneous eruptions, and hepatic and hematologic abnormalities occur frequently, especially when these drugs are used in combination. The patients must be monitored very closely.

The bactericidal drugs are isoniazid, rifampin, streptomycin, and pyrazinamide, which are all considered to be "first line" antituberculous drugs. The atypical mycobacteria are generally resistant to isoniazid (with the exception of *M. kansasii*); however, this drug can be effective when used in combination treatment. Of the remaining drugs, rifampin is the best choice and causes the least number of side effects. It does give the bodily secretion a reddish discoloration, and patients must be forewarned of this effect. Drug interactions can cause major problems. Rifampin is a potent inducer of hepatic microsomal enzymes and can result in the acceleration of metabolism of digoxin, quinidine, ketoconazole, and coumadin. It also enhances the catabolism of steroids and can cause a decrease in the effectiveness of orally administered contraceptives. Isoniazid, on the other hand, inhibits the parahydroxylation process and can produce phenytoin (dilantin) toxicity. Isoniazid also causes peripheral neuritis, which is avoidable with the concurrent administration of pyridoxine (100 mg per day). Table 2 outlines the appropri-

TABLE 2 Bactericidal Antituberculous Drugs

Drug	Route	Adult Dosage (mg/kg/day)	Side Effects	Major Complications	% Patients Developing Serious Adverse Effects
Isoniazid	PO, IM	5	Jaundice, arthritis, vasculitis	Chemical hepatitis, peripheral neuritis, toxic encephalopathy, drug induced systemic lupus erythematosus	5–7
Rifampin	PO	10	Gastrointestinal symptoms, flulike symptoms	Hepatitis, interstitial nephritis, hemolytic anemia	3–4
Streptomycin, kanamycin, capreomycin	IM	15–25	Nephrotoxicity	Neurotoxicity of VIII cranial nerve	8–10
Pyrazinamide	PO, divided doses	30	Gastrointestinal symptoms, hyperuricemia, dysuria, arthritis	Hepatitis, gout attacks	15

Adapted from Moschella SL, Hurley JH. Dermatology 1985; 924.

TABLE 3 Bacteriostatic Antituberculous Drugs

Drug	Route	Adult Dosage (mg/kg/day)	Side Effects	Major Complications	% Patients Developing Serious Adverse Effects
Ethambutol	PO	10–20	Pruritus, gastrointestinal upset, hyperuricemia	Retrobulbar neuritis, gout attacks	1–2
Ethionamide	PO, divided doses	15–25	Metallic taste, gastrointestinal irritability, hypertension, alopecia, acne	hepatitis, impotence, neurotoxicity	20–30
Para-aminosalicylic acid	PO, divided doses	150	Gastrointestinal distress, malaise, arthritis, sore throat	Hemolytic anemia, exacerbation of peptic ulcer disease, colitis	20–30
Cycloserine	PO, divided doses	10–15	Headache, personality changes	Psychosis, convulsions	10–30

Adapted from Moschella SL, Hurley JH. Dermatology 1985; 925.

ate dosages, indicated routes of administration, side effects, and major complications of the bactericidal drugs.

The bacteriostatic drugs are ethambutol, para-aminosalicylic acid, cycloserine, and ethionamide. Table 3 outlines the appropriate dosages, routes of administration, side effects, and major complications of these drugs. Ethambutol is the only "first line" drug in this group and is also the least toxic. Because of the well recognized complication of retrobulbar neuritis with associated loss of visual acuity and color vision, it is important that the patient undergo a complete ophthalmologic examination prior to beginning this drug and bimonthly during therapy. All the other drugs in this category are considered to be "second line" therapy, in addition to kanamycin and capreomycin.

ADJUNCTIVE THERAPY

In the overall treatment plan for these infections, adjunctive surgical therapy has a definite place. In patients with superficial infections that are not responding to medical management, simple surgical excision or local destruction by electrodesiccation and curettage is advised. However, if the lesion is not completely removed, surgery can cause extension of the infection into the deeper tissues. In patients with large suppurative abscesses, incision and drainage are recommended. Other treatment modalities include cryosurgery with liquid nitrogen and localized heat therapy when the infection is caused by an organism that grows at 30° C.

CONCLUSION

Undoubtedly the guidelines for the duration of therapy in these infections and for alternate or concomitant surgical intervention need to be individualized, depending on the infecting agent, drug sensitivities, and the immune status of the infected patient. Time, patience, persistance, and reassessment of the treatment program and patient response are the necessary components for therapeutic success.

ROCKY MOUNTAIN SPOTTED FEVER

JAY S. GOODMAN, M.D.

Rocky Mountain spotted fever is the most serious of all rickettsial diseases. In the United States this infection is actually much more common in the eastern part of the country than in the Rocky Mountain states. The illness is seasonal, with a summer peak corresponding to man's increased contact with the tick vector. The causative microorganism, *Rickettsia rickettsii*, spreads throughout the body via the blood and invades endothelial cells of capillaries, venules, and arterioles as well as the smooth muscle cells of the latter. The rash of Rocky Mountain spotted fever is only part of a diffuse vasculitis that occurs in other organs as well, most commonly the central nervous system and myocardium. Microinfarctions, gangrene of the acral portions of the body, and fluid extravasation with edema and hypovolemia are not uncommon.

THERAPEUTIC RATIONALE

Specific therapy greatly alters the impressive morbidity and mortality of this infection. Untreated Rocky Mountain spotted fever is fatal in 20 to 80 percent of the cases; the wide variation is probably related to the differing virulence of rickettsia in localized geographic pockets. Although treatment should theoretically eliminate mortality from this infection, the fatality in the antibiotic era persists at 5 percent. Nearly all deaths can be traced to a delay in treatment caused by failure to suspect the disease early in its course. Because laboratory confirmation requires a delay of several days to weeks, treatment of Rocky Mountain spotted fever must be initiated on the basis of clinical suspicion. This is not difficult when the disease presents as a febrile illness with a centripetally progressing rash, occurring in an endemic area and associated with a recent tick bite. However, there may be no obvious tick exposure or the patient may be noncommunicative. The rash in black patients can be difficult to

see, and in unusual cases a rash may not occur at all. Reports of tragic outcomes related to atypical presentations of Rocky Mountain spotted fever have sensitized some physicians to the point of recommending antirickettsial therapy for any individual presenting with a fever in the warmer months of the year. This approach is extreme and more likely to perpetuate a diagnostic dilemma than to prevent fatalities from Rocky Mountain spotted fever.

SPECIFIC ANTIMICROBIAL THERAPY

The tetracyclines and chloramphenicol are highly effective antibiotics for Rocky Mountain spotted fever (and other rickettsial infections as well; Table 1). The tetracyclines prevent rickettsial protein synthesis by inhibiting the binding of transfer RNA-amino acid complexes to ribosomes. Chloramphenicol inhibits protein synthesis at the 50S ribosome site.

The older tetracyclines (tetracycline HCl, chlortetracycline, oxytetracycline) can be administered in a dose of 2 g per day (500 mg every 6 hours) to adults or 25 to 50 mg per kilogram per day to children. These drugs are incompletely absorbed from the upper gastrointestinal tract; inadequate absorption occurs when they are given with food, milk, or antacids. Intravenous formulations are available. In children in the first decade of life, interference with tooth development and dental staining may occur; the risk of this is small when only a single course of therapy is given. Tetracyclines can cause hepatic damage, especially when used in large doses intravenously and particularly in pregnant women. Azotemia may also be seen as well as gastrointestinal intolerance and photosensitization.

Although the older tetracyclines have the longest "track record" in the treatment of Rocky Mountain spotted fever, a newer analog, doxycycline, appears to be equally effective. It is more convenient to administer and may have fewer side effects. Doxycycline's longer half-life allows for twice daily dosing. Since it is not excreted by the kidneys, the dose does not have to be modified, as it does for other tetracyclines, when there is renal insufficiency. The drug is well absorbed orally and may be administered in the presence of food or milk. Probably because of its decreased tendency to bind to calcium and its smaller dose

TABLE 1 Therapeutic Alternatives for Rocky Mountain Spotted Fever

	Route	Usual Adult Dose	Serum Half-Life (hr)		Side Effects and Comments
			Normal	Oliguria	
Tetracycline HCl	PO, IV	500 mg q 6 h	8.5	100	GI, allergy, primary dentition staining, liver toxicity, ↑BUN, poor absorption with food and milk, photosensitivity
Chlortetracycline	PO, IV	500 mg q 6 h	5.6	11	
Oxytetracycline	PO, IV	500 mg q 6 h	9.6	100	
Doxycycline	PO, IV	100 mg q 12 h	16	16	Better absorbed, less dental staining, may be used in renal failure
Chloramphenicol	PO, IV	750 mg q 6 h	1–2	3–5	Rare aplastic anemia

compared to other tetracyclines, doxycycline produces little detectable dental staining in children. Doxycycline should be given in a dosage of 200 mg per day in two divided doses for adults or 2 mg per pound of body weight per day for children. Intravenous doses of doxycycline are stable and well tolerated; it can also be administered twice daily in the same dose as in the oral regimen. Most cases of Rocky Mountain spotted fever can be treated by the oral route, but intravenous therapy for the first 48 hours of illness is advisable in any patient sick enough to be hospitalized. Since this is a life threatening infection, intravenous therapy avoids vicissitudes of intestinal absorption during this critical period.

Chloramphenicol is equal in efficacy to the tetracyclines in the treatment of Rocky Mountain spotted fever. Intestinal absorption of chloramphenicol is quite predictable, and so oral therapy is appropriate in most instances. The dose of chloramphenicol should be 50 mg per kilogram of body weight daily (four doses per day) for the same period of time as recommended for the tetracyclines. The use of chloramphenicol does have a serious drawback. In addition to this drug's dose-related suppressive effect on the bone marrow, it may cause a nondose-related idiosyncratic marrow aplasia, which is usually fatal. This catastrophic event occurs in approximately one in 40,000 patients receiving chloramphenicol. Although the risks of alternate therapies must be balanced, the relatively low incidence of important side effects should not receive disproportionate attention in the face of a life threatening infection.

A tetracycline, especially doxycycline, is the preferred therapy in most cases. Some patients, however, cannot tolerate these drugs. Other patients may have a clinical syndrome compatible either with Rocky Mountain spotted fever or meningococcemia; thus chloramphenicol would be a better choice. Both infections may present with a similar rash and central nervous system involvement. Rocky Mountain spotted fever is frequently accompanied by cerebrospinal fluid pleocytosis, which can lead to further confusion. When the distinction between these two infections is difficult, it is best to treat for both. Tetracycline cannot be relied upon to enter the cerebrospinal fluid in amounts adequate to produce levels bactericidal for the meningococcus. Chloramphenicol, on the other hand, crosses the blood-brain barrier effectively and is bactericidal against this micro-organism. The other alternative is to give large intravenous doses of penicillin along with a tetracycline to cover both meningococci and rickettsiae. This approach carries the theoretic drawback of antagonism by tetracycline of penicillin's bactericidal action on the meningococcus.

It must be stressed that empiric antibiotic regimens for suspected sepsis, which usually include a cephalosporin or broad spectrum penicillin along with an aminoglycoside, are completely ineffectual against rickettsiae. Valuable time can be wasted in patients receiving such regimens who are found later to have Rocky Mountain spotted fever. Empiric regimens containing sulfonamides are particularly dangerous because these drugs may cause deterioration of the clinical status of patients with rickettsial infections.

Interestingly, one of the earliest effective and now obsolete drugs used for the treatment of Rocky Mountain spotted fever was para-aminobenzoic acid, for which sulfonamides are a metabolic antagonist.

When treatment for Rocky Mountain spotted fever is initiated early in the course of illness, marked improvement generally occurs within the first 2 days, and fever is gone by the third or fourth day. After clinical improvement is evident, there is no reason to continue intravenous medication if oral therapy can be tolerated. Therapy should be continued for at least 2 days after the patient becomes afebrile or for a total of 1 week. If specific antimicrobial therapy is begun extremely early, as might occur in laboratory acquired infection, a relapse is possible. This is because none of the available antibiotics is rickettsiacidal. Their rickettsiastatic nature implies that ultimate cure is dependent on the development of specific immunity by the host. Relapses are early managed with a second course of therapy. Resistance of rickettsiae to tetracycline and chloramphenicol has not occurred. Patients treated late in the course of illness, or after tissue damage due to vasculitic infarction has occurred, may have a prolonged febrile course. Even so, the antibiotic need not be continued for longer than 1 week since, by this time, fever is related to factors other than rickettsiae multiplying in tissues. For most patients with Rocky Mountain spotted fever, antibiotics such as doxycycline, tetracycline, or chloramphenicol suffice for complete recovery. Improvement usually occurs rapidly; thus the latter portion of the antimicrobial course can be self-administered at home. Mild cases treated early in the course of illness can be adequately managed on an outpatient basis.

SUPPORTIVE CARE

Severe cases of Rocky Mountain spotted fever present special problems requiring supportive care in addition to specific chemotherapy. Extensive damage to small blood vessels may lead to extravasation of fluid, electrolytes, and protein from the intravascular space, resulting in edema and a reduced blood volume. Shock, with oliguria and increasing azotemia, may supervene, and fluid replacement may be complicated by cardiac failure. Myocarditis is probably common in Rocky Mountain spotted fever but is usually subclinical. Efforts to reverse hypotension or shock with fluid or colloid administration may unmask underlying myocardial damage and lead to pulmonary edema. Therefore, maintenance of adequate organ perfusion by volume replacement in the critically ill patient with this disease is best carried out in an intensive care unit, where monitoring of pulmonary capillary wedge pressure by Swan-Ganz catheterization is possible.

Some unresolved therapeutic questions in the management of Rocky Mountain spotted fever include the use of corticosteroids and anticoagulants. Corticosteroids definitely shorten the febrile period and induce an early feeling of well-being in patients receiving antirickettsial antibiotics. This early defervescence could be important in severely ill patients. Corticosteroids are probably not harmful when used for 1 or 2 days in this setting, but their administration should not be prolonged. These agents are not recommended as routine therapy in mild or even moderately severe cases.

The use of heparin presents a more difficult question. Rocky Mountain spotted fever is often associated with some degree of thrombocytopenia, probably due to diffuse endothelial injury and subsequent platelet consumption. Some patients develop low platelet counts (less than 50,000 per cubic millimeter with accompanying hypofibrinogenemia, prolonged prothrombin and partial thromboplastin times, and circulating fibrin split products. This is due to disseminated intravascular coagulation, which in some instances can be severe. Purpura fulminans with massive skin necrosis may develop. If the patient survives, plastic surgery may be necessary. Heparin is sometimes recommended, but there is no evidence that this drug improves the clinical status of such patients. In fact, a number of patients with Rocky Mountain spotted fever accompanied by full-blown disseminated intravascular coagulation have been cured by treatment with antirickettsial drugs alone. This would appear to be the preferred approach.

MANAGEMENT OF THE PATIENT WITH AN ATTACHED TICK

In the warmer months of the year, physicians practicing in endemic areas are often consulted by patients who are otherwise well, but have discovered an attached tick. The temptation to give an antirickettsial antibiotic as chemoprophylaxis should be avoided for the following reasons: (1) only a minority of ticks in most endemic areas are infected with virulent *Rickettsia rickettsiae*; (2) transmission of this disease from tick to man usually requires several hours of attachment; and (3) tetracycline and chloramphenicol are rickettsiastatic; (4) administration of these drugs during the incubation period interferes with the development of an immune response and probably only delays the onset of clinical infection.

Patients who have attached ticks should be advised to remove the tick with a pair of forceps by exerting steady gentle traction, allowing the mouth parts to be pulled intact from the skin. The temperature should be recorded by the patient morning and evening for 2 weeks. If fever develops, the physician should obtain a blood specimen for acute serology and begin specific antirickettsial therapy, as already outlined. A convalescent blood titer for confirmation of diagnosis can be obtained 2 to 4 weeks later.

VIRAL INFECTIONS

ACQUIRED IMMUNO-DEFICIENCY SYNDROME (AIDS)

ANTOINETTE F. HOOD, M.D.
THOMAS T. PROVOST, M.D.

ETIOLOGY

No treatise on dermatologic treatment in 1988 can be considered complete without a discussion of the cutaneous manifestations of the acquired immunodeficiency syndrome (AIDS). Our knowledge of the spectrum of cutaneous manifestations and etiopathogenesis of AIDS is in a rapid state of evolution. At the time of the writing of this article, three retroviruses (two have yet to be officially designated) of putative simian origin have been found to cause AIDS in man. The virus most commonly associated with the disease has been designated the human immunodeficiency virus (HIV). Several other closely related retroviruses have been described in addition to the three associated with AIDS. Human T cell lymphotrophic virus type I (HTLV-I) is a cause of human T cell leukemia, cutaneous T cell lymphoma, and adult T cell leukemia. Human T cell lymphotrophic virus type II (HTLV-II) causes hairy cell leukemia.

The HIV virus is cytotropic for the T4 (helper-inducer) cell lymphocyte. The virus binds to a specific protein T4 molecule on the T helper cell, initiating the infection. The HIV virus is also capable of infecting Epstein-Barr virus infected B-lymphocytes, Langerhans cells, and other macrophage-like cells. Because the virus integrates itself in a latent form into the host DNA, the infection persists for a lifetime.

EPIDEMIOLOGY

In 1979 AIDS, the newest and perhaps the worst epidemic in the history of mankind, was heralded by the recognition of the occurrence of unusual bacterial, protozoan, and fungal infections and Kaposi's sarcoma in homosexual males, Haitians, hemophiliacs, and intravenous drug addicts. Epidemiologic studies have subsequently revealed that the HIV infection is widespread in Africa, affecting an estimated 40 percent of individuals living in the sub-Saharan basin. It must be emphasized that in Africa AIDS is a heterosexual disease. Indeed the recent International Congress on the Acquired Immunodeficiency Syndrome held in Washington in June 1987 focused on the heterosexual transmission of this epidemic. Particularly at risk for spreading the disease is the intravenous drug abusing prostitute. In one recent study of a large eastern United States city, 50 percent of randomly screened prostitutes possessed the HIV antibody. Other studies have indicated that 50 to 75 percent of intravenous drug abusers are HIV antibody positive. Thus, two of the greatest social dilemmas of our era, drug abuse and AIDS, are intimately linked.

It is now known that homosexual men, especially those with many partners and those who practice rectal intercourse, are at greatest risk for infection, as the transmission of the virus sexually is via infected seminal fluid. Male to female infection frequently occurs; the authors of one study estimate that approximately 70 percent of the female sexual partners of HIV positive males are infected with the virus. However, female to male transmission occurs less frequently. One preliminary report estimates that female transmission to a male sexual partner occurs following intercourse approximately one in every 50 times. The infected female also can transfer the virus to her unborn child. An infected child develops poorly and generally dies within the first year of life.

In the recent past, contaminated blood supply has been a significant source of infection. This risk has been reduced by vigorous screening of donated blood. It has been estimated that approximately 85 percent of hemophiliacs have contracted the HIV infection from contaminated factor VIII cryoprecipitate.

In contradistinction to the high degree of infectivity associated with sexual contact, blood transfusions, and intravenous drug abuse, the virus has a low degree of infectivity among medical personnel inadvertently injured by needle stick and in individuals who come into close but nonsexual contact with AIDS patients. Apparently the AIDS retrovirus does not survive for long periods of time outside the body.

The clinical features of the AIDS syndrome are many and varied. In general, the development of the opportunistic infections corresponds to the development of a profound lymphopenia. Initially this lymphopenia is indicated by a reversal of the helper T cell/suppressor T cell (T4/T8) ratio. As the T helper-inducer lymphocytes disappear from the peripheral circulation, the host becomes more and more susceptible to the development of opportunistic infections. In general, as the T helper lymphocyte count falls below 100 cells per cubic millimeter of blood, significant opportunistic infections occur.

The cutaneous manifestations of the initial viremia are protean and are frequently not observed or correctly diagnosed. It has been demonstrated however, that following a documented infection several patients have developed a macular and papular (morbilliform) rash accompanied by fever and myalgia. Other patients have developed a mononucleosis-like syndrome, and on rare occasions urticaria has been described. The time lapse between infection and seroconversion ranges from 3 weeks to 6 months after infection. Following the initial infection, most patients develop generalized lymphadenopathy with hypergammaglobulinemia, and some develop thrombocytopenia. This form of the disease is known as the acquired immunodeficiency syndrome related complex (ARC). With the development of tumors such as Kaposi's sarcoma or opportunistic infections with such organisms as *Candida albicans* and *Pneumocystis carinii*, the disease is considered to have evolved into AIDS. The length of time between the initial infection and the development of AIDS is unknown, but it appears to be longer than 3 years. Some seropositive patients have not developed AIDS after 7 years of follow-up.

The cutaneous manifestations of AIDS can be divided into the following categories: infections, nonspecific dermatoses, and neoplasia (Tables 1 and 2).

INFECTIOUS MANIFESTATIONS

The infectious dermatoses associated with AIDS include manifestations of viral, bacterial, fungal, and protozoan infections. Herpes simplex infections are often seen as unusually severe, persistent, or recurrent erosions or ulcerations around the mouth or perineum. They may become secondarily infected with bacteria and if untreated can result in scarring. It is important to note that these lesions frequently do not develop the classic appearance of grouped vesicles on the erythematous base. Identification of these lesions usually can be made with either a Tzanck smear preparation or a herpes culture. Most infectious disease physicians caring for large groups of HIV infected individuals treat these herpes simplex infections with oral doses of acyclovir.

Herpes zoster infections may be severe in AIDS patients. In most instances the varicella-zoster affliction represents a secondary infection (that is, a recurrence following childhood chickenpox). These patients may develop a generalized cutaneous eruption associated with pneumonia. Like their herpes simplex counterparts, the individual lesions of varicella zoster may be clinically atypical in appearance, failing to demonstrate the usual segmental dermatomal eruption or erythema surrounding the vesicles. The Tzanck smear and viral culture are helpful confirmatory diagnostic tests. In general, oral acyclovir treatment is only partially effective in these patients, and intravenous acyclovir therapy is often necessary for patients with disseminated varicella-zoster infection.

Molluscum contagiosum infections are frequently seen in AIDS patients. These lesions can involve any area of the body but most commonly occur in the genital and perioral regions. The lesions have a tendency to become very large (i.e., larger than 1 cm in diameter). The lesions tend to persist and to recur following therapy. Surgical removal of the viral core with curettage or a shave biopsy technique is recommended, although cryosurgery has also been successfully employed.

Epstein-Barr virus infections may act synergistically with the HIV virus to produce unusual lymphoproliferations and lymphomas in the AIDS patient. Infectious mononucleosis with a generalized macular dermatitis and a severe hemolytic anemia associated with cold agglutinin antibodies has been described. The diagnosis of this type of dermatosis is difficult; biopsies are of little help. However, serologic studies to examine the patient's serum for antibody responses to early and late Epstein-Barr virus antigens may provide confirmatory data. At this time there is no effective treatment for this Epstein-Barr virus induced disease.

Papillomavirus infections are very frequent in AIDS patients, who may develop warts involving the oral mucosa as well as the genital region. These lesions may be large, recurrent, and very resistant to conventional therapy.

A distinctive leukoplakia of the tongue (oral hairy leukoplakia) has been described in ARC and AIDS patients. The lesions, varying in size from 2 mm to 2 cm, are poorly demarcated, irregular white areas on the lateral surfaces of the tongue, which demonstrate a corrugated or "hairy" appearance. They are generally asymptomatic and clinically may be confused with oral changes seen in cigarette smokers. Histologically the lesions resemble warts, but they are thought to be caused by the Epstein-Barr virus. Because of their asymptomatic nature, they usually do not require treatment.

Fungal infection, especially candidiasis, is common in patients with AIDS. *Candida albicans* is a normal saprophyte–commensal organism present in approximately 70 percent of normal individuals. The *Candida* infection in AIDS patients may take the form of plaques on the buccal mucosa and tongue; extension of oral candidiasis to involve the throat and esophagus may produce dysphagia. When *Candida* infections of the mucosa become deep and erosive, they may produce a great deal of discomfort and become difficult to treat. Vaginal candidiasis occurs frequently in women with AIDS and like oral candidiasis may be both extensive and intractable. The diagnosis of candidiasis can be suspected from the physical examination and confirmed using either potassium hydroxide examination of scrapings from lesions or fungal cultures.

The treatment of AIDS related oral candidiasis involves the use of nystatin oral suspension, 1 teaspoon, three to four times a day. The patient is instructed to swish the material around in the mouth and then to swallow. Amphotericin B, 50 mg suspended in 4 ounces of wild cherry syrup, 1 teaspoon four times a day (swish and swallow), has also been shown to be an effective alternative therapy for the treatment of candidiasis in immunosuppressed patients. (Note: It is important to place the amphotericin B in an acid pH to prevent its deactivation;

TABLE 1   Mucocutaneous Findings in AIDS

Infection
  Viral infections
    Herpesvirus infection (herpes simplex, herpes zoster varicella)
    Cytomegalovirus
    Human papillomavirus
    Epstein-Barr virus
    Molluscum contagiosum
    Oral hairy leukoplakia
  Fungal infections
    Oral candidiasis
    Dermatophytosis
    Tinea versicolor
    Cutaneous manifestations of disseminated systemic infection
      Cryptococcus neoformans
      Histoplasma capsulatum
      Coccidioides immitis
      Sporothrix schenckii
  Bacterial infections
    Pyoderma, folliculitis, secondary impetiginization
    Mycobacterium
    Syphilis
  Protozoal infections
    Acanthamoeba castellani
Inflammatory dermatoses
  Seborrheic dermatitis
  Papular (pruritic) eruption
  Drug eruptions
  Exacerbation of pre-existing skin disease, especially psoriasis
  Granuloma annulare-like lesions
  Xerosis, ichthyosis
Neoplasm
  Kaposi's sarcoma
  Lymphoma
  Other vascular proliferation
    Angiomas
    Telangiectasia

hence, the use of wild cherry syrup.) Vaginal candidiasis is treated with nystatin, miconazole, or clotrimazole suppositories daily. Finally, ketoconazole, 200 mg by mouth daily for 10 to 14 days, may be necessary in order to control the most severe forms of mucosal candidiasis. Patients receiving long-term treatment with ketaconazole must be monitored for hepatotoxicity (see chapters on treatment of fungal infections); it should also be mentioned that ketaconazole interferes with the metabolism of rifampin.

Dermatophyte infections can be extensive, severe, and symptomatic in patients with AIDS. These infections classically involve the genital areas, feet, and toenails but also have been described involving the face and other skin surfaces. The lesions are occasionally very extensive and have a tendency to be hyperkeratotic and may produce little or no erythema. Potassium hydroxide examination of scrapings from these lesions as well as fungal cultures establishes the true nature of the infection. These lesions generally respond poorly to topical treatment with miconazole and clotrimazole. Systemic therapy in the form of griseofulvin or ketoconazole may be necessary, but the infections may be refractory to this aggressive treatment.

Tinea versicolor has been commonly reported in patients with AIDS. These lesions are commonly refractory to topical applications of selenium sulfide, miconazole, or clotrimazole and may require systemic treatment with ketoconazole. Relapses are frequent.

Disseminated deep fungal infections with cutaneous manifestations have been reported in AIDS patients. We have seen several patients with a cutaneous cryptococcal infection that resembled molluscum contagiosum. Histoplasmosis presenting as papulonecrotic plaques on the trunk and extremities in an AIDS patient has also been reported.

Bacterial infections are common in AIDS patients. Perirectal ulcerations are frequently infected with *Staphylococcus aureus*. These infections respond well to the appropriate antibiotics. Finally, it should be noted that genital ulcerations in AIDS patients may be a manifestation of syphilis. Therefore, in addition to culturing ulcers for viruses and bacteria, a darkfield examination and a serologic test for syphilis should be obtained with all perineal ulcerations.

Cutaneous mycobacterial infections have been described in patients with AIDS, including *Mycobacterium avium-intracellulare*, *M. scrofulaceum*, and *M. marinum*.

Protozoal infections are highly unusual in patients with AIDS. Recently, however, a disseminated protozoal infection caused by *Acanthamoeba castellani* was associated with the development of a papule on the thigh of an AIDS patient.

NONSPECIFIC DERMATOSES

In addition to these viral, fungal, bacterial, and protozoal infections, AIDS patients may develop nonspecific inflammatory disorders of the skin. For example, seborrheic dermatitis is very common, occurring in approximately 80 percent of AIDS patients. The severity of the seborrheic dermatitis appears to correlate with the severity of the disease. AIDS patients with an explosive onset of erythematous recalcitrant seborrheic dermatitis appear to have the worst prognosis. Xeroderma appears to be frequently associated with the seborrheic dermatitis. Acquired severe ichthyosis has also been described in many patients.

A clinically characteristic papular eruption has also been described in the acquired immunodeficiency syndrome and the related complex. This condition consists of discrete skin colored papules occurring on the head, neck, and upper trunk. These lesions are usually pruritic, and although the condition waxes and wanes, the course of the disease is usually chronic. In many of the patients the lesions persist longer than 9 months. There appears to be no correlation between the severity of the eruption and systemic signs and symptoms of HIV infection. The histology of the lesions is nonspecific but characteristically demonstrates a superficial perivascular mononuclear cell infiltrate with or without eosinophils.

In addition to these cutaneous manifestations of the AIDS syndrome, there is evidence to indicate that AIDS patients may have an increased frequency of cutaneous drug reactions. A high frequency of a generalized macular and papular erythematous dermatitis has been described

TABLE 2 Frequency of Cutaneous Manifestations in AIDS

	Common	Less Common	Rare
Infections	Herpesvirus infection Warts and condyloma acuminata Molluscum contagiosum Oral candidiasis	Dermatophytoses Tinea versicolor Oral hairy leukoplakia	Cutaneous lesions associated with disseminated systemic fungal infection
Inflammtory dermatoses	Seborrheic dermatitis Drug eruptions (Bactrim)	Papular eruption Ichthyosis	Granuloma annulare-like lesions Exacerbation of preexisting dermatoses
Neoplasms	Kaposi's sarcoma	Lymphoma Angiomas	Telangiectasis

in AIDS patients treated for *Pneumocystis carinii* pneumonia with trimethoprim-sulfamethoxazole.

Finally, persons with pre-existing dermatoses such as psoriasis may experience severe exacerbation of the cutaneous disease as an early manifestation of HIV infection. We have recently seen and cared for two patients who presented with widespread erythrodermic psoriasis. The history of a preceding coronary artery bypass graft requiring blood transfusions alerted the attending physicians to the possibility of HIV related disease; both patients were antibody positive, and one has subsequently died of the sequelae of HIV infection.

NEOPLASIA

Immunocompromised patients develop a spectrum of malignant diseases, and it has been estimated that approximately 40 percent of AIDS patients develop neoplasms. The most common tumor is an aggressive form of Kaposi's sarcoma occurring in homosexuals with AIDS. In addition to involving the skin (25 percent of the patients with homosexually transmitted AIDS have cutaneous Kaposi's sarcoma), Kaposi's sarcoma lesions in these patients often develop in other organs. In one autopsy series more than 90 percent of AIDS patients had Kaposi's sarcoma involving internal organs. The observation that Kaposi's sarcoma occurs almost exclusively in homosexuals who develop AIDS raises important questions about the etiology of this tumor and its relationship to the human immunodeficiency virus.

Typically the cutaneous lesions of Kaposi's sarcoma occur in AIDS patients as small, round, oval papules or plaques on the upper trunk, face, and proximal extremities. The lesions tend to be reddish brown to violaceous and may be extremely subtle in the early stages. Often lesions are oriented along the long axis of skin tension lines on the trunk, in a pityriasis rosea-like pattern. Kaposi's sarcoma has been described developing a dermatomal distribution following an episode of herpes zoster. Kaposi's sarcoma may be rapid in onset and oral lesions may be prominent. Its treatment is discussed elsewhere in this book.

In addition to Kaposi's sarcoma, lymphomas develop in individuals with AIDS. These lymphomas have a peculiar disposition to occur in the oral and genital regions.

CONCLUSION

It is evident that as the AIDS epidemic continues and spreads, dermatologists will play an increasing role in the early diagnosis of this disease. It should be emphasized that many of the characteristic inflammatory features of bacterial, fungal, and viral lesions are muted or nonexistent owing to the underlying immune suppression in these patients. Dermatologists must develop a healthy suspicion that any individual lesion may represent an opportunistic infection in an AIDS patient. Therefore, viral cultures, Tzanck smears, bacterial cultures (including those for atypical mycobacteria), and punch biopsy become increasingly important tools in the diagnosis of infections and malignant disease in these patients. If an opportunistic infection is detected, the patient should be referred to an appropriate medical facility for further investigation and treatment. At the present state of development of the medicolegal ramifications in AIDS testing, it is recommended that physicians obtain written permission from the patient prior to obtaining an HIV antibody determination.

Because of the magnitude of the AIDS epidemic, we currently recommend that dermatologists glove for all invasive diagnostic or therapeutic procedures, including venipuncture. Careful hand washing with an antiseptic soap before and after each invasive procedure is also advised. If one is inadvertently exposed to a patient's blood, for example, via a needle stick, we recommend that the following serologic tests be obtained on the patient's blood (with his permission): hepatitis antibody and antigen screen, cytomegalic virus antibody screen, and HIV antibody. An infectious disease consultation should also be obtained for up to date recommendations regarding follow-up evaluation.

Finally, from a philosophic point of view, it is important to remember that physicians in previous generations have also been placed in potentially dangerous situations. The infectivity and danger to medical personnel posed by an AIDS patient are far less than the high infectivity danger to physicians in previous eras who cared for patients with tuberculosis. Good common sense and a healthy respect for the inherent dangers in handling blood and bodily secretions and for performing invasive procedures are of paramount importance for self-protection.

Dermatologists must realize that they are now, and will remain, in a "front line" position in dealing with

AIDS, and that in this position they are responsible for the recognition and diagnosis of cutaneous diseases that may be early manifestations of AIDS. As newer therapies become available for the treatment of HIV infection, early recognition and treatment may be of paramount importance in controlling this epidemic.

For those readers interested in obtaining detailed information about the cutaneous manifestations and immunology of the AIDS infection we recommend the following articles:

1. Ho DD. N Engl J Med 1987; 317:278–268.
2. Kaplan MH, et al. J Am Acad Dermatol 1987, 16:485–506.
3. Pennys NS, Hicks B. Arch Dermatol 1987; 16:485–506.

WARTS

BARBARA M. ROCK, M.D.

Warts are caused by infection of the skin and mucous membranes with human papillomavirus, a nonenveloped, double-stranded DNA virus of the Family Papovaviridae. The papillomas induced by the wart virus infection are entirely intraepithelial. The infectious particles, called virions, are produced in the host cells in conjunction with the maturation of normal epithelium. Warts are contagious and are generally spread by direct contact. Spread by fomites is also implicated, particularly in plantar warts, which may be spread through contact with shower floors. Warts may be autoinoculated by scratching or otherwise traumatizing the involved skin. The incubation time may be weeks to years.

There have been as many as 42 human papillomavirus types identified to date. Each has been shown to be generally body site specific. Most verrucae are benign, but some types of viruses, particularly those of the genital tract, have been found in association with malignant disease. This is an important consideration in the treatment of warts involving various body sites. An abbreviated list of common types of papillomavirus is presented in Table 1.

One large study has shown that most common warts are self-resolving in 2 years. Both cell mediated and humoral types of immunity are involved in the host defense against viral infection. Recurrence incidences may be high in any individual patient in spite of the usual self-resolving nature, and that will be the patient most often encountered in the physician's office. Furthermore, extensive and recalcitrant warts may be seen in specific disorders of immunity, such as epidermodysplasia verruciformis, IgM deficiency, inherited T cell immunodeficiency syndromes, and acquired immunodeficiency of any type that is associated with treatment related immunosuppression, such as renal transplantation and primary biliary cirrhosis. There is also preliminary evidence that there is an increased incidence of wart virus infection in the acquired immunodeficiency syndrome (AIDS).

PRINCIPLES OF TREATMENT

Several factors should be considered when treating warts; each of these is discussed when appropriate in the therapy section. Since most common warts are benign and self-limited, the simplest and least traumatic treatment should be used. This may avoid complications of treatment such as painful or disfiguring scarring, which may be more troublesome than the original wart. Alternatively warts that may be associated with malignant disease, even if only in small numbers of patients, should be treated more aggressively. This principle specifically applies to genital tract infection in both men and women. The flat warts of epidermodysplasia verruciformis and immunosuppression secondary to renal transplantation have been shown to be associated with Bowen's disease and squamous cell carcinoma and should be followed more carefully as well.

Other factors to consider in the treatment of warts include the age of the patient, pain tolerance, compliance, anatomic site, and the number of lesions. One of the most helpful adjuncts to treatment involves patient education. The physician should explain to the patient the infectious nature of warts, the benignity (if appropriate), the natural history of wart infection, what to expect from treatment, and the possibility of recurrence.

Wart treatment generally involves destructive methods and care must be taken to avoid overtreatment. It is better to exercise caution at the risk of the need for retreatment than to cause unnecessary scarring or discomfort to the patient.

TREATMENT MODALITIES

Verruca Vulgaris

The common hand or finger warts are frequently seen in dermatologic practice. They are entirely benign lesions with no known malignant potential. They are most often seen in children and young adults. The advantages of several of the most common treatment modalities are outlined in Table 2. The treatment should be tailored to the individual patient's needs.

Cryotherapy

In general, the preferred treatment is cryotherapy with liquid nitrogen because of its ease of use and the lack of associated scarring. If there are multiple lesions, it is best to limit the number treated per visit to about five, depending on the patient's pain tolerance. Liquid nitrogen is applied with either a continuous cryospray or a cotton ball wrapped loosely around a Q-tip or proctoscopic swab. The

TABLE 1 Common Types of Papillomavirus

HPV 1, 2, 4	Plantar warts, verruca vulgaris, filiform warts
HPV 3, 10	Verruca plana, epidermodysplasia verruciformis
HPV 5	Macular lesions of epidermodysplasia verruciformis and renal transplant recipients, Bowen's disease, squamous cell carcinoma
HPV 7	Butcher's warts
HPV 6, 11, 16, 18	Genital tract papillomas, laryngeal papillomas, female genital tract carcinoma, conjunctival papillomas
HPV 13	Oral focal epithelial hyperplasia

TABLE 2 Comparison of Common Treatment Modalities

	Advantages	*Disadvantages*
Cryotherapy	Simple, well tolerated procedure Minimal scarring No anesthesia required	May require more than one treatment
Electrodessication	Wart is completely treated at time of office visit	Requires local anesthesia Risk of scarring greater than with other modalities
Shaving or curettage	Biopsy material available if diagnosis is in doubt	Requires local anesthesia Risk of scarring greater than with other modalities
Duofilm	Little discomfort Patient may apply at home	Multiple treatments required Patient compliance essential Failure incidence high
Cantharidin	No discomfort in doctor's office	"Halo" warts after treatment
Trichloroacetic acid	Minimal discomfort with application	Depth of tissue destruction difficult to predict

liquid nitrogen should be applied until the frosted area extends 1 to 2 mm beyond the wart periphery. The duration of freezing should allow for a 30 second thawing time. Upon thawing, a second, repeated application of liquid nitrogen should be carried out. It is the freeze-thaw cycling that results in the controlled destruction of the tissue containing the wart. The patient should be instructed to expect blistering to occur within the first day after treatment and that hemorrhage into the blister is common. Unroofing of the blister is unnecessary, but should it rupture, the blister roof may be removed. The patient should be instructed then to clean the area twice a day with hydrogen peroxide and apply bacitracin ointment. The patient should be seen at 1- to 2-week intervals for retreatment if necessary. At follow-up visits all necrotic tissue should be pared down before retreating. The entire procedure is generally well tolerated, even by children. The patient experiences only a brief painful burning sensation at the time of liquid nitrogen application and to a far lesser extent for several hours thereafter.

Electrodesiccation

If the number of lesions is limited and none are over joints or in cosmetically significant areas, light electrodesiccation with a monopolar current is an acceptable treatment. This treatment should be avoided in patients with pacemakers. Local anesthesia with 1 or 2 percent Xylocaine is indicated. After desiccation, the wart tissue can be easily removed with an appropriately sized curette. Hemostasis is obtained with pressure and the application of 10 percent aluminum chloride. Some scarring may result from this treatment, but if patient selection has been appropriate and the lesions are small, this is acceptable.

Shaving and Curettage

When biopsy material is needed for diagnosis, this is the preferred technique. Local anesthesia with 1 or 2 percent Xylocaine is indicated. The lesion is then shaved or curetted flush with the skin. The curette may be used to scrape the base to be sure that the lesion has been totally removed. Hemostasis is obtained with pressure, aluminum chloride (10 percent solution), or light electrodesiccation.

Keratolytics (Duofilm)

For patients (particularly children) who prefer a less painful technique for wart treatment, keratolytic topical agents are the treatment of choice. Duofilm (16.7 percent salicylic acid and 16.7 percent lactic acid in flexible collodion; Stiefel Laboratories) or its generic equivalent is the product we generally use, although others on the market are equally efficacious. Duofilm is applied daily to the wart only after soaking for 5 minutes in warm water and allowed to dry. A Band-Aid is then applied. The next day the patient is instructed to remove the Band-Aid and soak the affected area in warm water for 5 to 10 minutes. This is followed by gentle debridement of the wart tissue with a nail file. The Duofilm is then reapplied, and the whole process is repeated daily until the wart is gone. The process may take 2 to 6 weeks for removal of the wart. If significant irritation or inflammation occurs, treatment should be discontinued until the patient is seen by the physician.

Cantharidin (Cantharone, Verrusol)

An alternative to keratolytic treatment is the application of cantharidin, a blister beetle extract. After paring down of the lesion, the physician applies the solution carefully only to the wart. The solution is allowed to dry; then occlusive tape is applied. The patient is instructed to remove the tape in 24 hours and wash with soapy water. A blister forms that lifts the wart off, as in liquid nitrogen treatment. There is no need to unroof the blister. The patient is seen in 1 to 2 weeks to evaluate the response and to retreat if necessary. A disadvantage of treatment is the possibility of halo or doughnut warts appearing at the periphery of the treatment site. An advantage, particularly in children, is that the discomfort is felt 12 to 24 hours after application rather than in the doctor's office.

Trichloroacetic Acid

Application of 50 to 70 percent trichloroacetic acid may be used to treat verrucae either as the primary therapy or in conjunction with keratolytic drugs. The trichloroacetic acid should be applied by the physician only to the wart with the stick end of a Q-tip. A white discoloration of the treated tissue develops after application. Neutralization is not necessary because the acid is neutralized by the protein hydrolization that it causes. The patient should be followed weekly for paring down and retreatment as needed. The disadvange of this treatment is the unpredictability of the depth of tissue destruction.

Filiform Warts

Filiform or beard warts are a variant of verruca vulgaris, generally seen on the face or neck. They are often multiple. Because of the stalk or filiform projection, light desiccation with monopolar current after local anesthesia with 1 or 2 percent Xylocaine is simple and effective. Equally effective is shaving flush with the skin with light curettage of the base, but this is more time consuming. Liquid nitrogen is effective, but it is difficult to control the application and avoid damage of the surrounding skin. Care must be taken to be as atraumatic as possible on the face to avoid postinflammatory pigment changes.

Periungual Warts

Verruca vulgaris appearing in the cuticle or under the nail may be difficult to treat. Treatment should begin as outlined in the section on verruca vulgaris. If unsuccessful, treatment with a carbon dioxide laser may be indicated. In experienced hands, results are excellent, with minimal or no nail damage. The incidence of recurrence is high.

Verruca Plana

Flat warts often occur in extensive crops and frequently involve the face. They are benign lesions in normal individuals.

Cryotherapy-Retin A

A combination of weekly light liquid nitrogen application with twice daily Retin A application is very effective. The liquid nitrogen spray should be used for about 5 to 10 seconds or less each lesion. The patient is then instructed to apply 0.025 percent Retin A gel to affected areas twice daily. The patient should be seen weekly for evaluation and refreezing, increasing the Retin A application if necessary. The patient is instructed to expect some irritation and peeling with this treatment. Men are advised to use disposable razors or electric razors to prevent autoinoculation.

Efudex (5-FU)

Application of 5 percent Efudex cream twice daily to limited areas of flat warts may be effective. The duration of treatment varies according to the response, but generally 2 to 4 weeks should suffice. This treatment is not recommended for children or pregnant patients.

Formaldehyde

Ten to 20 percent formaldehyde in petrolatum applied twice daily to individual warts is an effective treatment. It is also useful for extensive verrucae that may be seen on the lower legs of women who have autoinoculated warts secondary to shaving. The duration of treatment depends on the response. This treatment should be used only after the more traditional Retin A treatment has failed. Not all warts need to be treated; this therapy seems to elicit a more generalized immunity to the wart virus, resulting in the disappearance of both treated and untreated warts. An irritant effect is expected. Allergic sensitivity to formalin may develop, and formalin is sometimes a component of clothing.

Condyloma Acuminatum

Venereal warts are seen most often in the sexually active population. A woman with vulvar condylomata acuminata should be examined by a gynecologist for the presence of cervical flat warts or vaginal condylomata. As mentioned earlier, human papillomavirus infection of the vulva has been associated with vulvar intraepithelial neoplasia and squamous cell carcinoma. Human papillomavirus infection of the cervix has been associated with cervical carcinoma. In men an association with malignant disease has been established with Bowen's disease, verrucous carcinoma, and squamous cell carcinoma of the penis all having papillomavirus DNA present. If extensive perianal warts are seen, an anoscopic examination is indicated. When condyloma acuminatum is seen in a child, sexual child abuse must be considered and investigated.

Podophyllin

Particularly for moist verrucous warts, application of 25 percent podophyllin in tincture of benzoin is the treatment of choice. Podophyllin is an antimitotic and cytotoxic preparation and should not be used in pregnant patients or on internal mucous membranes. The area of treatment should be limited to 2 sq cm to avoid excessive irritation and potential absorption. The liquid is applied by the physician only to the warts and allowed to air dry. Cornstarch powder then may be applied to the area to prevent spread of the medication to normal skin. The patient is instructed to wash the area with warm soapy water in 4 to 8 hours, depending upon discomfort. Cooling sitz baths may be helpful to ease discomfort in the healing phase. The patient is seen weekly for repeated applications as needed. For resistant warts a light freeze with liquid nitrogen before application of the podophyllin may increase efficacy.

Electrodesiccation or Laser

If after four treatments with podophyllin the warts are not responding satisfactorily, electrodesiccation under local anesthesia with 1 to 2 percent lidocaine may be helpful for the residual lesions. If the lesions are extensive, carbon dioxide laser therapy should be considered because a large number of lesions can be treated at one time in a more controlled setting.

Cryotherapy

Liquid nitrogen may be used to treat venereal warts, particularly on the penile shaft. Generally shorter freezing times are indicated. Pain is greater in the genital area than on glabrous skin. The patient should always be in the reclining position for this treatment in order to avoid a vasovagal response.

Trichloroacetic Acid

Careful application of 50 to 70 percent trichloroacetic acid may be useful in the genital area, particularly for flat lesions. The drawback is the lack of predictability of the depth of tissue destruction (see verruca vulgaris).

Verruca Plantaris

Plantar warts, particularly the mosaic type, may be difficult to treat. Aggressive treatment may result in a long recovery period or permanent painful scarring, particularly if the wart is over a pressure point. For this reason a longer, more gradual treatment program is indicated.

Salicylic Acid Plasters

A 40 percent salicylic acid plaster is cut slightly larger than the wart to be treated and applied after the wart and calloused tissue have been pared down. The plaster is taped in place and allowed to stay for at least 24 hours. The patient then removes the plaster and soaks the foot in warm soapy water before paring the wart with a nail file. The plaster is then reapplied after an 8 hour "break." If the patient can tolerate it, the plaster may be left on for 48 to 72 hours before removal and soaking. The physician should see the patient approximately every 2 weeks to paredown the wart and evaluate the efficacy of therapy. Trichloroacetic acid, cantharidin, or a single application of liquid nitrogen may be added as an adjunct to treatment if needed (see previous instructions). After adjunctive treatment with the foregoing, the plaster is reapplied and treatment proceeds as before. If the patient experiences too much discomfort, treatment is interrupted.

Blunt Enucleation

The plantar wart may be dissected using blunt technique under local anesthesia by an experienced physician. Excision of the plantar wart with a scalpel is generally contraindicated because of the risk of painful scarring.

Recalcitrant Warts

Recalcitrant warts are best treated by referral to a specialist in these techniques.

Dinitrochlorobenzene

Dinitrochlorobenzene treatment may be effective for multiple veruccae that have failed to respond to alternative treatment. A sensitizing dose of 0.1 ml of 2 percent dinitrochlorobenzene is applied in a 3 sq cm area on the inner aspect of the upper arm and covered for 24 hours. An eczematous response indicates sensitization. Several weeks later a 0.1 percent solution of dinitrochlorobenzene in acetone is applied to each lesion, and the area is kept dry for 24 hours. Wart regression along with inflammation begins in 1 to 2 days. Repeated application to the lesions may be needed to continue the inflammatory process. Widespread allergic contact dermatitis may occur as a side effect of this therapy.

Bleomycin

Large resistant warts in small numbers can be treated intralesionally with the antineoplastic drug bleomycin sulfate. A 0.1 percent solution (1 mg per milliliter) of bleomycin sulfate in normal saline is injected in volumes of less than 0.2 ml into each lesion. Pain may be experienced by the patient for several days. A repeat injection may be needed in 3 weeks. Warts on digits should be avoided because of the possibility of permanent Raynaud's phenomenon after injection.

Interferon

Clinical trials of interferon are under way in the treatment of recalcitrant vulvar warts. Preliminary reports have demonstrated some efficacy. This drug is not available for general use at this time.

HERPES SIMPLEX

MARK H. SAWYER, M.D.
STEPHEN E. STRAUS, M.D.

There is no better example of the progress made to date in the treatment of viral infections than the current therapy available for infections caused by herpes simplex virus (HSV). The need for specific antiviral treatments for HSV infections has become increasingly apparent for two major reasons. First, the prevalence of genital herpes infection in the United States has increased approximately 10-fold over the last decade: by early adulthood 70 to 80 percent of the people in the United States will harbor either HSV-1 or HSV-2. One-fourth of these individuals will experience recurrent infections. Second, increasing indications for the use of immunosuppressive therapies expand the settings in which HSV infections are problematic.

Specific antiviral therapy has been available for ocular HSV infections since the early 1960s. However, until recently no effective treatments were identified for the more common mucocutaneous forms or the rare visceral forms of HSV disease. Over the past 10 years a large number of clinical trials have documented a range of useful treatment strategies for these HSV infections. Now the practitioner can design therapeutic plans for HSV infections in both normal and immunocompromised patients.

The two types of HSV, HSV-1 and HSV-2, cause mucocutaneous infections that are typically localized to the oral and genital regions, respectively. Although limited areas of skin and mucous membranes are most commonly affected by HSV, infection may involve diffuse areas of skin, as well as the eye, esophagus, lung, liver, and central nervous system. Widespread disease and visceral involvement carry a substantial morbidity and are occasionally fatal.

In this chapter we outline the development of specific antiviral drugs for HSV infections, with an emphasis on their role in the treatment of mucocutaneous disease. We review drug pharmacology as it relates to appropriate drug dosing schedules and routes of administration. We discuss known drug toxicities as well as the importance of assessing host immune competence as a factor in tailoring therapy for the immunocompromised patient. Practical approaches to initial and long-term suppressive therapy for HSV infections are outlined. Our treatment approaches should be considered as general guidelines for the design of individual treatment plans and may need to be modified on the basis of the clinical or virologic response. Finally we touch on current research regarding new approaches to therapy and the prevention of HSV disease.

TREATMENT ALTERNATIVES

Over the last 20 years many compounds were studied as treatments for herpes infections. These have fallen into three general classes—topically applied detergents and other nonspecific chemical agents that can be applied to lesions, drugs said to modulate the immune response, and inhibitors of viral replication. The first two classes of compounds have produced little clinical success. The most effective therapies for mucocutaneous and systemic infections caused by HSV are drugs that specifically inhibit viral replication.

Topical applications of detergents, ether, chloroform, and the photoactive dyes, neutral red and proflavine, have been of no value in the management of mucocutaneous HSV infection. However, a recent study with Inter-Vir A, a mixture of the topical surfactants p-diisobutylphenoxy polyethoxyethanol and polyoxyethylene-10-oleyl ether, showed modest improvement in the lesion healing time and a dramatic reduction in symptoms in a study of oral and gentital herpes infections. Further studies with this drug must be performed to determine whether this type of topical therapy is useful.

The immune response, particularly the cellular immune response, is critical to the control of herpesvirus infections. It has been postulated that even in the absence of a demonstrable immune defect in patients who have recurrences of HSV infection, the very fact that such recurrences occur suggests that such a defect may exist. Hence, augmentation of the immune response has been attempted as a therapy for these diseases. Interferon alpha has been the most effective drug used for this type of therapy and is known to inhibit HSV replication in vitro. It is effective in some patients when given prospectively prior to contact with known inducers of reactivation, such as surgical manipulation of the trigeminal ganglion. The use of interferon is limited, however, by toxicity, cost, and the need for parenteral administration. Recent in vitro studies suggest that a combination of interferon and a detergent, nonoxynol-9, administered topically, may prove more effective and less toxic than parenterally administered interferon. Nonspecific stimulators of cell mediated immunity such as cimetidine, isoprinosine, and vaccines for bacillus Calmette-Guerin (BCG), vaccinia, polio, and influenza have been studied, and all are ineffective in the treatment of HSV infections.

The most effective therapies for mucocutaneous and systemic infections caused by HSV have been compounds that specifically inhibit viral replication. The majority of such drugs are nucleoside analogues, which inhibit viral DNA synthesis and thereby arrest viral replication. Idoxuridine (5'-iodo-2'-deoxyuridine) was the first such compound to be licensed in this country in the 1960s. Because of poor tissue penetration and weak activity, topical therapy with idoxuridine has been ineffective in the treatment of mucocutaneous herpes. Its very low therapeutic ratio reflects substantial toxicity when given systemically; hence its only useful role is in the topical treatment of herpes keratitis.

The first substance to significantly ameliorate severe mucocutaneous or visceral HSV infections was vidarabine (adenine arabinoside). When administered intravenously, this purine analogue decreases the morbidity and mortality of HSV encephalitis in children and adults and HSV infections of the skin, eye, mouth, brain, or viscera in the neonate. Recently the guanosine analogue, acyclovir, has been proven superior to vidarabine for all HSV infections except for those in the neonate, in which both drugs appear comparable. Currently vidarabine remains a treatment alternative in neonatal herpes infections, in the topical treatment of HSV keratitis, and perhaps in the rare immunocompromised individual who appears to fail to benefit from acyclovir therapy. Another nucleoside analogue, triflurothymidine, is also effective for herpes keratitis, but like idoxuridine is limited to topical use. Investigational nucleoside analogues for herpes infections include bromovinyldeoxyuridine (BVDU), phosphonoformate, fluroiodoaracytosine (FIAC), and ribavirin. Preliminary data regarding these substances indicate that they are either more toxic or less effective than acyclovir.

Acyclovir is by far the most effective antiviral compound developed to date. It is the drug of choice for the majority of HSV infections and can be given topically, orally, and intravenously. Acyclovir therapy for primary and recurrent outbreaks of mucocutaneous herpes is discussed extensively in the following sections.

PHARMACOLOGY AND MECHANISM OF ACTION OF ACYCLOVIR

Acyclovir is available in several forms: as a 5 percent ointment in polyethylene glycol for topical use, as 200 mg orally administered capsules, and as a sodium salt for intravenous use. Blood levels following topical application are negligible, except when the drug is applied to very large areas of denuded skin. A single 200 mg oral dose of acyclovir results in a peak serum level of approximately 1 μg per milliliter, which averages three and 10 times the level required in vitro for a 50 percent inhibition of HSV-2 and HSV-1, respectively. Levels obtained with the usual intravenous dose of 5 mg per kilogram are five to 10 times higher than those obtained orally.

Once inside virus infected cells, acyclovir is phosphorylated by the viral enzyme thymidine kinase and is thus activated. The phosphorylated form interferes with the viral DNA polymerase and blocks further synthesis of the viral DNA chain. These virus specific steps of activation and chain termination are the reasons for acyclovir's specificity for HSV. Most other viruses do not activate acyclovir. Furthermore, because acyclovir is not a good substrate for cellular enzymes, it is remarkably free of toxicity to human cells. This gives acyclovir the highest therapeutic ratio of any currently available antiviral drug.

THERAPY

The ultimate goals of treatment in HSV infections include speeding recovery from individual outbreaks, decreasing symptoms, preventing recurrences, preventing complications (dehydration in severe oral infection, aseptic meningitis, dissemination of infection, postherpetic neuralgia), decreasing transmission of disease, and blocking or eradicating latent infection. Unfortunately only a few of these goals are attainable at present. The impor-

tant goal of preventing or eliminating the latent state of HSV remains beyond our grasp.

The diagnosis of mucocutaneous HSV infection is usually based upon recognition of the typical symptoms and lesions. At the first available opportunity, or when atypical lesions appear, the diagnosis should be confirmed by culture. The approach to confirmed mucocutaneous herpes infections is divided into two categories: treatment of acute primary or recurrent infection and suppression of recurrent disease.

The initial treatment of primary and recurrent mucocutaneous outbreaks of HSV infection has been studied using topical, oral, and intravenous forms of acyclovir. Parameters used to measure the effectiveness of such therapy include the duration of viral shedding, the duration and severity of symptoms, and the rate of lesion healing. By these criteria all forms of acyclovir are effective in certain infections of normal and compromised hosts.

In the normal host the clinical responses are most dramatic in the treatment of first episodes of genital herpes. Untreated first episodes of genital herpes typically require 14 to 21 days for healing. Using an oral acyclovir dose of 200 mg five times daily for 10 days, one notes, on the average, a 70 to 80 percent decrease in the duration of viral shedding, a 40 to 50 percent decrease in the duration of symptoms, and a 30 to 40 percent decrease in the time to healing. Oral therapy appears to be as effective as intravenous therapy in this setting and obviously has the advantage of convenience, outpatient use, and decreased cost. In the rare patient who cannot tolerate oral medication, or whose primary attack is complicated by urinary retention or aseptic meningitis, intravenous therapy may be indicated, and doses of 5 mg per kilogram every 8 hours should be used for 7 days. Topical acyclovir therapy should be reserved for very mild first episodes of genital herpes; oral therapy is well tolerated and is more effective. No studies have been performed to determine the efficacy of acyclovir therapy of primary labial herpes, but oral acyclovir treatment probably would be helpful. It is important to note that the therapy of first episodes of HSV infection does not prevent the establishment of latent infection in neural ganglia and therefore does not prevent later recurrences. Recurrent genital infections in normal individuals are inherently milder than first infections, requiring an average of only 7 to 10 days for healing. Intravenous treatment is not indicated and topical therapy is inadequate. Oral acyclovir therapy is effective, but the degree of benefit is modest, with only a 40 to 50 percent decrease in viral shedding, a 15 to 25 percent decrease in the duration of symptoms, and a 20 to 30 percent decrease in the time to lesion healing.

Initiation of therapy early in the course of recurrent disease is critical if any benefit is to be obtained. Therefore, reliable patients with established recurrent disease patterns should be given acyclovir and instructed to begin therapy at the onset of symptoms, preferably during the prodromal stage of the disease. We reserve such therapy of recurrent disease for patients who tend to have longer or more severe episodes, because the benefit in patients with mild or short lived recurrences is minimal. For recurrent disease in normal individuals the usual oral dosage of acyclovir is 200 mg five times daily for 5 days.

The treatment of recurrent labial herpes has been less well studied. However, the usual episode resolves so quickly (4 to 7 days) and is associated with such mild symptoms that acyclovir is not likely to be of benefit.

The duration of therapy in primary or recurrent disease may have to be altered, depending on the clinical or virologic response. If lesions remain ulcerated or if new lesions continue to develop, treatment should continue until all lesions are crusted. Therapy also can be monitored by viral culture, and treatment should be continued for at least 2 to 3 days after the last positive culture.

The management of mucocutaneous herpes in immunocompromised hosts is more complex, because patients present with a broad spectrum of disorders of immune impairment and in these patients HSV infections can be mild or remarkably aggressive. The most severe infections with HSV occur in patients with congenital cellular immune defects, in those undergoing treatment for malignant disease, and in organ transplant recipients. Patients with AIDS tend to develop protracted mucocutaneous HSV infections. These are generally less painful or destructive than the infections in other immunodeficient patients but may progress over long periods of time to involve large areas of skin.

For the treatment of HSV disease in virtually all immunodeficient patients, both intravenous and oral doses of acyclovir are effective. For the management of aggressive infections in severely ill patients or those with profound immunosuppression, acyclovir in intravenous doses of 5 mg per kilogram every 8 hours should be used. However, unless mucositis or gastrointestinal upset precludes the oral use of acyclovir, a dosage of 400 mg five times daily may also be tried. Topical applications of acyclovir can also be used to treat small superficial lesions. The duration of treatment depends on the virologic and clinical response, as already discussed, but typically extends from 7 to 10 days. Less severely immunosuppressed patients, such as those taking alternate day steroid therapy or patients who have completed cancer chemotherapy, usually can be treated like normal hosts, using oral doses of acyclovir, 200 mg five times daily for 5 days. For AIDS patients with prolonged indolent mucocutaneous herpes infections, long courses of oral doses of acyclovir for up to many weeks may be necessary for healing. The standard dosage may have to be increased on an individual basis to achieve a virologic and clinical response; we have used oral dosages totaling as much as 4 g per day.

Perhaps the most salutary use of acyclovir is in long-term administration to prevent the reactivation of HSV infection. This approach was first used in immunocompromised hosts during periods of high risk for reactivation, such as during chemotherapy induced leukopenia and for the first 5 to 6 weeks after organ transplantation. Both oral (200 to 400 mg five times daily) and intravenous (5 mg per kilogram every 8 hours) doses of acyclovir are highly effective when used in this manner.

Symptomatic reactivation of HSV infection in normal patients also can be prevented by the prolonged administration of acyclovir. Divided doses totaling 400 to 1,000 mg daily for 4 months prevent recurrent genital disease in about 70 percent of the patients. In our research, patients who prior to therapy experienced eight to 12 recurrences per year have been treated for periods of up to 1 year without any episodes of reactivation. Patient selection is important for this form of therapy, and it should be reserved for those with particularly troublesome infections or those with an established pattern of frequent recurrences (more than six to eight per year). It should be recognized that many patients have several recurrences immediately following the primary infection, but this does not necessarily portend a continuing problem with very frequent infections. It is important to reassess the need for long-term therapy every several months, because in some patients the disease fails to be reactivated for extended periods after treatment is stopped. These patients should not be retreated over long periods unless the recurrences become frequent once again. Unfortunately such patients are the exception. Most patients revert to the usual pretreatment pattern of reactivation when taken off therapy. Thus our practice is to initiate sequential 6 month courses of acyclovir with an assessment of the time to recurrence between each course. The potential complications of sustained acyclovir use are still not completely known, and patients taking such therapy should be followed closely.

Some individuals report stimuli that predictably lead to reactivation of HSV infection. Ultraviolet light, trauma, the onset of menses, and emotional stress are frequently cited. One recent study has shown that oral doses of acyclovir given prior to intense sun exposure can prevent reactivation of oral herpes, and other studies are currently under way using acyclovir in an anticipatory fashion prior to other known causes of reactivation. In carefully selected individuals this would obviate the need for prolonged daily treatment. Table 1 summarizes our approach to initial and long-term treatment of mucocutaneous HSV infections in normal and immunocompromised hosts.

There are other clinical situations in which systemic acyclovir therapy may be effective, but these have not been well studied. In herpes induced erythema multiforme, prolonged or very early use of acyclovir appears to prevent this complication. Once erythema multiforme has developed, acyclovir is without benefit. It would also seem reasonable to attempt acyclovir therapy in herpes gladiatorum or eczema herpeticum to prevent the spread of lesions to wide areas of skin. Severe eczema herpeticum may warrant intravenous therapy. Frequent herpetic whitlow, particularly in health care workers in whom the risk of transmission is high, might also be an indication for oral acyclovir therapy. Other unusual herpes infections, such as culture proven zosteriform simplex or the frequent cutaneous recurrences that follow neonatal infection, could also benefit from acyclovir. Doses similar to those used in genital herpes should be effective in these conditions, but more detailed studies are needed before the indications for acyclovir in these herpes infections are established.

TABLE 1 Acyclovir for Treatment of Mucocutaneous HSV Infections

Infection	Dose	Route	Dose Regimen	Duration (days)*	Comments
Normal host, genital herpes, first episode	5% ointment	Topical	6× per day	7	For mild external lesions only
	200 mg	Oral	5× per day	10	Route of choice for most patients
	5 mg/kg	IV	q8h	5–7	For some patients requiring hospitalization
Genital herpes, recurrence	200 mg	Oral	5× per day	5	May not benefit all patients
Genital herpes, suppression	200 mg	Oral	3× per day	Up to 6 months	For patients with frequent and troublesome recurrences (>6–8 per year)
Immunocompromised host, oral or genital herpes, first or recurrent episode	5% ointment	Topical	6× per day	7–10	For mild external lesions
	200–400 mg	Oral	5× per day	7–10	Route of choice for most patients
	5 mg/kg	IV	q8h	7–10	For extensive disease or prolonged shedding or delayed healing with oral therapy
Prophylaxis against recurrent herpes	200–400 mg	Oral	5× per day	Period of risk	Short-term prophylaxis for profoundly immunosuppressed patients (transplant recipients, neutropenic patients)
	5 mg/kg	IV	q8h	Period of risk	

* The durations listed have been found effective in clinical studies and represent general recommendations. As discussed in the text, the duration of therapy may need to be extended as dictated by clinical and virologic responses. (From Felser JF, Straus SE. In: Mills J, Corey L, eds. Antiviral chemotherapy. New York: Elsevier, 1986, Reproduced with permission.)

TREATMENT FAILURES

Treatment failures have been seen with acyclovir, even when properly used. When such failures occur, a number of issues need to be addressed. First the diagnosis of herpes simplex virus infection should be confirmed by culture. We have been referred many patients for supposed acyclovir treatment failure in whom we have been unable to document HSV infection despite numerous cultures. Second, in the immunocompromised host the failure to respond to acyclovir is almost always the result of immune deficiency and is not related to the antiviral treatment of HSV. However, in the immunocompromised host, in particular, infections with varicella-zoster virus may mimic HSV infection. This virus also produces latent and recurrent infections and is 10- to 30-fold less sensitive to acyclovir than HSV; hence it may appear refractory to acyclovir in the oral doses already recommended. Third, one must be alert to the development of viral drug resistance as a cause of treatment failure. Acyclovir resistant mutants of HSV have been isolated from patients taking such therapy. These viruses possess mutations in the viral thymidine kinase gene, which prevent the activation of acyclovir and render it ineffective. Fortunately these virus strains have not been a great clinical problem to date, and in most patients the infections resolve without further therapy. Additionally these drug resistant viruses do not seem to persist as well as the natural virus. Subsequent recurrences in patients from whom drug resistant viruses have been isolated are caused by reactivation of the original drug sensitive virus. Nevertheless the emergence of drug resistant strains should continue to be sought and the indiscriminate or erratic use of acyclovir must be discouraged.

Recurrent infections during long-term suppressive therapy occur even in patients with none of the foregoing factors. In a few of our patients who have established a pattern of frequent "breakthrough" recurrences of this type, we have found that dosage escalation to as much as 1,200 mg daily is effective in suppressing the disease. Viruses isolated from some of these individuals prove slightly less sensitive to acyclovir and presumably require higher dosages for inhibition in vivo.

Now that effective antiviral therapy exists, the local and symptomatic care of herpes infections should not be neglected. Saline or dilute peroxide rinses decrease the likelihood of bacterial superinfection in oral gingivostomatitis. Cutaneous lesions should be kept clean and dry. The use of occlusive dressings and tight garments should be discouraged. Analgesics for pain, such as aspirin or acetaminophen, are helpful. Occasionally narcotics are necessary for severe pain, particularly in primary disease. The topical application of anesthetics, such as 5 percent lidocaine, may be helpful for the temporary relief of pain in gingivostomatitis. Antihistamines such as diphenhydramine and hydroxyzine may relieve the pruritus associated with herpetic lesions.

Finally patients need to be educated about factors important in the transmission of HSV. They should avoid contact with others while they have active lesions and should practice careful handwashing. They should be made aware that shedding of virus can occur while taking acyclovir therapy and that transmission is possible. Furthermore, shedding of virus in the absence of symptoms occurs and is another possible means of transmission.

TOXICITY

The most important requirement of a specific antiviral drug is that it must effectively inhibit viral replication without exhibiting significant toxicity to eukaryotic cells. There is extensive experience with the use of acyclovir, both intravenously and orally, and it is very well tolerated. The most serious known side effect of acyclovir is the development of acute renal failure associated with crystalluria. This uncommon complication has been seen only with high dose intravenous therapy and appears to be completely reversible if the drug is discontinued promptly. Because of this severe adverse effect, patients taking intravenous doses of acyclovir should be very well hydrated, and serum creatinine levels should be monitored at least every 3 days. Even more frequent monitoring is necessary in patients whose creatinine level is elevated prior to therapy. Nomograms are available for the appropriate adjustment of the acyclovir dosage in patients with impaired renal function. The adverse renal effects of acyclovir appear to be dose related, for patients have been rechallenged with oral doses after recovery and have tolerated it well. No cases of renal toxicity have been reported with oral use of the drug.

Rare central nervous system toxicity with lethargy, myoclonic jerking, tremors, and confusion has been reported with intravenous administration of acyclovir. With oral doses of 200 mg, about 5 percent of the patients report mild gastrointestinal upset, which often can be overcome by administering the drug with meals. Less frequent side effects include diarrhea, dizziness, arthralgias, and headache. Rash due to drug allergy also occurs. In studies that we have conducted, patients receiving oral acyclovir therapy continuously for 1 year showed no adverse effects. Because of its mechanism of action (the inhibition of DNA synthesis), the use of acyclovir should be strongly discouraged in pregnancy, even though no teratogenic effects have been seen in man or experimental animals. In addition, males and females should be counseled to practice effective birth control while taking therapy. Similarly, acyclovir use in children for other than serious disease has not been studied systematically and for the present should be discouraged.

FUTURE ALTERNATIVES IN THE MANAGEMENT OF HSV INFECTIONS

The greatest hope for the future management of HSV infections is that an effective method of prevention will be discovered. The development of a herpes vaccine is an active research area and involves a variety of approaches, including live attenuated herpes strains, viral subunit vaccines, synthetic peptide vaccines, and recombinant vaccinia virus strains that express immunogenic glycoproteins of HSV. Because of the capacity of HSV to establish latent infection and to cause transformation of eukaryotic cells in vitro, concerns exist about most of the potential herpes vaccines. Obviously many trials will have to be made before any such vaccine could become generally available. Such vaccines will have to be targeted for individuals at risk for exposure to herpes simplex virus, since vaccination after the establishment of neural latency has little effect on subsequent reactivation.

ORF

FRANK W. CROWE, M.D.

Orf is an infectious viral disease of the mucous membrane and skin of sheep and goats (scabby mouth disease). The orf virus is a member of the poxvirus group. The disease is characterized by a vesiculopustular eruption of the lips and mouth in the animal, but may occur on any part of the human body by accidental inoculation of the causative virus. In man the disease is relatively mild despite the clinical appearance, and it is self-limited.

The initial small red papules rapidly progress to vesicles and hemorrhagic bullae, usually with an umbilicated center. These rupture within 48 hours to form thick eschar-like crusts. Although usually seen on the fingers, hands, and forearms, they may appear anywhere, including the face. The lesion may appear like a primary smallpox inoculation, but it is rarely painful and only occasionally pruritic. Regional lymphadenopathy is minimal and there may be mild fever. A transitory erythema multiforme-like eruption has been reported during the second week in a few cases. Orf is relatively common in rural areas, but patients seldom seek medical care, since most herdsmen and grandmothers are aware of the benign self-limited nature of the disease.

TREATMENT

Minimizing the possibility of secondary bacterial infection is the main concern. I have found that the use of a drying shake lotion with 2 percent chloramphenicol added is effective (Table 1). This lotion is painted on the areas with a small paint brush twice daily. No attempt is made to remove the paint, but the patient may wash and bathe as needed. As noted earlier, the eruption is self-limited, and no therapy is really necessary. I have not found the oral use of antibiotics to be needed or beneficial. After the crusts have dried and sloughed, the use of any bland lubricant is helpful. A residual scar may be noted, but the patient now has a life-long immunity.

TABLE 1 Formula for White Shake Lotion

Amylum	24	g
Glycerine	18	cc
Zinc oxide	24	g
Bentonite magma, USP	30	g
Chloramphenicol	2.4	g
Distilled water qs	120	cc

MOLLUSCUM CONTAGIOSUM

BONNIE S. EPSTEIN, M.D.

Molluscum contagiosum is a disease primarily seen in childhood and adolescence. It is caused by the molluscum contagiosum virus, a member of the pox virus group.

Clinically the lesions present as dome shaped, firm, umbilicated papules, usually less than 5 mm in diameter. The number of papules in an individual usually ranges from one to twenty although rarely a patient may have hundreds. Lesions can be spread either by direct contact or by fomite to skin transmission. The diagnosis of molluscum contagiosum is clinically usually apparent—an asymptomatic array of umbilicated papules on normal skin. If the diagnosis is uncertain, it can be confirmed most easily by expressing the core and crushing it on a slide. The homogeneous cytoplasmic inclusion bodies can be identified with either Wright's or Giemsa's stain. Biopsy of the lesion for diagnosis is usually not necessary. If done for other reasons, it would show the characteristic inclusion bodies.

Once the diagnosis is established, all therapeutic decisions should be made with the recognition that the disease is self-limited. Individual papules that are untreated resolve spontaneously in 2 months. If left untreated, all the lesions on a patient clear 6 months to 3 years after their onset. Because the disease resolves spontaneously, treatment should be painless and not leave scars. The benign self-limited nature of the lesions should be stressed to both parents and child. Emphasis should be placed on the possible psychological as well as physical trauma that could occur in treatment. Patients should be reassured that although new lesions could crop up, the disease as a rule usually runs its course (on the average) in about 16 months. The number of lesions is not prognostic of the time course of the disease (i.e., children with few lesions may have them for a long period of time and vice versa). It is important to wait for 4 months after the appearance of a new lesion in order to state that the disease has run its course. New lesions can crop up at intervals of less than 4 months.

If treatment is deemed necessary, it is important to realize that it is not necessary to treat every lesion. Minimal trauma to a few lesions appears to induce a generalized immune response, which hastens resolution of the remaining lesions.

A good technique for the young child is to prick the surface of the skin and express the central contents. This can be done with either a sterile needle or a number 11 blade and the core expressed with a tongue blade.

Curettage followed by light electrodesiccation or application of an agent such as aluminum chloride, which controls any bleeding, is also very effective. A Band-Aid is applied over the area, which can be removed the next day. The area then can be washed with soap and water subsequently, with no further postoperative care needed. Since it can be difficult for the child to tolerate this procedure, numbing the area with lidocaine can be valuable. This in itself is painful and may produce psychological trauma.

If it is decided to infiltrate with lidocaine, two helpful tricks are (1) to apply an ice cube to the area first for a local numbing effect, and (2) to inject the lidocaine very slowly, as this is less painful than a few fast bursts.

Cryotherapy is also effective for the child who is old enough to cooperate. It can be a somewhat painful procedure, and it is necessary for the child to be still and not move. No special care is required after this procedure.

An alternative method that is not as frightening for the child is the application of Duofilm (a combination of salicylic and lactic acid), trichloroacetic acid, or cantharidin. I do not recommend cantharidin because it is hard to predict the size of the resulting blister. The liquid is applied using a dropper provided or the wooden edge of a Q-tip applicator. One drop is placed on the lesion. Larger lesions then may be covered with tape. The parent must be instructed to wash the area thoroughly in 4 to 6 hours or earlier if the lesion is very painful.

VENEREAL DISEASE

SYPHILIS

PETER E. DANS, M.D.

Syphilis is a sexually-transmitted disease resulting from infection by *Treponema pallidum*. Since the introduction of penicillin, its prevalence has declined sharply. Although currently overshadowed in severity by AIDS and in incidence by gonorrhea and genital herpes, it remains an important sexually-transmitted disease. Because accurate diagnosis and disease staging are essential to appropriate management, a brief discussion of these aspects is warranted.

The principal stages of acquired syphilis are primary, secondary, early and late latent, and tertiary. Primary syphilis is characterized by the development of a "chancre"—an indurated and ulcerated papule that appears 10 to 90 days after infection. Secondary syphilis, which occurs 6 weeks to 6 months after infection, usually manifests itself by a generalized nonpruritic and usually maculopapular rash often involving the trunk, palms, and soles. Accurate diagnosis is made by darkfield microscopy of exudate from an ulcer or any moist lesion (except in the mouth where normal flora may mislead the observer).

Latent syphilis, the period after infection with no clinical signs and symptoms, is the most frequently-encountered stage. The only clue to its diagnosis is a positive serologic test. The most commonly-used tests are the RPR (rapid plasma reagin) and the VDRL (Venereal Disease Research Laboratory) tests. Called nontreponemal because of their nonspecificity, they are useful for screening, but must be followed by more specific treponemal tests, such as the FTA-ABS (fluorescent treponemal antibody absorption) test. Approximately one-third of untreated patients develop tertiary syphilis involving primarily the heart and brain 10 to 30 years after infection.

A careful history of sexual contacts and sexual practices as well as of the dates, types, and results of serologic tests is essential. The motto should be to look carefully before leaping from test results to diagnostic closure, since the therapeutic and social consequences of this diagnosis are far from trivial.

The remainder of this article is devoted to the treatment of syphilis. This is discussed in the context of overall management, which includes not just antibiotic therapy but also follow-up of patients and their contacts as well as patient education.

ANTIBIOTIC REGIMENS

Early Syphilis

Penicillin is clearly the drug of choice, but there is some controversy about preferred treatment schedules. This is because most treatment studies were done shortly after the introduction of penicillin when the prevalence of syphilis was high but penicillin availability was limited in both amount and type. *T. pallidum* is very sensitive to small concentrations of penicillin (in the range of 0.03 unit of penicillin per milliliter); this level must be maintained for about 7 to 10 days for the effective treatment of early syphilis. Using benzathine penicillin (Bicillin) fulfills these criteria, but there have been few controlled studies of varying dosage schedules. The Centers for Disease Control (CDC) periodically convenes experts to assess the current state of treatment of sexually transmitted diseases. Most of what is outlined here is based on the 1985 treatment guidelines. Readers should be alert to the possibility of future revisions.

The generally accepted treatment of choice for primary, secondary, and early latent syphilis, as well as of known contacts of patients with infectious syphilis, is 2.4 million units of benzathine penicillin G intramuscularly. In one study of this regimen for the treatment of primary and secondary syphilis, the cumulative incidence of retreatment because of failure or reinfection was 7.5 percent for primary syphilis and 11.9 percent for secondary. Other studies have shown slightly lower incidences.

Fiumara has strongly advocated that a second injection of 2.4 million units of benzathine penicillin G be given 1 week later to all patients with early syphilis. He has reported an uncontrolled study of this regimen as having a zero percent failure incidence. Although I adhere to the CDC recommendations, I am more apt to use a second injection of benzathine penicillin G in patients with secondary syphilis, especially if they have systemic manifestations such as hepatitis or the nephrotic syndrome. The recommended regimen in patients who are allergic to penicillin is 500 mg of tetracycline or erythromycin by mouth four times a day for 15 days. Although less well-studied than penicillin, these regimens are somewhat less effective. In the best controlled study the retreatment incidence for the erythromycin regimen was 12.3 percent and that for tetracycline, slightly lower.

Late Syphilis

Before assigning a seropositive patient with syphilis of more than 1 year's duration a diagnosis of late latent syphilis, the CDC recommends a lumbar puncture to exclude asymptomatic neurosyphilis. I do not adhere to this recommendation in patients who have no neurologic or psychiatric signs on careful examination and who are not allergic to penicillin. My reasons are two-fold: (1) the majority of such patients (probably 90 percent or more) have negative cerebrospinal fluid findings; and (2) whatever the results, I would use a regimen of 2.4 million units of benzathine penicillin G weekly for 3 weeks. My rationale is based on the most extensive study to date of the treatment of asymptomatic neurosyphilis in which Hahn et al. showed that only one of 765 patients treated with penicillin in doses equivalent to this regimen went on to develop clinical neurosyphilis. For many years, in fact, this regimen was the recommended treatment schedule even for clinical neurosyphilis and still remains an option, although other regimens are more advisable for overt neurosyphilis. It is worth noting, however, that there are a few investigators who advise a lumbar puncture be done in all asymptomatic preoperative patients and who would treat patients with asymptomatic neurosyphilis with the intravenous penicillin regimen, which will be outlined for symptomatic neurosyphilis. One group for which this may be an apparent strategy is patients with concurrent human immunodeficiency virus (HIV) infection.

Assessing the effectiveness of treatment for latent syphilis is extremely difficult because of the absence of clinical markers and consists of long-term follow-up to demonstrate the arrest of progression to the tertiary stage. Thus, it is reassuring to note that in a multicenter review of use of penicillin equivalent to the schedule just given, all 469 patients with late latent syphilis were symptom free 12 years later.

For patients who have documented penicillin allergy, the argument for a lumbar puncture is somewhat more persuasive. The primary reason is that the usual alternative antibiotics, erythromycin and tetracycline, do not diffuse well into the cerebrospinal fluid. However, benzathine penicillin G seems to be effective even though its penetrance into the spinal fluid is also low; this raises serious questions about the relationship of cerebrospinal fluid antibiotic levels to therapeutic success. If one elects not to perform a lumbar puncture in a penicillin-allergic patient, I would advise validating the penicillin allergy by a skin test, since most patients giving such a history are not sensitive to penicillin on rechallenge. If the patient is truly penicillin allergic and a lumbar puncture is not done, one still can use the recommended alternative for the treatment of latent syphilis—500 mg of tetracycline or erythromycin by mouth four times daily for 30 days.

In seropositive patients with neurological and psychiatric signs, a lumbar puncture is mandatory, and the spinal fluid should be tested for cells and protein as well as VDRL or RPR and FTA-ABS tests. Since the spinal fluid FTA-ABS test is not approved for use in routine laboratories, it is advisable to have this test performed at the CDC or at the state health department or other regional reference laboratory. If clinical neurosyphilis is confirmed, a more intensive course of penicillin is recommended because of case reports of failure of the benzathine penicillin G regimen to eradicate the organism and to arrest the disease. The following schedule is recommended:

Twelve to 24 million units of aqueous crystalline penicillin G given intravenously each day for 10 days followed by benzathine penicillin G; 2.4 million units intramuscularly weekly for three doses.

Alternate regimens considered potentially effective are:

a. Aqueous procaine penicillin G; 2.4 million units intramuscularly once daily, plus to probenecid, 500 mg by mouth four times a day, both for 10 days, followed by benzathine penicillin G, 2.4 million units intramuscularly weekly for three doses and

b. Benzathine penicillin G, 2.4 million units intramuscularly weekly for three doses.

Because of the seriousness of clinical neurosyphilis, it is extremely important to document penicillin allergy before using an alternative regimen. When allergy is confirmed, the therapeutic choice is difficult. On the basis of a single case report, some experienced investigators recommend ceftriaxone, 1 g intra-muscularly daily for 14 days. However, when treating such a patient, it is advisable to consult an infectious disease expert to determine the most current recommendation.

The results of treatment for neurosyphilis vary directly with the extent of disease and inversely with its duration. Thus, one usually sees reversal of acute meningovascular syphilis, stabilization of tabes dorsalis, and lesser effects on general paresis, especially if treatment is given late in its course.

The recommended treatment for cardiovascular syphilis is the same as for late latent syphilis, i.e., three injections of 2.4 million units of benzathine penicillin G 1 week apart. Although the effectiveness of this therapy is uncertain, it is generally believed that treatment arrests the disease but does not reverse it. Ascending aortic aneurysms, characteristic of this stage, usually continue to enlarge, even after adequate treatment, because of the already weakened media.

Congenital Syphilis

Traditionally the term congenital syphilis refers to infection of a fetus in utero (prenatal). However, the child can be infected during passage through the birth canal (neonatal). Prenatal congenital syphilis is usually severe and often fatal. Neonatal congenital syphilis is characterized by prematurity, low birth weight, anemia, and jaundice. Meningitis is present in half the cases. Congenital syphilis may manifest itself later in childhood by keratitis, long bone and teeth deformities, and deafness.

The diagnosis of congenital syphilis in a child born to a woman with a positive serology is difficult. This is because infants born to even adequately-treated mothers are seropositive at birth because of passive transfer of IGG across the placenta. If the infant appears healthy and the mother was apparently adequately treated, regular examinations should be performed at 4 to 6 week intervals until serologic tests are negative (usually in 3 to 6 months). When there are signs and symptoms suggestive of syphilis or the baby's serologic titer as tested on venous (not cord) blood using the VDRL or RPR test is equal to or higher than that of the mother, congenital syphilis should be diagnosed and treatment instituted. When there is no history of adequate treatment of the mother for infectious syphilis during pregnancy, the child should be treated because of the possibility of delayed onset disease. Treatment should also be instituted if there is any question about the treatment status or if adequate follow-up of the infant cannot be insured. Many believe that any patient born to a mother treated with erythromycin should be retreated using penicillin (see next section).

The following are the current recommendations for treatment: Children with abnormal spinal fluid results should receive aqueous crystalline penicillin G (50,000 units per kilogram intramuscularly or intravenously daily in two divided doses) for a minimum of 10 days or aqueous procaine penicillin G (50,000 units per kilogram intramuscularly daily) for a minimum of 10 days. Asymptomatic children with normal spinal fluid test results should receive benzathine penicillin G (50,000 units per kilogram intramuscularly in a single dose with a maximum, of 2.4 million units). Only penicillin regimens are recommended for neonatal congenital syphilis. In older children, if penicillin allergy is suspected, the patient should be skin tested before diagnosing allergy to penicillin. In cases in which the skin test is positive, expert consultation should be sought regarding treatment, since tetracycline is contraindicated in children less than 8 years of age.

Special Treatment Considerations

1. Patients who were treated for syphilis with heavy metals before the penicillin era are now rarely encountered. When they are, questions arise as to the need for further treatment. Most experts do not recommend retreating such patients whose syphilis acquisition dates back 40 years or more in the absence of clinical signs or of exposure to infectious syphilis in the interim.

2. In pregnant patients with syphilis treatment should be the same as for nonpregnant patients (i.e., penicillin). In patients who are definitely penicillin allergic, tetracycline is contraindicated and erythromycin is the preferred alternative. Since it is more likely to cause nausea and vomiting in pregnant patients, erythromycin should be used in the enteric coated form. Even so, there is concern about how effective erythromycin is in treating both fetus and mother. This is an area of active research, and consultation with experts at the CDC is advisable to ascertain the most current treatment recommendation.

3. Concern has been raised recently regarding the effect of concurrent infection HIV on the efficacy of syphilis treatment schedules. This is especially important given the higher prevalence of both HIV infection and syphilis in male homosexuals. Although there is nothing yet to suggest that treatment schedules should be altered when the HIV test is positive, one might wish to err on the side of giving, for example, the second injection of benzathine penicillin G, as Fiumara recommends, in cases of early syphilis.

Complications

Any physician's office or clinic must be equipped to handle emergencies, especially penicillin anaphylaxis or a reaction to procaine following the use of procaine penicillin. It is advisable to ask the patient to wait in the waiting room for 20 to 30 minutes after intramuscular administration of penicillin to detect potential reactions. A properly-equipped emergency cart with ventilation equipment (e.g., epinephrine, intravenous fluids) should be readily accessible. Since these events are rare, the staff must be regularly retrained in life support procedures to be used in the event of such occurrences. Additionally each staff member should know the process for expediting the transfer of patients to an emergency facility when necessary.

Vasovagal reactions are episodes of syncope during or shortly after drawing blood or injections. They are not usually serious in themselves, because the hypotension usually responds quickly after the patient has been in the reclining position for a short period of time. However, such episodes can become serious if the patient falls and hits his head on a hard object. To prevent this, it is best to insure that precautions have been taken to prevent or cushion a fall when drawing blood or administering injections.

Jarisch-Herxheimer Reaction

The Jarisch-Herxheimer reaction is characterized by a mild temperature elevation within 6 to 8 hours after the first injection of penicillin. The reaction occurs primarily in patients with early syphilis but can also occur in those with latent disease. It can consist of slight fever, chills, headache, muscle and joint pains, and sore throat. In patients with secondary syphilis the skin lesions become transiently more prominent. Because it is so common, patients should be informed of its possible occurrence and that, if it occurs, it is invariably mild and should last only a few hours. If necessary, aspirin or acetaminophen may be taken. Patients should be instructed to notify you in the rare cases in which serious side effects, such as transient hypotension, occur. Since the Jarisch-Herxheimer reaction has been reported to exacerbate neurological signs in a small percentage of patients treated for neurosyphilis, concurrent use of steroids has been recommended when administering the first dose of penicillin, although their utility has not been established. The Jarisch-Herxheimer reaction does not occur with subsequent antibiotic administration.

FOLLOW-UP

The necessity for regular follow-up must be stressed. Since signs and symptoms are usually absent or disappear even without treatment, the nontreponemal test titer is the most useful index of the response to treatment. Most patients with early syphilis exhibit substantial reactivity in tests such as the VDRL or RPR (i.e., titers of 1:8 or greater). A serologic response to treatment is considered to be a four-fold or greater decrease in titer (e.g., from 1:16 to 1:4 or lower). If the expected fall in titer does not occur within 9 to 12 months, the patient should be retreated according to the same treatment schedule. It is important to remember that the RPR is a more sensitive test than the VDRL, and when they are done simultaneously, the titer of the RPR often is at least a one dilution higher than that of the VDRL. Thus, when comparing nontreponemal test titers, it is preferable to use the same test done in the same laboratory. Patients who are treated later in the course (e.g., late secondary syphilis) have slower serologic responses than those treated at an earlier stage.

Patients with persistently high titers of 1:8 or higher after 1 year may represent either treatment failures or undetected reinfections and should be retreated. A spinal fluid examination to rule out neurosyphilis is indicated in such patients if one has not already been done. Patients who have a four-fold or greater rise in titer at follow-up should be considered to be reinfected and staged and treated accordingly.

The follow-up in patients with late latent syphilis is difficult, not only because of the absence of signs, as noted, but also because the serologic titer is low (e.g., 1:1 or 1:2). Thus, one must be alert to the development of signs or symptoms of tertiary syphilis on routine revisits. In following patients who have neurosyphilis, the CDC recommends periodic serologic testing and clinical evaluation at 6-month intervals with repeat spinal fluid-examinations until they are negative or for at least 3 years.

Contact Tracing

In addition to following patients, the physician is obligated to initiate the process of contact tracing. In most states physicians must report the patient's name and stage of disease to the health department. Some patients may ask the physician not to report them. This presents a conflict between the obligation of the physician to the patient regarding confidentiality and the binding legal requirement to report the patient. The obligation to report must take precedence. The patient should be advised that health department investigators are trained to insure that the patient's name is not divulged. In certain circumstances especially in small towns, the physician can help coordinate the contact tracing in a way that further insures confidentiality. Situations such as this require great sensitivity on the part of the physician and are the paradigm of the art of medicine.

Most patients are increasingly comfortable in having their contacts notified and brought in directly; thus, the physician often can help expedite contact tracing by insuring proper evaluation. All identified contacts of patients with infectious syphilis or of syphilis of less than 1 year's duration should undergo the same thorough investigation as the patient. This should involve a pertinent history and physical examination, serologic testing, disease staging, and treatment when indicated. If there are no signs or symptoms, contacts of someone with syphilis of less than 1 year's duration should be treated epidemiologically anyway with 2.4 million units of benzathine penicillin G intramuscularly or the alternative regimens if the patient is penicillin allergic. If early syphilis is detected, the patient's contacts must also be traced.

Education

Any patient with a sore or rash must be advised to abstain from sexual activity until these have resolved. Education should focus primarily on the prevention of not only syphilis but other sexually transmitted diseases. Since most patients with syphilis are engaging in sexual relations with multiple partners, they should be counseled about the signs and symptoms of syphilis and other diseases and their risk of contracting them and passing them on to others. A nonjudgmental approach to managing patients with sexually transmitted diseases is advisable because it encourages openness and compliance. However, such an approach is not incompatible with serious discussion of the implications of the patient's behavior for his own health and that of partners and society. Since the advent of AIDS, most patients are increasingly responsive to such admonitions and are changing their life styles. Psychiatric counseling is sometimes indicated. Those who plan to continue such activity, e.g., those engaged in prostitution, should be cautioned to insure the use of protection such as a condom. To be effective, these must be used during foreplay, must be properly worn, and must be intact. Contraceptive jellies and creams also may provide some protection. Such patients also should be advised to attend sexually transmitted disease clinics regularly for checkups as well as at the first sign of infection.

GONOCOCCAL INFECTIONS

EDWARD W. HOOK III, M.D.

At the present time there are four regimens recommended for the treatment of uncomplicated urogenital gonorrhea by the Centers for Disease Control:

1. Single doses of 4.8 million units of aqueous procaine penicillin G intramuscularly and probenecid, 1.0 g orally, as well as tetracycline, 500 mg orally four times daily for 7 days.

2. Single doses of ampicillin, 3.5 g (or amoxicillin, 3.0 g), and probenecid, 1.0 g, in addition to tetracycline, 500 mg four times daily for 7 days, all taken by mouth.

3. A single dose of ceftriaxone, 125 to 250 mg intramuscularly, in addition to tetracycline, 500 mg orally four times daily for 7 days.

4. A single dose of spectinomycin, 2.0 g intramuscularly, in addition to tetracycline, 500 mg orally four times daily for 7 days.

Each of these recommended regimens is composed of single dose therapy directed at uncomplicated infection with *Neisseria gonorrhoeae* in addition to 7 days of tetracycline therapy for the treatment of possible coexistent *Chlamydia trachomatis* infection. In the United States today approximately 20 percent of the men and 30 to 50 percent of the women with uncomplicated gonorrhea are coinfected with *C. trachomatis* and, unless treated, are at risk for the development of complications such as postgonococcal urethritis, cervicitis, pelvic inflammatory disease, or epididymitis. Given the relatively high probability of coinfection, the risks of development of complications, and the relatively high cost of chlamydia testing, it is currently more efficient, and probably more cost-effective, to provide patients with simultaneous cotherapy aimed at both *N. gonorrhoeae* and *C. trachomatis* than to treat acute gonococcal infections, test for the presence of *C. trachomatis*, and await results. Although previously effective for gonorrhea therapy as well, tetracycline alone can no longer be relied upon to cure gonorrhea owing to increasing levels of gonococcal tetracycline resistance.

Doxycycline, 100 mg orally twice daily for 7 days, is a preferred alternative to tetracycline because of equal efficacy, the convenience of twice daily dosing, and better tolerability (in terms of gastrointestinal upset), but it costs more than tetracycline. For patients who are pregnant, nursing, or have difficulty in taking tetracyclines, erythromycin, 500 mg orally four times daily for 7 days, is an effective substitute for tetracycline or doxycycline. Patients who experience gastrointestinal upset while taking tetracycline do not necessarily experience similar problems with erythromycin despite the fact that both antibiotics cause gastrointestinal upset in approximately 10 percent of the patients.

Although each of the regimens listed is considered to be equally effective for the therapy of uncomplicated urogenital gonorrhea, there are advantages and disadvantages to each of the single dose components, which should be weighed in choosing therapy for patients with gonorrhea. Factors that should influence the choice of regimen include the possibility of infection with antibiotic resistant strains of *Neisseria gonorrhoeae*, probable sites of infection (sites of sexual exposure), the sexual preference of the patient, and patient variables such as drug allergies and tolerance for swallowing pills versus injectable therapy.

ANTIMICROBIAL RESISTANCE

In North America today, antibiotic resistance in *Neisseria gonorrhoeae* is usually due to one of three potentially coexistent mechanisms: high level penicillin resistance due to plasmid-mediated beta-lactamase production (penicillinase producing *N. gonorrhoeae*, PPNG); high level, plasmid-mediated tetracycline resistance; or gonococci with antimicrobial resistance resulting from the cumulative effect of multiple chromosomal mutations, which may mediate resistance to a variety of antimicrobial drugs by a number of different mechanisms. Although antibiotic resistant gonococci were (and still are) most common in other parts of the world and should be suspected in individuals who have recently traveled outside the United States, they have also steadily increased in number and prevalence within the United States. The prevalence of each form of antimicrobial resistance varies geographically within North America, and consequently the choice of therapy should vary on the basis of local experience and antibiotic susceptibility patterns. In areas where chromosomal resistance is common, failure rates in patients treated with oral ampicillin-probenecid-tetracycline regimens are often unacceptable, exceeding 3 to 5 percent. Although aqueous procaine penicillin G is also more effective than ampicillin, the ceftriaxone or spectinomycin containing regimens are often preferred for patients who are likely to be infected with chromosomally resistant gonococci. High level tetracycline resistance has not been a major problem for patients treated with recommended therapy to date, since the beta-lactam or spectinomycin components of each of the regimens listed are effective for gonococci with plasmid-mediated tetracycline resistance. For patients in or from regions where beta-lactamase producing *N. gonorrhoeae* account for more than 3 to 5 percent of the isolates, neither the ampicillin nor aqueous procaine penicillin G containing regimens should be used, and treatment utilizing either spectinomycin or ceftriaxone is preferred.

POTENTIAL SITES OF INFECTION AND SEXUAL PREFERENCE

Potential sites of infection and the sexual preference of men with gonorrhea should also be considerd in choosing gonococcal therapy. In general, strains of *N. gonorrhoeae* isolated from homosexual or bisexual men are more resistant to antibiotics than isolates from purely heterosexual men or women. In addition, owing to the somewhat lower efficacy of the ampicillin or amoxicillin containing regimens for rectal gonorrhea, the use of one of the three recommended parenteral regimens, which are more effective for resistant gonococci, is preferred to oral therapy. In patients with pharyngeal gonorrhea, the spectinomycin or ampicillin (or amoxicillin) containing regimens have unacceptably high incidences of failure, and therapy with aqueous procaine penicillin G or ceftriaxone is preferred.

PATIENT FACTORS

A final major consideration in the choice of antimicrobial regimens for uncomplicated gonorrhea is patient related factors. Although penicillin should not be used for the therapy of patients who give a history of penicillin allergy, related cephalosporin antibiotics such as ceftriaxone are often safe. Occasional hypersensitivity reactions may occur, however, and as a result, caution in using these therapies is indicated.

Some patients prefer parenteral therapy because of difficulty in swallowing the eight to nine pills required for oral therapy. However, when possible and not otherwise contraindicated, most patients prefer oral therapy using the ampicillin or amoxicillin regimens. These oral therapies are not only more convenient for most patients, but generally are cheaper and easier to administer as well. Among the three recommended parenteral therapies, aqueous procaine penicillin G, the traditional therapy of choice, has recently become less popular because of its diminished activity against antibiotic resistant *N. gonorrhoeae*, the large volume of the injections (nearly 10 cc total volume), the need for two injections in most cases (divided doses), and the possibility of procaine reactions.

Spectinomycin is given as a single injection and generally is somewhat better tolerated than aqueous procaine penicillin G (volume of injection, about 5 ml), but at present many believe that the intramuscular administration of ceftriaxone is the therapy of choice for patients requiring parenteral therapy. Ceftriaxone appears to be highly efficacious at all sites of therapy, is effective in a relatively small volume of injection (0.5 ml for 125 mg, or 1 ml for 250 mg), and has been effective to date against all strains of antimicrobial resistant gonorrhea.

The optimal dose of ceftriaxone for gonorrhea therapy is a subject of some debate. Initial studies and indications used the 250 mg dose, but there is now a large amount of both published and nonpublished data suggesting that in most instances the 125 mg dose is equally effective, but is less costly and is effective in a smaller injection. The author's preference is to use the 125 mg dose of ceftriaxone in all cases in which parenteral therapy is used, including those caused by gonococci with high level, chromosomally mediated antimicrobial resistance or beta-lactamase production.

PARTNER THERAPY

An often overlooked but essential component of therapy for acute gonococcal infections is the treatment of patient partners, irrespective of the presence or absence of symptoms. Informing patients of the possibility that their partners are likely to be infected with gonorrhea, even in the absence of symptoms, is an important message. Partners of the patient with acute symptomatic gonorrhea are often asymptomatic and should be treated with the same regimen as the patient whenever possible. Partner treatment prevents reinfection through reexposure to untreated asymptomatic partners.

COMPLICATED GONOCOCCAL INFECTIONS

For the treatment of patients with disseminated gonococcal infection, a variety of therapeutic options are currently available. In most instances, however, the recommended initial therapy is high doses of penicillin using intravenously administered aqueous penicillin G, 10 to 20 million units daily in divided doses. Following a response to therapy or the establishment of a microbiologic diagnosis and the availability of antimicrobial sensitivity data, completion of therapy on an outpatient basis using orally administered drugs such as ampicillin or amoxicillin for the duration of a 10 to 14 day course is usually acceptable. Most experts agree that it is highly desirable to hospitalize patients with acute disseminated gonococcal infection. The reason for hospitalization is not so much the severity of the clinical disease (disseminated gonococcal infection often is a relatively mild illness) as the potential for severe complications, such as gonococcal endocarditis, meningitis, or septic arthritis requiring irrigation or surgical drainage, and the possibility of compliance problems. In addition, although most gonococci currently causing disseminated gonococcal infection in North America are relatively sensitive to penicillin; increasing numbers of cases of disseminated gonococcal infection caused by either beta-lactamase producing *N. gonorrhoeae* or *N. gonorrhoeae* with high level chromosomal resistance are being reported. Thus it is important to observe patients and document clinical and bacteriologic improvement following therapy in those treated for disseminated gonococcal infection. All patients with disseminated gonococcal infection, like other patients with gonorrhea, have a high probability of coinfection with *C. trachomatis* and should also receive concomitant therapy using either tetracycline or doxycycline.

Discussion of therapy of other complications of gonococcal infection such as pelvic inflammatory disease is beyond the scope of this article. In general, the antibiotics used to treat pelvic inflammatory disease or epididymitis should reflect the fact that these infections are most often caused by *N. gonorrhoeae* and *C. trachomatis* irrespective of primary culture results. Patients with pelvic inflammatory disease and one pathogen isolated at the cervix may have other organisms present at deep tissue sites. Thus, because primary genital cultures may not accurately reflect all microorganisms present in the endometrium, fallopian tubes, or peritoneal cavity, combined therapy directed against both organisms is recommended. In addition, particularly for patients with recurrent pelvic inflammatory disease, in whom there is an increased likelihood of anaerobic bacteria, drugs with anaerobic activity are often included. The currently favored approach for the treatment of pelvic inflammatory disease is hospitalization and initial parenteral therapy using either cefoxitin and doxycycline or clindamycin and gentamicin. Following a clinical response, oral therapy with doxycycline may be substituted for completion of 14 days of therapy on an outpatient basis.

GRANULOMA INGUINALE

HERMAN S. MOGAVERO Jr., M.D.

Granuloma inguinale is a chronic inflammatory disease caused by *Calymmatobacterium granulomatis*. It is a disease characterized by a genital or perirectal chronic progressive ulcerative granulomatous process demonstrating little or no tendency toward spontaneous healing. The causative organism produces characteristic intracellular inclusions in macrophages taken from the lesions (Donovan bodies).

Granuloma inguinale is worldwide in distribution but is most common in the tropical and subtropical regions. It is very uncommon in the United States and appears to occur most frequently among blacks. It is still a moot point whether this is solely a venereal disease. Indeed the frequent occurrence of granuloma inguinale in the genitalia, the prominence of perirectal disease, especially in male homosexuals, and the occurrence of this infection in young sexually active individuals all suggest a venereal transmission. However, there is evidence to suggest that there also may be a nonvenereal transmission. For example, the occurrence of the disease process in children, the apparent low frequency of transmission of infection to sexual partners of infected individuals, and the low frequency of occurrence in prostitutes in endemic areas suggest caution in classifying granuloma inguinale solely as a sexually transmitted disease.

The disease manifests itself as a small papule, subcutaneous nodule, or ulcer. Experimentally the disease occurs approximately 3 weeks after inoculation. Clinically the incubation period has been reported to range from 2 weeks to 3 months. The papules and nodules quickly ulcerate, frequently producing red "cobblestone appearing" granulation tissue. The subcutaneous nodules may be mistaken for lymph nodes. However, true lymphadenopathy is unusual. Although the disease process predominantly involves the penis and scrotum in males and the labia minora in females, the disease frequently spreads to the inguinal and perianal regions. On unusual occasions extragenital lesions occur. These frequently involve the gastrointestinal tract and bones and show a peculiar tendency to involve the skin and bones in the orbital region. These lesions may demonstrate an increased frequency for the development of squamous cell carcinoma.

The differential diagnoses of granuloma inguinale include squamous cell carcinoma of the penis, condylomata lata for the perirectal lesions, and cutaneous amebiasis. The diagnosis is confirmed by scraping, curetting, or studying the lesion by biopsy. Giemsa or Wright's staining of the biopsy material demonstrates large mononuclear cells containing deeply basophilic staining, safety pin shaped Donovan bodies.

THERAPY

Antimicrobial therapy is the appropriate treatment for granuloma inguinale. Traditionally tetracycline, 500 mg four times a day, is the most widely employed drug. The treatment should continue for 3 to 4 weeks. Weekly clinical follow-up is necessary to monitor healing, which usually occurs by the end of the first week. Therapy should be continued until the lesions are fully healed and re-epithelialized. The Donovan bodies generally disappear within the first 5 to 10 days of therapy, but if therapy is discontinued at this time, there is a high incidence of relapse. It should be noted that resistance to therapy was observed in United States military personnel during the Vietnam War. Ampicillin, 500 mg four times a day for 3 weeks, was found to be a successful therapeutic alternative. In individuals with penicillin allergy, lincomycin (500 mg four times a day) was found to be effective.

In addition, chloramphenicol (500 mg orally every 8 hours) and gentamicin (1 mg per kilogram intramuscularly twice daily) are probably more effective drugs in terms of low incidences of relapse and shortened duration of therapy. However, their utilization has been tempered by concern about the risk of aplastic anemia with the former drug and renal toxicity and ototoxicity with the latter. Recently co-trimoxazole (80 mg trimethoprim, 400 mg sulfamethoxazole), two tablets orally every 12 hours for 10 to 15 days, has been found to be a highly effective form of therapy. Streptomycin (1 mg intramuscularly twice daily) also has been used because of apparent resistance in certain endemic areas. In pregnant patients a combination of erythromycin (500 mg orally every 6 hours) and lincomycin (500 mg orally every 6 hours) has also been reported to be effective.

In treating this condition, the coexistence of additional venereal diseases must not be overlooked, and appropriate diagnostic techniques should be used (e.g., VDRL and Gram's staining of urethral discharge). In cases in which there has been irreparable tissue destruction, radical surgery (total excision and grafting) may be necessary. Genital erosion, urethral stricture, or rectal stricture may develop, requiring appropriate surgical intervention as well as medical therapy. It is important to emphasize that the effectiveness of antimicrobial therapy is great if the antibiotics are introduced early in the course of the infection.

Finally if a lesion, considered to be granuloma inguinale, fails to respond to antimicrobial therapy, biopsy should be repeated and specimens stained with Giemsa or Wright's stain in a search for Donovan bodies.

LYMPHOGRANULOMA VENEREUM

NICHOLAS J. FIUMARA, M.D., M.P.H.

Lymphogranuloma venereum is an acute and chronic infection of the lymphatic nodes and lymphatic channels caused by *Chlamydia trachomatis* serotypes L1, L2, or L3. The acute phase is characterized by an evanescent papule or pustule, fever, lymphadenitis with or without nodal abscess, or abdominal pain with bloody diarrhea from hemorrhagic proctitis or colitis. The treatment at this stage is specific and effective. The following antibiotics are recommended:

1. Tetracycline hydrochloride, 500 mg orally four times daily for 14 days. The antibiotic should be taken 1 hour before meals, or 2 hours after meals. No milk or cheese or antacids should be ingested. Some patients develop gastrointestinal upsets with nausea, vomiting or diarrhea; others may develop monilial glossitis or vaginitis. Although tetracycline hydrochloride is effective, there is a problem of compliance in some patients. Therefore, I prefer to start my patients with doxycycline.

2. Doxycyline, 100 mg orally every 12 hours for 14 days.

3. Minocycline, 100 mg orally every 12 hours for 14 days.

4. Trimethoprim (160 mg)-sulfamethoxazole (800 mg) double strength tablets orally every 12 hours for 14 days. An occasional patient may develop a maculopapular rash or urticaria or erythema multiforme. In such cases one should switch to another antibiotic once the adverse reaction is under control.

5. Erythromycin, 500 mg orally four times daily for 14 days. The problems here are noncompliance by some patients and gastrointestinal upsets in others.

Some of the patients may develop an inguinal node abscess either before treatment or after treatment has been initiated. Node aspiration is preferred over incision and drainage. The normal looking skin above the abscess is infiltrated with a 1 percent lidocaine solution, and the abscess is aspirated with a 15-gauge needle and syringe superior to the abscess to prevent continuous dependent drainage.

Chronic lymphogranuloma infection may result in rectal or vaginal strictures, fistulas, intestinal obstruction, polypoid growths from chronic inflammation of the genitals and perianal areas, as well as obstructive lymphangitis with elephantiasis of the genitals. These are surgical problems, and surgical repair should be accompanied by administration of one of the antibiotics already mentioned.

CHANCROID

JAMES E. FITZPATRICK, M.D., LT. COL.,
M.C., U.S.A.

Chancroid is a sexually transmitted disease typically characterized by single or multiple genital ulcers that may be accompanied by enlarged or suppurative inguinal lymph nodes. The causative organism is *Haemophilus ducreyi*, a fastidious gram negative coccobacillary organism.

Chancroid has previously been believed to be endemic in Asia and Africa, with only sporadic cases appearing in North America, but recent outbreaks in Canada, California, Georgia, Washington, and Massachusetts suggest that it is a more common cause of genital ulcers than previously appreciated. Recent studies have documented that *H. ducreyi* is resistant to several previously recommended treatment modalities because of the capacity of the organism to pass resistance by plasmids. The difficulty in managing suspected cases of chancroid is further complicated by the fact that it may coexist with a second sexually transmitted disease, such as syphilis or herpes progenitalis. Because of the difficulty in culturing the organism in routine laboratories, treatment is usually instituted on the basis of clinical impression alone.

TREATMENT

The management of chancroid should be considered in terms of prophylaxis, systemic antibiotic therapy, local care, adjunctive surgical treatment, and evaluation of sexual partners.

PROPHYLAXIS

Prophylactic measures are infrequently addressed in modern studies, but the older literature suggests that other than the use of condoms, most topical prophylactic measures, including soap and water following sexual intercourse, are not effective in the prevention of infection. Males in endemic or epidemic areas should be advised to use condoms, and females should be advised to require that their male sexual partners use condoms.

Antibiotic Therapy

Systemic antibiotic therapy is the treatment of choice in the management of chancroid and should be given to each patient. Since chancroid is capable of plasmid coded resistance to several antibiotics, ideally cultures should be taken in each patient and the susceptibilities to different antibiotics determined. However, this information is not available during the initial visit when treatment should begin and may not become available because of the difficulty most routine microbiological laboratories experience in isolating *H. ducreyi* owing to the fastidious nature of the organism.

On the basis of in vitro evaluations of the minimal inhibitory concentrations during recent outbreaks, clinical studies, and personal experience, the treatment of choice is erythromycin base or stearate given in a dose of 500 mg by mouth four times daily for 7 days. The patient should be reevaluated in 3 days for subjective and objective responses. Most patients report a decrease in pain and tenderness in the ulcer within 48 hours, while objective evidence including absence of ulcer enlargement, decreased erythema, and dryness of the ulcer bed is usually detectable within 72 hours but may take longer. Buboes typically take longer to respond both subjectively and objectively, and failure to demonstrate improvement at this point is not indicative of treatment failure. Buboes may actually become fluctuant during adequate therapy even as the ulcer or ulcers improve.

If the clinical impression is that the patient has not responded to these parameters 3 days after institution of therapy or in vitro antimicrobial susceptibilities indicate evidence of resistance, therapy should be switched to a more sensitive antibiotic or to one of the alternative regimens. In practice this is rarely necessary, since erythromycin resistant strains have not been reported in North America and only rarely in Asia. More commonly patients must be switched to alternative antibiotics because of intolerance to gastrointestinal reactions. Patients should be reevaluated 7 to 10 days after beginning therapy to document continued improvement or resolution. By the tenth day the ulcer should be healed except for residual crust, although there may still be residual lymphadenopathy with minimal discomfort, which may take up to 1 month to resolve entirely.

The advantages of erythromycin over other antibiotics include excellent in vitro sensitivity, several documented clinical studies demonstrating efficacy, availability, low cost, and the rarity of severe adverse reactions. The disadvantages of this regimen include the four times per day dosage schedule, which may affect patient compliance, the relatively high percentage of patients who are unable to tolerate erythromycin induced gastrointestinal side effects, and the possibility that coexistent syphilis may be masked by partial treatment with an erythromycin schedule that is not considered adequate for the management of primary syphilis. Patients with significant gastrointestinal side effects should be switched to erythromycin enteric coated tablets or erythromycin ethylsuccinate.

When an alternative drug is needed either because of a poor clinical response, adverse reactions, or a history of allergy to erythromycin, the alternative drug of choice is trimethoprim-sulfamethoxazole, one double strength tablet (160 mg–800 mg) by mouth twice daily for 7 to 10 days. Studies comparing the efficacy of a 7 day and a 10 day regimen have not been done, but personal experience indicates that the longer course is preferable. This combination antibiotic is far superior to sulfonamides alone, which were formerly recommended as the drugs of choice by some authors as recently as 5 years ago.

A large number of recent in vitro studies have documented the worldwide emergence of sulfonamide resistant strains of *H. ducreyi*. Similarly, numerous studies have established frequent clinical failures with sulfonamides alone. The trimethoprim-sulfamethoxazole combination has been documented in several studies and by epidemics in the United States to be an effective treatment. However, the recent appearance of trimethoprim resistant strains in Thailand threatens its future usefulness if these strains spread to North America.

The advantages of the trimethoprim-sulfamethoxazole combination in addition to its documented clinical efficacy include the facts that it is the least expensive antibiotic choice for the management of chancroid, it will not mask underlying syphilis, and the twice per day dosage regimen is more likely to promote patient compliance. Various authorities, including the Center for Disease Control (CDC), have recommended a single oral dose of four double strength or eight single strength tablets (640 mg–3,200 mg) of trimethoprim-sulfamethoxazole as an acceptable alternative. This regimen was developed to treat populations in underdeveloped countries where patient compliance is a significant problem. Because of slightly lower cure rates reported in some studies, this schedule is not recommended.

The disadvantages of trimethoprim-sulfamethoxazole are the relatively high incidence of severe adverse reactions, including drug-induced toxic epidermal necrolysis, which may be life threatening, and the fact that in vitro antibiotic sensitivity studies have demonstrated that *H. ducreyi* is somewhat less sensitive to this combination than erythromycin.

The future value of this combination in the treatment of chancroid is somewhat in doubt because of the increasing resistance of the organism to sulfonamides and the recent emergence of trimethoprim resistance in Thailand. The efficacy of trimethoprim alone in the treatment of chancroid has not been evaluated, although it should be effective as indicated by antimicrobial sensitivity studies and the fact that patients with strains of *H. ducreyi* resistant to sulfonamides appear to respond to trimethoprim-sulfamethoxazole in combination. More recently trimethoprim has also been tried successfully in combination with rifampin, but further evaluations are necessary to see whether the combination provides additional advantages over currently recommended therapies.

For the rare patient who can take neither erythromycin nor trimethoprim-sulfamethoxazole, three alternatives remain, including ceftriaxone, amoxicillin in combination with clavulanic acid, and streptomycin. Ceftriaxone is a third generation cephalosporin recently recommended by the CDC as an acceptable alternative drug when given in a dose of 250 mg intramuscularly. Because of a longer half-life, it appears to produce a higher incidence of cures than other third generation cephalosporins, such as cefotaxime, which had been advocated as an alternative therapy. The single dose regimen eliminates patient compliance as a problem, but significant objections include the fact that it is not readily available at this time, it has undergone only limited evaluation in the management of chancroid, it may mask coexistent syphilis, and its usefulness in penicillin allergic patients is limited, particularly when the drug must be administered intramuscularly.

A 7-day course of oral doses of amoxicillin (500 mg) taken in conjunction with clavulanic acid (125 mg) three times daily has also been recommended by the CDC because of in vitro studies demonstrating synergistic antibacterial activity of this combination against *H. ducreyi*. Experience with this combination is limited, and it has not been evaluated in North America. The disadvantages of this regimen include potentially poor patient compliance because of the relative complexity of the regimen, the very high cost, the potential for cross reactions in patients who are allergic to penicillin, and the potential for masking syphilis.

Streptomycin has been used successfully for decades in the management of chancroid. Despite in vitro susceptibility and documented clinical success, it has fallen into relative disuse because of the potential for nephrotoxicity and ototoxicity. Personal experience indicates that it is effective in a dosage of either 1.0 g administered intramuscularly daily for 6 days or 2.0 g administered intramuscularly for 3 days.

Several additional antibiotics, including kanamycin, spectinomycin, gentamicin, choramphenicol, and minocycline, have been recommended, but experience with these antibiotics is limited and they do not offer additional advantages over the previously discussed treatments. Tetracline, doxycycline, penicillin, and ampicillin have previously been advocated as suitable treatments, but they are not recommended because of widespread plasmid coded resistance.

Local Care

The value of local adjunctive therapy has not been studied to determine whether it is of benefit. Smaller ulcers usually do not require topical management, but personal experience indicates that larger lesions reepithelialize more quickly if cleaned gently twice daily with hydrogen peroxide, followed by a thin application of 1 percent silver sulfadiazine cream.

Surgical Treatment

The management of suppurative lymph nodes has been somewhat controversial in the past, although the trend

TABLE 1 Summary of the Treatment of Chancroid

Systemic therapy	
Antibiotic of choice	Erythromycin, 500 mg PO q.i.d. for 7 days
Alternative antibiotic	Trimethoprim-sulfamethoxazole (160 mg - 800 mg) PO b.i.d. for 7 to 10 days
Topical therapy	None, or optional hydrogen peroxide cleansing followed by 1% silver sulfadiazine cream
Suppurative lymph nodes	Aspirate contents through normal skin with 16 or 18 gauge needle; repeat prn
Management of contacts	Treatment of symptomatic and asymptomatic partners with oral antibiotic therapy

has been toward the use of less aggressive procedures. The older literature suggests that incision and drainage may result in the formation of ulcers or draining fistulas in the site of drainage, and for this reason they are not recommended. Fluctuant lymph nodes are best managed by lateral aspiration through normal skin with a 16 or 18 gauge needle after appropriate preparation of the skin surface. Aspiration may be repeated if necessary. Foreskin surgery to relieve phimosis is contraindicated because of the relatively frequent occurrence of secondary inoculation.

Sexual Partners

Sexual partners of the patient should be contacted, examined, and treated with systemic doses of antibiotics even in the absence of lesions because of the apparent existence of asymptomatic carriers (Table 1). Few studies regarding the role of asymptomatic carriers have been done, but preliminary information suggests that *H. ducreyi* may reside within the vagina, beneath the prepuce, and within the oropharynx without causing symptoms.

OTHER DISORDERS

DRUG REACTIONS

ANTOINETTE F. HOOD, M.D.

MAGNITUDE OF THE PROBLEM

Drugs are ubiquitous in our society. In the United States millions of people regularly ingest aspirin and other anti-inflammatory drugs, antibiotics, contraceptives, anti-hypertensives, diuretics, and tranquilizers. The exact incidence of adverse reactions to these and other medications is unknown. According to the Boston Collaborative Drug Surveillance Program, 30 percent of medical service inpatients had one or more complications as a result of drugs administered during hospitalization; 2 to 3 percent of the patients developed a "skin rash." Among hospitalized patients the incidence of cutaneous reactions per course of therapy has been reported to be 3 per 1,000. It has been estimated that 60,000 to 90,000 inpatients develop cutaneous drug reactions each year. Fortunately these reactions are rarely life-threatening; nonetheless they may produce significant morbidity and expense, especially in the form of prolonged hospitalization.

The Boston collaborative study reflects the incidence of drug reactions on an inpatient medical service. These figures may not accurately reflect the problem in other units of the hospital, such as surgery, pediatrics, and oncology. We casually surveyed one oncology ward in our hospital for a 2-month period and discovered that 50 percent of the patients developed one or more cutaneous eruptions that clinically were consistent with drug eruptions. These reactions often resulted in great discomfort to the patient and necessitated complex therapy manipulations on the part of the attending physicians.

Even less is known about the frequency of cutaneous reactions occurring in an outpatient setting. Attempts to monitor drug reactions are obviously fraught with difficulties. However, the American Academy of Dermatology has made an important effort to do this by sponsoring the Adverse Drug Reaction Reporting System. This system permits dermatologists to share their experience with adverse cutaneous reactions to drugs, and to obtain information about such reactions as contained in the registry and in the medical literature.

PATHOGENESIS

Adverse drug reactions can be divided simplistically into two major categories: type A reactions, which are normal but augmented responses; and type B reactions, which are totally abnormal or bizarre responses. Type A reactions are pharmacologically predictable and dose dependent. They generally are of high incidence and morbidity but low mortality. Examples of type A reactions in the skin include aspirin induced purpura, mucositis, and alopecia caused by antimitotic chemotherapeutic drugs, striae associated with corticosteroid administration, and perhaps demeclocycline-induced phototoxicity. Type B (bizarre or idiosyncratic) reactions are less common, are pharmacologically unpredictable, and are not dose dependent. They may be produced by a variety of chemicals, including the active constituent in the medication, decomposition or byproducts of the active ingredient, or the various additives, solubilizers, stabilizers, and colorizers in a preparation.

The pathobiology of most cutaneous drug reactions is not well understood; the overused terms "hypersensitivity" and "allergic" should be limited to describing reactions that are immunologically mediated or that can reasonably be presumed to be immunologically mediated. True allergic reactions usually affect a small percentage of the population receiving the drug, require a prior exposure or latent period for the development of an immune response, can occur at subtherapeutic or very low doses, and usually simulate other known hypersensitivity reactions. Examples of cutaneous allergic drug reactions are listed in Table 1.

Rashes of unknown etiology but that are presumed to be allergic include morbilliform-exanthematous eruptions, fixed drug eruptions, erythema multiforme, toxic epidermal necrolysis, exfoliative erythroderma, and erythema nodosum.

Few controlled or stringent studies have been done on drug reactions, and for practical purposes it is not convenient to categorize them by etiology. Traditionally drug reactions are classified morphologically. In terms of the frequency of types of drug rashes, the morbilliform pattern is seen most commonly, followed by urticarial eruptions, fixed drug eruptions, erythema multiforme, and others. There is a clinical dictum that states that any drug may produce any reaction, and although this may be true, it is also accepted that certain drugs are more likely to

TABLE 1 Allergic (Immunologically Mediated) Drug Eruptions*

Type	Immunologic Mechanisms	Clinical Expression in Skin	Laboratory Testing
Type I anaphylactic	IgE mediated reactions to allergic haptens; involve mast cell activation and subsequent release of histamine, leukotrienes, and eosinophil-chemotactic factors of anaphylaxis; Neutrophil chemotactic factors, platelet activating factor, serotonin, and kinins may be involved	Urticaria Angioedema Transient cold urticaria Generalized pruritus	Radioallergosorbent test (RAST) Enzyme-inked immunosorbent assay (ELISA) Skin testing
Type II antibody mediated (cytotoxic) injury	IgG or IgM antibodies activate complement through the classic pathway; under certain conditions antigens and antibodies localized on circulating erythrocytes, leukocytes, or platelets cause drug-induced, antibody-dependent lysis of these cells	Thrombocytopenic reactions	
Type III antigen-antibody immune complex	IgG or IgM antibodies form circulating immune complexes with antigen and complement, activating complement-derived chemotactic factors and producing localized tissue inflammation	Serum sickness Leukocytoclastic vasculitis ?Drug induced lupus erythematosus	Direct immunofluorescence performed on skin biopsy specimen
Type IV cell mediated injury	Sensitized T-lymphocytes react with allergen and thereby generate lymphokines	Allergic contact dermatitis Photoallergic reactions Granuloma formation following topical use of zirconium	Lymphocyte transformation Patch test

* Based on the Coombs and Gell classification.

produce particular morphologic cutaneous reactions than others. Table 2 lists the various types of drug reactions and some of the more common drugs responsible for the eruptions. (For further listings and references, the reader is referred to a pocket-sized compendium of cutaneous drug reactions by Dr. W. Bruinsma entitled *A Guide to Drug Eruptions*.)

PRACTICAL APPROACH TO THE DIAGNOSIS OF A SUSPECTED DRUG ERUPTION

As dermatologists we are all aware that there are undoubtedly many more adverse reactions to drugs than are suspected and that, conversely, many reactions suspected of being drug induced actually may be caused by other agents. In evaluating a suspected drug reaction, every effort should be directed toward diagnosis, discovery, and discontinuation.

Diagnosis requires a high index of suspicion, a detailed and directed history, careful examination, classification of the eruption by morphologic characteristics, evaluation of accompanying signs and symptoms, collection of adjuvant laboratory test results, and elimination of other causes of similar eruptions. Important historical information includes the onset and evolution of the eruption, any history of drug reactions, and detailed descriptions of all medications being taken, including proprietary drugs and vitamins. If a true allergic reaction is suspected, a history of similar medications taken systemically or applied topically may be important. Note any

accompanying symptomatology, such as pruritus (favors a drug reaction), sore throat (against a drug eruption), fever, and malaise (neither pro nor con). Categorizing the eruption by the morphologic appearance of the lesions is helpful in determining the type of reaction (allergic versus nonallergic) and in limiting the possible etiologic agents responsible for the eruption (see Table 2). Other physical findings such as mucosal involvement, lymphadenopathy, and temperature elevation are important.

Adjuvant tests may be helpful by pointing either toward or away from the diagnosis of drug induced eruption (Table 3). Routine studies should include a complete blood cell count with a differential count urinalysis, and a multiphasic screening panel; other tests such as skin biopsy, and patch and light testing are also important in categorizing the type and sometimes the cause of the reaction. Realistically, although not necessarily practically, challenge by reintroduction of the suspected drug is still the most useful means of definitively diagnosing a drug eruption.

TREATMENT

The treatment of a drug reaction depends on the type of reaction, the severity and the presumed etiologic mechanism. With few exceptions, use of the suspected offender should be discontinued and the eruption treated symptomatically with antihistamines or antipruritics, compresses, and soothing lotions as needed. If the patient is taking multiple medications that are important to his health and well-being, I generally select the most likely causa-

TABLE 2 Drugs Associated with Various Morphologic Cutaneous Patterns

Morbilliform-exanthematous eruptions
* Allopurinol
* Antibiotics (especially penicillin, penicillin derivatives, and sulfonamides)
  Anticonvulsants
* Barbiturates
  Benzodiazepines
* Gold salts
* Isoniazid
  Meclofenamate sodium
  Para-aminosalicylic acid
  Phenylbutazone
  Phenothiazines
  Piroxicam
  Quinidine
  Thiazide diuretics
Urticaria
  Enzymes (L-asparaginase)
  Indomethacin
  Insulin
  Opiates
  Penicillin and related antibiotics
  Salicylates
  Sulfonamides
  X-ray contrast media
Fixed drug eruptions
* Barbiturates
  Chlordiazepoxide
  Phenacetin
* Phenophthalein
* Phenylbutazone
  Salicylates
* Sulfonamides
* Tetracycline
Erythema multiforme
* Barbiturates
  Chlorpropamide
  Griseofulvin
  Hydantoins
* Penicillin
  Phenothiazines
* Sulfonamides
  Thiazide diruetics
Leukocytoclastic vasculitis
* Allopurinol
  Gold salts
  Hydantoins
  Iodides
* Penicillin and penicillin derivatives
  Phenothiazines
* Sulfonamides
  Thiazide diuretics
  Thiouracils
Photosensitivity eruptions
  Griseofulvin
  Indomethacin
* Nalidixic acid

* Phenothiazines
  Piroxicam
  Sulindac
* Sulfonamides
* Tetracycline (demeclocycline)
* Thiazide diuretics
Toxic epidermal necrolysis
  Allopurinol
* Barbiturates
* Hydantoins
  Penicillin
  Phenylbutazone
* Sulfonamides
  Tetracycline
Lichenoid and lichen planus-like eruptions
  Antimalarials (chloroquine, hydroxychloroquine, quinacrine)
  Chlordiazepoxide
  Gold salts
  Hydroxyurea
  Para-aminosalicylic acid
  Penicillamine
  Quinidine
  Thiazide diuretics
Exfoliative dermatitis
  Allopurinol
  Carbamazepine
* Gold salts
  Hydantoins
  Isoniazid
  Para-aminosalicylic acid
  Phenindione
  Phenylbutazone
* Sulfonamides
  Streptomycin
Eczematous eruptions (topical sensitizer, systemic medication)
  Ampicillin
  Chlorbutanol, chloral hydrate
  Diphenhydramine (Caladryl, Benadryl)
  Ethylenediamine, aminophylline, antihistamines
  Iodine, iodides
  Neomycin sulfate, streptomycin, kanamycin
  Para-amino aromatic benzenes, para-aminobenzoic acid, sulfonamides, tolbutamide
  Penicillin
  Thiuram, Antabuse
Erythema nodosum
  Bromides
  Codeine
  Iodides
* Orally administered contraceptives
  Penicillin
  Salicylates
  Sulfonamides

* Drugs that are frequent offenders.

tive drug and stop its administration. If the eruption persists or progresses over the next 48 hours, the next most likely medication is discontinued, and so on. Another approach is to discontinue all medications until the rash fades or clears completely and then reinstitute the medications one at a time at 48 to 72 hour intervals. This approach is not recommended in the treatment of IgE mediated urticarial or angioedema episodes (since the challenging

might induce a life threatening anaphylactic reaction) or drug reactins, which concomitantly may involve the liver, or kidneys.

Severe widespread or extremely symptomatic drug eruptions may require a short course of prednisone therapy to reduce inflammation and shorten the natural course of the reaction. Assuming that there are no medical contraindications, prednisone can be administered orally, 40 to 60

TABLE 3   Diagnostic Procedures

History
Physical examination
Laboratory tests
   Complete blood cell count with differential count
   Multiphasic screening panel
   Serum IgE RAST
Skin biopsy
Patch tests
Ultraviolet light testing

mg per day, in divided doses. As soon as it is apparent that the eruption is receding, the dosage may be tapered to 10 mg per day and discontinued.

At times it may be necessary to treat through a drug-induced eruption. This may occur when the suspected medication is absolutely necessary and there are no unrelated drug substitutes of similar efficacy. We have occasion to do this on the oncology ward or when treating other immunocompromised patients for life threatening infections. In these situations the severity of the reaction may be diminished by switching modes of administration from intermittent to continuous intravenous administration of drugs (ticarcillin) or from daily administration to treatment three times a week (trimethoprim-sulfamethoxazole). Once a drug has been implicated in a drug reaction, especially an allergic or presumed allergic reaction, the patient should be given the name of the drug and a list of similar chemical compounds to avoid in the future. The front of the chart should be clearly labeled, other physicians caring for the patient should be informed, and the manufacturers of the medication should be notified.

MASTOCYTOSIS AND URTICARIA PIGMENTOSA

NICHOLAS A. SOTER, M.D.

Mastocytosis is an uncommon disease of mast cell proliferation that occurs in both cutaneous and systemic forms. The skin lesions may be isolated mastocytomas or generalized, multiple red-brown papules and plaques, which are designated urticaria pigmentosa. When a cutaneous lesion is stroked firmly, it becomes edematous with erythema (Darier's sign).

Individuals with urticaria pigmentosa should be evaluated for systemic disease. Systemic symptoms and signs reflect either a sudden and elevated blood level of released mast cell-derived mediators or infiltration of various organs with increased numbers of mast cells. An acute systemic episode, which tends to be transient and lasts for only a few hours, is characterized by headache, flushing, dizziness, tachycardia, hypotension, and syncope. Gastrointestinal manifestations include nausea, vomiting, abdominal pain, and diarrhea. More chronic features include a mixed organic brain syndrome accompanied by the cognitive manifestations of depression with affective components, such as poor attention span, irritability, difficulty in concentration, and inability to work effectively. Infiltration of organs can result in lymphadenopathy, hepatomegaly, and splenomegaly, as well as anemia and thrombocytopenia. Osseous lesions may be associated with bone pain. Malignant disorders of the reticuloendothelial system may occur with progression to leukemia or lymphoma. Prognosis in individuals with mastocytosis varies with the clinical form of the disease.

PREFERRED THERAPEUTIC APPROACH

Since the clinical features either reflect infiltration of various organs by mast cells or are related to the pharmacologic release of mediators, the choice of therapy depends on the pathobiology of the clinical manifestations. The more common clinical symptoms and signs are the result of the release of chemical mediators, and therapy usually is directed toward modifying the effects of mediators. None of the medical therapeutic measures affects permanent involution of either cutaneous or visceral lesions.

Patients should avoid circumstances that precipitate attacks. For example, drugs known to cause mast cell degranulation, such as morphine and codeine, are to be prohibited. Alcohol is well known to exacerbate the gastrointestinal diarrhea. Trauma to the skin lesions should be minimized. In addition, d-tubocurarine and decamethonium in high doses should be avoided in patients with mastocytosis owing to their ability to release histamine.

X-irradiation has been administered without therapeutic benefit. The use of histamine liberators has not proved effective. Attempts to increase the rate of histamine destruction or to decrease histamine production with histidine decarboxylase inhibitors have been unsuccessful.

Moreover, controlled clinical trials examining various therapeutic regimens often are lacking. A substantial amount of information is generated from isolated case reports.

Treatment of Cutaneous Manifestations

Isolated cutaneous mastocytomas in infants commonly involute spontaneously before the age of 10. When this does not occur, the single lesion may be removed surgically. When urticaria pigmentosa arises in childhood, spontaneous regression before adulthood occurs in approximately 50 percent of cases.

Pruritus and whealing usually are treated initially with the oral administration of H_1 antihistamines. There is often amelioration, but not total ablation of these manifestations. The addition of an H_2 antihistamine may be helpful. The therapeutic efficacy of such a combination of H_1 and H_2 antagonists in relieving pruritus and whealing has been established by one controlled study. The oral administration of disodium cromoglycate (cromolyn), to be discussed has been of benefit in the reduction of pruitus and whealing. The formation of bullous lesions in infants has been controlled by the administration of H_1 and H_2 antihistamines or oral cromolyn in isolated case reports.

Ketofiten, which is not yet available in the United States, was reported to be of benefit in relieving the pruritus and whealing. One patient has reported relief of whealing and flushing after the administration of nifedipine.

Mechanism of Action and Pharmacokinetics of H_1 Antihistamines

The H_1 antagonists compete with histamine at a specific tissue receptor site. In addition to their antihistaminic actions, there are a number of additional effects, including sedation, anticholinergic activity, local anesthesia, antiemetic activity, and activity against motion sickness. The H_1 antagonists have been divided into subgroups depending on their chemical structure. Although the therapeutic superiority of individual agents has not been well substantiated, the aforementioned effects can be important in deciding which drug class works best for an individual patient.

The H_1 antihistamines are readily absorbed from the stomach and small intestine, beginning within 20 minutes and reaching peak plasma levels within 1 hour. The duration of action ranges from 2 to 6 hours. For prolonged, uniform therapeutic drug levels to be achieved, it is necessary to administer such antihistamines in divided doses on a daily basis. Biotransformation of the H_1 antihistamines occurs chiefly in the liver, and the conjugated glucuronide metabolites then are cleared through the kidneys with complete excretion by 24 hours after administration.

Side Effects of H_1 Antihistamines

About 25 percent of individuals receiving H_1 antihistamines experience an adverse reaction. Sedation is the most common problem associated with these drugs. Some tolerance to this sedative effect occurs in most individuals within a few days of continual drug administration. If tolerance does not occur, the drug may be administered in smaller doses or a trial of another therapeutic agent can be undertaken. Other central nervous system (CNS) effects that may be experienced include dizziness, tinnitus, incoordination, blurred vision, and diplopia. Occasionally the CNS effects can be stimulatory and include nervousness, insomnia, tremor, and irritability. Gastrointestinal manifestations include nausea, vomiting, diarrhea, anorexia, and epigastric distress. Some H_1 antihistamines also have anticholinergic properties and may be associated with dry mucous membranes, difficulty in micturition, urinary retention, dysuria, urinary frequency, and impotence. The cardiovascular effects of H_1 antihistamines usually are not experienced after oral administration.

Mechanism of Action and Pharmacokinetics of H_2 Antihistamines

H_2 antagonists act as competitive inhibitors of histamine at a specific tissue receptor site. Cimetidine hydrochloride, which is the most frequently used example, is absorbed mainly from the small intestine with maximal blood concentrations being achieved within 80 to 90 minutes. The drug is eliminated unchanged in the urine with complete clearance within 24 hours. Effective concentrations are present for 4 to 6 hours after an oral dose. The absorption and duration of therapeutic effect may be prolonged by administering dose with meals. Clinical experience with newer H_2 antagonists, such as ranitidine hydrochloride, in mastocytosis has not yet been reported.

Side Effects of H_2 Antihistamines

Cimetidine hydrochloride is well tolerated and side effects are rare. Occasional instances of headache, dizziness, eruptions, and gastrointestinal symptoms have been noted. Cimetidine hydrochloride binds to androgen receptors, and this antiandrogen effect is presumably responsible for the occasional cases of gynecomastia and azoospermia in male patients. An important side effect of cimetidine hydrochloride is its interference with hepatic microsomal enzymes that metabolize drugs. Such alterations may lead to potentiation of the effects of numerous drugs, including warfarin, diphenylhydantoin, phenobarbital, diazepam, and propranolol. A prominent effect of cimetidine hydrochloride is its inhibition of histamine-induced gastric acid secretion. It is important to remember that cimetidine decreases the absorption of tetracycline because of the requirement of an acid pH for dissolution of the capsule. Although cimetidine was initially thought to have no effect on the bone marrow, a reversible granulocytopenia may occur.

Use of Psoralens and Ultraviolet Light

Oral 8-methoxypsoralen and ultraviolet A (PUVA)

have been used in a small number of instances and have effected relief of pruritus and decreased whealing. Relapses occur 3 to 6 months after the cessation of therapy. In some instances, there is a temporary reduction in lesional mast cell numbers after this form of therapy. Long-term follow-up information is unavailable. The use of photochemotherapy should be reserved for extensive cutaneous disease unresponsive to other forms of treatment.

Exposure to natural sunlight has been associated with a diminution in cutaneous lesions in an occasional patient. Controlled trials with ultraviolet B, however, have not been reported.

Use of Corticosteroids

Systemic corticosteroids have been administered without therapeutic benefit. The application, however, of potent topical corticosteroid preparations, such as 0.05 percent betamethasone diproprionate ointment under plastic-film occlusion for 8 hours daily for 8 to 12 weeks was associated with a decrease in the numbers of mast cells and clearing of the cutaneous lesions. The mean follow-up time was 11.5 months without recurrence.

Treatment of Gastrointestinal Manifestations

For the gastrointestinal tract symptoms and signs, the oral administration of disodium cromoglycate (cromolyn) or of H_1 and H_2 antihistamines has been of value in double-blind controlled trials.

Mechanism of Action and Pharmacokinetics of Disodium Cromoglycate

Although the mechanism of action of cromolyn is incompletely defined, it is thought to prevent mast cell degranulation by interfering with calcium transport across the cell membrane. It thus inhibits mast cell release of histamine and other inflammatory mediators. Inasmuch as less than 1 percent of the drug is absorbed, a local action on the gastrointestinal mast cell seems likely.

The half-life of cromolyn is about 80 minutes, and it is excreted unchanged via the renal and biliary systems. Use of this medication should be carefully considered when hepatic or renal function impairment exists. Patients sensitive to lactose, milk, or milk products may be allergic to the capsule dosage form since the capsules contain a lactose vehicle. Although it is not known whether cromolyn is excreted in breast milk, cromolyn reaches very low concentrations in maternal serum.

Dosage of Disodium Cromoglycate

Cromolyn capsules for inhalation are the dosage form being used for oral administration because a capsule for oral use is not commercially available in the United States. The usual adult dose is 100 to 200 mg four times daily up to 40 mg per kilogram of body weight per day. The usual pediatric dose is 40 mg four times daily up to 40 mg per kilogram of body weight per day. The oral solution may be prepared by dissolving the contents of the capsules in water.

Side Effects of Disodium Cromoglycate

Side effects reported with the oral use of cromolyn are rare, although some adverse effects have occurred with cromolyn formulations used for inhalation. There is a lag of 2 to 3 weeks before beneficial effects on the skin and gastrointestinal tract are noted. A lag of about 6 weeks occurs before beneficial effects on the CNS occur. Exacerbation of the clinical manifestations is noted within 2 weeks of cessation of drug therapy.

Treatment of Flushing and Hypotensive Episodes

Therapy with combined H_1 and H_2 antagonists alone is ineffective in preventing recurrent life-threatening episodes of flushing and hypotension; however, the judicious use of aspirin is of value. The use of cromolyn in controlling this manifestation is unreported. Since aspirin and other nonsteroidal anti-inflammatory drugs inhibit prostaglandin synthesis and since the human mast cell can generate prostaglandin D_2, it is reasonable to reconsider the previous prohibition of aspirin use in mastocytosis. Owing to the theoretic possibility of causing mast cell histamine release with nonsteroidal anti-inflammatory agents, it is advisable to administer therapeutic doses of both H_1 and H_2 antihistamines prior to the use of aspirin. Therapy can be initiated with 8 mg of chlorpheniramine maleate and 300 mg of cimetidine hydrochloride four times daily. After 2 days, aspirin can be added at an initial dose of 40 mg per day; the dose is doubled on each subsequent day until symptomatic relief is obtained or a plasma salicylate level between 20 and 30 mg per deciliter is achieved. The minimum therapeutic aspirin dose, in combination with the antihistamines, is maintained chronically. It is advisable to initiate the use of aspirin while the patient is in the hospital, since an attack may be evoked in a small number of individuals.

The subcutaneous and intravenous administration of epinephrine has been of value in the treatment of hypotension. Patients with a history of syncope should carry supplies of epinephrine.

Treatment of Malignant Mastocytosis

Malignant transformation in mastocytosis is a rare event with a high mortality. No particular cytotoxic drug protocol has been established, and a variety of agents has been used with limited success.

PROS AND CONS OF TREATMENT

The choice of therapy in patients with mastocytosis depends on the clinical manifestations. It is important to note that this disorder may spontaneously resolve, especially in infants and children. The use of H_1 receptor antagonists alone or in combination with an H_2 receptor antagonist usually is the initial therapy used. In individuals with severe gastrointestinal manifestations, cromolyn is an alternative therapeutic choice. For life-threatening episodes of hypotension, epinephrine and aspirin, in addition to combined H_1 and H_2 receptor antagonists, may be lifesaving.

ZINC DEFICIENCY SYNDROME: ACRODERMATITIS ENTEROPATHICA

RISE M. JAMPEL, M.D.

Acrodermatitis enteropathica is an autosomal recessive disorder of zinc deficiency characterized by dermatitis, diarrhea, and irritability. Although it was first described in 1942 by Danbolt and Closs, it was not until 1974 that zinc deficiency was shown to be fundamental in the pathogenesis of the disorder, and that clinical improvement was shown to be directly related to the restoration of normal serum zinc levels. Although the cause is still unknown, there appears to be a defect in zinc absorption in the small intestine, which may be overcome by the oral administration of large amounts of zinc.

In addition to the inherited form of acrodermatitis enteropathica, there have been many reported cases of transient "acrodermatitis enteropathica" occurring in clinical situations associated with zinc deficiency. Some of these include parenteral hyperalimentation without zinc supplementation, malabsorption syndromes such as cystic fibrosis and lactose intolerance, bowel resections, adolescents ingesting high phytate containing diets in the Middle East, alcoholism, premature infants; and general nutritional deficiency. These entities are also treated with zinc supplementation.

DIAGNOSIS

The first step in the treatment of zinc deficiency is its recognition. The serum zinc level is the accepted means of making the diagnosis and monitoring the effect of treatment. I do not recommend hair and nail analysis because it is not practical and does not correlate with the total body level of zinc. Normal serum zinc levels change with age (Table 1). However, in most laboratories the normal range is 55 to 150 μg per deciliter. There are, however, several limitations to the use of the serum zinc level. First, the serum zinc level does not necessarily reflect the degree of total body zinc depletion, which is the critical factor

in establishing the disease state. Thus a normal serum zinc level does not constitute assurance of an adequate total body zinc level. In fact there are several case reports of zinc deficiency syndromes in which patients with normal serum zinc levels responded to treatment. However, in patients with profound symptomatic zinc deficiency, serum zinc levels are usually less than 40 to 50 μg per deciliter. In addition, there are a number of factors that influence serum zinc levels; these factors include the serum albumin level, infection, hemolysis, and the use of test tubes containing extraneous metal. For this reason the use of metal-free test tubes is imperative.

TREATMENT

The treatment for zinc deficiency is zinc supplementation. In the inherited form of the disease, treatment may be necessary on a long-term basis, whereas in the acquired form, if the underlying deficiency is corrected, treatment may be necessary only to replace zinc stores. The oral dose of zinc is based on the recommended dietary allowance (RDA) of 15 mg of elemental zinc per day for an adult. Dietary needs for zinc are higher during periods of rapid growth—the neonatal period, adolescence, pregnancy, and lactation—and therefore zinc supplementation during these periods should be modified according to the RDAs in Table 2.

The orally administered zinc preparations most commonly used are zinc sulfate and zinc gluconate. Although both preparations are safe, the Food and Drug Administration has endorsed zinc sulfate as the choice for supplementation, since most absorption, bioavailability, and toxicity studies have been conducted with zinc sulfate. Zinc sulfate is available as Zinc-220 Capsules (Alto Pharmaceuticals Inc., Tampa, Florida), which contain 220 mg of zinc sulfate and provide 55 mg of elemental zinc. Zinc gluconate is available as Zinc "50" Tablets (Solgar Vitamin Company, Inc., Lynbrook, New York), which contain 409 mg of zinc gluconate and provide 50 mg of elemental zinc. Zinc products that do not specify the amount of elemental zinc provided should be avoided. Zinc preparations should be taken with a light meal to avoid gastric irritation (see discussion of side effects).

The most useful way to diagnose and follow disorders of zinc deficiency is through careful observation of clinical signs and symptoms combined with monitoring of

TABLE 1   Age Related Serum Zinc Levels[*]

Age	μg/dl $\pm$ SD
5 days	88±12
3 months	68±9
6–12 months	76±12
1–5 years	97±19
5–12 years	101±16
20–40 years	118±16
>50 years	95±19

[*] From Shaw JCL. Trace elements in the fetus and young infant. I. Zinc. Am J Dis Child 1979; 133:1260-1268.

TABLE 2   Recommended Dietary Allowance for Zinc[*]

Age	Elemental Zinc per Day (mg)
0–6 months	3
6–12 months	5
1–10 years	10
>11 years	15
Pregnancy	20
Lactation	25

[*] From Neldner KH. Zinc deficiency syndromes. In: Provost TT, Farmer ER, eds. Current therapy in dermatology. Toronto; B.C. Decker, 1985:247.

serum zinc levels. Improvement in clinical parameters occurs rapidly, usually in 2 to 3 days, with rapid healing of the characteristic skin rash, decrease in diarrhea, and decreased irritability. Other signs and symptoms of improvement include reversal of alopecia, restoration of taste and smell sensations, improved gonadal function, and a return to the normal growth rate in children.

Zinc levels should be determined at the initiation of therapy and then every 2 to 3 days until both a normal level is achieved and signs and symptoms have improved. Patients with the inherited zinc deficiency need a maintenance dosage, whereas patients with transient zinc deficiency need only a limited course of treatment. Initial replacement is about three to seven times the RDA level; for adults this is 50 to 100 mg of elemental zinc per day. The dosage is altered according to the clinical response and the serum zinc level. The maximal dosage is 10 times the RDA level (150 mg in an adult).

There are a few special situations that may require intravenous zinc therapy. First, occasionally a patient with a known zinc deficiency does not respond to oral supplementation even after dietary adjustment (see discussion of side effects) and trying different oral preparations. Second, premature infants may have acquired zinc deficiency because of their decreased body stores and increased needs. Lastly, hospitalized patients with multiple medical problems may develop zinc deficiency. Zinc chloride is the salt most commonly used for intravenous supplementation (Zinctrace, Armour Pharmaceutical Company, Tarrytown, New York). This salt may be very irritating if not sufficiently diluted. The recommended doses are listed in Table 3. The intravenous administration of zinc should be entrusted only to those familiar with its use.

Serum copper levels also should be monitored during the course of zinc supplementation because one expects to see a resolution of the hypercupremia that may accompany zinc deficiency. Failure of the hypercupremia to resolve should prompt further investigation. In addition all patients with zinc deficiency should be evaluated and treated for other nutritional deficiencies.

SIDE EFFECTS

An overdose of zinc may result in serious toxicity or even death, although the lethal dose is unknown. There

TABLE 3 Daily Intravenous Zinc Dosage*

Premature infants (1.5–3.0 kg)	300 μg/kg
Full term infants and children through age 5	100μg/kg
Stable patients over age 5	2.5–4.0 mg
Acute catabolic states in patients over age 5	4.5–6.0 mg

* From Solomons NW. Zinc nutriture in total parenteral nutrition. Clin Nutrit 1983; 3:8-13.

is a case report of a 72 year old woman who accidentally received 1.6 g of zinc parenterally over 2½ days (about 150 times the RDA level) and died 47 days later with severe kidney, lung, pancreas, and liver damage. Rapid intravenous infusion has been associated with transient flushing, blurred vision, profuse sweating, tachycardia, and hyperamylasemia. As mentioned previously, intravenous zinc therapy should be undertaken only by experienced physicians.

Oral zinc therapy may also be associated with toxicity. The accidental or purposeful ingestion of excess zinc produces fever, nausea, vomiting, diarrhea, lethargy, and muscle pain and stiffness. In rats prolonged ingestion of excess zinc leads to a reduced growth rate, anemia, impaired reproduction, copper deficiency, and hypertrophy of the adrenal cortex and pancreatic islets. There are no human diseases in which hyperzincemia occurs. Hyperzincemia may be associated with hypocupremia, which in turn may lead to microcytic anemia and leukopenia. In any patient receiving zinc supplementation for as long as 3 months hematologic parameters, ceruloplasmin, and serum copper levels should be monitored. The treatment of acute intoxication would require both hemodialysis with a zinc-free dialysate and the administration of chelating agents.

The most annoying side effects of oral zinc supplementation are gastrointestinal upset and gastritis. Even though zinc is most effectively absorbed from an empty stomach, I recommend that zinc be taken with a light meal in order to avoid the gastrointestinal symptoms and subsequent noncompliance. Many foods can impair zinc absorption, especially those high in fiber that contain the zinc chelator, phytate. Therefore, breads and probably also dairy products should not be taken with the zinc. Meats and fish are good sources of zinc and should be encouraged in the diet.

LEG ULCERS

DONALD P. LOOKINGBILL, M.D.

Leg ulcers can be due to a wide variety of etiologies, but the most common is stasis. This section deals primarily with the therapy of venous (stasis) ulcers, although some of the therapeutic measures can be applied to other types of leg ulcers as well.

PATIENT EVALUATION

Stasis ulcers result from sustained elevations in venous pressure in the lower extremities. Frequently there is a history of thrombophlebitis. The ulcers typically occur above the malleolus, usually on the medial side of the leg. Venous ulcers are often accompanied by petechiae and a brownish discoloration ("stasis changes") of the surrounding skin. Dermatitis may be present as well and is due either to the stasis itself or to secondary contact dermatitis. Dermatitis, if present, is sometimes confused with cellulitis in that both are manifested by erythematous skin; but dermatitis is often vesicular and almost always pruritic, whereas cellulitis is warm and tender and sometimes is accompanied by fever.

In patients with venous ulcers, leg and pedal edema is usually present and is a critical factor that must be addressed if treatment is to succeed. In the general evaluation of the patient, consideration should be given to other possible causes of edema, including congestive heart failure and kidney disease. The blood pressure should also be obtained and pedal pulses examined to screen for other vascular causes or factors contributing to the leg ulcer. If pedal pulses are absent, a vascular surgery consultation is recommended. In chronic nonhealing ulcers, a biopsy specimen should be taken from the edge of the ulcer to rule out other etiologies, particularly malignant disease.

MEDICAL THERAPY

The preferred therapy for venous ulcers is medical. Surgical treatment may be needed if medical management fails or becomes unduly prolonged. The foremost consideration in medical management is to control edema. If this is not achieved, other measures will be of little value. The other measures include treatment of infection (if present), debridement, and wound dressings.

Edema Reduction

Edema control is more easily said than achieved, especially in an outpatient. For patients with severe disease, hospitalization may be necessary. In the hospital setting the patient is put at strict bed rest with the foot of the bed slightly elevated. Pneumatic compression devices such as the Jobst extremity pump can also be used to reduce edema and lymphedema more quickly. In our hospital this is done once or twice daily in the physical therapy department.

For most outpatients, strict bed rest is impossible to achieve, but patients are encouraged to maximize the amount of time they spend lying flat with their legs slightly elevated and minimize time spent sitting in a chair. We have found that in patients who comply with bed rest instructions the ulcers are much more likely to heal than those in patients who are noncompliant.

The judicious use of diuretics may help reduce edema in some patients, but this is not a mainstay of therapy. Unna boots and elastic stockings are also helpful for edema control (to be discussed).

Treatment of Infection

Most ulcers contain potentially pathogenic bacteria, which can be recovered on routine culture. However, cultures are not usually performed, and antibiotic treatment is not instituted, unless there is evidence of cellulitis around the ulcer. If cellulitis is present, a culture is taken empiric antibiotic therapy is begun to cover gram positive organisms. Erythromycin is most frequently employed. If there is no clinical response, the culture results may be of help in selecting alternative antibiotic therapy. When the cellulitis subsides, antibiotics are discontinued. Sterilization of the ulcer is an unrealistic goal; long-term antibiotic therapy only selects out resistant organisms.

Debridement

Necrotic debris enhances bacterial growth and impairs ulcer healing. Physical debridement can be done with a curette or scissors and forceps. Viscous lidocaine is often helpful for local anesthesia. We have not found the topical application of enzymatic preparations to be very useful and they can cause irritiation.

Medical measures for debridement include wet-to-dry dressings and Debrisan dressings. Occlusive dressings also provide for debridement and are discussed separately.

Wet Dressings

Wet dressings are most useful in the initial stages of treating ulcers that have abundant debris. Wet dressings are most conveniently used in patients who are at bed rest. For the "wetness" we use saline or quarter strength Burow's solution (aluminum acetate). Full strength Burow's solution is not used because evaporation can result in an ultimate concentration that will cause irritation. Since patients with venous ulcers have a predilection for developing contact dermatitis in the area of involvement, the use of potentially sensitizing chemicals should be avoided. This includes antiseptics such as povidone-iodine (Betadine) and topically applied antibiotics such as neomycin.

Wet dressings are applied as follows: Several layers of wet gauze are placed over the ulcer and held in place with tubular gauze. Since evaporation is desired, the dressing should not be occluded. Depending upon the amount of wetness to begin with, it takes 30 minutes to several hours for the dressings to dry. The dressings should be changed every 4 hours. At the time of removal, some of the debris will have stuck to the dressing and hence will have been removed. The ulcer base is then gently cleaned and another dressing applied. Wet-to-dry dressings are used mainly in the initial stages of ulcer therapy or in preparation for grafting.

Dextranomer (Debrisan)

Dextranomer is a hydrophilic dextran polymer that has been formulated into small spherical beads (Debrisan). It is of use in debriding moist ulcers, wherein fluid is absorbed into the beads and particulate matter is trapped between the swollen beads. Edema in the ulcer area may also be reduced by the hydrophilic action. Debrisan is available in loose beads or in a paste, either of which is applied to the moist ulcer in a ¼ inch layer and covered with a gauze dressing, closed on all four sides. Dressings are changed twice daily at which time the ulcer is thoroughly irrigated. Since Debrisan often tends to adhere to the ulcer base, vigorous irrigation is frequently needed, sometimes accompanied by gentle swabbing. Debrisan should be used only on moist ulcers; if they become dry, the medication should be discontinued. This method is relatively effective in treating ulcers, but it is expensive.

Occlusive Dressings

Occlusive dressings exploit the theory of "moist wound healing." A number of these dressings are now on the market, including Bioclusive, Duoderm, Op-Site, Synthaderm, Tegaderm, and Vigilon. Most are made of polyurethane, and all but Tegaderm and Vigilon are self-adhesive. All have in common the property of occlusion, which causes an accumulation of exudate (which aids debridement) and accelerates wound healing. We have mainly used either Duoderm or Op-site. Duoderm is easier to handle than Op-site, but Op-site is more adhesive. The dressing is applied to the ulcer and surrounding skin. With Duoderm, tape is used to further secure the edges. The dressing should not be removed until it loosens naturally or drainage leaks out from under the edges. Most dressings stay in place for at least several days (up to 1 week), but in ulcers with copious exudate, more frequent dressing changes may be necessary. Patients need to be advised that fluid will accumulate under the dressing and that the drainage may have a foul odor. Patient instruction booklets are available for some occlusive dressings (for example, Duoderm). The dressings are moderately expensive, and some patients need help in applying them. Development of cellulitic infection under the occlusive dressing is a theoretical concern, but surprisingly rarely occurs. A major advantage of occlusive dressings is that they usually provide excellent pain relief. Elastic stockings can be used over Op-site or Duoderm dressings. The use of occlusive dressings can be continued until complete healing occurs.

Unna Boot

The time tested Unna boot still has a place in the treatment of leg ulcers. It is best used after debridement and edema reduction. It protects the ulcers, provides partial occlusion, and helps to prevent edema. We use a Dome-Paste dressing, which is applied in accordance with the directions on the package. With the foot in a flexed position, the leg is wrapped from the forefoot to just below the knee, including the heel. Wrinkles and reverse turns should be avoided. The dressing should be applied in a "pressure gradient" fashion with more pressure at the ankle than at the knee, but care must be taken not to make the dressing too tight. The entire dressing is used and covers the leg in about three layers. It is then wrapped with a Kling bandage, which is held in place with tape applied to the top, bottom, and sides. Removal is accomplished by carefully cutting the dressing with bandage scissors on the side of the leg opposite the ulcer. At dressing changes, the ulcer and leg are gently cleaned, but no medications are applied except for the fresh dressing.

The Unna boot dressing is changed weekly until healing occurs (often months) or until no further progress is made. The Unna boot method has the advantage of requiring infrequent dressing changes with relatively inexpensive materials, but it is somewhat bulky and requires weekly office (or home) visits and a nurse skilled in its application.

SURGICAL THERAPY

With medical therapy many ulcers heal, albeit slowly. At each office visit the ulcer should be measured or traced so that progress can be monitored. The surrounding skin should be checked for edema, and if it is present, that aforementioned measures should be readdressed. If, in the absence of edema, the ulcer is enlarging or not improving over time, surgery should be considered. This is a time to also re-evaluate the original diagnosis. For example, if a biopsy had not been done initially, it might now be considered to rule out malignant disease.

In our hospital ulcer surgery is done by either plastic surgeons or vascular surgeons. An accurate assessment of the patient's vascular status is important prior to leg surgery. Some venous ulcerations occur over incompetent perforating veins in the lower legs, and sclerosing one or several of these vessels may be helpful. The arterial blood supply of course must also be adequate for successful grafting.

If the ulcer bed is clean, the ulcer may be covered directly with a split thickness skin graft. For necrotic ulcers with poor granulation tissue, excision is needed before grafting.

Properly performed and cared for, skin grafting can result in excellent coverage of long standing venous ulcers.

POSTULCER TREATMENT: ELASTIC SUPPORT STOCKINGS

The successful management of venous ulcers does not end with ulcer healing. Prevention is important. For this, the use of elastic stockings is strongly recommended. Several types are manufactured, and kits are now available for measuring patients in the office. We use knee length stockings and fit patients for either Jobst Fast-Fit or T.E.D. stockings. The Jobst Fast-Fit stockings are more expensive, but are flesh colored and provide venous pressure gradient support. Measurements are made at the calf and ankle, and the patient is fitted with one of six sizes.

The T.E.D. stockings are white and are available in two lengths, each in small, medium, large, and extra large sizes. They are fitted on the basis of calf circumference and leg length measurements. Fitting measurements are preferably made when the patient has no or minimal edema; once fitted, patients are instructed to put the stockings on each morning before getting out of bed.

PRURITUS

MARCIA G. TONNESEN, M.D.

Pruritus, or itching, has been defined as an unpleasant cutaneous sensation that evokes the impulse to scratch. As the cardinal symptom in dermatology, it may vary from localized to generalized, from very mild to extremely intense. Frequently it has a major effect on the quality of life of its sufferers. Pruritus presents a particular challenge to the dermatologist because of its common occurrence, frequent association with numerous cutaneous and systemic diseases, and relative intractability. Appropriate management of the itching patient requires an understanding of the pathophysiology of the itch sensation, a thorough search to identify the underlying cause, and a clear knowledge of the therapeutic modalities available for intervention.

PATHOPHYSIOLOGY OF PRURITUS

Despite extensive investigation, the pathophysiology of itch is not well understood, owing in part to the subjective nature of the sensation and the multitude of environmental, cultural, and emotional factors that influence its perception. The receptor apparatus for itch is believed to be a finely arborizing network of free nerve endings located at the dermal-epidermal junction of the skin. A variety of stimuli and noxious agents are presumed to liberate diffusable chemomediators that stimulate these receptors. The pathologic itch stimulus is then transmitted by unmyelinated, slowly-conducting C-fibers to the spinal cord and thence to the thalamus and sensory cortex. Although knowledge of the biochemical events that elicit pruritus is incomplete, a number of mediators of inflammation have been implicated as inciting agents.

Histamine present in skin mast cells is believed to be the most important mediator. Inoculations of histamine produce itching in human skin, which can be successfully blocked by antihistamines. However, the fact that antihistamines are usually only minimally to moderately effective in many pruritic diseases suggests that histamine is not the only clinically relevant mediator of itch. Endopeptidases, released from skin and blood during inflammation, may contribute to the generation of pruritus, since experimental introduction into skin of a variety of proteases (such as trypsin, papain, kallikrein, and epidermal protease) can induce itching. However, the mechanism of action may not be related to their proteolytic activity, since no new potent itch-producing peptide has yet been isolated from human skin. Many known biologically active peptides, including vasoactive intestinal peptide, substance P, and neurotensin, have been shown to cause not only a vascular response but also varying degrees of itch, apparently at least in part via release of histamine from cutaneous mast cells. In addition, synergism between different mediators is an important and well-recognized factor contributing to the induction of pruritus. For example, prostaglandin E_1, although not itself pruritogenic, has been shown to be present in increased amounts in inflamed skin and to potentiate experimental itch induced by histamine.

The central nervous system may modulate the perception of itch. Morphine can provoke generalized pruritus not only by directly releasing histamine from cutaneous mast cells but also through a central mechanism, probably via binding to opiate receptors in the brain. Naloxone, an opiate antagonist, has been reported to attenuate pruritus induced by either cholestasis or the local cutaneous application of histamine, suggesting that enkephalins, opioid peptides that function as neurotransmitters within the peripheral and central nervous systems, may play a regulatory role by modulating the perception of pruritus. Psychologic and physical factors are known to modify the itch threshold. Feelings of stress, anxiety, frustration, fear, boredom, guilt, anger, or depression as well as stimuli such as touch or elevation in temperature may magnify itch, while competing mental distractions or cutaneous sensations may serve to reduce or competitively inhibit its perception. The multiplicity of chemomediators and the complexity of potentially modulating influences emphasize the need for a multifaceted therapeutic approach to the individual patient with pruritus.

EVALUATION OF THE ITCHING PATIENT

Pruritus is a symptom, not a disease. Therefore, a complete investigation into the cutaneous or underlying systemic cause of the itch is of critical importance to the successful evaluation and treatment of the patient with pruritus. Since itching is the most common symptom of diseases affecting the skin, characteristic cutaneous lesions are often present to enable the ready diagnosis of one of a variety of pruritic dermatoses (such as scabies, dermatitis herpetiformis, atopic or contact dermatitis, urticaria, psoriasis, lichen planus, and bullous pemphigoid).

The itching patient without an apparent skin eruption poses a diagnostic challenge. Initially a search should be undertaken for subtle evidence of cutaneous disease and for identification of any diagnostic primary lesions. Although useful as indicators of the severity of the itch, the myriad cutaneous manifestations of acute and chronic scratching (including linear excoriations, erythematous wheals, ulcers, eczematization, impetiginization, lichenification, pigment alteration, scars) may mask or obliterate the primary lesion—perhaps a patch of mild dermatitis, a scabetic burrow, the vesicle in dermatitis herpetiformis, the lice and nits of pediculosis, the scale of xerosis. The primary lesion may be transient, such as the wheal of chronic or papular urticaria, or may be delayed in onset, such as the blister of bullous pemphigoid.

A detailed history may be essential to uncover evidence of exposure to fiberglass, scabies, drugs, or infested animals. Since animal carriers of mites, fleas, and lice may be symptom free, all animals, especially dogs and cats, with which a pruritic patient has had contact should be examined by a veterinarian. If the itching is described as unbearable and interrupts sleep, a skin biopsy specimen sent for immunofluorescence studies may demonstrate dermatitis herpetiformis or bullous pemphigoid, or a therapeutic trial of lindane may cure the patient of scabies. Cellophane tape samples from skin and clothing may reveal fiberglass spicules acquired from handling fiberglass or not infrequently from wearing clothing washed with fiberglass curtains. Careful inspection of clothing may demonstrate an infestation with lice. Stroking of the skin may indicate the presence of dermographism.

Possible environmental causes of pruritus must also be explored. Extremely high humidity may produce sweat retention, irritation, and itch. Xerosis, particularly in the elderly, may be exacerbated by environmental factors (low humidity, high altitude, dry cold wind, central heating, frequent washing with soap and hot water). The itch of xerosis should be relieved by adequate hydration and appropriate topical therapy (to be discussed); if it persists, further diagnostic studies are indicated.

The patient with persistent generalized itching in whom there is no detectable cutaneous or environmental cause for pruritus must be evaluated for the presence of a possible underlying systemic disease. The incidence of the association of generalized pruritus with significant internal disease has been estimated to range from 10 to 50 percent. The most commonly associated diseases are listed in Table 1. Thorough assessment of the patient with generalized pruritus should include a complete history, a review of systems, and a physical examination as well as a basic laboratory evaluation as outlined in Table 2. More complex investigations should follow as appropriate.

TABLE 1 Systemic Diseases Associated with Generalized Pruritus

Hepatic diseases:
  obstructive biliary disease,
  intrahepatic cholestasis (pregnancy)

Renal diseases:
  chronic renal failure

Endocrine and Metabolic diseases:
  thyroid disease, ? diabetes mellitus,
  hypoparathyroidism, carcinoid syndrome

Hematologic diseases:
  polycythemia rubra vera, iron deficiency

Parasitic diseases:
  pediculosis, scabies, hookworm,
  onchocerciasis, filariasis

Neoplastic diseases:
  Hodgkin's disease, leukemia, lymphoma,
  mycosis fungoides, multiple myeloma,
  visceral tumors

Psychogenic diseases:
  depression, stress, delusions of parasitosis,
  psychosis, neurosis

Drug induced pruritus:
  opium derivatives, subclinical drug sensitivity

Miscellaneous diseases:
  mastocytosis, xerosis

Neurologic diseases:
  multiple sclerosis, central nervous system
  lesions

TABLE 2 Basic Laboratory Evaluation for Generalized Pruritus without Primary Skin Lesions

Complete blood count with differential
Erythrocyte sedimentation rate
Liver, renal, and thyroid function tests
Serum iron, total iron binding capacity
Serum protein electrophoresis
Fasting blood glucose
Urinalysis for albumin, glucose, cells, casts
Stool test for occult blood, ova, and parasites
Chest roentgenogram
Papanicolaou smear

TREATMENT

Therapy directed at the elimination or alleviation of the causative disorder, whether cutaneous or systemic, often results in resolution of the associated pruritus. During the evaluation period, and particularly if the cause cannot be determined or eliminated, effective symptomatic management is essential but usually only variably successful owing to the paucity of specific antipruritic drugs. Patients may nevertheless benefit from attempts to avoid exacerbating factors, the institution of a good skin care regimen with appropriate topical treatment, a trial of systemic therapy, phototherapy when indicated, and psychologic assessment as necessary.

Avoidance of Exacerbating Factors

Factors that are known to exacerbate pruritus and possible ways to avoid them must be thoroughly reviewed with the itching patient. Scratching, although often a source of transient relief, usually perpetuates the itch. Attempts should be made to interrupt the "itch-scratch cycle" by decreasing the urge to scratch with the local application of cool compresses or a cooling emollient, such as Lubriderm with 0.25 percent menthol, and by trying to break the scratch habit, aided by helpful reminders from caring friends or by the presence of physical barriers such as gloves or mitts. Fingernails should be kept short to avoid further damage to the skin. Since xerosis may either cause or exacerbate pruritus, institution of a good skin care regimen to reduce dry skin is essential, particularly in the elderly. Although excessive washing with hot water and harsh soaps may contribute to xerosis, adequate hydration is mandatory. One bath or shower per day for 10 to 20 minutes with warm water and a mild soap, such as Dove or Tone, should be immediately followed by the application of an emollient to prevent evaporation of water from the hydrated epidermis. Since moisture is lost from the skin when the ambient humidity is low (dry cold air, central heating, high altitude), humidifiers or open pans of evaporating water in the bedroom may be helpful.

Clothing may be a source of irritation and itch, either from the friction of tight-fitting garments or from the rough surface of wool and certain synthetics. Such clothes should be removed, or a protective nonirritating liner should be worn close to the skin. Heat, presumably through vasodilation and increased cutaneous blood flow, enhances itch. Therefore patients should avoid excessive environmental heat, overdressing, vigorous exercise, hot baths or showers, hot drinks, and excessive alcohol intake. Stress and anxiety intensify the perception of itch, and refractory itch with concomitant sleeplessness and discomfort heightens stress and anxiety. Patients should be encouraged to pursue means to minimize stress and anxiety with the assistance of psychologists, counselors, and social workers.

Topical Therapy

As discussed, application of an emollient, particularly immediately after a bath or shower, helps to prevent xerosis and with added menthol (0.25 percent), urea (10 percent), or lactic acid (12 percent) may itself bring relief from itching. The particular emollient selected really depends on patient preference. Lotions such as Lubriderm, Curel, and Moisturel have an advantage in that they can be applied to a large surface area in a reasonably short time. Bath oils, although useful, may make a tub or shower slippery enough to increase the risk of injury. Many patients obtain relief from colloidal oatmeal added to the bath. Topically applied antihistamines and anesthetics are relatively ineffective and are best avoided since they can be potent allergic sensitizers. Use of fluorinated topical steroid therapy should be reserved for the treatment of a specific steroid-responsive dermatosis. Long term application may result in dermal atrophy with associated telangiectasia, striae, and easy bruising.

Systemic Therapy

Antihistamines, competitive pharmacologic antagonists of histamine, have been clearly shown to inhibit experimental histamine-induced pruritus and to provide symptomatic relief of itching in disorders in which histamine is the principal mediator, such as urticaria. They are less effective in other pruritic conditions, and any relief obtained may be due in part to their sedative and placebo effects. Sedation is a significant but transient side effect, since most patients eventually develop tolerance with prolonged use. While the sedative effect is still present, patients should be cautioned about driving and the intake of alcohol. Sedation may be beneficial for nights made sleepless by itching and scratching.

A therapeutic trial of antihistamines (H₁ blockers) in an adequate oral dosage is usually worthwhile for symptomatic treatment. Several studies have suggested that hydroxyzine (Atarax) is superior to other antihistamines in decreasing pruritus, and since it may be less sedating, it probably deserves to be the antihistamine of choice at least initially. Chlorpheniramine (Chlor-Trimeton) and diphenhydramine hydrochloride (Benadryl) are reasonable alternatives. A typical regimen would be hydroxyzine (10 to 25 mg), chlorpheniramine (4 mg), or diphenhydramine (25 to 50 mg) by mouth every 4 to 6 hours. The dosage may be doubled with caution. Patients who cannot tolerate daytime sedation or whose itch is consider

ably worse at night may prefer to take up to twice the dosage only at bedtime. If no relief is obtained with one drug, it may be useful to switch to an antihistamine of a different chemical class or to use several in combination.

The addition of an H₂ blocker (cimetidine, ranitidine) has not proven to be as beneficial as initially hoped. Since recent experimental evidence indicates that only H₁ and not H₂ receptors are involved in histamine-evoked itching, there does not appear to be any rational basis for the use of histamine H₂ antagonists in the treatment of itching.

The tricyclic antidepressants doxepin hydrochloride (Adapin, Sinequan) and amitriptyline hydrochloride (Elavil) have a high binding affinity for histamine H₁ receptors and, when applied topically, suppressed histamine-induced pruritus. These drugs may prove to be additional therapeutic tools, particularly in patients who would benefit from the antidepressant as well as the antipruritic effect. The recommended dosage of doxepin is 10 to 25 mg three times daily for 2 weeks, after which the entire daily dosage (75 mg) may be taken in the evening. The maximal daily dosage is 300 mg. Doxepin and other antihistamines with anticholinergic activity are contraindicated in patients with narrow-angle glaucoma or urinary retention. A clinical role for the opiate antagonist naloxone in the treatment of itching has not yet been elucidated.

Systemically administered drugs also have been reported to be of benefit in the pruritus associated with specific diseases. Activated charcoal has been used successfully in relieving itching in patients with renal failure given maintenance hemodialysis. The recommended dosage is 6 g of activated charcoal in capsule form daily for 8 weeks. Oral doses of cholestyramine (5 g twice daily) have been variably effective in pruritus associated with renal and hepatic (cholestasis) disease, presumably acting by binding and removing pruritogenic substances in the gut. The nature of such substances is controversial. In hepatobiliary disease no direct relationship appears to exist between the degree of itching and the concentration of bile acids or salts in serum, skin, or interstitial fluid. In renal failure, pruritus is not directly correlated with levels of blood urea or with the duration of dialysis.

Phototherapy

Ultraviolet phototherapy is of therapeutic benefit in relieving uremic pruritus in some patients. Ultraviolet B therapy is administered three to five times a week, the initial dose being 75 to 80 percent of the minimal erythema dose as determined for each individual patient. Each subsequent dose can be increased by 10 to 20 percent as tolerated. Improvement usually occurs within 2 to 3 weeks (six to eight exposures) and appears to be related to the total dosage administered, without need for maintenance therapy. Lack of response after 15 to 20 treatments constitutes a therapeutic failure. Patients may experience remissions lasting weeks to months, and those who relapse may benefit from a second course of treatment. The mechanism of action of ultraviolet B therapy in pruritus is unclear but may involve the inactivation of a circulating pruritogenic substance or the formation of an antipruritic photo product. A role for ultraviolet B therapy and for PUVA (ultraviolet A and oral therapy with 8-methoxypsoralen) in the treatment of idiopathic pruritus shows promise but has yet to be well documented. PUVA unfortunately may be of limited usefulness, since it induces pruritus in the early stages of therapy.

Psychotherapy

Attributing generalized pruritus of unclear etiology to a psychologic disturbance is hazardous. However, as indicated in Table 1, such conditions may exist. In addition, since such emotional factors as stress, anxiety, fear, and depression may intensify the perception of itch, and severe intractable itching may itself induce secondary emotional reactions, many patients may benefit from a psychologic assessment and from attempts to help them to cope better. Unconventional therapies such as biofeedback, acupuncture, and transcutaneous nerve stimulation ultimately may become clinical adjuncts in the treatment of chronic idiopathic pruritus.

Assessment of the therapeutic effectiveness of any of the treatment modalities outlined is difficult because pruritus is extremely subjective. However, if despite all diagnostic and therapeutic attempts, significant itching persists unabated without apparent cause, periodic reevaluation should be performed, since generalized pruritus is a symptom that may herald the onset of such serious disorders as Hodgkin's disease, bullous pemphigoid, and mycosis fungoides.

KELOIDS

LEONARD M. DZUBOW, M.D.

A keloid is usually regarded as a scar of inappropriate dimensions relative to the precipitating traumatic event. Hypertrophic scars, although similar in appearance to keloids, are distinguished primarily by the confinement of their involvement to the exact area of initial injury. Although hypertrophic scars are typically self-resolving, keloids not only fail to improve with time but also may continue to enlarge and express "activity" (pain, pruritus, drainage) far beyond the period of initial trauma. A keloid, in simplistic terms, appears to be an expression of a malfunction in the inhibition of the wound healing process. The actual pathophysiology of keloid formation is unfortunately unkown.

The treatment of keloids is nothing less than frustrating. The ability to improve the appearance of a keloid is related to the anatomic site of occurrence, the possibility of utilizing a treatment that will minimize the factors that predispose to re-formation (tension, thermal injury), and the unpredictable genetic variations in the wound healing process. Therapy may incorporate combinations of medical, surgical, and physical modalities.

MEDICAL THERAPY

The initial approach to either hypertrophic scars or keloids relies upon the use of intralesional injections of corticosteroid suspensions. Intralesional steroid therapy not only promotes collagen breakdown and shrinkage in size, but may also inhibit the inflammatory component of the process and relieve pain and pruritus. Triamcinolone acetonide suspension (Kenalog) is usually employed in concentrations varying from 2 to 40 mg per milliliter. The larger concentrations are used initially to promote resolution. Injections are spaced at intervals of 4 to 5 weeks. As soon as change in size and relief of symptoms are evident, the concentration is tapered gradually. Even after the final result is attained, injections of 2 to 5 mg per milliliter may be continued as a maintenance program in an attempt to prevent recurrence.

The most common complications of intralesional steroid therapy are atrophy and pigmentary alteration. Atrophy may be caused by continued injection of steroids for too long a period or at too elevated a concentration. It is obviously critical to adjust the frequency and concentration of steroid therapy to the residual mass of the keloid as it decreases. Atrophy also may be due to incorrect placement of the steroid depot. The injection must be within the substance of the keloid. Unfortunately, this is the path of greatest resistance. It is inappropriate to inject the steroids below the keloid within the subcutaneous tissues because this will surely contribute to atrophy. Fortunately, this phenomenon is usually not permanent. Resolution is to be expected after a period of months to several years.

Intralesional steroid therapy also may cause hypopigmentation. This is particularly of concern in dark skinned individuals and may be a permanent alteration. The only prevention is to limit the extent and concentration of injections.

The injection technique is a key to success. Steroids must be placed within the substance of the keloid. A 27- to 25-gauge needle is often simpler to use in a high pressure delivery system. Similarly a 1 cc tuberculin syringe requires less force of injection than any larger size. A closed Luer-Lok system prevents separation of the needle from the syringe during delivery of the steroid suspension. Occasionally the density of the keloid prevents instillation of the steroid. The keloid may be briefly sprayed with liquid nitrogen using a cryosurgical delivery unit. The subsequent edema usually causes enough softening to permit successful injection.

Intalesional corticosteroid therapy may be utilized as the initial mode of therapy in all keloids. However, it may be the only available modality in such unfavorable anatomic sites as the presternal area, deltoid region, and back. Surgery in these regions, even in combination with compression dressings, frequently is unsuccessful. Unfortunately even after prolonged periods of remission following termination of intralesional steroid therapy, keloid regrowth may occur.

SURGICAL THERAPY

Surgical therapy of keloids may be undertaken utilizing conventional cold steel or a carbon dioxide laser as the cutting device. With either approach the surgery must be performed to minimize all types of trauma (tension, heat) to the wound bed. In general, it is prudent not to design a surgical procedure that potentially could eventuate in a keloid larger than the original. It also must be realized that residual keloidal tissue following surgical removal is capable of providing a nidus for regrowth. Empirically, any keloid demonstrating an inflammatory component (redness, pain, pruritus) should be pretreated weeks to months prior to surgery with intralesional corticosteroid therapy.

Excision

Excision is a reasonable approach for keloids in low risk anatomic sites—principally the head and neck region. Excision of keloids located in the presternal area or in sites subject to movement and tension frequently fails. In fact, if total removal of the keloid is attempted with one excision, the resulting scar and possibly the subsequent keloid will be larger than the original. Therefore, serial staged excisions within the substance of the keloid are prudent and advisable. The surrounding normal skin should be subject to minimal trauma (electrocoagulation) and tension. Three to 6 months should pass prior to a second staged excision to assess the success of the first attempt. Intralesional steroid therapy may be used as both pre- and post-treatment means to lower the risk of recurrence. Contoured, form-fitted compression dressings (obtainable through the Jobst company) may or may not be of ancillary help.

Proper technique includes removal of the keloid down to normal subcutaneous tissue. Undermining should be limited in order to minimize trauma. Neither cutaneous nor subcutaneous sutures should be tied under tension. If tension is required for closure, the chances for success are slim. Simple excision with low tension closure works best on the face, especially with keloids involving the ear lobe. As an exception to the philosophy of always cutting within a keloid, i.e., staged excisions, ear-lobe keloids often may be totally excised in a single step without adverse consequence. So-called "dumb-bell" shaped or through and through ear-lobe keloids may be totally "cored-out" and the resulting low-tension defect simply closed.

If serial staged excisions are employed, the patient must be aware that a line of residual keloid will always remain. Flattening of this residual keloidal line may be attempted with continued intralesional steroid injections.

If staged excision of the keloid is deemed unlikely to succeed owing to the realization of adverse tension, a "hinge-flap" or "keloid-graft" procedure may be considered. The philosophy of not exceeding original wound dimensions and utilizing pre- and postsurgical intralesional steroid therapy continues to apply. A hinge flap is created by incising the tissue at the junction of the keloid and normal skin approximately one-half to three-quarters of the way around the perimeter. The incision extends in depth to uninvolved subcutaneous tissue. The keloid flap, with pedicle intact, is gently separated from the base. Hemostasis is attempted using pressure and topical hemostatic drugs prior to resorting to electrocoagulation. Keloidal tissue is then removed from the undersurface of the flap. Some tissue must remain under the flap to insure a viable vascular supply. The flap is then replaced on the base and gently sutured to the adjacent skin.

This is only a debulking procedure. A keloidal nidus remains on the deep surface of the flap and is capable of regenerating the original lesion. Postsurgical steroid therapy is therefore a must if improvement is to occur. If the keloidal tissue is totally debulked, the flap is transformed essentially into a free graft. The pedicle then may be completely severed to gain access to any residual keloidal tissue. The graft is then sutured to the bed and covered with a compression dressing. The success of take of the graft varies with the adequacy of the blood supply of the bed. Failure of graft take is not a total catastrophe. The wound is left to heal by second intention (as one would following laser excision). Since wound contraction is so gradual, tension during the healing process may be less than the threshold needed for re-formation.

Carbon Dioxide Laser Excision

The carbon dioxide laser has been used for the treatment of keloids because of its purported capacity to excise tissue with minimal thermal damage to adjacent normal skin. Theoretically this minimizes the risk of reformation. As with other modalities, laser excision is most effective in treating keloids of the facial region, although areas at high risk for recurrence may be approached as well.

Postlaser and possibly even prelaser intralesional injections of the keloid with steroids are useful for all anatomic sites. The laser is used in the "cutting mode" with a small aperture lens to achieve precise separation of the keloid from the underlying bed. The keloid should be removed in its entirety down to a plane of uninvolved tissue. Bleeding not controlled by laser coagulation should be approached in as nontraumatic a fashion as possible. The wound is allowed to heal by secondary intention with attention to standard wound care, using hydrogen peroxide cleansing and an antibiotic ointment on a daily basis. Either simple or form-fitted compression dressings may be used during the healing period. Intralesional steroid injections are continued at monthly intervals and then slowly tapered, depending on the progress of the healing and the tendency for the keloid to recur.

Although laser therapy has been touted as a significant breakthrough in keloid treatment, no study has compared similar atraumatic excision using standard techniques and secondary intention healing. It is clear, however, that keloids of the presternal and deltoid regions often recur following laser excision.

Physical Modalities

Compression of the surgical site following keloid excision is often considered an adjunctive measure. Special compression earrings as well as form-fitted garments are available at reasonable cost. The effectiveness of compression has not been definitely demonstrated, however.

Postsurgical radiation therapy has been shown to be effective in preventing re-formation. However, the fear of potential carcinogenesis has damped the enthusiasm for this time-proven modality.

The treatment of keloids is clearly frustrating and the potential for success is somewhat unpredictable. The anatomic site of involvement and the dynamics of force and tension on the wound predefine the chances for resolution regardless of the modality chosen. Atraumatic technique and total extirpation of keloidal tissue appear to be the keys to a favorable outcome.

ICHTHYOSIS AND PALMOPLANTAR KERATODERMAS

MIGUEL R. SANCHEZ, M.D.
IRWIN M. FREEDBERG, M.D.

The ichthyoses and palmoplantar keratodermas are two groups of genetically determined or acquired cutaneous diseases traditionally classified as disorders of keratinization. The best current evidence suggests that the unifying feature among these dermatoses is enhanced corneocyte adhesion.

Ichthyotic skin is readily recognized by the presence of noninflammatory fishlike scales. Because the response to treatment, associated physical features, and inheritance patterns differ, it is important to determine the correct diagnosis before proceeding.

The primary ichthyoses are recognized at birth or in early childhood, (Table 1), although individuals with the milder forms may be aware of only dry skin. Acquired ichthyosis has been reported with several diseases and drugs (Table 2). Congenital syndromes in which ichthyosis is a prominent feature often exhibit a combination of ophthalmologic, neurologic, and skeletal manifestations with or without mental retardation. Since no therapy currently available completely restores the skin to a normal appearance or induces a permanent remission, the dermatologist should clarify the patient's expectations.

WATER AND EMOLLIENTS

The water content of the stratum corneum influences the flexibility of this layer and affects the degree of desquamation. Studies in some ichthyoses suggest that the degree of water binding is abnormally low. With a reduced water content the stratum corneum becomes drier and cracks more easily. Baths hydrate the statum corneum and facilitate desquamation. Some patients remove scales with a Buff-Puff type of sponge and may add dispersible oils to the bath water. The stratum corneum takes up water but does not retain it for long periods of time. Therefore an emollient should be applied after the bath, when the skin is moist, to prevent evaporation. Patients with more severe ichthyosis often choose petrolatum, whereas those with milder disease may prefer more appealing, but less effective, lubricating agents. In general, application of emollients to exposed body areas throughout the day is simple and this practice should be encouraged. Hydration and lubrication are the therapeutic modalities with which the efficacy of other treatments should be compared.

SALICYLIC ACID

Salicylic acid is a strong keratolytic drug that promotes desquamation. Since it causes rapid peeling, salicylic acid is especially useful at the initiation of a therapeutic program.

TABLE 2   Diseases and Drugs Associated with Acquired Ichthyosis

Diseases
Acquired immunodeficiency syndrome
Carcinoma (lung, breast, cervix)
Hansen's disease (borderline and lepromatous)
Hypothyroidism
Kaposi's sarcoma, classic type
Leiomyosarcoma
Leukemia
Lymphoma (especially Hodgkin's disease)
Malabsorption
Malnutrition
Multiple myeloma
Sarcoid
Systemic lupus erythematosus
Drugs
Cimetidine
Clofazimine
Haloperidol
Lipid lowering drugs
Niacinamide

TABLE 1   Primary Ichthyoses

Name	Inheritance*	Scale	Characteristic Physical findings	Associated Features
Ichthyosis vulgaris	AD	Small, fine, light, adherent scale	Flexural areas are not involved; palms and soles demonstrate increased linear markings	Atopy Keratosis pilaris
X-linked ichthyosis	X-linked	Larger dark scales prominent over flanks and neck	Flexural areas are involved; palms and soles are normal	Corneal stippling
Bullous congenital ichthyosiform erythroderma (epidermolytic hyperkeratosis)	AD	Coarse, verrucous scales accentuated over flexural areas	Blisters in childhood; offensive odor	Frequent cutaneous infections
Nonbullous congenital ichthyosiform erythroderma	AR	Fine, white scales	Skin appears erythrodermic; palms, soles, and flexural areas are abnormal	Mild ectropion or increased periorbital skin tension
Lamellar ichthyosis	AR	Large, dark scales	Face often involved; palms, soles, and flexural areas are abnormal	Moderate to severe ectropion

*AD, autosomal dominant. AR, autosomal recessive.

Salicylic acid is well absorbed percutaneously and as a result salicylism may occur. Therefore widespread use should be avoided in young children, and patients should be warned about ingesting salicylate containing products. The most common presentation of salicylism is tinnitus. Keralyt gel contains 6 percent salicylic acid in 40 percent propylene glycol and gives excellent results, especially when applied to moist skin under occlusion. Because this product is relatively expensive and difficult to compound, we suggest to patients that they use it regularly only over exposed areas. Sometimes dramatic desquamation occurs and the medication needs to be applied only every 2 to 3 days. Propylene glycol alone in a 40 to 60 percent concentration used with occlusion once daily is an inexpensive and effective treatment.

UREA

Urea enhances desquamation by breaking intercorneocyte bonds and reversibly denatures keratin by breaking hydrogen bonds. Urea may also improve scaling by binding water, therefore producing a softening and moisturizing effect and promoting skin flexibility.

Urea is available commercially in a variety of concentrations up to 25 percent (Utramide). Pharmacists can mix higher concentrations, but the irritant effect seems to increase in direct proportion to the concentration. Urea–lactic acid combinations are available, although it is not clear that these two agents have synergistic properties. If a mixture of urea and salicylic acid is not compounded correctly, the texture is gritty.

ALPHA-HYDROXY ACIDS

Alpha-hydroxy acids decrease corneocyte cohesion, reportedly by interfering with the formation of ionic bonds. In contrast to other keratolytics, disaggregation of cells occurs at the lower levels of the stratum corneum. There are many agents in this group, and it is not clear whether any is superior, although pyruvic acid has been recommended for epidermolytic hyperkeratosis and glycolic acid is occasionally preferred because of the theoretical advantages of its smaller molecular size.

The most commonly prescribed alpha-hydroxy acid is lactic acid. It can be purchased in lotion form with a 5 percent concentration, or it can be compounded alone or in combination with other agents.

Lac-hydrin lotion, a newer product, contains 12 percent ammonium lactate and significantly improves the appearance of ichthyotic skin. We have been impressed by its rapid beneficial action when used once daily, but the effects of alpha-hydroxy acids, particularly at lower concentrations, may not be evident for weeks.

TOPICAL RETINOIC ACID THERAPY

Topical therapy with retinoic acid may afford improvement in some cases of ichthyosis, but patients often discontinue treatment because of irritation. Even when this side effect is diminished by mixing Retin A with a corticosteroid, a problem still exists since the cost of daily application to the body is considerable.

ORAL RETINOID THERAPY

Retinoids are more effective than their parent compound, vitamin A. Isotretinoin (Accutane) has been studied most widely in this country, but etretinate (Tigason) has provided superior results in the conditions under discussion in this chapter.

The effect of retinoids on the harlequin fetus, epidermolytic hyperkeratosis and X-linked and lamellar ichthyosis is well documented. There is a rapid reduction in scaling and enhanced cutaneous flexibility. The skin surface is improved cosmetically, and patients with lamellar ichthyosis again develop the ability to sweat. In epidermolytic hyperkeratosis, however, the improvement is variable.

The dosage of isotretinoin required is between 1 and 3 mg per kilogram per day, and although side effects at these dosages are common, most patients with severe ichthyosis gladly endure them in return for the improved appearance and texture of the skin. However, in view of the high incidence of hyperostosis of the anterior spinal ligaments and the lack of permanent remissions, ichthyosis should not be routinely treated with isotretinoin. Etretinate therapy is initiated at a dosage of approximately 0.6 mg per kilogram per day, which is raised to 2.0 mg per kilogram per day. Both isotretinoin and etretinate are teratogenic and should be used only with extreme caution in patients with the potential for becoming pregnant.

In the future, topical preparations of these drugs probably will be introduced and may have a beneficial effect without serious complications.

CLINICAL CONSIDERATIONS

Offensive odor is particularly common in congenital bullous ichthyosiform erythroderma and results from bacterial overgrowth. This is treated with antiseptic cleansers, such as chlorhexidine (Hibiclens), wide spectrum topically applied antibiotics (Polysporin, Silvadene), and occasionally systemic antibiotic therapy. Patients may need to bathe with antiseptic agents indefinitely.

Fungal infections occur commonly with some forms of ichthyosis, and respond well to griseofulvin or ketoconazole.

Patients with ichthyosis vulgaris and ichthyosis linearis circumflexa may have atopic dermatitis, which responds to phototherapy or topical corticosteroid therapy. However, neither of these treatments probably benefits the ichthyosis itself unless secondary eczematization from rubbing or irritation has occurred.

A few cases of lamellar ichthyosis and bullous congenital ichthyosiform erythroderma have been treated successfully with methotrexate, although this drug may induce new blisters in the latter disorder. Cytoxan has been reported to improve ichthyosis linearis circumflexa, but the use of potentially dangerous immunosuppressants is not indicated in these chronic cutaneous conditions.

Pruritus is a frequent complaint with ichthyosis, and it is treated in the usual manner. Patients should be warned that the application of urea, salicylic acid, lactic acid, or retinoic acid to excoriated or fissured areas will induce a burning sensation. Topically applied antibiotic ointments are preferred on these areas to promote healing and reduce bacterial growth.

Although the ectropion associated with lamellar ichthyosis can be surgically corrected, this is rarely necessary.

The treatment of newborns with collodion membranes involves the management of temperature regulation, fluid and electrolyte balance, and infection. The infant should be placed in an incubator with high humidity and the weight, serum electrolyte levels, and temperature monitored. Maintaining the membrane moist and pliable prevents respiratory difficulty. The skin is cultured regularly, and systemic doses of antibiotics are prescribed as required. Spontaneous remission may result.

PALMOPLANTAR KERATODERMAS

Palmoplantar keratodermas are easily recognized by the characteristic firm, thickened skin. Differentiation among acquired keratodermas, psoriasis, and pityriasis rubra pilaris is essential, since the treatment and prognosis are different.

Although the compounds already mentioned are effective in treating keratodermas, distinct considerations related to the very thick stratum corneum should be remembered:

1. Debridement of excess keratin facilitates penetration and the action of medications. The feet and hands can be soaked in water or a 25 percent urea solution; the macerated, soft horny layer is pared with a blade.

2. Higher concentrations of therapeutic drugs are required in most patients. We prescribe salicyclic acid in concentrations of 10 to 20 percent. This concentration may be increased as needed. Salicylic acid plaster can be very beneficial on plantar surfaces. Keralyt gel and Lachydrin lotion may be efficacious. The keratin should be kept soft with topical applications of preparations containing lactic acid, urea, or both throughout the day.

3. In order to improve drug penetration, occlusion is particularly important.

Oral retinoid therapy clearly improves these conditions. Once again, etretinate is superior to isotretinoin. However, until safer retinoids are developed, there are few indications for use in chronic disorders. One exception is keratoderma mutilans of Vohrwinkel in which disappearance of the constricting band and normalization of digital circulation are induced, thus preserving the digits. Systemic retinoid therapy also may be considered in situations in which disability is severe.

Some severe keratodermas have been treated by the excision of abnormal skin and split thickness grafting. Except for the most extreme debilitating cases, surgery is rarely justified.

In persons with tyrosinemia II (Richner-Hanhart syndrome), a tyrosine and phenylalanine restriction diet (Mead-Johnson 3200 AB) restores the normal appearance of the skin.

Patients with keratoderma punctata often stop treatment and prefer to pick out the lesions when these become uncomfortable. "Space shoes" with rubber insoles help patients with fissured or painful soles. As discussed with reference to ichthyosis, dermatophyte infections are common with congenital palmoplantar keratodermas; an incidence as high as 40 percent was reported in one series of patients with the Unna Thost type. Rapid improvement occurs with systemic antifungal therapy, but relapses frequently occur and patients may need to be maintained on prophylactic doses for prolonged periods.

HYPERPIGMENTATION AND VITILIGO

THOMAS B. FITZPATRICK, M.D., Ph.D.
DAVID B. MOSHER, M.D.
MADHUKAR A. PATHAK, M.B., Ph.D.

Vitiligo is an idiopathic, acquired, patterned, circumscribed hypomelanosis of skin and hair in which other causes of hypomelanosis (e.g., following inflammation, exposure to chemicals) have been excluded. There is an absence of melanocytes in fully developed hypomelanotic vitiligo macules. The disease is important not only because the disfigurement can result in psychologic problems, especially in brown and black patients, but because it may be a marker for thyroid disease and, much less frequently, certain other diseases, such as diabetes mellitus, pernicious anemia, and Addison's disease. Iritis also may be seen occasionally.

One to 2 percent of the population are affected, with no sexual predilection. The average age of onset is 10 to 30 years, but congenital cases (rare) and onset in old age has been described. The onset may follow physical trauma (the Koebner or isomorphic phenomenon), severe sunburn, surgery, abrasions, skin pressure (such as the belt line and bra straps), or emotional stress. Patients with any skin type may be affected, but vitiligo is most apparent in those who tan well (skin types IV, V, VI). The family history is positive in 30 percent of the patients.

The macules are sharply marginated and typically pure "snow white" (newly developing areas being "off white" or light tan), often with hyperpigmented margins. The macules may be small and round to oval or large. Lesions may be isolated, segmental (unilateral, quasi-dermatomal), generalized, symmetrical (especially periorificial, extensor aspects of the elbows and knees, and bony prominences), or universal. The latter type is sometimes associated with the multiple endocrinopathy syndrome (including hypoparathyroidism, Addison's disease, thyroid disease, mucocutaneous moniliasis, and alopecia areata).

Vitiligo is usually slowly progressive, but rapid evolution may occur. Spontaneous repigmentation may occur in up to 30 percent but rarely to a satisfactory degree. Pigmented or depigmented hairs may be present in a vitiligo macule; white streaks may occur in scalp hair, eyelashes, and beard hair. Iritis, present in 10 percent or more, may not be clearly symptomatic; changes consistent with healed chorioretinitis occur in up to 30 percent of the patients.

Conventional skin biopsy usually shows only the absence of melanocytes (and mild lymphohistocytic infiltration in an active margin). The differential diagnosis includes chemical leukoderma, lupus erythematosus, tinea versicolor, pityriasis alba, piebaldism, and nevus depigmentosus. Laboratory investigations should include a complete blood count with indices, thyroid studies (T_3, T_4, TSH), and a fasting blood sugar determination.

Treatment

Sunscreens

Waterproof SPF 15–30 sunscreens are particularly important for sun-exposed areas of the face, arms, and hands to prevent acute and chronic effects of ultraviolet radiation (dermatoheliosis), including koebnerization (Table 1).

TABLE 1 Vitiligo Treatment Options

Method of Treatment	Advantages	Disadvantages
Sunscreens	Prevent sunburn Prevent photoaging	Daily (or more frequent) application required
Cosmetics Examples: Dermablend, Covermark	Relatively inexpensive Usually good color match	Daily application required Not a cure; rubs off
Dyes Examples: Dy-O-Derm, Vitadye	Relatively inexpensive Ease of use	Usually mediocre color match Only one color; washes off
Repigmentation Topical steroids (e.g., hydrocortisone acetate, 2.5%)	Relatively inexpensive Ease of use	Variably effective; risk of telangiectasia, atrophy, and striae, even with hydrocortisone acetate
PUVA Topical therapy (0.1% 8-methoxypsoralen cream solution) small areas only	No systemic phototoxicity; eye protection required	Requires careful application by physician or trained technician; high phototoxicity risk for up to 24 hours; temporary hyperpigmentation in margins; useful for small areas only
Oral therapy (8-methoxypsoralen, trimethylpsoralen)	Ease of treatment of all macules simultaneously	Minor side effects—giddiness, nausea, gastrointestinal upset; eye protection required; variable phototoxicity (lasts up to 8 hours after pill ingestion)
Depigmentation Monobenzylether of hydroquinone (Benoquin)	Permanent and irreversible	Universal chalk-white color;* skin irritation, dryness (during use); patient must forever abandon hope of repigmentation (tanning); depigmentation not necessarily localized to area of application; sunscreens required for life

* Can be modified satisfactorily by oral therapy with beta-carotene capsules.

Cosmetic Cover-up

Good camouflage techniques are often helpful regardless of what other options patients select. These include make-ups, such as Dermablend (Flori Roberts) and Covermark (Lydia O'Leary), and dyes, such as Dy-O-Derm (Owen Labs) and Vita Dye (Elder). Dyes are available in only one color and may wash off; cosmetics are more adaptable but may rub off.

Repigmentation

Corticosteroids used topically for only 6 to 8 weeks are occasionally effective for small macules and are especially helpful in children. Since telangiectasia and atrophy may develop, regular monitoring by a dermatologist is required. Hydrocortisone acetate 2.5 percent, is useful but is weak. Clobetasol propionate (Temovate) may be effective for small macules in adults, but there is a high risk of atrophy and telangiectasia if it is used for more than a few weeks. The general risks are those of topically applied steroids. Two months are normally required for the initial response; treatment is discontinued once the areas have filled in.

Topical application of 8-methoxypsoralen (8-MOP) may be used in carefully selected patients; application of the 0.1 percent 8-MOP solution or ointment (petrolatum) is followed in one-half hour by controlled artificial ultraviolet exposure (0.05 to 0.25 J per treatment initially) once weekly. The psoralens must be washed off thoroughly after treatment. Topically applied psoralens are extremely phototoxic, and this treatment should be administered by a physician with experience using this technique. Hyperpigmentation at the margins is a common occurrence. Phototoxicity may persist for 24 hours after application. Months of treatment are required for a response.

Oral photochemotherapy may be efficacious in up to 70 percent of carefully selected patients with vitiligo. Schedules include 0.3 to 0.6 mg per kilogram of 8-MOP followed by exposure to artificial ultraviolet A. One should treat only patients over age 12 (when the eyes are adequately mature) and insist on eye protection (sunglasses) outdoors for at least 24 hours after pill ingestion. A complete ophthalmologic examination and an anti-nuclear body (ANA) examination are required before treatment and then yearly during therapy. Treatments are given twice weekly—never 2 days in a row. A response begins after 15 to 25 treatments, but 100 to 300 or more treatments may be necessary to achieve a satisfactory conclusion. Treatment of the face and neck produces a 60 to 70 percent incidence of response; the responses on the trunk, arms, and legs are nearly as good, but the dorsal areas of the hands and feet respond poorly. Side effects are listed in Table 2. Treatments are stopped when repigmentation has occurred; no maintenance treatments are required. The incidence of retention in fully repigmented macules is 85 percent. Good patient compliance and careful physician supervision seem to be part of the formula for success. PUVA may be combined with topical steroid therapy in very closely monitored patients.

TABLE 2 Potential Problems Associated with Oral Psoralen Therapy of Vitiligo

Acute problems
  Subjective complaints of nausea, giddiness, gastrointestinal upset, or itching (often dose related)
  Phototoxicity of vitiligo skin
  Darkening of normal skin (objectionable to some)
  PMLE-like eruption (uncommon)
  Possibility of koebnerization
Chronic problems
  PUVA lentigines
  Chronic ultraviolet degenerative cutaneous changes
  Enhanced risk of nonmelanoma skin cancer (rare, because treatments are finite, i.e., less than 300)
  Possible premature cataract production in unprotected eyes
  Treatment failure or reversal of repigmented macules

Depigmentation

Benoquin (20 percent monobenzylether of hydroquinone, MBEH) is indicated only in patients who have tried and failed, or refused PUVA therapy and who can accept the irreversible nature of this method of treatment. Relative criteria include age over 40 and over 40 percent involvement of the body with vitiligo. Application is carried out twice daily. Transient irritation is common, but contact dermatitis is relatively uncommon. Treatment requires 1 year for complete depigmentation. Depigmentation may not be confined to sites of application but can appear in remote areas; therefore the patient must not attempt to use MBEH to depigment one area and hope to retain nomal pigment in another. Leukotrichia is a rare complication. Depigmentation is permanent and irreversible (the occasional reappearance of some pigmented macules may occur but usually can be eliminated with reapplication of Benoquin). Regular use of sunscreens (SPF 15–30) is required to prevent sunburn reaction of white (depigmented) skin.

MELASMA

Melasma is an acquired hypermelanosis that occurs primarily on the face and is exacerbated by sunlight. Melasma traditionally is associated with pregnancy or the oral administration of contraceptives but may be idiopathic and can occur in men. Typically the disease involves the forehead, cheeks, upper lip, nose, and chin. Lesions are characteristically tan to brown and are enhanced with Wood's light examination in skin types I to IV. Epidermal, dermal, and mixed types of melasma occur. The course may be chronic, but melasma may disappear following parturition or the discontinuation of oral contraceptive therapy. No medical work-up is normally required.

Treatment Options

The treatment of melasma of the epidermal type includes the topical use of 3 percent hydroquinone in combination with tretinoin gel, 0.01 percent, and opaque

TABLE 3 Melasma Treatment

Treatment	Duration	Complication
Tretinoin 0.01% + Hydroguinone 3% + Opaque sunscreen	2+ months required	Erythema, desquamation, contact dermatitis (rare) Failure in dermal melasma (partial failure in mixed type)

sunscreens (Table 3). Without the assiduous daily use of a sunscreen opaque to ultraviolet light and visible radiation (the action spectrum of melasma) the treatment of epidermal melasma will be unsuccessful. Two months may be required to initiate a response. If the response is inadequate, a 4 percent hydroquinone cream may be substituted; if this is inadequate, a stronger tretinoin gel, 0.025 percent may be used. Many months are usually required for clearing to occur. Upon achieving successful results, sunscreen use is usually required in the post-treatment period. (Dermal melasma is unlikely to respond.) Uniformity of pigmentation is the accepted endpoint of therapy.

Complications from treatment include erythema and desquamation, which are most likely with higher concentrations of hydroquinone (5 percent) and tretinoin (0.025 percent). Prolonged treatment with 5 percent hydroquinone may produce ochronosis.

Alternatives to depigmentation with the foregoing drugs include only the use of opaque masking preparations, such as Dermablend or Covermark. Monobenzylether of hydroquinone is absolutely contraindicated in melasma because leukomelanoderma may result (see Table 3).

SOLAR LENTIGINES

Solar lentigines are 1.0 to 3.0 cm, flat, brown macules resulting from localized proliferations of melanocytes in chronically ultraviolet light-exposed skin. These occur with all skin types but particularly with types I and II. Cryotherapy (liquid nitrogen) for a 5-second freeze results in clearing for about 2 years and is particularly effective for solar lentigines on the dorsal surface of the hands and face. Overtreatment could cause hypopigmentation and scarring. Topical hydroquinone therapy is ineffective.

POSTINFLAMMATORY HYPERPIGMENTATION

Postinflammatory hyperpigmentation may be associated with eczema, acne, lichen planus, drug eruptions, and exanthems. This may respond to topical therapy with 2 percent hydroquinone cream in an oil in water emulsion or 3 percent hydroquinone lotion.

HYPERHIDROSIS

MERVYN L. ELGART, M.D.

There are two types of sweat glands, apocrine and eccrine. Apocrine sweat is found in areas where apocrine glands persist, such as the axilla and groin. Hyperhidrosis of apocrine glands is rarely a problem. The most common symptom associated with apocrine gland secretion is odor. A huge cosmetic industry has arisen in response to this perceived difficulty. The sweat produced by these glands contains nitrogen compounds, which, when decomposed by bacteria, produce the characteristic "locker room" odor. Antibacterial drugs therefore are extremely successful in removing that odor.

Deodorants that are available over the counter are those that generally contain aluminum chlorhydroxide. However, some patients have odor problems that do not respond to this product. In addition, many patients find aluminum chlorhydroxide irritating.

Other antibacterial drugs may be useful in these areas. Neomycin cream or Neosporin can be very valuable, since the gram positive organisms are the ones that generally are responsible for this odor and neomycin has an excellent spectrum of activity against these organisms. Some people, however, develop allergies to neomycin and this must be kept in mind. Another modality is the use of the antiacne antibiotics, which are used topically in alcoholic solutions. Cleocin T, Erymax, and T Stat are solutions of clindamycin and erythromycin that are effective against gram positive bacteria and are useful in controlling axillary odor problems. They are also useful when deeper penetration is required, as in pateints who have incipient axillary hidradenitis suppurativa.

The remainder of this presentation deals with eccrine hyperhidrosis. Eccrine glands are phylogenetically new and have a major role in temperature regulation. Patients whose eccrine glands are not functioning well or who have no eccrine glands from birth have great difficulty in maintaining normal temperature. There are, however, areas in which sweat has no relation to temperature regulation. Sweating of the palms and soles, for example, is much more often seen in response to stress than in response to heat. Similarly axillary eccrine sweat may occur in response to heat but more often occurs in response to stress. Excessive sweating in the axillas, palms, and soles is a problem for many patients. The control of that problem would not seriously affect temperature regulation.

In addition to being a personal problem (e.g., patients being unwilling to shake hands with others), there are other difficulties associated with hyperhidrosis. Clothing is destroyed more readily in the presence of increased moisture, and allergic contact dermatitis may be more frequent. The presence of copious amounts of eccrine sweat may allow material to be leeched from shoes and from rings and other jewelry. This material readily produces contact dermatitis. Patients with hyperhidrosis find difficulty working in certain industries such as the electronics industry where sweat interferes with fine electronic insulation. Similarly in other metal working industries, copious moisture may produce corrosion, and hyperhidrotic individuals are known as "rusters."

THERAPY

The therapy of hyperhidrosis has many variations. The first has to do with psychotherapy. Since many of the problems we have discussed have to do with sweating in response to stress, psychotherapy and biofeedback have been used. In some instances the use of mild tranquilizers such as Valium may prove beneficial.

More often, however, tranquilizers produce only a partial remission. For this reason a physiologic approach is used. Eccrine sweating is stimulated by activation of postganglionic sympathetic fibers, which behave as if they were parasympathetic or cholinergic. Therefore, anticholinergic drugs may be useful. Pro-Banthine in a dose of 15 mg every 4 to 6 hours may diminish sweating. Liquid forms of atropine such as tincture of belladonna may be used to titrate the dose to stop sweating. The problem with these medications is the other anticholinergic effects that occur are frequently more bothersome than the sweating. Tachycardia, dry mouth, and reduced intestinal motility may vitiate whatever effect can be seen on the sweat glands. All these other complications seem to occur before sweating is affected. For this reason the anticholinergic drugs have only a limited place in the treatment of hyperhidrosis.

Some individuals have used medications such as Atarax, which has both a tranquilizing and an anticholinergic effect. In my experience they are a little better than either the tranquilizers or the anticholinergics, and the response has been relatively limited.

The most effective approach to treating hyperhidrosis has been to limit the delivery of sweat to the surface of the skin. This type of approach is one in which we participate every day by the use of antiperspirants in the axilla. The antiperspirant generally used, aluminum chlorhydroxide, has a minimal inhibitory effect on the production of sweat. The mechanism seems to be the production of a plug in the distal portion of the gland. The plug consists of a homogeneous eosinophilic material, and this plug is lost a week or 2 after stopping aluminum chlorhydroxide application. Aluminum chlorhydroxide is found in most of the commercial antiperspirants and is present in a higher concentration in antiperspirants than in deodorants.

Aluminum chlorhydroxide is clearly not the best antiperspirant available; indeed aluminum chloride works much better than aluminum chlorhydroxide. The problem with aluminum chloride is that it is much too acidic for general use and that if left in contact with clothing, it destroys many types of fibers. For this reason, aluminum chloride is not present in over-the-counter deodorants. However, it can be found in a product called Drysol as a 20 percent solution in absolute alcohol.

Aluminum chloride must be used in a particular manner. The axillae hands, or feet should be cleansed and thoroughly dried. When this has been accomplished, the aluminum chloride is applied and then the area is covered with an occlusive material. In the axilla a plastic wrap is used; on the hands and feet gloves or Baggies may be used. This occlusion is left in place for several hours or overnight and removed in the morning. The process is repeated for 2 to 3 nights, and many individuals find that the sweating is diminished for the next several days. The aluminum chloride must be reapplied every few days to maintain the diminished sweating. The effect may be dramatic. It must be remembered that if it is used in the axilla, this use is for diminished sweating but not for odor and a deodorant must be used in addition. Furthermore, aluminum chloride may be irritating and must be used with care.

Glutaraldehyde and formaldehyde are sometimes useful in the treatment of hyperhidrosis. Formaldehyde may be painted on the area once daily. The formaldehyde used is the 10 percent formalin as used for biopsies.

Formalin is a saturated solution of formaldehyde gas in water and contains 39 percent formaldehyde; therefore 10 percent formalin contains 3.9 percent formaldehyde. This aqueous solution produces some hardening of the keratin and some reduction in sweating. There is, of course, a significant incidence of allergy to formaldehyde, and this may develop with use. A 10 percent aqueous solution of glutaraldehyde works somewhat better than formaldehyde but produces a rather disturbing brownish coloration of the skin. Both glutaraldehyde and formaldehyde seem to work better on the hands and feet and are more difficult to use in the axilla.

Perhaps the most encouraging advance in the treatment of hyperhidrosis over the last several years has been the concept of tap water iontophoresis. This concept began in the late 1940s with the realization that a galvanic current passed through water in contact with skin produced some diminution of sweating. The exact mechanism for this is unknown. When diminished sweating is produced by this electronic method, tape stripping with Scotch tape can restore the sweating after several layers of epidermis are removed. This suggests that the blocking that occurs with tap water iontophoresis is close to the surface of the skin at the distal end of the eccrine duct.

The Drionic device has recently been approved by the FDA for patient use at home. It is available only by prescription and only by mail through the company, General Medical Corporation, 1935 Armacost Avenue, Los Angeles, California 90025. The device is a method of applying a battery supplied galvanic current to counteract hyperhidrosis of the palms, soles, or axillas. This current is processed through an electronic system, which has a current reversal device so that current does not build up in only one area. In addition, there are thick felt pads that are moistened to provide the tap water to the area. The pad at the negative pole is much thicker to attempt to retard the passage of hydroxides produced at that pole to the skin. The hydroxides are clearly somewhat irritating.

On the palms and soles this process works well. The patient moistens the pads and puts his hands or feet in contact with them. Using a rheostat he turns the current to the highest comfortable level. He then lets the current flow for 20 minutes and turns the machine off. He does this daily for 14 days, by which time sweating is considerably diminished.

Sweating remains diminished over a period of 6 weeks, by which time the effect is apparently lost and the patient must undergo retreatment. When treating with this machine it is important that jewelry be removed, since this makes a much better contact in some areas and may cause burns. Similarly it is important that the hands or feet be placed flat against the pads to allow for good contact. If there are splits or cuts in the skin, they should be covered with petrolatum or some other heavy ointment, since open cuts produce more pain and tingling.

The Drionic device for the axilla is somewhat more difficult to use because the tissues in the axilla are more tender. A lower intensity of treatment must be used, and it may be necessary to use the device longer than the established 2 weeks. Also the acid generated at the positive pole may irritate the delicate skin of the axilla, whereas it does not seem to affect the hands and feet. Therefore, for patients who have irritation, the small pad is soaked in sodium bicarbonate to neutralize the acid.

Results with the Drionic device have been very good in patients who have hyperhidrosis; 80 percent or more have shown some improvement and have continued its use. For these patients the knowledge that they can finally control sweating of the hands, feet, or axillas produces enough biofeedback so that, after some time, they have less requirement for the device.

If the chemical and electronic methods fail, surgery is a possibility. In the axilla the largest number of sweat glands can be excised. Excision of the axillary vault removes most of the eccrine and apocrine glands and therefore stops both odor and hyperhidrosis. An alternative procedure has been proposed by a Japanese surgeon in which an incision is made and the glands are destroyed on the underside of the skin. The limited results have been excellent, but I am unaware of other surgeons attempting this procedure.

On the hands and feet excision of the sweat glands themselves is impractical. However, for hyperhidrosis of the hands, dorsal sympathectomy has been used. In many individuals this produces diminished sweating but there are several problems. First, this is a major operation and has numerous side effects. Second, the nerves sometimes regrow after 2 to 3 years, and a return of sweating in these areas occurs in 50 percent of the patients. Therefore sympathectomy must be considered a measure of last resort to control hyperhidrosis.

LYME DISEASE (ERYTHEMA CHRONICUM MIGRANS)

JAMES W. PATTERSON, M.D.

Lyme disease is an infection characterized by erythematous annular skin lesions (erythema chronicum migrans) and systemic involvement that may include as target organs the joints, heart, and central or peripheral nervous system. It is now known to be caused by a spirochete, *Borrelia burgdorferi*, that is transmitted by the bite of an ixodid tick. The disease was initially reported as a cluster of cases occurring in the areas of Old Lyme, Lyme, and East Haddam, Connecticut (hence the designation Lyme disease), but it has since been recognized in other regions of the United States (northeast, midwest, and west) corresponding to locations of the tick vectors, *Ixodes dammini* or *I. pacificus*. A similar disease that has been recognized for a number of years in Europe is associated with the bite of a tick of the same *Ixodes ricinus* complex. The disorder also has been reported in Australia and other countries.

Lyme disease most often occurs in the summer and in its complete form, like other spirochetoses, progresses through three stages. Stage 1 is characterized by erythema chronicum migrans, an often intense annular erythema with partial central clearing occurring about a central papule that marks the site of a tick bite. The skin lesion may be accompanied by regional lymphadenopathy as well as headache, stiff neck, fever, malaise, fatigue, arthralgias, and myalgias. Stage 2, occurring weeks or months later, involves the nervous system (meningoencephalitis, cranial or peripheral neuropathies) or the heart (atrioventricular nodal block, myocarditis). Still later, in stage 3, there develops an acute recurrent monoarticular or asymmetric oligoarticular arthritis. Large joints are usually involved, especially the knees, but others, such as the temporomandibular joint and small joints of the hands and feet, may also be affected. Although often there is no significant joint damage, the arthritis may become chronic, with pannus formation and damage to cartilage and subchondral bone. Patients with severe forms of the disease are often found to have the B cell alloantigen DR 2.

There is a characteristic antibody response to the organism: IgM titers peak between the third and sixth weeks of the illness, while IgG titers are highest later in the course of the disease when arthritis is present. In addition, spirochetes occasionally can be recovered from blood, skin lesions, or cerebrospinal fluid.

The diagnosis is made by recognition of the typical signs and symptoms, especially when they occur in a patient from an endemic area, and is supported by appropriate serologic studies. Isolation of the spirochete may also be helpful.

TREATMENT

It has been gratifying to observe the rapid advances in our understanding of this disease since it was first recognized in 1975. Treatment has correspondingly evolved from an initial, largely symptomatic approach to the more specific antimicrobial therapy of today. For much of the information about treatment, we are indebted to the pioneering work of Steere and his colleagues.

Early Disease

The treatment of choice for early Lyme disease is tetracycline hydrochloride, 250 mg by mouth four times daily for 10 days. This course can be extended to 20 days if symptoms persist or recur. The evidence indicates that this regimen instituted early in the course of the disease shortens the duration of erythema chronicum migrans and prevents or attenuates subsequent arthritis. In one study none of the patients receiving tetracycline developed major late complications of the disease.

Also effective is phenoxymethyl penicillin, 250 mg orally four times daily for 10 days. Erythromycin in an oral dose of 250 mg four times daily for 10 days is somewhat less effective, since symptoms tend to resolve more slowly and retreatment for persistent disease is necessary more often than with the other drugs. Minor late complications are common with all three regimens; these include headaches, myalgias, arthralgias, and lethargy. Some patients treated with penicillin or (more frequently) erythromycin develop major late complications such as meningoencephalitis, carditis, or recurrent arthritis. In addition to the usual side effects associated with each of these drugs, a Herxheimer type of reaction may develop during the first 24 hours of therapy; symptoms include fever, pain, and intensification of erythema in skin lesions. These symptoms are somewhat more common with tetracycline or penicillin therapy than with erythromycin.

Early Disease in Childhood

The recommended therapy for children under 7 years of age is phenoxymethyl penicillin, 50 mg per kilogram per day orally (between 1.0 and 2.0 g per day) in divided doses for 10 to 20 days. For patients who are allergic to penicillin, an alternative treatment is erythromycin, 30 mg per kilogram per day by mouth in divided doses for 15 to 20 days. However, it should be recognized that erythromycin may not be as efficacious as penicillin, and at this dosage it may not be tolerated owing to gastrointestinal side effects.

For children over 7 years of age, the preferred therapy is tetracycline hydrochloride, 40 mg per kilogram per day by mouth in four divided doses (up to 250 mg four times daily) for 10 to 20 days.

Therapy of Later Manifestations of Lyme Disease

In all likelihood the protocols just recommended should promote disease resolution and prevent the occurrence of major late manifestations. Occasionally a second course of therapy, or extension of therapy from 10 to 20 days, is necessary for recurrent or persistent disease. This may be especially true when erythromycin has been administered. However, despite full courses of therapy, an occasional patient progresses to stage 2 (meningoencephalitis, carditis) or stage 3 (arthritis). Patients with severe initial symptoms are more likely than others to develop major late complications. Furthermore, the clinician may first see a patient at a more advanced stage of the disease, at a point at which late complications have already begun.

In these circumstances the recommended treatment consists of high intravenous doses of penicillin—penicillin G, 20 million units per day in divided doses (3.3 million units intravenously every 4 hours) for 10 days. This regimen is effective in the treatment of patients with established Lyme arthritis as well as those with neurologic abnormalities such as meningitis, pleocytosis of cerebrospinal fluid, or cranial or peripheral neuropathy. Headache, stiff neck, and radicular pain tend to resolve rapidly with this therapy, but some patients continue to have attacks of arthritis, and motor deficits resolve more slowly (over a period of several months). A longer duration of therapy may prove to be necessary for some patients; clinicians are advised to follow the current literature for new information about this aspect of therapy.

Lyme arthritis has also been treated with benzathine penicillin, 2.4 million units intramuscularly each week for 3 weeks (a total of 7.2 million units), with good results, although some patients also fail to respond to this regimen. Treatment of late manifestations in patients who are allergic to penicillin is not well established, but alternative regimens such as those used in tertiary syphilis have been recommended, e.g., tetracycline, 500 mg by mouth four times daily for 30 days.

Other Aspects of Management

Oral doses of corticosteroids generally do not hasten the resolution of neurologic abnormalities, but patients with neurologic involvement limited to facial palsy and no history of therapy can be treated orally with antimicrobial drugs and a short course of prednisone if seen within 24 hours after the onset of facial palsy.

Carditis is usually of short duration, but it may develop despite early antimicrobial therapy. The rare patient with high degree AV block or first degree block with a PR interval greater than 0.30 second requires in-hospital observation for the possible development of complete heart block. Such a patient may benefit from insertion of a temporary transvenous pacemaker, which can be removed in about 1 week. Aspirin, 3.6 g per day in divided doses, is also administered.

The use of corticosteroids in these circumstances is controversial. Although the degree of AV block is rapidly diminished and other abnormalities tend to diminish, corticosteroid therapy must be continued for 2 to 4 months, with slow tapering of the dosage to prevent recurrence of neurologic symptoms or arthritis. Corticosteroids may still be indicated for patients who have had complete AV block for over 1 week, or for those with markedly compromised cardiac function and cardiomegaly. The treatment then consists of prednisone, 40 to 60 mg per day, tapered by 5 to 10 mg per week once improvement is established. If joint symptoms flare while tapering prednisone, a nonsteroidal anti-inflammatory drug can be added.

The acute arthritis of Lyme disease is self-limited and should respond to antimicrobial therapy, but the short term use of acetaminophen or a nonsteroidal anti-inflammatory drug may provide symptomatic relief. These drugs are also helpful in the management of chronic arthritis. Partial weight bearing and avoidance of strenuous activity are sometimes necessary in chronic disease, and synovectomy is useful for patients with persistent joint effusions. Because of possible interference with the host immune response and, therefore, inhibition of spirochetocidal activity, intra-articular administration of corticosteroids concurrently with antibiotics is not advised.

VULVAR DERMATOSIS

MARIA L. TURNER, M.D.

When a young woman presents to a dermatologist because of a vulvar problem, it is either because she can see a rash or because she has persistent pain or burning for which relief has not been found after repeated visits to numerous physicians. In such an instance it is generally the last stop before seeing a psychiatrist and finally admitting that, indeed, the pain may be "psychogenic" in origin. I thus find it useful to classify the vulvar problems that I see into those giving rise to pruritus vulvae and those giving rise to vulvodynia or the burning vulva syndrome.

PRURITUS VULVAE

Pruritus vulvae means itching in the vulvar area, occasionally accompanied by itching in the perianal area as well. It may be acute or chronic and is almost always associated with a visible rash or a discharge. It is useful to categorize the causes of pruritus vulvae, as in Table 1.

Preferred Approach for Diagnosis

Since the conditions we are considering in this section occur in a physically sensitive area in an emotionally sensitive patient, one must first try to make the patient comfortable and instill in her a feeling of confidence in the physician's ability to help alleviate the problem. A history of the presenting problem as well as related systemic, dermatologic, and medication information is generally all that is necessary before proceeding to an examination of the vulvar area.

The external genitalia are examined for signs of rubbing (broken hairs, erythema, excoriations, lichenification,

TABLE 1 Causes of Pruritus Vulvae

Infections
  Vaginitis, e.g., Candida, Trichomonas,
    Gardnerella, Chlamydia
  Pediculosis
  Dermatophyte
  Erythrasma
  Warts

Dermatologic conditions
  Seborrheic dermatitis
  Psoriasis
  Contact dermatitis
  Lichen planus
  Lichen simplex chronicus
  Lichen sclerosus et atrophicus

Miscellaneous disorders
  Systemic disorders, e.g., as diabetes
  Atrophic or senile vaginitis
  Neoplasia, e.g., Bowen's disease, Paget's disease,
    basal cell epithelioma, and invasive squamous
    cell carinoma of the vulva

and scaling), nits, lice, pustules, pigment changes, and swelling. The labia minora and vulvar vestibule are examined for mucosal changes, growths, and abnormal secretions. A potassium hydroxide mount of a vaginal discharge yields information about the presence of Candida, "clue cells," and the fishy amine odor associated with Gardnerella vaginitis. A potassium hydroxide smear of the advancing border of a serpiginous upper inner thigh rash should also be obtained. Wood's light examination showing a uniformly hyperpigmented, finely scaling eruption in the same area that fluoresces coral red indicates erythrasma. When appropriate, the rest of the body should be examined for evidence of atopic dermatitis, psoriasis, seborrheic dermatitis, lichen planus, and lichen sclerosus et atrophicus. Since the oral mucosa is covered by the same type of epithelium, it should not be missed in the examination. Patch testing with the screening tray when indicated, or when a good therapeutic regimen does not work in a reasonable length of time, is strongly recommended.

The presence of discrete red, white, black or atrophic patches call for a biopsy. This is done under local anesthesia (Xylocaine with epinephrine) with iris scissors or a Keyes punch. The biopsy site is closed with 4-0 silk sutures. The specimen is laid over filter paper, epidermis side up, before inserting it gently into formalin. Atrophic or senile vaginitis is confirmed by a Gram's stain of the vaginal secretion demonstrating rounded epithelial cells with nuclei and a paucity of long gram positive rods (Döderlein bacilli).

Treatment

Candida

Acute vulvitis due to Candida in the absence of a history of recent antibiotic therapy requires that one check for evidence of diabetes. The vaginal problem should be treated topically with one of the imidazole compounds according to the manufacturer's directions. I prefer to treat the external genitalia with a mixture of 1 million units of Mycostatin powder in 1 ounce of 1 percent hydrocortisone lotion three to four times a day. This mixture is nonirritating and has the advantage of drying up into a powder, thus not contributing to the moisture and maceration that accompany this condition. Discomfort is markedly decreased in 48 hours and there is generally complete clearing in 1 week.

Gardnerella

Metronidazole, 250 mg four times daily for 5 to 7 days.

Trichomonas

Metronidazole, 500 mg twice daily for 5 days.

Pediculosis

Kwell shampoo applied for 4 minutes. Treatment is repeated after 1 week.

Tinea

One of the imidazole lotions or solutions twice daily for 2 to 3 weeks and whenever necessary thereafter.

Erythrasma

Erythromycin, 250 mg four times daily for 10 days, and maintenance treatment with Cleocin T twice daily. Because of its alcohol vehicle, Cleocin T is too irritating to use during the acute phase.

Warts

Minimize the secretion that frequently accompanies this condition. Orally administered contraceptives increase normal vaginal secretions, hence, I generally discontinue them. A smear and postassium hydroxide preparation should be obtained to diagnose accompanying infection so that specific therapy can be instituted. If warts are not keratinized and the patient is not pregnant, 20 percent podophyllin may be used. I generally apply a thick coat of zinc oxide ointment over the treated areas to prevent contact with normal tissue. The patient is instructed to wash the medication off in 5 hours and is advised about pain and discomfort, which peak 2 to 4 days after application. Soaking in a tub and the use of analgesics may be helpful during this period. Other modes of therapy include the application of liquid nitrogen, desiccation and curettage under local anesthesia, and, for the most resistant cases, laser surgery. The cervix and vagina should be examined for possible involvement and treated accordingly.

With all the foregoing conditions, sexual partners should be examined and treated if indicated.

Seborrheic Dermatitis

Two percent sulfur in 1 percent hydrocortisone lotion twice a day on a whenever-necessary basis is generally sufficient.

Psoriasis

Two percent sulfur in 0.05 percent flurandrenolide (Cordran) lotion is applied twice daily until clearing occurs and whenever necessary thereafter. A fluorinated steroid is often necessary, but seldom have I had to use anything stronger than flurandrenolide. When the scales are thick, I incorporate 2 to 3 percent salicylic acid in the formulation.

Contact Dermatitis

The patient should be given a list of contactants that contain the substances to which she had reacted on patch testing. These may take the form of topical medications, over the counter lotions, and creams, including douches, contraceptive jellies, and lubricants.

Paper products, in the form of toilet tissue and pads, should be avoided by formaldehyde sensitive individuals. To reverse chronic skin changes, I prefer to use 0.025 percent Synalar ointment because this steroid preparation is free of preservatives. If the offending agent has been eliminated, a 2-week course of therapy should be more than sufficient.

Lichen Sclerosus et Atrophicus

A biopsy is necessary in the management of this condition. Preferably, adjacent atrophic and hypertrophic areas should be included in an excisional biopsy. Although rare, squamous cell carcinoma has been seen in association with hypertrophic areas in about 5 percent of the cases. I use 0.025 percent Synalar ointment to flatten out the hypertrophic areas because these tend to be the most pruritic. For the atrophic stage, a 2 percent concentration of testosterone propionate (in oil) mixed with white petrolatum, applied thinly twice daily for 2 to 6 months, reverses the atrophy and decreases the itching. Ground-up testosterone tablets mixed in petrolatum tend to be too granular and uncomfortable to apply to an already irritated vulva. Maintenance therapy with testosterone ointment once or twice a week is generally necessary to maintain the beneficial effects. Side effects, in the form of increased libido, facial hirsutism, acne, and voice change, have been reported although they are rarely seen. In general, prepubertal children improve at menarche and therefore do not need treatment. Regular follow-up is needed to monitor testosterone side effects and to watch for dysplastic changes.

Lichen Planus

Lichen planus may present as white or gray, flat papules and small plaques or as widespread erythematous erosions of the vulva. The diagnosis is generally not difficult to make because often there is evidence of lichen planus elsewhere. Treatment, however, is another matter. In my experience, just about nothing works, particularly for the erosive phase. Systemic steroid therapy when used for widespread involvement clears up this area as well. Topical and systemic retinoid therapy has been reported to be beneficial, but these preparations have not been useful in my experience. I have never found griseofulvin to work. Intralesional steroid therapy followed by applications of the stronger fluorinated steroids is palliative. This form of therapy invariably becomes complicated by vulvar candidiasis and burning.

Lichen Simplex Chronicus

Because this is a chronic pruritic condition, the entire cutaneous surface of the external genitalia is hyperpigmented and lichenified, with broken-off hairs and even prurigo-like lesions. In addition to chronicity, there is frequently a history of atopy. In my experience this is not a sign of undiagnosed diabetes. It is in these instances that mild irritation or allergic reactions to contactants should be searched for. This condition best exemplifies the itch-scratch-itch cycle, and this must be carefully explained to the patient.

After the initial work-up, the program I recommend is as follows: (1) Discontinue all previous creams, lotions, and topical applications. (2) Wash the area with nothing but plain cool water and wear only 100 percent cotton underwear. (3) Apply 0.025 percent Synalar ointment thinly over the involved area two to three times daily. (4) Take hydroxyzine hydrochloride 10 to 50 mg before bedtime.

(5) Do not scratch or rub. Because itching is often most bothersome at night, I tell the patient to take an ice bag to bed for relief of pruritus. A follow-up at 2 weeks is necessary to evaluate progress, which should be substantial if the diagnosis is correct and the patient has followed directions carefully. At this point topical steroid therapy should be tapered and the patient re-educated about the problem. If there is not marked improvement, proceed with further work-up such as patch testing and biopsy.

Atrophic or Senile Vaginitis

My preference is to manage the patient in concert with a gynecologist. Systemic estrogen therapy is considered a better form of treatment than topically applied creams because one is unable to judge how much is being absorbed.

Neoplasia

I cannot overemphasize the importance of biopsy examination in chronic cases that do not respond to good care. Multiple Bowen's disease, which may initially present as difficult-to-see flat papules or hyperpigmented macules, often presents as pruritus vulvae. The incidence of this entity is increasing, especially in younger women. The current consensus is that this is related to human papillomavirus infection, and because extremely rare cases of invasion have been reported, management is somewhat controversial. However, "skinning vulvectomy" is no longer the treatment of choice for this particular variant of Bowen's disease. Local excisions, laser surgery, and topical 5-fluorouracil therapy are all acceptable. Close follow-up examination of the vulvar, perineal, and perianal skin with selective biopsy using 1 percent toluidine solution as a guide (reveals parakeratotic epidermis) is mandatory.

Paget's disease may have the appearance of a chronic eczematous process but, unlike lichen simplex chronicus, is more erythematous and is asymmetric with eroded areas. A work-up for internal malignant disease is necessary and surgical treatment is indicated.

Basal cell carcinoma, although rare, can occur in the vulva, and the half-dozen cases I have seen presented with localized pruritic areas. The treatment is surgical excision, which can be done in the office without any trouble.

VULVODYNIA AND THE BURNING VULVA SYNDROME

In any vulvar disease clinic there is a small but distinct group of women who complain of chronic disabling pain and burning with a paucity of physical and laboratory findings and whose complaints defy therapeutic intervention. They are a demanding and difficult group, no doubt because of the enigma that surrounds their problem. In 1983 the ISSVD (International Society for the Study of Vulvar Diseases) proposed the term vulvodynia to describe the chronic discomfort characterized by the patient's complaint of burning, stinging, irritation, or "rawness." The condition may have multiple etiologies. The term burning vulva syndrome, on the other hand, has been reserved for an end stage condition for which no physical cause can be found. Psychogenic factors have been strongly implicated (Table 2).

Preferred Approach for Diagnosis

Since by definition we are dealing with an overtreated patient with a chronic disease who is also difficult and demanding, one must be sure to reserve enough time for a complete evaluation. It is, in fact, wise to do the evaluation in stages. Taking a thorough history aided by a questionnaire designed by the ISSVD Task Force on Vulvar Pain is a good way to start. A thorough gentle examination taking special note of small ulcers and erythematous plaques in the vestibule and around the orifices of the minor vestibular glands is the next step. At this point smears are taken for hanging drop, potassium hydroxide mount, Gram staining, Tzanck smears (when indicated), and pertinent cultures. Papillations and erythematous plaques should be subjected to biopsy study.

Steroid Withdrawal

Just as one sees steroid induced rosacea on the face, the same occurs in the vulva with grouped pinhead pustules on brightly erythematous bases noted over the labia majora and minora. The intertriginous folds between the labia majora and minora may be smooth and atrophic or erythematous with macerated scales.

Vestibular Papillomatosis

Although most consider this a normal variant, when velvety papillations extend to the hymenal ring and when it is accompanied by a copious sticky gray secretion, the condition is more likely to be symptomatic. Some biopsy specimens have histologic features consistent with condyloma.

Pudendal Neuralgia

Pudendal neuralgia is characterized by increased sensitivity to touch over the entire genital area such that even light pressure, as from clothing, becomes intolerable. There is great discomfort on sitting and, needless to say, bike riding and intercourse are impossible. The condition frequently is accompanied by pain around the rectum, the lower back, the gluteal areas, and down the legs. This may be seen after herpes zoster and with recurrent genital herpes simplex, silent slipped disc, as well as other neurologic and metabolic diseases. In one of my recent cases, a woman with a 1½ year duration of symptomatol-

TABLE 2　Causes of Vulvodynia

Atrophic vaginitis
Lichen sclerosus et atrophicus
Steroid withdrawal
Vestibular papillomatosis
Pudendal neuralgia
Minor vestibular gland syndrome

ogy consistent with this entity came for evaluation during a period of acute exacerbation, with her first positive physical finding—a 3 mm erosion that was Tzanck positive.

Minor Vestibular Gland Syndrome or Valvar Vestibulitis

This entity is a symptom complex encountered in sexually active women with a history of culture proven Candida infection but without evidence of active infection. They complain mainly of introital dyspareunia and on examination have exquisitely tender erythematous plaques on the vestibule and around the openings of the minor vestibular glands. Biopsy shows a lymphohistiocytic infiltrate with plasma cells in the subcutis, especially around simple tubular glands lined by a single layer of columnar epithelium (minor vestibular gland).

Treatment

The therapy for atrophic vaginitis and lichen sclerosus et atrophicus has been considered. Vestibular papillomatosis is treated only when no other cause for vulvar pain is found or if the biopsy findings are consistent with condyloma acuminatum. Laser surgery is the treatment of choice in this instance.

The treatment for pudendal neuralgia depends on the etiology. Recurrent herpes simplex is treated with a 5-day course of acyclovir, 200 mg five times a day. Nonsteroidal anti-inflammatory drugs, such as ibuprofen (Motrin), 300 mg four times daily, have been of some use. In recalcitrant cases diphenylhydantoin (Dilantin), 300 mg a day, or carbamazepine (Tegretol) can be tried.

The only treatment for the minor vestibular gland syndrome with an 80 percent incidence of success is vulvar perineoplasty. Laser therapy has yielded an unsatisfactory number of recurrences. It has been my experience that in the less chronic cases (less than 2 years' duration), careful avoidance of topical irritants and immediate treatment of proven vaginal infections result in resolution of the problem.

Burning Vulva Syndrome

Anti-inflammatory drugs, antidepressants, Dilantin, and Tegretol have been tried with uneven results. Because the cause remains unknown, strong psychologic support must be given for these patients. Ascribing the condition to a psychosomatic disorder should be a last resort, done only after a thorough work-up and periodic re-evaluations.